DERMATOLOGICAL SIGNS OF SYSTEMIC DISEASE

DERMATOLOGICAL SIGNS OF SYSTEMIC DISEASE

FIFTH EDITION

Jeffrey P. Callen, MD, FACP
Professor of Medicine (Dermatology)
Chief, Division of Dermatology
Department of Medicine
University of Louisville
Louisville, KY, USA

Joseph L. Jorizzo, MD
Professor and Former (Founding) Chair
Department of Dermatology
Wake Forest University
Winston-Salem, NC;
Professor of Clinical Dermatology
Weill Cornell Medical College
New York, NY, USA

John J. Zone, MD
Professor and Chairman
Department of Dermatology
University of Utah School of Medicine
Salt Lake City, UT, USA

Warren W. Piette, MD
Chair, Division of Dermatology
John H. Stroger Jr. Hospital of Cook County;
Professor, Department of Dermatology
Rush University Medical Center
Chicago, IL, USA

Misha A. Rosenbach, MD
Assistant Professor
Department of Dermatology and Internal Medicine
Perelman School of Medicine
University of Pennsylvania
Philadelphia, PA, USA

Ruth Ann Vleugels, MD, MPH
Director, Autoimmune Skin Disease Program
Brigham and Women's Hospital
Department of Dermatology;
Co-Director, Rheumatology-Dermatology Clinic
Boston Children's Hospital;
Associate Professor of Dermatology
Harvard Medical School
Boston, MA, USA

For additional online content visit http://expertconsult.inkling.com

ELSEVIER

Edinburgh   London   New York   Oxford   Philadelphia   St Louis   Sydney   Toronto   2017

ELSEVIER

© 2017, Elsevier Inc. All rights reserved.
First edition 1988
Second edition 1995
Third edition 2003
Fourth edition 2009

No part of this publication may be reproduced or transmitted in any form or by any means, electronic or mechanical, including photocopying, recording, or any information storage and retrieval system, without permission in writing from the publisher. Details on how to seek permission, further information about the Publisher's permissions policies and our arrangements with organizations such as the Copyright Clearance Center and the Copyright Licensing Agency, can be found at our website: www.elsevier.com/permissions.

This book and the individual contributions contained in it are protected under copyright by the Publisher (other than as may be noted herein).

Chapters 32, Bacterial and Rickettsial diseases and 34, Protozoal Diseases are in the public domain.

Notices

Knowledge and best practice in this field are constantly changing. As new research and experience broaden our understanding, changes in research methods, professional practices, or medical treatment may become necessary.

Practitioners and researchers must always rely on their own experience and knowledge in evaluating and using any information, methods, compounds, or experiments described herein. In using such information or methods they should be mindful of their own safety and the safety of others, including parties for whom they have a professional responsibility.

With respect to any drug or pharmaceutical products identified, readers are advised to check the most current information provided (i) on procedures featured or (ii) by the manufacturer of each product to be administered, to verify the recommended dose or formula, the method and duration of administration, and contraindications. It is the responsibility of practitioners, relying on their own experience and knowledge of their patients, to make diagnoses, to determine dosages and the best treatment for each individual patient, and to take all appropriate safety precautions.

To the fullest extent of the law, neither the Publisher nor the authors, contributors, or editors, assume any liability for any injury and/or damage to persons or property as a matter of products liability, negligence or otherwise, or from any use or operation of any methods, products, instructions, or ideas contained in the material herein.

ISBN: 978-0-323-35829-3
E-ISBN: 978-0-323-35831-6

Content Strategist: Russell Gabbedy
Content Development Specialist: Joanne Scott
Project Manager: Srividhya Vidhyashankar
Design: Miles Hitchen
Illustration Manager: Emily Costantino
Illustrator: Graphic World Inc.
Marketing Manager: Kristin Koehler

Printed in the United States of America

Last digit is the print number: 9 8 7 6 5 4 3 2

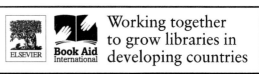

*Dr. Callen dedicates this book to his wife Susan,
his children Amy Maidenberg and David Callen,
their Spouses Dan and Laura, and his grandchildren
Judah and Noa Callen, Aviva and Eden
Maidenberg and Liam Sondreal.*

*Dr. Jorizzo dedicates his contribution to this edition to
Irene Carros, John, Michael, Melina, to the late Joseph
and Margaret, and to Johanna and Paul.*

*Dr. Zone dedicates his contribution to his wife Judy,
and children Joe, Sara and Stephanie.
Stephanie has honored him by pursuing
a career in Academic Dermatology.*

*Dr. Piette dedicates this book to his wife Michelle,
son Evan, and daughter Lauren, and thanks them
for their patience and support.*

*Dr. Rosenbach dedicates this book to Anna, Lara, and
Jake, and thanks them for their patience and support.*

*Dr. Vleugels dedicates her contribution
to her husband Keith and to the rest of her family
for their many years of support.*

Contents

Preface, ix

List of Contributors, xi

Acknowledgments, xv

1 **Lupus Erythematosus**, 1
Christopher B. Hansen • Jeffrey P. Callen

2 **Dermatomyositis**, 13
Ruth Ann Vleugels • Jeffrey P. Callen

3 **Scleroderma, Raynaud's Phenomenon, and Related Conditions**, 22
Stephanie T. Le • Nicole Fett • Anna Haemel

4 **Vasculitis**, 31
Miguel A. González-Gay • Trinitario Pina

5 **Neutrophilic Dermatoses**, 39
Joanna Harp • Joseph L. Jorizzo

6 **Psoriasis and Systemic Disease**, 45
Jashin J. Wu • Johann E. Gudjonsson

7 **Other Rheumatologic–Dermatologic Conditions**, 51
Natalie A. Wright • Joseph F. Merola

8 **Autoinflammatory Syndromes**, 59
Kieron S. Leslie

9 **Eosinophil-Associated Diseases with Dermatologic Manifestations**, 69
Kristin M. Leiferman

10 **Urticaria**, 77
Julie B. Zang • Joseph L. Jorizzo

11 **Erythema Multiforme, Stevens–Johnson Syndrome, and Toxic Epidermal Necrolysis**, 87
Andrew Avarbock • Joseph L. Jorizzo

12 **Panniculitis**, 93
Ana M. Molina-Ruiz • Luis Requena

13 **Pruritus**, 99
Gil Yosipovitch

14 **Erythroderma**, 104
Megan H. Noe • Karolyn A. Wanat

15 **Purpura**, 109
Warren W. Piette

16 **Bullous Diseases**, 117
Anneli R. Bowen • John J. Zone

17 **Skin Signs of Internal Malignancy**, 131
Edward W. Cowen • Jeffrey P. Callen

18 **Dermatologic Adverse Events of Cancer Therapy**, 141
Zhe Hou • Viswanath Reddy Belum • Mario E. Lacouture

19 **Metastatic Disease**, 155
Courtney R. Schadt • Jeffrey P. Callen

20 **Cutaneous Lymphomas and Cutaneous Signs of Systemic Lymphomas**, 159
Lorenzo Cerroni

21 **Dysproteinemias, Plasma Cell Disorders, and Amyloidosis**, 171
Warren W. Piette

22 **Cutaneous Manifestations of the Histiocytoses**, 183
Warren T. Goodman • Joshua R. Bradish • Terry L. Barrett

23 **Vascular Neoplasms and Malformations**, 192
Julie V. Schaffer • Jean L. Bolognia

24 **Diabetes and the Skin**, 205
Christine S. Ahn • Gil Yosipovitch • William W. Huang

25 **Thyroid and the Skin**, 215
Elizabeth Ghazi • Ted Rosen • Joseph L. Jorizzo • Warren R. Heymann

26 **Cutaneous Manifestations of Lipid Disorders**, 222
Inbal Braunstein

27 **Adrenal, Androgen-Related, and Pituitary Disorders**, 228
Robert G. Micheletti

28 **Porphyrias**, 235
Maureen B. Poh-Fitzpatrick

29 **Cutaneous Diseases Associated with Gastrointestinal Abnormalities**, 243
Mark D. Herron • John J. Zone

30 **Hepatic Disease and the Skin**, 255
J. Mark Jackson • Jeffrey P. Callen • Kenneth E. Greer

31 **Viral Diseases**, 262
Ramya Kollipara • Sheevam Shah • Stephen K. Tyring

32 **Bacterial and Rickettsial Diseases**, 271
Dirk M. Elston

33 **Fungal Diseases**, 277
Scott A. Norton

34 **Protozoal Diseases**, 285
Dirk M. Elston

35 **Acquired Immunodeficiency Syndrome and Sexually Transmitted Infections**, 289
Eseosa Asemota • Carrie Kovarik

36 **Sarcoidosis**, 305
Misha A. Rosenbach • Joseph C. English III • Jeffrey P. Callen

37 **Cardiovascular Diseases and the Skin,** 315
Alisa Femia • Kathryn Schwarzenberger • Jeffrey P. Callen

38 **Renal Disease and the Skin,** 323
Mary P. Maiberger • Julia R. Nunley

39 **Cutaneous Manifestations Observed in Transplant Recipients,** 330
Fiona Zwald • Manisha J. Loss • Dennis L. Cooper • Jean L. Bolognia

40 **Neurocutaneous Disease,** 345
Sarah D. Cipriano • John J. Zone

41 **Pregnancy,** 359
Bethanee J. Schlosser

42 **Mast Cell Disease,** 370
Michael D. Tharp

43 **Hair Disorders in Systemic Disease,** 377
Kimberly S. Salkey • Amy McMichael

44 **Nail Signs of Systemic Disease,** 387
Shari R. Lipner • Richard K. Scher

45 **Oral Disease,** 397
Charles Camisa • Jeffrey P. Callen

46 **Leg Ulcers,** 402
Katherine L. Baquerizo Nole • Robert S. Kirsner

47 **Cutaneous Drug Eruptions,** 425
Kara Heelan • Neil H. Shear

48 **Principles of Systemic Drug Use,** 437
Cindy England Owen • Stephen E. Wolverton

Index, 443

PREFACE

This is the fifth edition of our book. We began this journey together in the mid-1980s having recognized a gap in the knowledge of practicing dermatologists and internists. We have somewhat altered our approach with each new edition and this one is no different. With this edition we said farewell to Jean Bolognia as an editor and welcome Misha Rosenbach and Ruth Ann Vleugels. Misha is one of the first people to train in a combined dermatology–medicine residency in the United States and has developed a focused interest in hospital medicine, with a specific research focus on granulomatous diseases. Ruth Ann began and runs one of the most successful rheumatology–dermatology clinics in the United States and has now successfully trained multiple others in a postresidency fellowship program. We have retained our collaboration with Warren Piette and John Zone.

In this revision of our book we added some additional chapters and have selected many new authors and co-authors to update and revise most of the chapters. We have continued our goal of providing the practicing physician, academic physician, or resident with a text that explores the relationship of the skin with internal diseases or conditions. Each chapter now has been reviewed by one of our associated editors as well as both of us. We continue our stance of providing suggested readings rather than an extensive reference list. These suggested readings have been updated so that the interested reader may delve into the most current literature. We have continued the use of color photographs throughout this edition of our text and in many cases have found new photographs for inclusion.

Contributors

Christine S. Ahn, MD
Resident Physician
Department of Dermatology
Wake Forest School of Medicine
Winston-Salem, NC, USA

Eseosa Asemota, MD, MPH
Clinical Research Fellow
Department of Dermatology
Perelman School of Medicine
University of Pennsylvania
Philadelphia, PA, USA

Andrew Avarbock, MD, PhD
Assistant Professor of Dermatology
Department of Dermatology
Weill Cornell Medical College
New York, NY, USA

Katherine L. Baquerizo Nole, MD
Resident Physician
Department of Medicine
Nassau University Medical Center
Long Island, NY, USA

Terry L. Barrett, MD
Director, ProPath Dermatopathology
Clinical Professor of Dermatology and Pathology
University of Texas Southwestern Medical Center
Dallas, TX, USA

Viswanath Reddy Belum, MD
Research Associate
Dermatology Service
Department of Medicine
Memorial Sloan Kettering Cancer Center
New York, NY, USA

Jean L. Bolognia, MD
Professor of Dermatology
Department of Dermatology
Yale School of Medicine
New Haven, CT, USA

Anneli R. Bowen, MD
Associate Professor of Dermatology
Department of Dermatology
University of Utah
Salt Lake City, UT, USA

Joshua R. Bradish, MD
Director of Dermatopathology
Midwestern Pathology;
Clinical Assistant Professor of Pathology
Western Michigan University
Kalamazoo, MI, USA

Inbal Braunstein, MD
Assistant Professor
Department of Dermatology and Pathology
Johns Hopkins School of Medicine
Baltimore, MD, USA

Jeffrey P. Callen, MD, FACP
Professor of Medicine (Dermatology)
Chief, Division of Dermatology
Department of Medicine
University of Louisville
Louisville, KY, USA

Charles Camisa, MD
Affiliate Associate Professor
Department of Dermatology and Cutaneous Surgery
University of South Florida School of Medicine
Tampa, FL, USA;
Director
Department of Phototherapy
Riverchase Dermatology and Cosmetic Surgery
Naples, FL, USA

Lorenzo Cerroni, MD
Associate Professor of Dermatology
Director of Dermatopathology
Department of Dermatology
Medical University of Graz
Graz, Austria

Sarah D. Cipriano, MD, MPH, MS
Visiting Instructor
Department of Dermatology
University of Utah School of Medicine
Salt Lake City, UT, USA

Dennis L. Cooper, MD
Professor of Medicine
Robert Wood Johnson Medical School
New Brunswick, NJ, USA

CONTRIBUTORS

Edward W. Cowen, MD, MHSc
Senior Clinician and Head
Dermatology Consultation Service
Center for Cancer Research
National Cancer Institute
National Institutes of Health
Bethesda, MD, USA

Dirk M. Elston, MD
Professor and Chairman
Department of Dermatology and Dermatologic Surgery
Medical University of South Carolina
Charleston, SC, USA

Joseph C. English III, MD
Professor of Dermatology
Department of Dermatology
University of Pittsburgh
Pittsburgh, PA, USA

Alisa Femia, MD
Assistant Professor
Director of Inpatient Dermatology
The Ronald O. Perelman Department of Dermatology
New York University Langone Medical Center
New York, NY, USA

Nicole Fett, MD, MSCE
Associate Professor
Department of Dermatology
Oregon Health and Science University
Portland, OR, USA

Elizabeth Ghazi, MD
Chief Resident of Dermatology
Department of Dermatology
Cooper University Hospital
Camden, NJ, USA

Miguel A. González-Gay, MD, PhD
Professor of Medicine
University of Cantabria
Rheumatology Division
Hospital Universitario Marqués de Valdecilla
Santander, Cantabria, Spain

Warren T. Goodman, MD
Medical Director of Dermatopathology
Regions Hospital;
Clinical Assistant Professor of Dermatology and Laboratory Medicine and Pathology
University of Minnesota
Saint Paul, MN, USA

Kenneth E. Greer, MD
Rick A. Moore Professor of the University of Virginia School of Medicine;
Professor of Dermatology
Chairman Emeritus (1993-2008)
University of Virginia
Charlottesville, VA, USA

Johann E. Gudjonsson, MD, PhD
Assistant Professor
Department of Dermatology
University of Michigan
Ann Arbor, MI, USA

Anna Haemel, MD
Assistant Professor
Department of Dermatology
University of California, San Francisco
San Francisco, CA, USA

Christopher B. Hansen, MD
Assistant Professor
Department of Dermatology
University of Utah School of Medicine
Salt Lake City, UT, USA

Joanna Harp, MD
Assistant Professor of Dermatology
Department of Dermatology
Weill Cornell Medical College
New York, NY, USA

Kara Heelan, MBBChBAO, MRCPI
Clinical Fellow
Department of Dermatology
University College London Hospital
London, UK

Mark D. Herron, MD
Private Practice
Montgomery, AL, USA

Warren R. Heymann, MD
Professor of Medicine and Pediatrics
Head, Division of Dermatology
Cooper Medical School of Rowan University
Camden, NJ;
Clinical Professor of Dermatology
Perelman School of Medicine
University of Pennsylvania
Philadelphia, PA, USA

Zhe Hou, MD, PhD
Resident Physician
Department of Dermatology
University of California at San Diego
San Diego, CA, USA

William W. Huang, MD, MPH
Assistant Professor and Residency Program Director
Department of Dermatology
Wake Forest University School of Medicine
Winston-Salem, NC, USA

J. Mark Jackson, MD
Clinical Professor of Medicine (Dermatology)
Division of Dermatology
Department of Medicine
University of Louisville
Louisville, KY, USA

Joseph L. Jorizzo, MD
Professor and Former (Founding) Chair
Department of Dermatology
Wake Forest University
Winston-Salem, NC;
Professor of Clinical Dermatology
Weill Cornell Medical College
New York, NY, USA

Robert S. Kirsner, MD, PhD
Chairman (Interim) and Harvey Blank Professor
Department of Dermatology and Cutaneous Surgery
University of Miami Miller School of Medicine
Miami, FL, USA

Ramya Kollipara, MD
Dermatology Resident
Texas Tech University Health Sciences Center
Lubbock, TX, USA

Carrie Kovarik, MD
Associate Professor
Departments of Dermatology and Medicine
Perelman School of Medicine
University of Pennsylvania
Philadelphia, PA, USA

Mario E. Lacouture, MD
Associate Professor
Director, Oncodermatology Program
Dermatology Service
Department of Medicine
Memorial Sloan Kettering Cancer Center
New York, NY, USA

Stephanie T. Le, MS
Eastern Virginia Medical School
Norfolk, VA, USA

Kristin M. Leiferman, MD
Professor of Dermatology
Department of Dermatology
University of Utah School of Medicine
Salt Lake City, UT, USA

Kieron S. Leslie, MB BS, FRCP
Associate Professor of Dermatology,
Department of Dermatology,
University of California
San Francisco, CA, USA

Shari R. Lipner, MD, PhD
Assistant Professor,
Department of Dermatology
Weill Cornell Medical College
New York, NY, USA

Manisha J. Loss, MD
Assistant Professor
Department of Dermatology
Johns Hopkins School of Medicine
Baltimore, MD, USA

Mary P. Maiberger, MD
Chief of Dermatology
Veterans Affairs Medical Center;
Assistant Professor of Dermatology
Howard University Hospital
Washington, DC, USA

Amy McMichael, MD
Professor and Chair
Department of Dermatology
Wake Forest School of Medicine
Winston-Salem, NC, USA

Joseph F. Merola, MD, MMSc
Assistant Professor
Departments of Dermatology and Medicine
Division of Rheumatology
Brigham and Women's Hospital
Harvard Medical School
Boston, MA, USA

Robert G. Micheletti, MD
Assistant Professor of Dermatology and Medicine
Perelman School of Medicine
University of Pennsylvania
Philadelphia, PA, USA

Ana M. Molina-Ruiz, MD, PhD
Associate Professor
Department of Dermatology
Fundación Jiménez Díaz
Universidad Autónoma
Madrid, Spain

Megan H. Noe, MD, MPH
Clinical Instructor and Post-Doctoral Fellow
Department of Dermatology
University of Pennsylvania
Philadelphia, PA, USA

Scott A. Norton, MD, MPH, MSc
Chief of Dermatology
Children's National Medical Center;
Professor of Dermatology and Pediatrics
George Washington University School of Medicine and Health Sciences
Washington, DC, USA

Julia R. Nunley, MD
Professor, Dermatology
Program Director, Dermatology
Medical College of Virginia Hospitals
Virginia Commonwealth University
Richmond, VA, USA

Cindy England Owen, MD, MS
Assistant Professor of Dermatology
University of Louisville
Louisville, KY, USA

Warren W. Piette, MD
Chair, Division Dermatology
John H. Stroger Jr. Hospital of Cook County
Professor, Department of Dermatology
Rush University Medical Center
Chicago, IL, USA

Trinitario Pina, MD, PhD
Rheumatologist
Rheumatology Division
Hospital Universitario
Marques de Valdecilla
Santander, Spain

Maureen B. Poh-Fitzpatrick, MD
Professor Emerita and Special Lecturer
Department of Dermatology
Columbia University College of Physicians and Surgeons
New York, NY, USA

Luis Requena, MD, PhD
Professor of Dermatology and Head
Department of Dermatology
Fundación Jiménez Díaz, Universidad Autónoma
Madrid, Spain

Ted Rosen, MD
Professor of Dermatology
Department of Dermatology
Baylor College of Medicine
Houston, TX, USA

Misha A. Rosenbach, MD
Assistant Professor
Department of Dermatology and Internal Medicine
Perelman School of Medicine
University of Pennsylvania
Philadelphia, PA, USA

Kimberly S. Salkey, MD
Assistant Professor
Department of Dermatology
Eastern Virginia Medical School
Norfolk, VA, USA

Courtney R. Schadt, MD
Assistant Professor of Medicine
Reisdency Program Director
Division of Dermatology
University of Louisville School of Medicine
Louisville, KY, USA

Julie V. Schaffer, MD
Pediatric Dermatology Program Director
Division of Pediatric Dermatology
Hackensack University Medical Center
Hackensack, NJ, USA

Richard K. Scher, MD, FACP
Clinical Professor
Department of Dermatology
Weill Cornell Medical College
New York, NY, USA

Bethanee J. Schlosser, MD, PhD
Assistant Professor
Departments of Dermatology and Obstetrics/Gynecology
Northwestern University Feinberg School of Medicine
Chicago, IL, USA

Kathryn Schwarzenberger, MD
Amonette-Rosenberg Chair and Professor of Dermatology
Kaplan-Amonette Department of Dermatology
University of Tennessee Health Science Center
Memphis, TN, USA

Sheevam Shah, BS
Texas A&M Health Science Center
College of Medicine
Temple, TX, USA

Neil H. Shear, MD, FRCP
Professor and Chief of Dermatology
University of Toronto
Toronto, ON, Canada

Michael D. Tharp, MD
The Clark W. Finnerud, MD Professor and Chair
Department of Dermatology
Rush University Medical Center
Chicago, IL, USA

Stephen K. Tyring, MD, PhD
Medical Director
Center for Clinical Stuies and Clinical Professor
Department of Dermatology
University of Texas Health Sciences Center at Houston
Houston, TX, USA

Ruth Ann Vleugels, MD, MPH
Director, Autoimmune Skin Disease Program
Brigham and Women's Hospital
Department of Dermatology;
Co-Director, Rheumatology-Dermatology Clinic
Boston Children's Hospital;
Associate Professor of Dermatology
Harvard Medical School
Boston, MA, USA

Karolyn A. Wanat, MD
Clinical Assistant Professor
Department of Dermatology and Pathology
University of Iowa Hospitals and Clinics
Iowa City, IA, USA

Stephen E. Wolverton, MD
Theodore Arlook Professor of Clinical Dermatology
Department of Dermatology
Indiana University School of Medicine
Indianapolis, IN, USA

Natalie A. Wright, MD
Dermatology-Rheumatology Fellow
Department of Dermatology
Brigham and Women's Hospital
Harvard Medical School
Boston, MA, USA

Jashin J. Wu, MD
Director of Dermatology Research
Kaiser Permanente Los Angeles Medical Center
Los Angeles, CA, USA

Gil Yosipovitch, MD
Professor and Chair
Department of Dermatology and Itch Center
Temple University School of Medicine
Philadelphia, PA, USA

Julie B. Zang, MD, PhD
Assistant Professor
Department of Dermatology
Weill Cornell Medical College
New York, NY, USA

John J. Zone, MD
Professor and Chairman
Department of Dermatology
University of Utah School of Medicine
Salt Lake City, UT, USA

Fiona Zwald, MD, MRCPI
Staff Physician
Piedmont Transplant Institute
Dermatology Consultants, P.C.
Atlanta, GA, USA

ACKNOWLEDGMENTS

Dr. Callen acknowledges and thanks the following physicians: Carol L. Kulp-Shorten, MD, Jyoti B. Burruss, MD, Kristin O. Donovan, MD, Shannon M. McAllister, MD, Alfred L. Knable, MD, Timothy S. Brown, MD, Janine Malone, MD, Anna Hayden, MD, Soon Bahrami, MD, Cindy E. Owen, MD, Courtney R. Schadt, MD, Sonya Burton, MD, and Michael W. McCall, Jr. for allowing him the time to write by providing care for his patients in his absence. In addition, he thanks all of the residents and staff at the University of Louisville for their academic stimulus and assistance with patients and their families.

Dr. Jorizzo acknowledges and thanks the faculty, residents, and staff at the Departments of Dermatology at both the Wake Forest University School of Medicine and the Weill Cornell Medical College for their ongoing support.

Dr. Zone acknowledges and thanks the faculty, residents and staff at the University of Utah Department of Dermatology for their support.

Dr. Piette thanks all of the dermatology residents and faculty at Cook County and at Rush Medical Center for their academic stimulus and assistance with patients and their families.

Dr. Rosenbach thanks his faculty, residents, staff, and mentors.

Dr. Vleugels acknowledges the continued support of the Department of Dermatology at Brigham and Women's Hospital and thanks her patients as well as her mentors, colleagues, staff, residents, and fellows.

Lupus Erythematosus

Christopher B. Hansen • Jeffrey P. Callen

KEY POINTS

- Lupus erythematosus is a multisystem disorder that frequently has cutaneous involvement
- Lupus-specific skin disease can be characterized as acute, subacute, or chronic based on clinical and laboratory features
- Other nonspecific cutaneous changes such as cutaneous vasculitis and Raynaud's phenomenon occur more commonly in lupus patients
- Prevention involves protection from ultraviolet radiation and smoking cessation
- Topical and intralesional corticosteroids and other topical immunomodulators may be effective for mild or localized disease
- Antimalarials are the first-line systemic treatment, with other systemic agents reserved for more severe or recalcitrant disease

Lupus erythematosus (LE) is a multisystem disorder that encompasses a spectrum from a relatively benign, self-limited cutaneous eruption to a severe, sometimes fatal, systemic disease. Prior to Hargraves' recognition of the LE cell, LE was diagnosed by a constellation of clinical findings. Ultimately, the American College of Rheumatology (ACR) developed a set of criteria that could be used for the classification of systemic lupus erythematosus (SLE). The criteria were revised in 1982 (Table 1-1). When a patient fulfills four or more of the ACR criteria, either concurrently or serially, during any period of observation, that patient can be classified as having SLE.

In the 1940s and 1950s, dermatologists first recognized that most of their patients with chronic, scarring discoid lupus erythematosus (DLE) lesions had few, if any, systemic findings, whereas those with malar erythema and/or photosensitivity frequently had systemic disease. They also recognized a middle group in whom the cutaneous lesions were more transient than in patients with DLE, but for whom the prognosis was not as poor as in those patients with SLE. These patients were later categorized as having subacute cutaneous LE (SCLE). The classification of cutaneous LE subsets was stressed by Gilliam and his coworkers. Gilliam proposed that cutaneous manifestations characterized by interface dermatitis (histopathologically-specific LE) be classified into one of three groups based on clinical features. An individual LE patient can present with more than one subtype of the disease. Gilliam also recognized that LE patients can have a skin disease that is not histopathologically specific (Table 1-2). Although each subset listed in Table 1-2 is generally predictive of outcome, it must be remembered that the full spectrum of LE-associated organ dysfunction is possible in any individual patient.

The prevalence of SLE is reported to be 17–48/100,000 people. The prevalence of cutaneous LE is not well established, but it appears to be at least as common as SLE. SLE has a strong female preponderance, with a 12:1 female-to-male ratio in the childbearing years. Cutaneous LE appears to be more common than SLE in males and older adults, but remains more common in women, with a 3:1 female-to-male ratio.

CHRONIC CUTANEOUS LUPUS ERYTHEMATOSUS

Chronic cutaneous LE can have several clinical manifestations. The most common subset is discoid lupus erythematosus (DLE). Patients with DLE may be classified as having either localized DLE, in which lesions are confined to the head and neck, or widespread DLE, in which lesions are found on other body surfaces in addition to the head and neck. DLE can also occur as a manifestation of SLE in approximately 20% of patients. Other less

---

TABLE 1-1 Revised ACR Criteria for the Diagnosis of Systemic Lupus Erythematosus

If four or more of the following criteria are present serially or simultaneously during any observation, the patient may be considered to have systemic lupus erythematosus:
1. Malar rash
2. Discoid lupus erythematosus lesions
3. Photosensitivity, by history or by observation
4. Oral ulcers, usually painless, observed by the physician
5. Arthritis, nonerosive, involving two or more joints
6. Serositis, pleuritic, or pericarditis
7. Renal disorder with proteinuria (>500 mg/day) or cellular casts
8. Central nervous system disorder with seizures or psychosis (absence of known cause)
9. Hematologic disorder, such as hemolytic anemia, leukopenia (<4000/mm^3), or thrombocytopenia (<100,000/mm^3)
10. Immunologic disorder, detected by positive lupus erythematosus preparation, abnormal titers of antinative DNA and anti-Sm, and false-positive Venereal Disease Research Laboratory or rapid plasma reagin results
11. Positive antinuclear antibody titers

From Tan EM, Cohen AS, Fries JF, et al. The 1982 revised criteria for the classification of systemic lupus erythematosus. Arthritis Rheum 1982;25:1271–7, with permission.

TABLE 1-2 A Classification of Mucocutaneous Lesions in Lupus Erythematosus

I. LE-specific histopathologic findings
   A. Chronic cutaneous LE
      1. DLE (localized versus generalized)
      2. Hypertrophic/verrucous LE
      3. Palmar/plantar LE
      4. Oral DLE
      5. LE panniculitis
      6. Tumid LE
   B. SCLE
      1. Polymorphous light eruption-type lesions
      2. Annular lesions (may be seen in Asian patients with SCLE [annular erythema of primary Sjögren's syndrome])
      3. Papulosquamous lesions
      4. Neonatal LE
      5. C2-deficient LE-like syndrome
      6. Drug-induced SCLE
   C. ACLE
      1. Malar erythema
      2. Photosensitivity dermatitis
      3. Generalized erythema
II. LE-nonspecific histopathologic findings
   A. Vasculopathy
      1. Urticaria
      2. Vasculitis
      3. Livedo reticularis/livedo racemosa/pyoderma gangrenosum-like leg ulcerations
   B. Mucosal lesions
   C. Nonscarring alopecia
   D. Bullous LE or epidermolysis bullosa acquisita
   E. Associated mucocutaneous problems
      1. Mucinous infiltrations
      2. Porphyrias
      3. Lichen planus
      4. Psoriasis
      5. Sjögren's syndrome
      6. Squamous cell carcinoma

LE, lupus erythematosus; DLE, discoid LE; SCLE, subacute cutaneous LE; ACLE, acute cutaneous LE.

common forms of chronic cutaneous LE include hypertrophic LE, tumid LE, lupus erythematosus panniculitis (LEP, or lupus profundus), oral DLE, as well as DLE lesions on the palms and/or soles.

Discoid Lupus Erythematosus

DLE lesions are characterized by erythema; telangiectasia; adherent scale, which varies from fine to thick; follicular plugging; dyspigmentation; and atrophy and scarring (Fig. 1-1). The lesions are usually sharply demarcated and can be round, thereby giving rise to the term discoid (or disc-like). The presence of scarring and/or atrophy is the characteristic that separates these lesions from those of SCLE. The differential diagnosis most often includes papulosquamous diseases such as psoriasis, lichen planus, secondary syphilis, superficial fungal infection, and sarcoidosis. A histopathologic examination is usually helpful in confirming the diagnosis, and only rarely is immunofluorescence microscopy necessary.

Patients with localized DLE have lesions located solely on the head, neck, or both. These appear to represent the majority of cases of DLE. These patients differ from those with widespread discoid lesions of LE in a number of ways. They have fewer manifestations that suggest systemic disease, and they less frequently demonstrate a positive antinuclear antibody (ANA) or leukopenia. It appears that patients with DLE who progress to develop SLE are generally not in the subset with localized discoid lesions of LE. Those patients with disease localized to the head and neck will frequently (roughly 50%) have a remission, whereas the disease rarely becomes clinically inactive (less than 10%) in those with widespread involvement. Lastly, it also appears that those with widespread disease respond less well to antimalarial treatment. Thus, it seems that it is prognostically worthwhile to separate patients with localized DLE and those with generalized DLE into different subsets.

Hypertrophic Lupus Erythematosus

Hypertrophic or verrucous DLE (HLE) is a unique subset in which the thick, adherent scale is replaced by massive hyperkeratosis, and the resulting lesions resemble verruca or squamous cell carcinomas (Fig. 1-2). These lesions usually occur in the setting of other, more typical DLE lesions. Patients with HLE tend to have chronic disease, to have little in the way of systemic symptoms or abnormal laboratory findings, and to be extremely difficult to treat with conventional therapy. They may respond to oral retinoids.

Palmar/Plantar Discoid Lupus Erythematosus

The lesions of DLE can occur on the palms and/or soles (Fig. 1-3). The frequency of this subset is low, and there is no specific clinical or serologic correlation. Patients with DLE of the palms or soles can have chronic cutaneous disease, or the lesions can be present in patients with SLE. Palmar and/or plantar lesions are often difficult to treat.

Oral Discoid Lupus Erythematosus

Oral DLE lesions are histopathologically and clinically similar to cutaneous discoid lesions of LE (Fig. 1-4). Oral DLE lesions are distinct from the oral and nasal ulcerations that occur in SLE, which are associated with active systemic disease and are histopathologically nonspecific. Lesions that look like those of discoid lesions of LE in the oral mucosa have associations similar to those seen with localized or widespread discoid lesions of LE.

Tumid Lupus Erythematosus

Tumid lupus erythematosus (lupus tumidus) is characterized by erythematous to violaceous papules, plaques (Fig. 1-5), or nodules, that usually occur on sun-exposed surfaces. The lesions classically have no epidermal changes and tend to heal with no residual scarring or atrophy. Patients with tumid LE are photosensitive. Serologic abnormalities are distinctly uncommon in these patients, and patients with tumid LE rarely meet criteria for SLE. The pathology of tumid LE reveals an increase in mucin and a periappendiceal and perivascular dermal

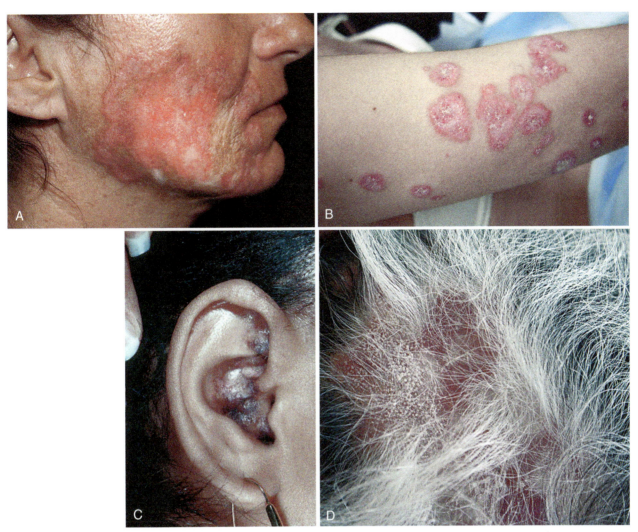

FIGURE 1-1 ■ Discoid lesions of lupus erythematosus. Erythematous to violaceous lesions with adherent scale, slight atrophy, and early scar formation. **A**, Facial lesion; **B**, lesions on the extensor surface of the arms; **C**, patulous follicles in the conchal bowl; **D**, scarring scalp lesion.

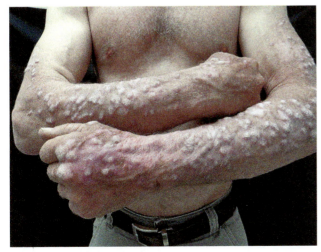

FIGURE 1-2 ■ Hypertrophic (verrucous) lupus erythematosus. These lesions simulate verruca, keratoacanthoma, or squamous cell carcinoma.

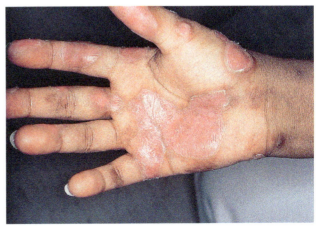

FIGURE 1-3 ■ Erosive lesions of discoid lupus erythematosus involving the palms. Typical lesions of discoid lupus erythematosus are present elsewhere.

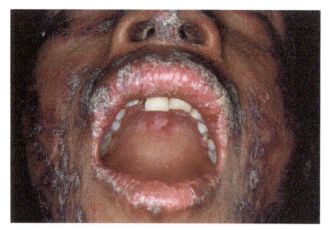

FIGURE 1-4 ■ Oral lesions in a patient with chronic cutaneous lupus erythematosus. Note the discoid lupus erythematosus lesion on the palate.

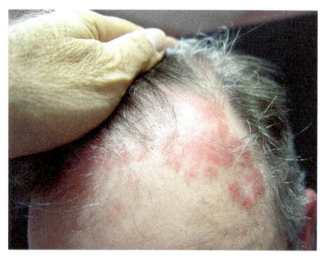

FIGURE 1-5 ■ Lupus tumidus. This patient has erythematous plaques on the forehead without surface change. Biopsy of these lesions revealed a perivascular and periadnexal lymphocytic infiltrate without an interface dermatitis. Extensive mucin deposition was also noted.

infiltrate composed of lymphocytes, but there is little if any change at the dermal–epidermal interface. It is possible that there is overlap, both clinically and histologically, between reticulated erythematous mucinosis and tumid LE.

There are several controversies regarding tumid LE: (1) some authorities believe that tumid LE is not a variant of lupus erythematosus; and (2) as there is no residual scarring or atrophy, it differs from other types of chronic cutaneous lupus. Some have argued that it would fit better as a variant of subacute cutaneous lupus or in a separate classification. Patients with tumid LE are usually responsive to photoprotection and antimalarials.

Lupus Panniculitis

Lupus erythematosus panniculitis (LEP, lupus panniculitis) is a lobular panniculitis that occurs rarely in patients with DLE or SLE (Fig. 1-6). Whether LEP is histopathologically distinct is controversial; thus, in the authors' opinion, the patient should have documented SLE or DLE to be classified as having LEP. The term lupus profundus is sometimes used as a synonym for LEP, while others reserve this term for LEP with overlying discoid lesions. LEP is often chronic, and it can lead to cutaneous and subcutaneous atrophy, calcification, and occasional ulceration. Lesions preferentially involve the face as well as areas with prominent subcutaneous tissue, such as the upper arms, thighs, and buttocks. Twice as many patients with LEP do not have systemic disease as have systemic disease. It has been postulated that in the patient with LEP, renal disease is rarely present, and when present, it is among the more benign forms.

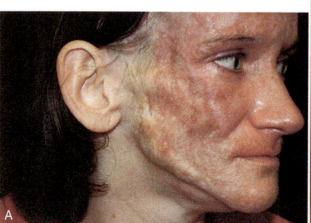
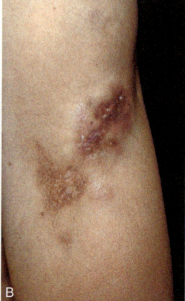

FIGURE 1-6 ■ Lupus panniculitis. **A,** This woman has inflammatory, subcutaneous nodules that have resulted in severe subcutaneous atrophy on the face. Typical lesions of discoid lupus erythematosus were present on other body sites. **B,** Calcified subcutaneous nodules and atrophy on the lateral arm.

Chilblains Lupus

Chilblains lupus is a rare manifestation of LE that typically presents as red or dusky papules or plaques in acral locations (Fig. 1-7) that are exacerbated by cold and may improve—but do not always resolve—in warmer weather. This entity can be extremely difficult to distinguish from "common" pernio in the absence of other features of LE, but lesions classically should have histological changes of LE, such as vacuolar interface changes. Lesions of chilblains lupus are often recalcitrant to typical treatments of cutaneous LE, such as antimalarials. Over time, lesions may develop an appearance of more typical DLE. In half of patients, chilblains may be the only presenting manifestation of LE. Long-term follow-up of these patients for signs of systemic disease is warranted.

DLE–SLE Subset

The DLE–SLE subset defines a small group of patients (about 5% to 15%) who, by the nature of their selection, have systemic disease in association with scarring cutaneous disease. Patients whose disease progresses from being purely cutaneous into this group are typically characterized by widespread DLE, the presence of clinically appreciable periungual telangiectases, persistent elevated erythrocyte sedimentation rates, leukopenia, and positive ANA titers. Patients in this group may have DLE alone at the onset, DLE with other symptoms or signs, or systemic disease without cutaneous lesions. The timeframe for developing SLE is variable—in one study, most patients with DLE developed the criteria for SLE within 1.3 years of diagnosis; in a more recent study, however, the mean time to developing SLE was 8.2 years. Patients in the DLE–SLE subset rarely have renal disease, and, when present, it is most often transient and mild. The DLE–SLE population is often considered to be a distinct LE subset because of its relatively benign, albeit chronic, course.

SUBACUTE CUTANEOUS LUPUS ERYTHEMATOSUS

The predominant skin lesion in patients with SCLE has all of the features of the DLE lesion without the scarring or atrophy. In addition, follicular plugging is only rarely observed in SCLE. Patients with such lesions as their major cutaneous manifestation have been classified as having a subset of LE called SCLE. It is important to understand, however, that a patient in the SCLE subset can also have the scarring lesions of DLE or lesions generally associated with SLE, such as a malar rash or vasculitic lesions. Many patients with SCLE fulfill four or more of the ACR criteria for SLE; thus, some authorities have not recognized these patients as forming a distinct subset. However, these patients differ from patients with DLE and from those with SLE, typically having a more benign disease course than those patients meeting SLE criteria based on findings other than skin manifestations. Therefore, the authors believe that SCLE should be considered a distinct LE subset.

There are two types of SCLE skin lesions: annular and papulosquamous. Annular SCLE (SCLE-A) lesions are characterized by erythematous rings with central clearing and peripheral scaling (Fig. 1-8). The lesions of SCLE-A must be differentiated from other figurate erythemas, such

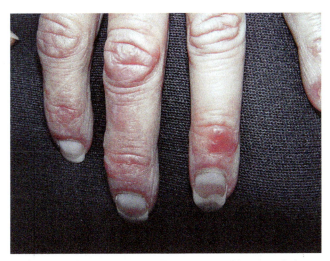

FIGURE 1-7 ■ Chilblains lupus. This woman with systemic lupus erythematosus has erythematous to violaceous papules on her hands.

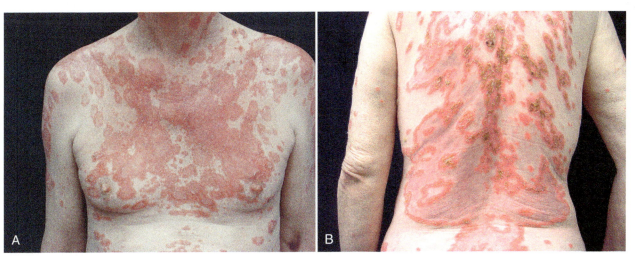

FIGURE 1-8 ■ Widespread annular scaly lesions of subacute cutaneous lupus erythematosus.

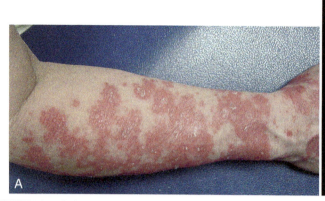
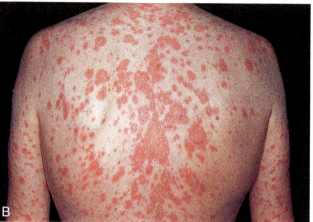

FIGURE 1-9 ■ Subacute cutaneous lupus erythematosus, papulosquamous variant. This patient developed an exquisitely photosensitive eruption after minimal sun exposure.

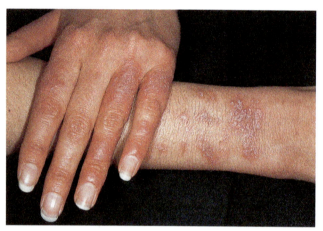

FIGURE 1-10 ■ Lichen-planus-like lesions of subacute cutaneous lupus erythematosus.

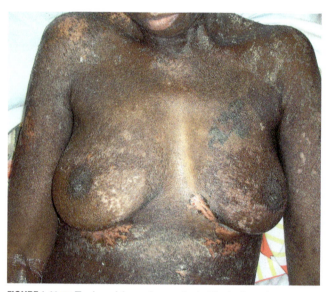

FIGURE 1-11 ■ Toxic epidermal necrolysis-like lesions in a patient with systemic lupus erythematosus.

as erythema annulare centrifugum, and from tinea corporis. Papulosquamous SCLE (SCLE-P) lesions are characterized by plaques and papules with scale (Figs 1-9 and 1-10). The differential diagnosis of SCLE-P lesions includes psoriasis and lichen planus. Patients with presumed psoriasis who flare following ultraviolet light therapy may in fact have SCLE. In both SCLE-A and SCLE-P, the lesions often begin as erythematous papules or plaques in a photosensitive distribution. In the early stage, the process may be difficult to distinguish clinically from polymorphous light eruption, and characteristic histopathologic findings may not be observed. Most often, a patient with SCLE has only one type of SCLE lesion, but in about 10% of cases, both annular and papulosquamous lesions can be present. DLE skin lesions, generally limited in number, can occur in up to 35% of patients in the SCLE subset. Rare cutaneous patterns include an erythroderma, a pityriasis rubra pilaris-like disease, a disease mimicking toxic epidermal necrolysis (Fig. 1-11), and an erythema gyratum repens-like disease.

About 50% of patients with SCLE have four or more of the ACR criteria for SLE. This takes into account the skin lesions as one criterion and photosensitivity as a second (more than 90% of patients with SCLE have these two criteria). Those with SCLE also frequently have serologic abnormalities, in particular the presence of anti-Ro (SS-A) antibody. Leukopenia is also observed in some SCLE patients. Approximately 40% to 50% of patients with SCLE have arthralgias or a nondeforming arthritis. Serositis, central nervous system disease, and renal disease are possible, but are uncommon in SCLE. The type of clinical skin lesion (annular vs papulosquamous) has not been related to specific organ system involvement.

The presence of SCLE has been described in association with other conditions, including Sjögren's syndrome, rheumatoid arthritis, idiopathic thrombocytopenic purpura, urticarial vasculitis, other cutaneous vasculitic syndromes, and/or deficiency of the second component of complement. An annular erythema has also been described in Asian or Polynesian patients with Sjögren's syndrome. In the authors' opinion this is a clinical variant of SCLE.

Anti-Ro (SS-A)-positive SCLE has been induced by hydrochlorothiazide, calcium channel blockers, terbinafine, anti-TNF (tumor necrosis factor) therapies, angiotensin-converting enzyme (ACE) inhibitors,

TABLE 1-3	Drugs Commonly Reported to Cause or Exacerbate Subacute Cutaneous Lupus Erythematosus

Thiazides—chlorothiazide, hydrochlorothiazide, triamterene
Terbinafine
Biologic therapy—etanercept, infliximab, adalimumab
Calcium channel-blocking agents—diltiazem, nifedipine, verapamil, nitrendipine
ACE inhibitors—captopril, cilazapril, enalapril, lisinopril
Proton-pump inhibitors

proton-pump inhibitors, and a growing list of other drugs (Table 1-3). Drug-induced SCLE (DI-SCLE) may account for as many as one-third of patients with new-onset SCLE. DI-SCLE may have a latency period of many weeks to months before the onset of the eruption. It may be reversible upon cessation of the triggering/exacerbating agent; however, some patients' lesions persist after withdrawal of the offending drug. There are no clinical or histopathological features that distinguish DI-SCLE from idiopathic cases. It is therefore a clinical distinction based on the timing of administration of the drug. DI-SCLE should be strongly considered in patients who initially develop the disease over the age of 55 years. Notably, these medications may also flare skin disease in patients with native SCLE.

Laboratory studies in patients with SCLE have focused on the finding of anti-Ro (SS-A) and anti-La (SS-B) antibodies. These antibody systems are poorly represented in rodent tissue substrates, and thus many of these patients were previously believed to have "ANA-negative LE." However, with the widespread use of HEp-2 (human epithelium) as a substrate, it has become apparent that many anti-Ro-positive patients are not ANA-negative. On a single determination in patients with SCLE, anti-Ro (SS-A) is present in 35% to 60% of cases. Repeated testing will demonstrate a positive anti-Ro (SS-A) test result in 60% to 95% of patients with SCLE. Despite this high percentage, we must keep in mind that the marker of the disease is not this serologic result but rather the clinical skin lesions. In addition, there is some controversy regarding the special relationship of anti-Ro (SS-A) with SCLE-A, several studies suggesting a stronger relationship with this variant than with SCLE-P. Furthermore, anti-Ro (SS-A) is found in many non-SCLE situations; thus, it is neither a sensitive nor a specific marker of SCLE.

NEONATAL LUPUS ERYTHEMATOSUS

Neonatal LE (NLE) is a syndrome in which cutaneous disease is frequently present. NLE can also manifest as congenital heart block. In addition, transient hemolytic anemia, thrombocytopenia, leukopenia, and hepatitis may be observed in NLE. Rarely, central nervous system involvement has been reported. For unknown reasons, patients with NLE uncommonly have both cutaneous disease and heart block. However, families in which one baby has had heart block can subsequently have normal infants, infants with heart block, or infants with cutaneous disease. These neonates have

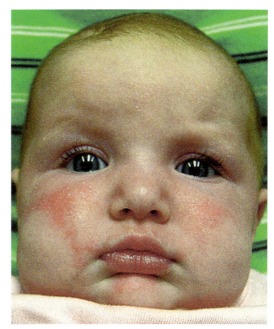

FIGURE 1-12 ■ Erythematous facial lesions of neonatal lupus erythematosus.

photosensitive cutaneous disease (often closely resembling SCLE-A) (Fig. 1-12), which begins shortly after birth and spontaneously resolves over a period of 4 to 6 months. In addition, neonates may have cytopenias, hepatitis, and neurologic disease. Data from a registry of NLE have demonstrated that the cutaneous eruption may be delayed in its onset and may not resolve for up to a year. The heart block is usually permanent and can result in fatal outcomes.

NLE has been linked to the presence of anti-Ro (SS-A), anti-La (SS-B), or, on rare occasions, anti-U_1RNP in the mother and infant. However, some babies with anti-Ro (SS-A) can be normal; thus, the presence of this antibody is not the only determining factor. The mother of a baby with NLE may be asymptomatic, may have photosensitivity, or may have a connective tissue disease (e.g., LE, rheumatoid arthritis, or Sjögren's syndrome). In one study, at the time of follow-up, half of those mothers who had initially been asymptomatic developed a connective tissue disease (usually SCLE or SLE). Women with anti-Ro (SS-A) antibodies who have not had a neonate with one of the manifestations of NLE have roughly a 1% risk of having a baby with NLE; however, once a mother has one child with NLE, the risk for a subsequent pregnancy is 25%. Patients with antibodies that may result in NLE should be followed by a high-risk obstetrician; monitoring includes fetal echocardiography in utero. In infants with NLE, there is some risk of developing a collagen vascular disease later in life.

ACUTE CUTANEOUS LUPUS ERYTHEMATOSUS

Acute cutaneous lupus erythematosus (ACLE) produces malar erythema, the classic "butterfly" rash from which the term LE (wolf-like redness) was coined

(Fig. 1-13). The eruption is induced by sun exposure, or by exposure to other sources of ultraviolet light. Patients with a butterfly rash usually have active systemic disease, but there is no specific correlation between the malar rash and the particular organ system involved. In addition patients with ACLE may develop a papular eruption on sun-exposed areas, including the dorsal arms and hands, which characteristically spares the knuckles.

Several cutaneous abnormalities were previously part of the ACR criteria for SLE, but have been found to be less specific than photosensitivity. Diffuse hair loss (alopecia) was one of the original criteria. Patients with SLE can develop a diffuse hair thinning, but this is most likely related to the presence of a severe episode of systemic illness. This type of hair loss is seen after major surgery, or can follow systemic infections or pregnancy. It is known as telogen effluvium because the trauma of the associated disease forces most hairs to cycle into the same phase, and they then all go through the telogen (resting) phase 3 to 6 months later, at which time the hair loss occurs. This hair loss is different than that resulting from the alopecic lesions of DLE.

Photosensitivity is a major factor in all types of cutaneous LE. It is one of the 11 ACR criteria for the classification of SLE. Photosensitivity implies that there is an abnormal reaction to sunlight. An abnormal reaction to sunlight occurs in all patients with LE; however, in general, most of those with DLE are not considered to have "true" photosensitivity, despite a worsening of their clinical disease in the spring and summer. Almost all patients with SCLE are photosensitive, and about 60% to 75% of those with SLE demonstrate photosensitivity. Studies have demonstrated that UVB, UVA, or both may exacerbate cutaneous disease in the lupus patient. In addition, polymorphous light eruption may be more common in LE patients, and also appears to be more common in their family members.

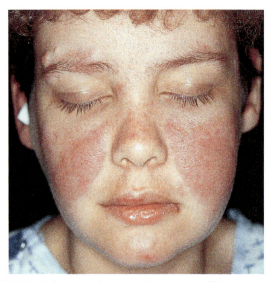

FIGURE 1-13 ■ Systemic lupus erythematosus. This young man has the typical malar rash of systemic lupus erythematosus. Note the prominent nasolabial sparing.

OTHER CUTANEOUS CHANGES ASSOCIATED WITH LUPUS ERYTHEMATOSUS

Any mucosal surface (oral, nasal, or vaginal) may be affected in LE. Occasionally the lesions may be histologically specific, but nonspecific erosions or ulcerations are seen in roughly 5% to 10% of patients with SLE. The presence of oral ulcers may correlate with active systemic disease.

Raynaud's phenomenon was one of the original 14 criteria for SLE. It occurs in otherwise healthy patients and in those with systemic sclerosis, cold-associated disorders, or other collagen–vascular diseases. There has been some suggestion that the presence of Raynaud's phenomenon is associated with a more benign SLE course, but this is controversial.

Palmar erythema and periungual telangiectases occur as nonspecific signs of SLE. Periungual telangiectases are an important finding in patients with DLE because they occur only in patients who are likely to have or to develop SLE. Nailfold capillaroscopy has also demonstrated abnormalities, but the use of this procedure to differentiate LE from other collagen–vascular diseases is controversial.

Secondary Sjögren's syndrome occurs in LE, and its incidence varies from 5% in chronic cutaneous LE to 10% to 30% in SCLE and SLE. The presence of Sjögren's syndrome has been linked to cutaneous vasculitis and central nervous system disease in patients with LE. Cutaneous vasculitis can also complicate LE. It can be manifested as urticaria-like lesions, nailfold infarcts, or palpable purpura. The presence of vasculitis in the patient with SCLE has been correlated with a positive anti-Ro (SS-A) titer, but not with active systemic disease. However, the presence of vasculitis in patients with SLE correlates with active disease and a poor prognosis. In particular, active renal disease or central nervous system disease has been reported in patients with vasculitis. In addition, approximately 50% of patients with hypocomplementemic urticarial vasculitis (HUV) have SLE. Notably, patients with HUV typically have more associated symptoms and are more challenging to treat than patients with normocomplementemic urticarial vasculitis.

Livedo reticularis, livedo racemosa, and/or pyoderma gangrenosum-like leg ulcerations may occur in patients with antiphospholipid antibodies (anticardiolipin and lupus anticoagulant). Many of these patients have LE, but some have a primary antiphospholipid antibody syndrome (Fig. 1-14). These patients may have arterial occlusion that can result in transient ischemic attacks, cerebrovascular accidents, and recurrent fetal loss; venous occlusion that can result in thrombophlebitis, renal or hepatic vein occlusion, and/or pulmonary embolism; thrombocytopenia; and cardiac valvular vegetations and dysfunction.

Bullous (or vesicular) lesions can complicate LE. Often, these lesions are present in the patient with active systemic disease. The lesions are often grouped (Fig. 1-15) and may occur on photoexposed and photoprotected skin. Bullous LE, which classically presents with a subepidermal split with neutrophils, is typically exquisitely responsive to therapy with dapsone. Both bullous

LE and epidermolysis bullosa acquisita (EBA) involve antibodies directed against type VII collagen; however, EBA typically presents with bullae on a noninflammatory base, scarring, and milia formation on trauma-prone areas, whereas bullous lupus lesions have an inflammatory base, do not result in scarring or milia formation, and do not favor trauma-prone areas. Notably, some patients with EBA either have or may develop SLE, and the presence of EBA may suggest more severe systemic LE, particularly lupus nephritis.

Various other cutaneous changes or diseases occur more commonly in patients with LE. Squamous cell carcinoma can complicate longstanding lesions of DLE. Cutaneous mucin deposition occurs in LE, but in some patients, nodules, mucinous plaques, or reticular erythematous mucinosis may occur. Various porphyrias can occur in those with LE. Lichen planus, psoriasis, and autoimmune bullous disorders may also occur with an increased frequency.

LABORATORY PHENOMENA IN PATIENTS WITH CUTANEOUS LUPUS ERYTHEMATOSUS

The full gamut of systemic disease manifestations of SLE can occur in patients with cutaneous disease, and thus these individuals can have any or all of the laboratory associations of the disorder. Serologic abnormalities are common in LE. They are less common in patients with "pure" cutaneous disease, such as DLE or HLE. The presence of serologic abnormalities in these patients correlates with the potential for progressive disease or with the criteria for SLE.

ANA is a system that represents many antibodies to multiple substrates. The frequency of a positive ANA titer correlates with the substrate used. The reported pattern of the ANA titer may also correlate with specific antibodies; however, except when interpreted by experts, the ANA pattern is not specific. Table 1-4 lists the antibody subsets and their clinical correlates. Table 1-5 presents the frequency of these antibodies in the subsets discussed. Antinative DNA (double-stranded) correlates with active SLE and, in particular, active renal disease. However, clinicians must be certain that the testing method used does not detect antisingle-stranded DNA, which is not

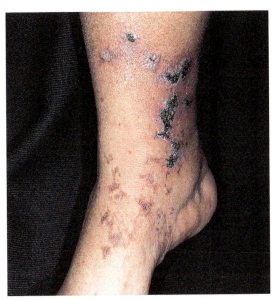

FIGURE 1-14 ■ Necrosing livedo racemosa in a patient with antiphospholipid antibody syndrome.

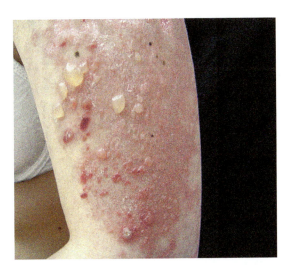

FIGURE 1-15 ■ Grouped vesicular lesions on an erythematous base on photoexposed and photoprotected skin of a patient with active systemic lupus erythematosus.

TABLE 1-4	Antibody Subsets in Lupus Erythematosus
Positive Titer/Finding	**Clinical Disorder**
Antinuclear antibody	Wide array of collagen–vascular diseases and some normal patients
HEp-2 (substrate)	Less specific
Mouse liver (substrate)	More specific
Antisingle-stranded DNA	Nonspecific, presence in patients with cutaneous LE suggests systemic disease
Antidouble-stranded DNA (antinative DNA)	SLE, active nephritis
Antihistone antibody	Drug-induced SLE
Anti-U_1RNP	Mixed connective tissue disease (low titer also present in some SLE patients)
Anti-Sm	SLE
Anti-Ro (SS-A)	SCLE, neonatal LE, Sjögren's syndrome, vasculitis, C2 deficiency-associated LE, drug-induced SCLE
Anti-La (SS-B)	Sjögren's syndrome
Antiphospholipid antibody–anticardiolipin antibody, and/or lupus anticoagulant	Thromboses (venous or arterial), cerebrovascular accidents, transient ischemic attacks, recurrent fetal loss, livedo reticularis, livedo racemosa, pyoderma gangrenosum-like leg ulcers, cutaneous necrosis, cardiac valvular vegetations, thrombocytopenia

LE, lupus erythematosus; SLE, systemic LE; SCLE, subacute cutaneous LE.

TABLE 1-5	Frequency of Antinuclear Antibody and Other Antibodies in Various Clinical Subsets of Lupus Erythematosus (%)						
Test	DLE	HLE	DLE/SLE	SCLE	NLE	ACLE	
ANA	5-10	5	75	50-75	60-90	95+	
Anti-ssDNA	35	25	75	20-50	?	90	
Anti-nDNA	5	5	10	10	10-50	70	
Anti-U$_1$RNP	<5	<5	?	10	?	40	
Anti-Sm	<5	<5	25	10	?	25	
Anti-Ro (SS-A)	5	5-10	5	40-95	90	30	
Anti-La (SS-B)	<5	<5	5	15	15-20	10	

ANA, antinuclear antibody; ss, single-stranded; n, native; RNP, ribonucleoprotein; DLE, discoid LE; HLE, hypertrophic LE; SLE, systemic LE; SCLE, subacute cutaneous LE; NLE, neonatal LE; ACLE, acute cutaneous LE.

SLE-specific. Anti-Ro (SS-A) was initially described in ANA-negative LE and Sjögren's syndrome. However, it is also present in SCLE, NLE, vasculitis, and C2-deficient LE syndromes. Thus, it is not specific for any one subset. Antibody testing must be carefully correlated with other laboratory findings and with clinical abnormalities. Neither diagnosis nor therapy should be based solely on these laboratory abnormalities.

Circulating immune complexes can often be found in patients with SLE and SCLE, but are rarely detected in patients with pure cutaneous disease. Circulating immune complexes tend to correlate with vasculitis, active renal disease, arthritis, or serositis. They may be pathogenetically important in vasculitis and renal involvement, but are probably not involved in the pathogenesis of the nonvasculitic cutaneous lesion. Complement activation is also a feature of SLE, and hypocomplementemia correlates with active systemic disease. Patients with persistent hypocomplementemia should be evaluated for complement component deficiencies, of which C2 deficiency is the most common.

Cutaneous immunofluorescence applied as a diagnostic and prognostic tool has led to a better understanding of LE. Lesional immunofluorescence may be helpful when the clinical and histopathologic diagnosis is in question. However, we must realize that normal facial skin can demonstrate false-positive reactions in 10% to 20% of cases. A positive lupus band test from noninvolved, "nonexposed" skin is believed to correlate with active renal disease. Refined antibody testing has reduced the need for immunofluorescence testing.

TREATMENT OF CUTANEOUS LUPUS ERYTHEMATOSUS

Before therapy is begun, it is necessary to evaluate the patient thoroughly to note the extent of disease, to consider the risk for progression to systemic disease, and to be able to counsel the patient appropriately regarding this risk. Table 1-6 lists the testing that should be ordered. This testing is costly, but if all results are negative, the value of the assurance that can be given regarding the benign nature of the disease process is inestimable.

The goals of management of cutaneous LE are to suppress disease activity, improve the patient's appearance, and prevent the development of deforming scars, atrophy, or dyspigmentation. Few randomized clinical trials have been performed, and hence the response to all therapies

TABLE 1-6	Evaluation of the Patient with Cutaneous Lupus Erythematosus

I. History
II. Physical examination
III. Standard tests
   A. Skin biopsy for routine processing
   B. Complete blood count with differential
   C. Tests of renal function
   D. Urinalysis
   E. Serologic tests—ANA, anti-nDNA, anti-Sm, anti-Ro (SS-A)
   F. Total hemolytic complement (if abnormal C2, C3, C4 levels)
   G. Serum protein electrophoresis
IV. Optional tests
   A. Immunofluorescence microscopy
   B. Antiphospholipid antibodies

has largely been determined only by a global assessment by the treating physician. An outcomes measure specific to cutaneous lupus, the Cutaneous Lupus Erythematosus Disease Area and Severity Index (CLASI), has been developed by Werth and colleagues. This tool can be used to quantify disease activity and damage over time, and has now been used in multiple clinical trials to demonstrate treatment response for existing and novel therapies.

The most important therapeutic intervention (Table 1-7) is the use of sunscreens, photoprotective clothing and wide-brimmed hats, and sun avoidance. This is a basic aspect of therapy that is frequently overlooked. Sunscreens with a sun protective factor of at least 30 are to be used every day. Some patients also react to ultraviolet A light and require a broad-spectrum sunscreen. The patient should be encouraged to apply the sunscreen each morning, and then again prior to sun exposure. Sunbathing, whether active or passive, is strongly discouraged. The use of sunbeds in tanning parlors should also be strongly discouraged. Artificial tanning from chemicals that do not involve UV activation is safe. Protective clothing and intelligent planning (e.g., early morning or late afternoon) with regard to sun exposure are encouraged. There are several companies that make clothing that has been demonstrated to have photoprotective properties. In addition, there are commercially available antioxidants such as *Polypodium leucotomos* that may offer additional protection against UV damage. The benefits of these supplements for LE patients have not yet been tested in appropriately controlled studies.

TABLE 1-7 Agents Used to Treat Cutaneous Lupus Erythematosus

Standard Therapy
Sunscreens, photoprotective clothing, sun avoidance
Smoking cessation
Topical corticosteroids
Intralesional corticosteroids
Antimalarials
    Hydroxychloroquine
    Chloroquine
    Quinacrine

Alternative Therapy
Topical agents—tretinoin, tazarotene, tacrolimus, pimecrolimus
Dapsone
Auranofin
Cytotoxic/immunosuppressive agents—azathioprine, methotrexate, mycophenolate mofetil
Thalidomide, lenalidomide
Systemic corticosteroids
Intravenous immune globulin

Although topical corticosteroids have been shown to be effective under experimental conditions, when prescribed in the clinic or office they may not be highly effective. Probably because of their expense, messiness, and the time involved in their application, they are not always used as directed. Despite these limitations, topical corticosteroids should be prescribed in conjunction with other agents. The choice of a specific agent is based on the clinical lesion and the area of the body that is affected. The prescribing physician must bear in mind that these agents can produce atrophy, which is also a sign of the disease. Other topical immunomodulators, such as tacrolimus ointment and pimecrolimus cream, have also been used with some success, particularly in ACLE. These agents appear to be a reasonable choice for longer-term treatment of lesions on the face in particular, to avoid atrophy, telangiectases, and steroid-induced acne.

Lesions that do not respond to topical agents can be injected with a corticosteroid, such as triamcinolone acetonide (3 to 4 mg/mL). Hypertrophic lesions, scalp lesions, palmar lesions, and recalcitrant DLE lesions are well suited to therapy with intralesional corticosteroids. Again, it is important to recognize that atrophy is dose-related, and that there is a fine line between effectiveness and this complication. Secondary infection can rarely occur at the injection site.

Antimalarials form a mainstay of systemic therapy of cutaneous LE. The mechanism of action of these agents is unknown, but may relate to photoprotection and/or to immunomodulation. The agents available include hydroxychloroquine sulfate, chloroquine phosphate, and quinacrine HCl (quinacrine is available, but only from a compounding pharmacy). In some studies, antimalarial agents have been shown to be less effective in patients who smoke. In addition, smoking cessation has resulted in improved efficacy in individual patients. It is not fully elucidated whether smoking is associated with a worsening of the LE, or whether it inactivates or blocks the action of the antimalarial, or both. Chloroquine and hydroxychloroquine may be associated with retinopathy, whereas the major side effects of quinacrine are bone marrow suppression and a reversible yellow discoloration of the skin. The authors' first choice is hydroxychloroquine because, despite possibly being less efficacious, it has less ocular toxicity than chloroquine. Hydroxychloroquine is given by mouth in a dose of 200 to 400 mg/day based on ideal body weight. When this regimen is less effective than desired, either quinacrine 100 mg once daily can be added, or the patient can be switched to chloroquine (250 to 500 mg/day). The risk of retinopathy from chloroquine and hydroxychloroquine is dose-related, and regular eye exams should be performed in these patients. The elderly and those with renal insufficiency may be at higher risk. Antimalarials are effective for DLE, SCLE, tumid LE, LEP, and the arthritis, malaise, and aches associated with LE, but are less effective for patients with hypertrophic DLE, palmar DLE, chilblains LE, or vasculitic lesions. Patients with the DLE–SLE subset may not respond as well to antimalarials as those without systemic manifestations.

The number of patients with cutaneous LE who have a good clinical response to antimalarials has not been systematically studied but has been estimated to be 75% to 90%. However, there is clearly a subset of patients who remain recalcitrant to the above-mentioned therapies. Many other systemic agents have been used for recalcitrant cutaneous LE. Systemic corticosteroids are generally less effective for the cutaneous disease, despite their dramatic effect on systemic symptoms and signs. Doses required to maintain control of cutaneous disease typically lead to steroid-related side effects; therefore, strong consideration should be given to steroid-sparing agents. Immunosuppressants such as azathioprine, mycophenolate mofetil, and methotrexate have been reported to be effective in recalcitrant cases. Perhaps the most dramatic clinical response to treatment comes from thalidomide at doses of 50 to 150 mg/day. Thalidomide prescribing is associated with a program to prevent pregnancy (STEPS program), and the physician and pharmacy must be registered with the company. In addition, there is real concern about the possibility of thalidomide-induced peripheral neuropathy that may not be reversible upon cessation of the drug as well as an increased risk of thrombotic events. A thalidomide analog, lenalidomide, has been reported to be effective for recalcitrant disease and appears to carry a lower risk of neuropathy.

Additionally, several other cytotoxic/immunosuppressive agents have been used in individual patients with some success. Dapsone 100 to 200 mg/day has been reported to be effective. It may be helpful in the rare patient with SCLE, in those with LE and cutaneous vasculitis syndromes, and in individuals with bullous LE. High-dose intravenous immunoglobulin has provided good but short-lived results in some patients. Apremilast, a newly approved agent for psoriasis and psoriatic arthritis, has been used in a small study of patients with cutaneous LE and might be another agent to consider in antimalarial-resistant patients.

There are several newer biological agents that have been approved or studied in systemic LE patients; however, their benefit specifically for cutaneous disease is not yet known. The use of TNF-α inhibitors is currently not widely recommended given reports of induction of antinuclear antibodies and lupus-like syndromes in some patients with rheumatoid arthritis, inflammatory bowel disease, and psoriasis using these medications. There are several reports of ustekinumab, which more specifically blocks IL-12/23, improving cutaneous lesions of LE, but larger studies are needed. Belimumab, although useful for SLE, has not been demonstrated to be effective in the management of cutaneous lesions.

SUGGESTED READINGS

Albrecht J, Berlin JA, Braverman IM, et al. Dermatology position paper on the revision of the 1982 ACR criteria for systemic lupus erythematosus. Lupus 2004;13:839–49.

Callen JP. Cutaneous lupus erythematosus: a personal approach to management. Australas J Dermatol 2006;47:13–27.

Jarukitsopa S, Hoganson DD, Crowson CS, et al. Epidemiology of systemic lupus erythematosus and cutaneous lupus in a predominately white population in the United States. Arthritis Care Res (Hoboken). http://dx.doi.org/10.1002/acr.22502, in press.

Krathen MS, Dunham J, Gaines E, et al. The cutaneous lupus erythematosus disease activity and severity index: expansion for rheumatology and dermatology. Arthritis Rheum 2008;59:338–44.

Kuhn A, Landmann A. The classification and diagnosis of cutaneous lupus erythematosus. J Autoimmun 2014;48–49:14–9.

Lowe GC, Henderson CL, Grau RH, et al. A systematic review of drug-induced subacute cutaneous lupus erythematosus. Br J Dermatol 2011;164:465–72.

Okon L, Rosenbach M, Krathen M, et al. Lenalidomide in treatment-refractory cutaneous lupus erythematosus: efficacy and safety in a 52-week trial. J Am Acad Dermatol 2014;70:583–4.

Petri M, Orbai AM, Alarcon GS, et al. Derivation and validation of the Systemic Lupus International Collaborating Clinics classification criteria for systemic lupus erythematosus. Arthritis Rheum 2012;64:2677–86.

Rothfield N, Sontheimer RD, Bernstein M. Lupus erythematosus: systemic and cutaneous manifestations. Clin Dermatol 2006;24:348–62.

Winchester D, Duffin KC, Hansen C. Response to ustekinumab in a patient with both severe psoriasis and hypertrophic cutaneous lupus. Lupus 2012;21:1007–10.

CHAPTER 2

DERMATOMYOSITIS

Ruth Ann Vleugels • Jeffrey P. Callen

KEY POINTS

- Classic dermatomyositis involves a proximal inflammatory myopathy with a characteristic cutaneous eruption. In patients with clinically amyopathic dermatomyositis, skin disease is the prominent feature.
- Pathognomonic cutaneous findings of dermatomyositis include the heliotrope eruption and Gottron's papules. In dermatomyositis, cutaneous disease is photoexacerbated.
- All adult patients with dermatomyositis require screening for malignancy and pulmonary disease, regardless of whether they have muscle involvement.
- Juvenile dermatomyositis is not associated with an increased risk of cancer, but does have an increased association with calcinosis cutis and vasculitis.
- In dermatomyositis, treatment for and therapeutic response of muscle and skin disease often differ. Cutaneous dermatomyositis is classically challenging to treat and negatively impacts patient quality of life.

DEFINITION AND CLASSIFICATION

Dermatomyositis is a condition that combines an inflammatory myopathy with a characteristic cutaneous disease. A closely related disease, polymyositis, has all the clinical features of the muscular disease of dermatomyositis but lacks the characteristic cutaneous findings. A third idiopathic inflammatory myopathy, inclusion body myositis, also lacks cutaneous disease, but has a unique pattern of weakness with prominent involvement of the wrist and finger flexors and quadriceps. The pathogenesis of these disorders is only partially understood, but immune-mediated muscle damage is believed to be important as a pathogenetic mechanism. Dermatomyositis appears to be characterized by an increased frequency of internal malignancy, whereas the association of polymyositis with malignancy is less well resolved. There is a female to male preponderance of approximately 2:1, with a peak incidence in the fifth and sixth decades. A juvenile form of dermatomyositis also exists, which is not associated with an increased risk of malignancy, but does have an increased incidence of calcinosis cutis and vasculitis. Because both dermatomyositis and polymyositis are associated with morbidity and occasional deaths, a prompt and aggressive approach to therapy is indicated.

Bohan and Peter first suggested the use of five criteria to diagnose dermatomyositis. These include (1) proximal symmetric muscle weakness that progresses over a period of weeks to months; (2) elevated serum levels of muscle-derived enzymes; (3) an abnormal electromyogram; (4) an abnormal muscle biopsy; and (5) the presence of cutaneous disease compatible with dermatomyositis. These criteria are useful for patient evaluation, but it is not necessary to perform all of the muscle testing in patients with characteristic skin disease, particularly those who have proximal muscle weakness and elevated muscle-derived enzymes.

The inflammatory myopathies may be subclassified into eight groups. The following system of classification has been useful in differentiating groups of patients with regard to their prognosis, potential for an associated process, and potential to respond to various therapies: (1) dermatomyositis; (2) polymyositis; (3) myositis in association with malignancy; (4) juvenile dermatomyositis (most often diagnosed before age 16); (5) myositis in association with another connective tissue disease; (6) inclusion body myositis; (7) dermatomyositis sine myositis (amyopathic dermatomyositis); and (8) drug-induced disease.

Given that the incidence and prevalence of amyopathic dermatomyositis appear to be increasing, Sontheimer has proposed a revised classification system that better recognizes the cutaneous manifestations of the inflammatory myopathies (Table 2-1).

PATHOGENESIS

The pathogenesis of the idiopathic inflammatory myopathies is not well understood. The pathogenetic mechanisms involved in the muscular disease are better understood than are those involved in the induction of cutaneous disease. Many agents and events have been associated with the appearance of dermatomyositis, including various infections (particularly viral or parasitic infections), vaccination, neoplasms, drug-induced disease, various types of stress, and trauma. In addition, dermatomyositis and polymyositis have been linked with various diseases associated with immunologic phenomena. The demonstration of the Jo-1 antibody in patients with myositis further supports a viral etiology because the antigen for the Jo-1 antibody has characteristics similar to those of viral and muscle proteins. Patients with active dermatomyositis or polymyositis have been demonstrated to have upregulation of type I interferon-α/β-inducible genes in blood samples, and

TABLE 2-1	The Idiopathic Inflammatory Myopathies

Dermatomyositis (DM)
  Adult-onset DM
    Classic DM
    DM with malignancy
    DM in a patient with another connective tissue disease
    Clinically amyopathic DM (also known as DM sine myositis)
  Juvenile-onset DM (JDMS)
    Clinically amyopathic JDMS
    Classic JDMS
Polymyositis
Inclusion body myositis

Adapted from Sontheimer RD. Cutaneous features of classical dermatomyositis and amyopathic dermatomyositis. Curr Opin Rheumatol 1999;11:475–82.

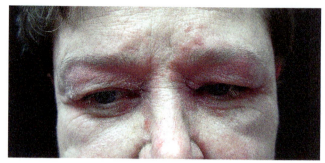

FIGURE 2-1 ■ Heliotrope eruption with violaceous erythema, scaling, and mild edema of the upper eyelids.

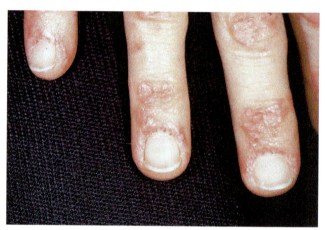

FIGURE 2-2 ■ Gottron's papules: This patient has typical erythematous to violaceous papules and plaques over the bony prominences on the extensor surfaces of the hands.

the level of type I interferons has been shown to correlate with disease activity. Despite having this upregulation of type I interferons in common, it is thought that the immunopathogenesis of dermatomyositis and polymyositis is different. In polymyositis, clonally expanded autoreactive CD8-positive T cells invade myocytes expressing major histocompatibility complex (MHC) class I antigens and cause necrosis via the perforin pathway. In dermatomyositis, autoantigens activate a humoral immune process in which complement is deposited in capillaries, causing capillary necrosis and ischemia. For both diseases, a genetic predisposition has also been suggested. Thus, under appropriate circumstances in an immunogenetically predisposed individual, an infection, drug, trauma, or neoplasm may be able to initiate an inflammatory reaction in the muscle and skin. Through a complex set of reactions involving immunologic phenomena, muscle damage and cutaneous disease may occur.

MANIFESTATIONS

Cutaneous Manifestations

The characteristic and possibly pathognomonic cutaneous features of dermatomyositis are the heliotrope eruption and Gottron's papules. Several other cutaneous features that occur in patients with dermatomyositis are characteristic of the disease but are not pathognomonic. These include midfacial erythema that involves the nasolabial folds (as opposed to the malar erythema in lupus erythematosus, which spares the nasolabial folds), poikiloderma in a photosensitive distribution on the chest ("V-neck" sign) or back (shawl sign), a violaceous erythema on the extensor surfaces, alopecia with or without scaly poikilodermatous changes, a scaly poikilodermatous rash on the lateral thighs (Holster sign), and periungual and cuticular changes. The cutaneous disease in dermatomyositis is photodistributed and often photoaggravated. In addition, pruritus may be a prominent feature in dermatomyositis, and may be helpful in clinically distinguishing this entity from lupus erythematosus. Quality-of-life impairment in dermatomyositis is greater than in other skin diseases, including both psoriasis and atopic dermatitis, based on its cutaneous manifestations alone. Notably, the cutaneous manifestations of dermatomyositis can follow the course of the myositis or can be discordant from the muscle disease activity. Reactivation of any skin manifestation of dermatomyositis in a patient otherwise considered to be in remission may signify a relapse of the myositis. Most often, however, the activity of the muscle disease is not reflected by that of the cutaneous disease.

The heliotrope eruption consists of a dusky erythematous to violaceous cutaneous eruption with or without edema involving the periorbital skin in a symmetric distribution (Fig. 2-1). Often only the upper lid is involved. Sometimes this sign is subtle and may involve only faint erythema along the eyelid margin. Gottron's papules are found over bony prominences, particularly the metacarpophalangeal joints, the proximal interphalangeal joints, and/or the distal interphalangeal joints. They may also be found over bony prominences such as the elbows, knees, and feet. The lesions consist of slightly elevated erythematous to violaceous papules and plaques (Figs. 2-2 and 2-3); they often contain telangiectases, and there may be hyper- and/or hypopigmentation. These lesions can be clinically confused with those of lupus erythematosus or, at times, with those of papulosquamous disorders such as psoriasis or lichen planus. In instances in which differentiation is difficult, a biopsy is warranted; however, the features of dermatomyositis are indistinguishable

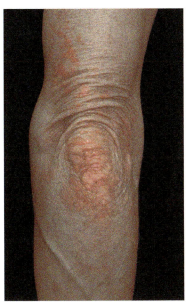

FIGURE 2-3 ■ Gottron's papules and sign. Violaceous papules and erythema over the elbow.

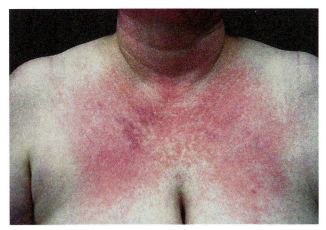

FIGURE 2-5 ■ Poikilodermatous eruption in a photosensitive distribution in a woman with malignancy and dermatomyositis.

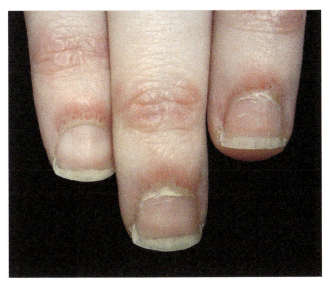

FIGURE 2-4 ■ Cuticular hypertrophy and periungual telangiectases (consisting of both dilated capillary loops and capillary dropout) in a patient with dermatomyositis.

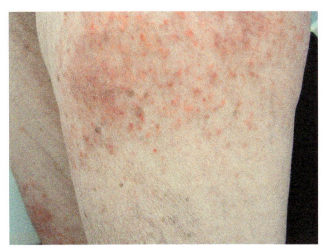

FIGURE 2-6 ■ Poikilodermatous changes on the lateral thighs, known as the "holster sign."

from those of cutaneous lupus erythematosus. Gottron's sign typically refers to violaceous erythema over the areas where Gottron's papules tend to occur.

Nailfold changes consist of periungual telangiectases (consisting of both dilated capillary loops and capillary dropout), cuticular hypertrophy, and small hemorrhagic infarcts within this hypertrophic area (Fig. 2-4). The periungual telangiectases may be clinically apparent or may be appreciated only by capillary microscopy. Clinically, they may closely resemble those seen in other connective tissue diseases. The cuticular overgrowth may be similar to that seen in scleroderma.

Poikiloderma can occur on any photodistributed site, most classically the upper chest and neck ("V-neck" sign) and the upper back (shawl sign) (Fig. 2-5), but also on the extensor surfaces of the arms and within Gottron's papules on the dorsal hands. This photosensitive poikilodermatous eruption must be differentiated from lupus erythematosus and from other diseases that cause poikilodermatous skin changes. In addition, poikilodermatous changes may also occur on the lateral thighs, known as the "holster sign" (Fig. 2-6).

Scalp involvement in dermatomyositis is relatively common. Mild to moderate nonscarring alopecia (Fig. 2-7) can occur in some patients and often follows a flare of the disease. In addition, the scalp is often diffusely affected by scaling and erythema with poikilodermatous features, which can result in intense scalp pruritus. The scalp pruritus is often severe, and the symptoms often are greater than one might appreciate from the clinical findings. Clinical distinction from seborrheic dermatitis or psoriasis may be challenging, but histopathologic evaluation is helpful.

Less common cutaneous findings include an exfoliative erythroderma as well as vesiculobullous, erosive, and ulcerative lesions. Patients with myositis can also develop the lesions of other collagen–vascular diseases. The presence of these types of lesions allows physicians to classify the patients into an overlap category. In general, sclerodermatous skin changes have been the most frequently

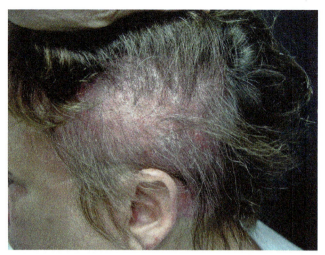

FIGURE 2-7 ■ Erythema, poikiloderma, psoriasiform scaling, and nonscarring alopecia in a patient with dermatomyositis.

seen in patients with overlap syndrome. However, cutaneous vasculitis, discoid lupus erythematosus, and rheumatoid nodules have also been known to occur in patients with dermatomyositis.

Skin biopsy may aid in differentiating dermatomyositis from other papulosquamous or eczematous diseases, but cannot be used to reliably distinguish dermatomyositis from lupus erythematosus. In addition, direct immunofluorescence microscopy is usually not helpful in differentiating lupus erythematosus and dermatomyositis. Classically, skin biopsy in dermatomyositis demonstrates a vacuolar interface dermatitis with mucin deposition in the dermis. Cutaneous lesions of dermatomyositis that do not demonstrate the interface change classically observed with the pathognomonic and characteristic skin lesions include mechanic's hands (hyperkeratosis of the lateral fingers and palms), panniculitis, cutaneous vasculitis, urticaria, a flagellate erythema, and follicular hyperkeratosis.

Although cutaneous lesions precede muscle disease in 30% to 56% of patients with classic dermatomyositis, myositis follows within 3 to 6 months in most cases. In a significant portion of patients, the myositis resolves with therapy, whereas the cutaneous disease persists and becomes the most salient feature of disease (postmyopathic dermatomyositis). Amyopathic dermatomyositis is provisionally diagnosed when typical cutaneous disease is present for at least 6 months without clinical weakness, with repeatedly normal serum muscle enzyme levels, and in patients who have not been treated with systemic corticosteroids or immunomodulatory agents for more than a few months. The diagnosis of amyopathic dermatomyositis is considered confirmed after skin disease has been present for 2 years in the absence of muscle involvement. Predictive factors for progression to classic dermatomyositis with muscle involvement have not yet been identified in this subset of patients.

Muscle Disease

Clinical and laboratory abnormalities that suggest muscle disease are characteristic features of polymyositis and dermatomyositis. Even in patients who have only cutaneous disease at presentation, myositis follows in the majority of patients. Myositis precedes the cutaneous findings in less than 10% of patients. The myositis occurring in dermatomyositis is indistinguishable from that occurring in polymyositis as assessed by clinical and laboratory features. Also, when considered alone, the individual features of myositis are not diagnostic of dermatomyositis or polymyositis; rather, the diagnosis is one of exclusion.

Clinically, the myopathy affects mainly the proximal muscle groups of the shoulder and pelvic girdle. In severe, progressive disease all muscles may become involved. The disease is usually symmetric. The initial complaints include weakness, fatigue, an inability to climb stairs, an inability to raise the arms for actions such as hair grooming or shaving, an inability to rise from a squatting or sitting position, or a combination of these features. The progression of disease is variable, but usually occurs over a period of weeks to months. Muscle aching is a common subjective complaint, but frank tenderness on palpation is variable. An inability to swallow and symptoms of aspiration may reflect the involvement of striated muscle of the pharynx or upper esophagus. Dysphagia often signifies a rapidly progressive course and may be associated with a poor prognosis.

Muscle enzyme levels are frequently elevated in patients with inflammatory myopathy. The enzymes that are commonly elevated are creatine kinase, aldolase, lactic dehydrogenase, and/or serum transaminases. In the vast majority of patients, creatine kinase is the most practical test available for measuring the activity of muscle disease. Other potential abnormalities include disturbances of electrical action on electromyography (EMG), histopathologic changes (muscle biopsy classically demonstrates type II fiber atrophy, necrosis, regeneration, a centralization of the nuclei, and a lymphocytic infiltrate in a perifascicular and/or perivascular region), and/or abnormalities on magnetic resonance imaging (MRI) or ultrasound. The use of MRI may improve yield when performed prior to muscle biopsy or may demonstrate clinically inapparent inflammation. In children, levels of factor VIII-related antigen or neopterin may predict a more severe dermatomyositis variant with vasculopathy.

Systemic Features

Dermatomyositis and polymyositis are multisystem disorders. This is reflected by the high frequency of other clinical features in patients with these diseases.

Arthralgias and/or arthritis may be present in up to one-quarter of patients with inflammatory myopathy. This percentage rises in patients with overlap syndromes. The usual picture is one of generalized arthralgias accompanied by morning stiffness. The small joints of the hands, wrists, and ankles may be involved with symmetric nondeforming arthritis. Patients with arthritis may have a lower frequency of malignancy than those who do not have arthritis.

Esophageal disease as manifested by dysphagia is estimated to be present in 15% to 50% of patients with inflammatory myopathy. The dysphagia can be of two types: proximal or distal. Proximal dysphagia is caused by the involvement of striated muscle in the pharynx or proximal esophagus. This involvement correlates well with the severity of the muscle disease and is corticosteroid responsive. Distal dysphagia is related to the involvement of nonstriated muscle and appears to be more frequent in patients who have overlap syndromes. Distal dysphagia may also be accompanied by symptoms of reflux esophagitis. In general, dysphagia portends a poor prognosis and is often associated with pulmonary involvement.

Pulmonary disease occurs in approximately 15% to 30% of patients with dermatomyositis and polymyositis. It can be characterized by a primary diffuse interstitial fibrosis that may be manifested radiologically, or by abnormalities seen on pulmonary function testing. Pulmonary disease may also occur as a direct complication of the muscular disease, such as hypoventilation or aspiration in patients with dysphagia, or it may be a result of treatment, such as with opportunistic infections or drug-induced hypersensitivity pneumonitis. It is important to note that patients with amyopathic dermatomyositis may have aggressive lung disease even in the absence of myositis. Overall, pulmonary complications have been associated with a poor prognosis. Data have suggested that patients with myositis who have Jo-1 antibodies are at a greater risk for pulmonary involvement. In fact, 70% of patients with Jo-1 antibodies have interstitial lung disease. The antisynthetase syndrome is the constellation of interstitial lung disease, myositis, polyarthritis, Raynaud's phenomenon, fever, and mechanic's hands in a patient with antitransfer RNA autoantibodies.

Cardiac disease may also occur in patients with inflammatory myopathy, as manifested by myocarditis or pericarditis. Pericarditis appears to be more common in patients with overlapping features of other connective tissue diseases. Myocarditis can result in conduction defects, arrhythmias, or, when severe, congestive heart failure.

Calcinosis of the skin or muscle is unusual in adults but may occur in up to 40% of children with dermatomyositis. Calcinosis cutis is manifested by firm, yellow-white, or skin-colored nodules, often over bony prominences. Occasionally, these nodules can extrude through the surface of the skin, in which case secondary infections may occur. Calcification of the muscles is often asymptomatic and may be seen only on radiologic examination. In severe forms, the calcinosis can cause loss of function, and, rarely, bone formation is possible.

Pregnancy has been shown to have an effect on the inflammatory myopathy. In addition, the inflammatory myopathy may produce profound effects on the neonate and/or the mother. Studies suggest that dermatomyositis and/or polymyositis may be activated during pregnancy, or that the initial manifestations may be appreciated during pregnancy. In addition, in a large group of women with multiple pregnancies, premature delivery, spontaneous abortions, perinatal deaths, and fetal loss were more common in patients with active myositis.

AMYOPATHIC DERMATOMYOSITIS

An evolving topic in the realm of dermatomyositis is how to classify and refer to patients with only or predominantly cutaneous disease. It is becoming more widely accepted that a subset of patients will have skin-limited disease, similar to patients with lupus limited to the skin rather than with systemic involvement. This is a change from the previous notion that all patients with dermatomyositis would by definition have some degree of muscle involvement if physicians simply investigated sufficiently to find it. In the current nomenclature, clinically amyopathic dermatomyositis includes patients with both amyopathic and hypomyopathic dermatomyositis, subgroups which comprise approximately 20% of the total population of dermatomyositis patients according to the best existing epidemiologic data.

Amyopathic dermatomyositis has been recognized to include a unique subset of patients with typical cutaneous disease for at least 6 months without weakness or abnormal muscle enzymes or testing. By definition, these patients must not have received 2 consecutive months or more of systemic immunosuppressive therapy in the first 6 months after skin disease onset, and must not have received medications known to cause dermatomyositis-like skin changes, including hydroxyurea and statins. These patients can be referred to as having provisional amyopathic dermatomyositis until 2 years after diagnosis, at which point their disease can be called confirmed amyopathic dermatomyositis. Although it presents with cutaneous disease indistinguishable from that of classic dermatomyositis, amyopathic dermatomyositis is a distinct entity rather than a group of patients in whom muscle abnormalities are not yet detectable. In the largest systematic review of adult-onset clinically amyopathic dermatomyositis, most patients had a normal EMG, muscle biopsy, and/or muscle MRI when performed.

Hypomyopathic dermatomyositis includes cutaneous findings and subclinical myositis evident on laboratory tests, EMG, biopsy, and/or MRI, but no clinical weakness or muscle tenderness. Importantly, these findings do not reliably predict the onset of clinically significant muscle disease at a later time, and should therefore not necessarily warrant more aggressive therapeutic intervention. Sontheimer reported that no patients with hypomyopathic dermatomyositis had developed clinically significant muscle weakness at the time of follow-up, despite an average duration of skin disease of 5.4 years.

Cutaneous lesions and histopathology are indistinguishable from those of classic dermatomyositis. Similar to classic dermatomyositis, there is a female preponderance, a peak onset in the fifth and sixth decades, and a pediatric population affected by amyopathic dermatomyositis. Laboratory results in amyopathic dermatomyositis are similar to those in classic dermatomyositis except for a relative lack of anti-Jo-1 antibodies, including in patients with pulmonary disease, and an increased prevalence of antimelanoma differentiation-associated gene or MDA-5 antibodies (previously referred to as anti-CADM-140 antibodies). In an American study, there was no significant difference in prevalence of interstitial lung disease between patients with amyopathic and classic dermatomyositis. In Eastern Asian populations, patients with skin-limited disease and MDA-5 autoantibodies have been shown to have a high risk of rapidly progressive lung disease and a poor prognosis despite a lack of muscle disease. In addition, an MDA-5 antibody-associated dermato-pulmonary syndrome has recently been reported in a non-Asian population. Finally, similar to classic dermatomyositis, amyopathic dermatomyositis also has an association with malignancy, mandating that these patients be followed for manifestations of both interstitial lung disease and cancer.

MYOSITIS AND MALIGNANCY

The issue of the relationship between dermatomyositis–polymyositis and malignancy has been clarified. The frequency of malignancy in dermatomyositis has varied from 6% to 60% in various studies. This variation is probably related to differing methods, and the best data suggest that 18% to 32% of patients with dermatomyositis have or will develop a malignancy. In 1992, Swedish investigators first documented the increased frequency of malignancy in patients with dermatomyositis over that in the general population. Although patients with polymyositis had a slight increase in cancer frequency, it was not highly significant and could be explained by a more aggressive cancer search creating a diagnostic suspicion bias. Subsequent studies from other Scandinavian countries have demonstrated similar findings. An Australian study demonstrated a relative risk of malignancy three to six times that of the general population in patients with dermatomyositis. Although this risk declines over time, it is highest in the first 3 years after diagnosis, and remains elevated for at least 5 years. Heightened surveillance for malignancy must therefore continue for at least 3 years from the onset of the disease.

Malignancies may occur prior to, concurrently with, or after the onset of dermatomyositis. In addition, the myositis may follow the course of the malignancy (a paraneoplastic course) or follow its own course, independent of treatment of the malignancy. Studies demonstrating the benefits of cancer treatment on the myositis and studies showing no relationship have been reported. Relapse of myositis and/or cutaneous manifestations of dermatomyositis may indicate cancer recurrence and warrant careful investigation. A wide variety of malignancies have been reported in patients with dermatomyositis. Gynecologic malignancy, in particular ovarian carcinoma, is clearly overrepresented, as are lung, pancreatic, colon, non-Hodgkin's lymphoma, and breast cancer. Furthermore, in a Southeast Asian population carcinoma of the nasopharynx is overrepresented.

Although advanced age has been demonstrated to be a risk factor for malignancy in patients with dermatomyositis, all adult dermatomyositis patients are considered to be at risk for cancer. This concept is supported by reports of young adults with malignancy-associated dermatomyositis. Malignancy in younger age groups occurs in tissues that are more commonly affected by malignancy in the absence of myopathy (e.g., a 30-year-old man would be more likely to harbor a testicular tumor, whereas a 70-year-old man would be more likely to have colon cancer). Overall, young age should not dissuade a clinician from completing a careful malignancy work-up in a patient with adult-onset dermatomyositis. Children with juvenile dermatomyositis are not considered to be at an increased risk of malignancy. In this group, formal cancer screening is not recommended. Rather, a full physical examination and review of systems are conducted at each patient visit.

Finally, the issue of whether the use of immunosuppressive medications is associated with an increased risk of subsequent malignancy in patients with myositis remains controversial. In several studies there has been no demonstrated increased risk of malignancy associated with the immunosuppressive therapy commonly given to control the inflammatory myopathy in dermatomyositis and polymyositis. On the other hand, there are several reports of Epstein–Barr virus-associated lymphomas arising in patients with systemic rheumatic diseases, including dermatomyositis, on immunosuppressive medications such as methotrexate. In some of these cases, the lymphoma resolved after discontinuation of immunosuppressive therapy without requiring the initiation of radiation therapy or chemotherapy.

EVALUATION OF THE PATIENT WITH MYOSITIS

The diagnosis of myositis is one of exclusion (Table 2-2). A complete history should be conducted, with particular attention to drugs or toxins that may be involved. It should include a history of previous malignancies, previous travel, changes in the diet, and any symptoms of associated phenomena, such as dysphagia, dyspnea, or arthritis. A thorough review of systems is necessary to aid in the evaluation of patients with dermatomyositis for malignancies.

A complete history and physical examination should be conducted. In women, a careful breast and pelvic examination should be included. These examinations should not be deferred. If the examiner does not feel confident in these areas, it is necessary to obtain a gynecologic consultation. Similarly, in men, examination of the rectum and prostate is necessary.

Routine evaluation in the adult patient with dermatomyositis includes a complete blood count and comprehensive metabolic panel, urinalysis, stool occult blood testing, tests for thyroid function, CA 19-9, an electrocardiogram, chest X-ray, age-appropriate gastrointestinal endoscopic studies, chest, abdominal, and pelvic computed tomography (CT) scans, and in women, mammography, transvaginal pelvic ultrasound, CA-125, and a Papanicolaou smear. Children should have a fasting glucose and lipid screening because of an increased risk of insulin resistance and lipoatrophy. In all adult patients, pulmonary function tests (PFTs), including diffusion studies, should be performed regardless of whether there are symptoms or abnormalities on the chest X-ray. Abnormal PFT findings, particularly reduced diffusing capacity of carbon monoxide (DLCO), should prompt evaluation with a high-resolution chest CT scan. An esophageal study is necessary to evaluate for dysmotility in all patients with muscle disease. Optional studies include a Holter monitor, echocardiography, and serologic tests. In addition to the tests above, screening should include age-, race-, and ethnicity-related testing. For

TABLE 2-2 **Evaluation of the Patient with Myositis**

I. History
   A. Previous malignancy
   B. Associated symptoms
   C. History of toxins, infections, travel, vaccinations, or drug intake
II. Physical examination
   A. Dermatologic evaluation
   B. Women: pelvic and breast examination
   C. Men: rectal and prostate examination
III. Evaluation of muscle disease
   A. Creatine kinase, aldolase
   B. Electromyography (if A is normal)
   C. Muscle biopsy (if A and B are normal)
   D. Magnetic resonance imaging (particularly if A is normal and B and C are declined)
IV. Skin disease evaluation
   A. Lesional biopsy for routine histopathologic evaluation
   B. Immunofluorescence in selected patients (rarely helpful)
V. Routine studies
   A. Complete blood count, comprehensive metabolic panel, and urinalysis
   B. Thyroid function
   C. Stool occult blood testing
   D. Electrocardiogram
   E. Women: Papanicolaou smear, CA-125
   F. CA 19-9
   G. Gastrointestinal endoscopy (age-appropriate)
   H. Fasting glucose and lipids (in children)
VI. Radiographic examination
   A. Chest X-ray, consider high-resolution chest computed tomography (CT)
   B. CT scan chest/abdomen/pelvis
   C. Women: pelvic ultrasound, mammography
VII. Pulmonary function tests (with diffusion studies)
VIII. Esophageal studies, e.g., barium swallow, manometry, or cineradiography (in patients with muscle disease)
IX. Optional
   A. Holter monitor
   B. Echocardiogram
   C. Autoantibody studies; e.g., Jo-1, Mi-2, MDA-5, TIF-1γ, NXP-2, PM, SRP, etc.
X. Further testing is based on abnormalities discovered in steps I–VII. Malignancy screening should be performed at the time of diagnosis and annually for at least 3 years

example, Southeast Asian patients should have a careful ear, nose, and throat examination to evaluate for nasopharyngeal cancer. We believe that malignancy screening should take place annually for 3 years, in addition to careful investigation of any new signs or symptoms. It is important to note that the current recommendations for malignancy screening are an evolving concept and may change if a reliable marker becomes available and is proven in evidence-based studies to be able to replace empiric screening methods.

Although they may be positive in pure cases of dermatomyositis, tests of antinuclear antibody have not traditionally been shown to influence the prediction of the course of the disease or its therapy. Antinuclear antibody is positive in approximately two-thirds of cases. Newer serologic studies, including myositis-specific autoantibodies, have become available, and include Jo-1, Mi-2, PL-7, PL-12, EJ, OJ, KS, Zo, YRS, and SRP. Three others, U_1RNP, Ku, and PM-Scl, have been found in myositis-overlap syndromes. Anti-MJ and -PMS1 have been found to correlate to cases of juvenile dermatomyositis, and the p155/140 antibody has also been associated and may correlate with more extensive cutaneous involvement in children. Although these tests correlate with subsets of patients, the correlations are imperfect. For example, anti-Jo-1 antibodies are linked to pulmonary disease and the antisynthetase syndrome, yet are not uniformly present in these circumstances. In patients with clinically amyopathic dermatomyositis, MDA-5, or anti-CADM-140, autoantibodies may be present. Cutaneous manifestations seen in patients with MDA-5 autoantibodies include palmar papules as well as cutaneous ulcerations. Most recently, it has been demonstrated that most patients with cancer-associated dermatomyositis have antibodies to either transcription intermediary factor 1γ (TIF-1γ) or nuclear matrix protein NXP-2. These novel autoantibodies may allow for a redefined classification of idiopathic inflammatory myopathies.

Currently, widespread use of autoantibody testing is discouraged because it neither confirms nor excludes the diagnosis, is an imperfect predictor of the prognosis, and is not helpful in monitoring therapy. The novel autoantibodies may, however, help identify patients requiring more aggressive malignancy or pulmonary work-up and surveillance in the future.

A subsequent evaluation is necessary following the initiation of therapy. Repeat testing of each abnormality is advised. Follow-up of the myositis generally includes a combination of the clinical examination and serial serum muscle enzyme testing. Repeat muscle biopsy or electromyography is reserved for unusual circumstances. The use of biomechanical assessment to quantify muscle strength may be of benefit in following a patient's course. Careful questioning with regard to new symptoms should occur at each follow-up visit, and if a symptom develops, careful evaluation is necessary.

COURSE AND TREATMENT

Several general measures are helpful in treating patients with dermatomyositis and polymyositis. Bed rest may be required in those with progressive weakness; however, this must be combined with an aggressive but passive range-of-motion exercise program to prevent contractures. Any patient with muscle disease should have an appropriate physical therapy regimen, and exercise and rehabilitation have been demonstrated to be beneficial, without inducing flares of the myositis, even in the course of active disease. Nutrition is important because of the negative nitrogen balance that exists in inflammatory myopathy. This is particularly important in children. Patients who have evidence of dysphagia should have the head of the bed elevated and should avoid eating meals before retiring.

The overall therapeutic plan is determined primarily by the presence or absence of myositis or other internal organ involvement. The mainstay of therapy for myositis is the use of systemic corticosteroids. There has been debate over low-dose versus high-dose therapy and alternate-day therapy. Traditionally, prednisone is given in a dose of 1 to 2 mg/kg/day as the initial therapy. This treatment should continue for at least 1 month and until after the myositis has become clinically and enzymatically inactive. At this point, the dose is slowly tapered, generally over a period 1.5 to 2 times as long as the period of active treatment. Approximately 25% to 30% of patients with dermatomyositis and/or polymyositis will not respond to systemic corticosteroids or will develop significant steroid-related side effects. In these patients, immunosuppressive agents (methotrexate, azathioprine, mycophenolate mofetil, intravenous immunoglobulin, cyclophosphamide, chlorambucil, or cyclosporine) may be an effective means of inducing or maintaining remission. In addition, most patients are treated with an immunosuppressive regimen at disease onset in order to help with corticosteroid-sparing. Roughly half to three-quarters of patients treated with an immunosuppressive agent respond, as evidenced by an increase in strength, a reduction in enzyme levels, or a reduction in corticosteroid dosage.

Methotrexate can be used on a weekly basis, given either orally, subcutaneously, or intravenously. It is administered in an empiric dose of 25 to 30 mg/week (oral doses above 15 mg should be split into two administrations as absorption is decreased). The drug usually becomes effective in 6 to 12 weeks and is therefore not recommended for rapid control of a fulminant disease process.

Azathioprine has been used in a double-blind controlled trial with prednisone versus a group with prednisone and placebo. In a short-term analysis of 3 months, there were no differences between these two groups. However, in the open follow-up study 3 years later, a significantly lower steroid dosage was needed and significantly greater muscle strength was found in the patients who had been treated with azathioprine. Azathioprine is administered orally in a dosage of 1 to 2 mg/kg/day, depending on the results of thiopurine methyl transferase testing in order to achieve efficacy yet avoid bone marrow suppression.

Mycophenolate mofetil has also demonstrated efficacy for refractory muscle involvement, typically in doses of 2 to 3 g per day in divided doses.

The use of immunosuppressive agents is to be undertaken with caution. A complete evaluation prior to prescribing immunosuppressive therapy is necessary, as are the usual measures for follow-up of these patients.

Some patients fail to respond to these agents, and in these individuals various other measures have been suggested. Single-case or open-trial reports support the benefits of pulse methylprednisolone therapy, combination immunosuppressive therapy, chlorambucil, cyclosporine, tacrolimus, sirolimus, stem cell transplantation, ruxolitinib and total body irradiation. High-dose intravenous immunoglobulin (IVIG) and rituximab are the only therapies that have been tested in randomized, placebo-controlled clinical trials. IVIG demonstrated benefit for both the myositis as well as the cutaneous disease when given at a dose of 1 g/kg/day on two consecutive days monthly. The largest randomized clinical trial to date in the inflammatory myopathies involved 200 patients with refractory dermatomyositis (adult or juvenile) or polymyositis treated with rituximab. The trial failed to meet its primary and secondary endpoints, which were muscle-based criteria. Despite this, a majority of patients had improvement of myositis and corticosteroid-sparing. No validated skin index was used in those patients with dermatomyositis.

A placebo-controlled study showed no benefit from plasmapheresis. Despite case reports demonstrating benefits from antitumor necrosis factor-α (anti-TNF-α) medications, a pilot study of infliximab for patients with refractory inflammatory myopathies demonstrated radiological and clinical worsening of muscle disease and activation of the type I interferon system in several cases. A series of patients treated with etanercept all had exacerbation of muscle disease. In addition, there have been reports of anti-TNF-induced dermatomyositis, polymyositis, and antisynthetase syndrome.

Therapy for cutaneous disease in patients with dermatomyositis is often difficult because, even though the myositis may respond to treatment with corticosteroids and/or immunosuppressants, the cutaneous lesions often persist. In one study, 50% of patients who received immunosuppressive therapy for muscle involvement showed no improvement in cutaneous manifestations. Although cutaneous disease may be of minor importance in patients with fulminant myositis, in many patients the cutaneous disease becomes the most important aspect of the disorder. Most patients with cutaneous lesions are photosensitive; thus, as in patients with lupus erythematosus, the daily use of a broad-spectrum sunscreen with a sun protective factor of at least 50, sun protective clothing, and a wide-brimmed hat is recommended. Topical modalities include corticosteroids, tacrolimus, or pimecrolimus. Hydroxychloroquine in doses of 200 to 400 mg/day is effective in select patients, providing some control of the cutaneous disease and allowing a reduction in corticosteroid dosage. Patients who do not respond well or fully to hydroxychloroquine can be switched to chloroquine 250 mg/day or can receive quinacrine 100 mg daily in addition given its lack of ocular toxicity. Quinacrine requires compounding and may not be available in all locations. The usual precautions regarding antimalarial therapy should be taken, including a careful ophthalmologic examination and follow-up. It appears that patients with dermatomyositis have a greater potential than those with lupus erythematosus to develop morbilliform drug reactions with hydroxychloroquine, and a pretreatment warning is helpful. Patients with dermatomyositis who develop a cutaneous reaction to hydroxychloroquine may go on to tolerate chloroquine.

Open-label studies support the usefulness of methotrexate in doses between 10 and 30 mg/week and of mycophenolate mofetil for the skin disease. Observations regarding retinoids, dapsone, thalidomide, adjuvant leflunomide, antiestrogens, cyclosporine, tacrolimus, sirolimus, total body irradiation, infliximab, etanercept, and ruxolitinib are anecdotal, but intravenous immunoglobulin appears to be effective and safe, albeit expensive. Although case reports and one small trial have shown improvement in skin manifestations of dermatomyositis with rituximab, the largest open trial to date as well as a randomized controlled trial demonstrated limited effects on cutaneous disease. Furthermore, some reports and series note flaring of dermatomyositis skin disease on anti-TNF therapy.

Although clinical studies supporting a particular treatment algorithm for cutaneous dermatomyositis are lacking, many experts use antimalarials, followed by methotrexate, mycophenolate mofetil, and subsequently IVIG for cases of refractory skin disease in dermatomyositis.

Pruritus can be particularly refractory in patients with dermatomyositis, interfering with sleep patterns and overall quality of life, and should therefore be treated accordingly. Notably, if traditional antipruritic regimens fail, altering a patient's immunomodulatory or immunosuppressive regimen is warranted given that the pruritus is a component of their inflammatory disease. Finally, studies have suggested that aggressive corticosteroid therapy is not warranted in patients without clinical evidence of myositis. Therefore, treatment for amyopathic dermatomyositis can differ significantly from that of classic dermatomyositis.

Calcinosis cutis is extremely challenging to treat, but may respond best to diltiazem or surgical excision. Various other therapies have been tried, including bisphosphonates, colchicine, low-dose warfarin, aluminum hydroxide, probenecid, IVIG, anti-TNF therapy, sodium thiosulfate, and electric shock wave lithotripsy, among others. Occasionally the calcinosis will regress without therapy. Early and aggressive therapy of juvenile dermatomyositis has been shown to reduce the risk of development of calcinosis in children.

Given the frequently refractory nature of skin disease compared to muscle disease in dermatomyositis, it is necessary to assess the severity of cutaneous disease accurately in order to design clinical trials that can reliably evaluate the efficacy of therapeutic interventions. A Dermatomyositis Skin Severity Index has been developed and validated as a severity measure in cutaneous disease. An additional index, the Cutaneous Dermatomyositis Area and Severity Index, has also been designed, and the Cutaneous Assessment Tool measures skin involvement in cases of juvenile dermatomyositis.

The prognosis of dermatomyositis and polymyositis varies greatly depending on the series of patients studied. Factors that affect the prognosis include the patient's age, the type and severity of the myositis, the presence of dysphagia, the presence of an associated malignancy, the presence of lung disease or clinically apparent cardiac disease, and the response to corticosteroid therapy. The concept that therapy alters the prognosis seems to be well established by retrospective reports on the benefits of corticosteroids and immunosuppressants.

SUGGESTED READINGS

Bohan A, Peter JB, Bowman RL, Pearson CM. A computer-assisted analysis of 153 patients with polymyositis and dermatomyositis. Medicine 1977;56:255.

Callen JP, Wortmann RL. Dermatomyositis. Clin Dermatol 2006;24:363–73.

Chaisson NF, Paik J, Orbai AM, Casciola-Rosen L, Fiorentino D, Danoff S, et al. A novel dermato-pulmonary syndrome associated with MDA-5 antibodies: report of 2 cases and review of the literature. Medicine (Baltimore) July 2012;91(4):220–8.

Dalakas M, Hohlfeld R. Polymyositis and dermatomyositis. Lancet 2003;362:971–82.

Edge JC, Outland JD, Dempsey J, Callen JP. Mycophenolate mofetil as an effective corticosteroid-sparing therapy for recalcitrant dermatomyositis. Arch Dermatol 2006;142:65–9.

Femia AN, Vleugels RA, Callen JP. Cutaneous dermatomyositis: an updated review of treatment options and internal associations. Am J Clin Dermatol August 2013;14(4):291–313.

Fiorentino DF, Chung LS, Christopher-Stine L, Zaba L, Li S, Mammen AL, et al. Most patients with cancer-associated dermatomyositis have antibodies to nuclear matrix protein NXP-2 or transcription intermediary factor 1γ. Arthritis Rheum November 2013;65(11):2954–62.

Hill CL, Zhang Y, Sigurgeirsson B, et al. Frequency of specific cancer types in dermatomyositis and polymyositis: a population-based study. Lancet 2001;357:96–100.

Morganroth PA, Kreider ME, Okawa J, Taylor L, Werth VP. Interstitial lung disease in classic and skin-predominant dermatomyositis: a retrospective study with screening recommendations. Arch Dermatol July 2010;146(7):729–38.

Oddis CV, Reed AM, Aggarwal R, Rider LG, Ascherman DP, Levesque MC, et al. Rituximab in the treatment of refractory adult and juvenile dermatomyositis and adult polymyositis: a randomized, placebo-phase trial. Arthritis Rheum February 2013;65(2):314–24.

Sontheimer RD. Cutaneous features of classic dermatomyositis and amyopathic dermatomyositis. Curr Opin Rheumatol 1999;11:475–82.

Walsh R, Kong S, Yao Y, et al. Type I interferon-inducible gene expression in blood is present and reflects disease activity in dermatomyositis and polymyositis. Arthritis Rheum 2007;56:3784–92.

CHAPTER 3

Scleroderma, Raynaud's Phenomenon, and Related Conditions

Stephanie T. Le • Nicole Fett • Anna Haemel

> **KEY POINTS**
>
> - The range of conditions presenting as "hard skin" is broad, including those diseases that cause cutaneous sclerosis (increased connective tissue with normal or decreased fibroblasts) and those that cause cutaneous fibrosis (increased connective tissue and increased fibroblasts).
> - The clinical differential diagnosis of "hard skin" can be divided into two main categories: morphea and morphea-like conditions and systemic sclerosis and sclerodermoid conditions.
> - Patients with morphea and morphea-like conditions tend to have more asymmetric, discontinuous skin involvement, while patients with systemic sclerosis and sclerodermoid conditions tend to have more symmetric, distal, and continuous skin involvement.
> - The presence of sclerodactyly, nailfold capillary changes, and Raynaud's phenomenon are useful in distinguishing systemic sclerosis from other causes of hard skin.

SCLERODERMA

The term "scleroderma" is frequently used in reference to both localized (morphea) and systemic (systemic sclerosis) conditions presenting with "hard skin." While both morphea and systemic sclerosis (SSc) share a common endpoint of cutaneous sclerosis with identical histologic features, key differences in their pathophysiology, autoantibody profile, and clinical presentation suggest they represent separate disease processes rather than a spectrum. Importantly, morphea does not evolve into SSc, and patients with morphea do not develop the specific internal organ manifestations of SSc. As a general rule, patients with morphea tend to have more asymmetric, discontinuous skin involvement, and patients with SSc tend to have more symmetric, distal, and continuous skin involvement. Thus, the differential diagnosis of "hard skin" can be separated into two main diagnostic categories: morphea and morphea-like conditions and systemic sclerosis and sclerodermoid conditions.

Morphea (Localized Scleroderma)

Clinical Manifestations

Morphea (localized scleroderma) occurs in both adults and children and may present as one or more edematous, indurated, or atrophic plaques. Morphea is typically erythematous or violaceous in its active (or inflammatory) phase (Fig. 3-1) and ivory-colored or hyperpigmented in its damage (or noninflammatory) phase. Morphea is distinguished from SSc based on the absence of sclerodactyly, Raynaud's phenomenon, and nailfold capillary changes. The term "morphea" may be preferred over "localized scleroderma" to emphasize the distinction from SSc and its specific end-organ complications. Extracutaneous manifestations of morphea can include involvement of underlying structures such as bone and, in cases of linear morphea affecting the head, the central nervous system. Arthralgias may also be present (e.g., 10% of pediatric patients) (Fett, 2013). ANA (antinuclear antibody) positivity is observed in 20% to 80% of patients with morphea, but is generally not indicative of an underlying systemic autoimmune connective tissue disease such as lupus erythematosus or SSc.

While the classification of morphea subtypes has been controversial, one of the more commonly used systems proposed by Laxer and Zulian describes five morphea variants based on clinical manifestations: circumscribed, linear, generalized, pansclerotic, and mixed variants. Circumscribed morphea, the most common subtype in adults, presents with up to three individual plaques. Active lesions often demonstrate a characteristic indurated lilac rim (Fig. 3-1); they may expand or burn out, becoming ivory-white or hyperpigmented and softening over several years. Both superficial (more common; limited to the epidermis and dermis) and deep (involving the deep dermis and subcutaneous tissues) variants of circumscribed morphea have been described.

Linear morphea presents as a band of sclerotic, depressed skin, frequently with overlying hyperpigmentation. Linear morphea is most common in children and affects the limbs, face, and/or scalp, typically as a single lesion (Fig. 3-2). In children, linear morphea of the limbs can cause focal growth arrest and limb length discrepancies due to disruption of the growth plate. Joint contractures are a particular concern when the lesion crosses a

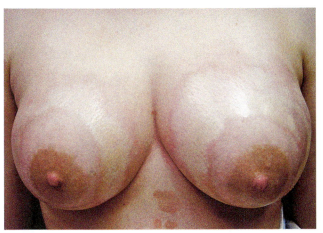

FIGURE 3-1 ■ Sclerotic plaques of morphea on the breasts with erythematous to violaceous borders.

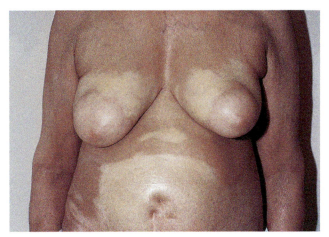

FIGURE 3-3 ■ Generalized morphea. The lesions are widespread and coalescent.

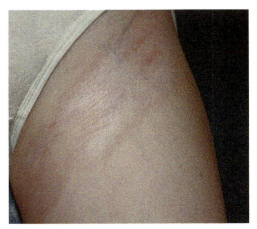

FIGURE 3-2 ■ Lichen sclerosus/morphea overlap in a child.

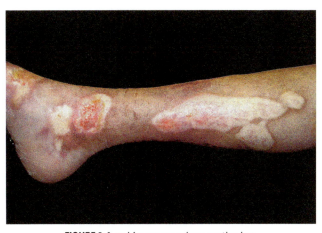

FIGURE 3-4 ■ Linear morphea on the leg.

joint. The head variant of linear morphea includes two subtypes: en coup de sabre (ECDS; frontoparietal linear morphea) and progressive hemifacial atrophy (PHA; Parry Romberg syndrome). En coup de sabre (Fig. 3-3) most often presents as a depressed and/or hyperpigmented plaque on the paramedian forehead; when the lesion extends into the scalp, prominent alopecia may be observed. Early in its course, ECDS can present as an erythematous patch mimicking a port wine stain. In contrast, PHA predominantly affects the subcutaneous tissues, sometimes with only subtle changes of overlying skin. Overlapping features of both ECDS and PHA in the same patient are not uncommon. Head variant linear morphea is associated with central nervous system and eye abnormalities. Central nervous system manifestations include seizures and headaches, reported in 13% and 9% of patients, respectively. The severity of skin findings is not predictive of CNS abnormalities, and a magnetic resonance image (MRI) with contrast is helpful to guide management. Ocular manifestations may be present in 3% of patients with head variant linear morphea, with common features including adnexal sclerosis and uveitis; detection by serial ophthalmologic examinations may help prevent permanent visual loss. Dental abnormalities may also be present, particularly in patients with PHA. Although most common in children, linear morphea may also present in adults.

Generalized morphea describes the presentation of four or more indurated plaques, larger than 3 cm each, involving two or more separate anatomical areas (Fig. 3-4). Arthralgias may be more prevalent than in other morphea subtypes. Patients with generalized morphea are more likely to have positive autoantibodies. Severe generalized morphea can be distinguished from SSc based on the absence of Raynaud's phenomenon, nailfold capillary changes, and sclerodactyly.

Pansclerotic morphea is a poorly defined, very rare, and aggressive morphea subtype, which has been proposed by some authors to be a variant of generalized morphea. Pediatric patients in particular may have circumferential and subcutaneous involvement, affecting nearly the entire body surface area. Pansclerotic morphea may also present with full-thickness involvement of the underlying muscle, tendon, and bone, with associated nonhealing ulcers and cutaneous squamous cell carcinoma.

Up to 15% of morphea patients present with a combination of two or more of the previously discussed subtypes, or the "mixed subtype" variant. Other entities that may fall along the morphea spectrum include lichen

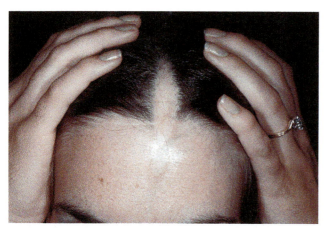

FIGURE 3-5 ■ En coup de sabre involving the forehead and scalp.

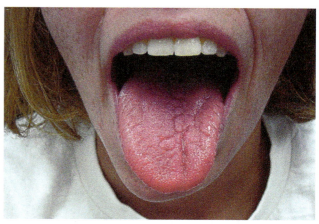

FIGURE 3-6 ■ Hemifacial atrophy (Parry–Romberg syndrome) with atrophy of the left jaw and tongue.

TABLE 3-1	Differential Diagnosis of Morphea—Key Entities to Consider
Morphea Group	**Morpheaform Conditions**
• Circumscribed • Linear • Generalized • Pansclerotic • Mixed variants • Lichen sclerosus (possibly)	• Radiation-induced morphea • Cutaneous malignancy • Sclerosis at injection sites • Lipodermatosclerosis

Adapted from Laxer, Ronald M., and Francesco Zulian. Localized scleroderma. Current Opinion in Rheumatology. 2006;18(6): 606–613.

sclerosus and eosinophilic fasciitis (discussed separately later in this chapter). Genital lichen sclerosus has been reported to occur with greater than average frequency in individuals with plaque, linear, and generalized morphea; a genital exam is ideally included in the care of patients with morphea. Whether lichen sclerosus truly falls along the morphea spectrum (Fig. 3-5) or is an associated condition requires further clarification.

Diagnosis

The diagnostic approach to morphea includes characterization of the extent and location of involvement as well as exclusion of other common morphea mimics or morpheaform disorders (Table 3-1). Morphea is generally a clinical diagnosis, and skin biopsy may not be required in typical cases. Morphea and SSc are indistinguishable on biopsy. Skin biopsy may nevertheless be useful when atypical findings are present and/or to assess the severity of active inflammation when considering treatment options. Biopsy specimens from well-developed lesions should include underlying subcutaneous tissue and are square in appearance histologically (the so-called "square biopsy"). The epidermis may be normal or atrophic, with thickened and densely packed collagen bundles in the dermis, atrophy or absence of the skin appendages, adnexal trapping, and replacement of the fat cells in the subcutaneous tissue by hyalinized collagen bundles. In the early inflammatory stages of morphea, a predominantly lymphocytic infiltrate, with or without plasma cells, is seen in the dermis and superficial subcutaneous fat (Fig. 3-6).

Differential Diagnosis

The differential diagnosis of morphea includes a number of morpheaform conditions or morphea mimics, some of the most clinically relevant including radiation-induced morphea, cutaneous malignancy, injection site reactions, and lipodermatosclerosis (Table 3-1).

Radiation-induced morphea may be a subtype of "true" morphea triggered by radiation-related immunologic aberration in the affected skin. Radiation-induced morphea typically presents within 1 year after completion of radiation treatment, though delayed presentations can occur. Radiation-induced morphea is most common in women following radiation for breast cancer, where it presents with shrinkage of the affected breast, distinguishing it from radiation dermatitis. In this clinical scenario, biopsy is indicated to rule out recurrent malignancy, primary malignancy (e.g., basal cell carcinoma), and metastatic disease (e.g., carcinoma en cuirasse).

Injection-site reactions and lipodermatosclerosis may also mimic morphea. Cutaneous sclerosis at injection sites has been reported with vitamin B_{12} and vitamin K injections, vaccinations, and other injectables. Lesions tend to slowly resolve without treatment. Lipodermatosclerosis, or sclerosing panniculitis, is a manifestation of venous insufficiency identifiable by its typical features of induration and hyperpigmentation along the lower medial aspect of the leg, with a classic "inverted champagne bottle" appearance. Findings may be either unilateral or bilateral and can occasionally simulate morphea or eosinophilic fasciitis. Lipodermatosclerosis is often a clinical diagnosis; biopsy may be deferred in typical cases due to compromised healing of affected regions.

Management

Several treatment algorithms for morphea have recently been proposed. Treatment for morphea is generally tailored to the condition's activity, severity, subtype, and potential functional and cosmetic implications. Of note, there is little evidence for the treatment of inactive morphea. Some treatment considerations with respect to disease subtype are as follows.

Circumscribed Morphea. Topical corticosteroid monotherapy is a common initial approach to treating circumscribed morphea in practice; while topical corticosteroids alone may indeed be beneficial, there are presently no data to specifically support this. Topical tacrolimus resulted in improved skin thickness in a small randomized controlled trial and is another reasonable approach. If lesions are unresponsive, other options include topical imiquimod, topical calcipotriene, a combination of calcipotriol and betamethasone dipropionate, or lesion-limited phototherapy (NB-UVB, UVA, or UVA-1). The accessibility and limited toxicity of NB-UVB make it a favorable initial form of phototherapy for many patients. Patients with deeper or recalcitrant disease may benefit from a UVA-based regimen—excimer laser.

Linear Morphea. Both prospective and retrospective data support the efficacy of methotrexate (e.g., 15 to 25 mg/week in adults, 1 mg/kg per week in children) in combination with systemic steroids (e.g., prednisone 1 mg/kg PO daily or IV pulse with or without subsequent oral prednisone taper) in the treatment of morphea (Fett and Werth, 2011b). In children with linear morphea, methotrexate plus systemic corticosteroids is the standard of care and is supported by data from a randomized placebo-controlled trial. If there is no improvement after 8 to 12 weeks, addition of or transition to phototherapy (UVA1 or PUVA for deeper lesions and a trial of NB-UVB for superficial lesions) or mycophenolate mofetil can be pursued. Pediatric rheumatologists frequently add mycophenolate mofetil in addition to methotrexate in refractory cases. Notably, assessing treatment response can be very challenging in cases of linear morphea. Appropriate counseling is critical in that the first goal of therapy is to halt disease progression; tissue that has already been damaged will not return to normal and should not lead to increasing the patient's treatment regimen. Reconstructive surgery can be considered for disfiguring facial atrophy, provided the disease has been quiescent for several years. Surgical intervention during active disease has caused rapid progression in individual patients.

Generalized Morphea. Phototherapy is typically considered first-line treatment for generalized morphea if the patient does not have functional limitations. If there is no response after 8 weeks, a combination of methotrexate and systemic corticosteroids can be implemented. If there is no improvement after an additional 8 to 12 weeks, mycophenolate mofetil can be considered.

Systemic Sclerosis

Clinical Manifestations

Systemic sclerosis (SSc) is an autoimmune connective tissue disease characterized by vascular dysfunction, autoimmunity, and sclerosis of end organs including skin.

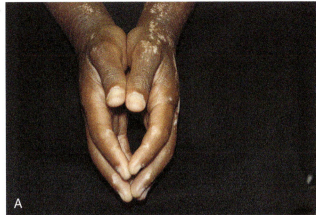
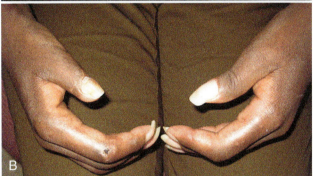

FIGURE 3-7 ■ Taut, bound-down skin on the digits and hands in systemic sclerosis. This symmetrical involvement of the digits is a clinical feature that helps distinguish systemic sclerosis from eosinophilic fasciitis. Note the "prayer sign" in **(A)**. Note the digital ulceration in **(B)**.

While SSc is most prevalent in middle-aged women, it can occur at all ages and in both genders. The etiopathogenesis likely involves both genetic and environmental factors. Disease subtypes include: (1) limited cutaneous systemic sclerosis (formerly known as CREST, i.e., calcinosis, Raynaud's, esophageal dysmotility, sclerodactyly, telangiectasia); (2) diffuse cutaneous systemic sclerosis; (3) overlap syndromes, including mixed connective tissue disease (discussed separately at the end of this chapter); and (4) systemic sclerosis sine scleroderma (lacking skin involvement).

Diffuse cutaneous systemic sclerosis (dSSc) and limited cutaneous systemic sclerosis (lSSc) are the most well-recognized clinical patterns of disease, differentiated based on the extent of skin involvement. Specifically, dSSc is defined by cutaneous sclerosis proximal to the elbows while lSSc is characterized by skin involvement only distal to the elbows and often limited to the most distal extremities. Early disease is characterized by an edematous phase in which patients may present with "puffy fingers" or "puffy hands." As the disease progresses, the areas of swelling become indurated, with findings progressing from distal to proximal (Fig. 3-7). In dSSc, hand and finger edema may present shortly after the first episode of Raynaud's phenomenon. In contrast, patients with lSSc may experience Raynaud's phenomenon for years before other manifestations develop, reflecting what is often a more protracted disease course.

The skin signs of SSc are diverse, not only including cutaneous sclerosis, but also nailfold capillary changes, mat telangiectases (Fig. 3-8), calcinosis cutis, and pigmentary changes. The pigmentary alteration of SSc may comprise diffuse hyperpigmentation simulating Addison's disease; patchy hypo/hyperpigmentation; or leukoderma with a "salt-and-pepper" appearance due to perifollicular sparing (Fig. 3-9). Internal manifestations are also varied, with potential involvement of multiple organ systems including the gastrointestinal tract (e.g., esophageal dysmotility, reflux, and gastric antral vascular ectasias), heart and lungs (e.g., interstitial lung disease and pulmonary hypertension), and kidneys (e.g., scleroderma renal crisis). The specific diagnostic criteria for SSc are discussed below.

Diagnosis

To help distinguish SSc from sclerodermoid conditions and other mimickers (Table 3-2) (Fett and Werth, 2011a), the American College of Rheumatology published new diagnostic criteria in 2013 (Table 3-3). Clinical skin findings are very important in this system and account for six out of the eight additive criteria. Cutaneous sclerosis is of paramount importance, with skin thickening proximal to the metacarpophalangeal joints alone being sufficient diagnostic

TABLE 3-2 Differential Diagnosis of Systemic Sclerosis—Key Categories to Consider

Systemic Sclerosis Group	Sclerodermoid Conditions
• Limited SSc • Diffuse SSc • Mixed connective tissue disease • Overlap syndromes	Inflammatory • Eosinophilic fasciitis • Sclerotic type GVHD Mucinoses • Scleredema • Scleromyxedema Paraneoplastic • POEMS • Carcinoid • Amyloid Genetic/metabolic • Progerias • Porphyrias • Others Drug • Bleomycin • Taxanes • Others Historical toxins • Nephrogenic systemic fibrosis (NSF) • Eosinophilia–myalgia syndrome • Toxic oil syndrome

Adapted from Connolly MK. Systemic sclerosis (scleroderma) and related disorders. In: Bolognia J, Jorizzo JL, Rapini RP, editors. Dermatology. 2nd ed. St. Louis, MO; 2008. p. 585–95.

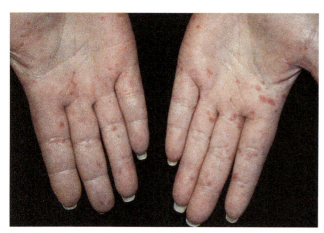

FIGURE 3-8 ■ Mat telangiectases of systemic sclerosis—CREST variant.

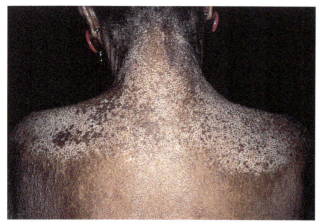

FIGURE 3-9 ■ Patchy hypo- and hyperpigmentation in systemic sclerosis.

TABLE 3-3 ACR 2013 Classification Criteria for Systemic Sclerosis

	Item	Subitems
Cutaneous sclerosis	Skin thickening of fingers of both hands extending proximal to MCPs	
	Skin thickening of fingers	• Puffy fingers • Sclerodactyly (distal to MCPs but proximal to PIPs)
Cutaneous vascular manifestations	Raynaud's phenomenon Abnormal nailfold capillaries Fingertip lesions Mat telangiectases	 • Digital ulcers • Pitting scars
Internal disease	Pulmonary arterial hypertension and/or ILD	• Pulmonary arterial hypertension • ILD
Autoantibodies	SSc-related autoantibodies	• Anticentromere • Antitopisomerase (Scl-70) • Anti-RNA pol III

Adapted from Hoogen F van den, Khanna D, Fransen J, Johnson SR, Baron M, Tyndall A, et al. 2013 Classification criteria for systemic sclerosis: an American College of Rheumatology/European League Against Rheumatism collaborative initiative. Ann Rheum Dis November 1, 2013;72(11):1747–55.

criteria. Other skin-related diagnostic criteria include vascular manifestations: Raynaud's phenomenon, abnormal nailfold capillaries, fingertip lesions, and mat telangiectases.

Cardiopulmonary manifestations of SSc, pulmonary arterial hypertension (PAH), and interstitial lung disease (ILD) are also included in the 2013 diagnostic criteria. These important complications currently account for the greatest SSc-related mortality. In PAH, vasoconstriction in the pulmonary vascular beds results in elevated right heart pressures. PAH affects up to 30% of patients and accounts for 26% of SSc-related deaths. PAH is more common in patients with the lSSc disease subtype, particularly as a late complication, though all patients with SSc are at risk. In ILD, inflammation and/or scarring in the pulmonary interstitium impair lung physiology and gas exchange. ILD affects 30% to 90% of patients with SSc and accounts for 35% of SSc-related deaths. ILD may be more common in patients with dSSc, particularly early in the disease course. Hypoxia from ILD can lead to pulmonary hypertension, which can be difficult to distinguish from the PAH associated with SSc itself.

Laboratory criteria for SSc diagnosis include SSc-specific autoantibodies. While ANA positivity is present in over 95% of cases, patients tend to have only one or no SSc-specific autoantibody (anticentromere, antitopoisomerase I (or Scl-70), or RNA polymerase III). Anticentromere antibodies, observed in ~30% of patients, are associated with lSSc and possibly PAH. Antitopoisomerase antibodies, occurring in ~20% of patients, are associated with dSSc and increased risks of ILD and mortality. RNA polymerase III antibodies, identifiable in ~10% of patients, are associated with dSSc, scleroderma renal crisis, and underlying cancer. Importantly, negative SSc-specific autoantibody studies should not dissuade the clinician from making a diagnosis of SSc in the presence of a supportive clinical examination.

Skin biopsy can be useful in atypical presentations to help differentiate SSc from sclerodermoid mimics. Most conditions producing "hard skin" can be categorized histologically by either sclerosis (increased connective tissue with normal or decreased fibroblasts, as seen in SSc and morphea) or fibrosis (increased connective tissue and increased fibroblasts, as seen in scleromyxedema and nephrogenic systemic fibrosis).

Differential Diagnosis

The differential diagnosis of SSc includes other cutaneous sclerosing/fibrosing disorders presenting predominantly with diffuse and/or symmetric disease (Tables 3-2 and 3-4) (Fett and Werth, 2011a). The differential diagnosis of sclerodermoid conditions is broad and includes entities in the following six disease categories: inflammatory, mucinoses, paraneoplastic, genetic/metabolic, drug, and historic toxins (Table 3-2) (Fett and Werth, 2011a); some of the most clinically relevant entities are highlighted below.

Inflammatory sclerodermoid conditions include eosinophilic fasciitis (discussed in a separate section below) and sclerotic type, or sclerodermoid graft-versus-host disease (GVHD), a form of chronic GVHD. In contrast to SSc, which predictably progresses from distal to more proximal sites, sclerotic type GVHD rarely affects the distal fingers, toes, and face. Raynaud's phenomenon and PAH are typically absent in sclerotic type GVHD, though patients may develop pulmonary fibrosis and pulmonary hypertension secondary to lung disease.

Both scleredema and scleromyxedema are mucinoses, which present with sclerodermoid features. Scleredema manifests as poorly defined indurated plaques typically affecting the upper back and sparing the hands/feet. Skin biopsy reveals mucin deposition between slightly expanded collagen bundles. Scleredema may occur in the setting of recent febrile illness, paraproteinemia, or poorly controlled diabetes. Scleromyxedema, also referred to as lichen myxedematosus, presents with linear arrays of small, waxy dermal papules and skin thickening, typically favoring the face, ears, neck, forearms, and hands. The palms are generally spared, and sclerodactyly is typically absent, helping to distinguish scleromyxedema from SSc. Diagnosis is based on typical skin findings, monoclonal gammopathy, absence of thyroid disease, and a skin biopsy demonstrating mucin deposition, fibroblast proliferation, and fibrosis. Extracutaneous manifestations may occur, including severe neurologic complications.

Other sclerodermoid disorders include paraneoplastic conditions, e.g., polyneuropathy, organomegaly, endocrinopathy, monoclonal gammopathy, and skin changes

TABLE 3-4 Distinguishing Features of Several Sclerosing/Fibrosing Skin Conditions

Features	LM	SSc	EF	Sd	Sm	NSF
Primarily children	++	–	–	+	–	–
Primarily women	++	++	+	–	–	–
Rapid onset	–	–	++	+	–	+
Symmetrical	–	++	++	+	+	+
Extremities	+	+	++	–	–	++
Face	+	+	–	–	+	–
Trunk	+	+	–	++	+	–
Raynaud's phenomenon	–	++	–	–	–	–
Sclerodactyly	–	++	–	–	–	–
Pigment changes	++	+	–	–	–	+
Telangiectasia	–	+	–	–	–	–
Calcinosis	+	+	–	–	–	–
Systemic disease	–	++	+	+	+	+
Blood eosinophilia	–	–	++	–	–	–
Fascial involvement	+	+	++	–	–	+/–
Autoantibodies	+	++	–	–	–	–
Monoclonal spike	–	–	+/–	+/–	++	–
Steroid responsiveness	+	–	++	–	–	–
Resolution in time	++	–	++	++	–	+/–

LM, linear morphea (localized scleroderma); SSc, systemic sclerosis; EF, eosinophilic fasciitis; Sd, scleredema; Sm, scleromyxedema; NSF, nephrogenic systemic fibrosis; –, rare; +, common; ++, very common.

(POEMS), carcinoid syndrome, and amyloidosis; genetic/metabolic conditions including progerias, porphyrias and others; reactions to drugs including bleomycin and taxanes; and historic toxin-related conditions including nephrogenic systemic fibrosis (NSF, discussed in a separate section later in this chapter).

While sclerodactyly is typically considered to be pathognomonic of SSc, the differential diagnosis of this finding includes other conditions involving joint pathology (e.g., diabetic cheiroarthropathy, joint ankyloses) or skin abnormalities (e.g., fibroblastic rheumatism, porphyria, exposure to drugs such as bleomycin). Diabetic cheiroarthropathy can be particularly challenging to differentiate from sclerodactyly due to thickening of periarticular skin as well as subcutaneous tissues; the typical ulnar to radial progression, initially involving the 5th and 4th digits, can be a helpful clue.

The differential diagnosis of other, nonsclerotic skin manifestations of SSc becomes particularly important when cutaneous sclerosis is subtle. Telangiectases are commonplace skin lesions, appearing with conditions as diverse as rosacea, photoaging, and liver disease. The telangiectases of SSc, frequently referred to as "mat" telangiectases, have a characteristic flat, square, or matlike appearance and frequently involve the oral mucosa, helping to distinguish them from other etiologies. While hereditary hemorrhagic telangiectasia can present with prominent mucosal telangiectases, they tend to be more rounded and raised.

Management

As there is no cure for SSc, management is directed toward limiting the impact of individual disease manifestations, often with the help of several specialists and manifestation-specific medications.

Skin Manifestations. Trials addressing the cutaneous sclerosis associated with SSc have generally been met with limited success. The European League Against Rheumatism recommends methotrexate (e.g., 15 to 25 mg weekly) as a first-line treatment based on two randomized controlled trials that have shown methotrexate to modestly improve skin scores in early dSSc. If there is inadequate response, expert opinion would support adding or switching to mycophenolate mofetil. There are also trial data to support the use of oral or IV cyclophosphamide for severe disease. Both PUVA and UVA-1 may help with cutaneous sclerosis in SSc and are favored over UVB due to deeper penetration. Hand phototherapy and occupational therapy may be helpful for maintaining hand function in the presence of sclerodactyly. In addition, many patients with SSc have severe multifactorial pruritus, particularly early in the disease course; treatment considerations include agents targeting neuropathic pain (e.g., gabapentin), opioid antagonists (e.g., naltrexone), as well as agents aimed at treating the cutaneous sclerosis itself.

Nonsclerotic skin manifestations are best addressed individually. Telangiectases generally respond well to vascular laser. Calcinosis cutis typically remains resistant to treatment. For discussion of the management of Raynaud's and digital ulcers, see the separate section dedicated to Raynaud's phenomenon later in this chapter.

Systemic Manifestations. Cardiopulmonary and other end-organ involvement in SSc is often managed in an interdisciplinary manner. All providers can make a major contribution by ensuring patients are screened appropriately. Screening for ILD is invaluable as disease is often asymptomatic until late in its course, and treatment (e.g., mycophenolate mofetil) has been shown to improve survival. Basic screening for ILD includes pulmonary function tests (PFTs) with DLCO every 6 to 12 months. Findings of a low DLCO and/or a restrictive pattern should trigger further workup for ILD, including a high-resolution chest computed tomography (CT). In addition to PFTs, some experts advocate a baseline high-resolution chest CT. Similarly, PAH may be asymptomatic until late in its trajectory, and early treatment may improve outcomes. Appropriate screening for PAH includes PFTs and cardiac echocardiography yearly; patients suspected to have PAH should be referred to cardiology for right heart catheterization for definitive diagnosis and ongoing management. Although scleroderma renal crisis is not included in the 2013 classification criteria for SSc, it was the major cause of mortality prior to the advent of ACE inhibitors and remains an important complication. Evaluation and treatment for scleroderma renal crisis should be prompted by systolic blood pressure 20 mm Hg above or diastolic pressure 10 mm Hg above baseline. Prednisone dose is often limited to ≤10 mg/day in patients with SSc due to retrospective data suggesting a possible association of doses ≥15 mg/day with scleroderma renal crisis.

EOSINOPHILIC FASCIITIS

Eosinophilic fasciitis (EF) is considered a morphea spectrum disorder by some authors, and lesions suggestive of circumscribed morphea may occur at distant sites (e.g., trunk) in up to 30% of patients. In contrast to many other morphea subtypes, EF tends to present symmetrically and is therefore considered in the differential diagnosis of sclerodermoid conditions (Table 3-2). EF is distinguishable from SSc based on sparing of the fingers and toes, and often of the hands and feet, and absence of Raynaud's phenomenon and nailfold capillary changes.

EF may initially present with sudden pain and edema in the extremities, occasionally following intense exercise or trauma; this rapidly progresses to symmetric sclerosis, often with a dimpled peau d'orange appearance. Patients may develop a characteristic "groove sign," consisting of linear depressions along the course of veins, which accentuate when the affected extremity is elevated against gravity. The "groove sign" of EF results from tethering of veins to deeper involvement, with relative sparing of the overlying epidermis and dermis. Laboratory features may include an elevated erythrocyte sedimentation rate with or without peripheral eosinophilia. An associated paraproteinemia is reported in some patients. Deep skin biopsy and/or MRI may be helpful to define fascial involvement. The response to high-dose prednisone (e.g., 1 mg/kg) tapered over several months is typically favorable, particularly when initiated early; however, tapering without a steroid-sparing agent may result in disease recurrence. The early addition of a steroid-sparing agent such as methotrexate may provide additional benefit, and is typically utilized by experts. As in patients with other sclerosing disorders overlying a joint, referral for physical therapy is imperative.

RAYNAUD'S PHENOMENON AND RELATED DISORDERS

Raynaud's phenomenon, presenting as color change of the affected digits, is reflective of paroxysmal vasospasm often in response to cool temperatures. While classic Raynaud's is triphasic (progressing from white to blue to red), biphasic attacks (white to blue) are consistent as well. Raynaud's phenomenon can be classified as either primary (idiopathic, a.k.a. "Raynaud's disease") or secondary (related to underlying conditions, including SSc).

Criteria for primary Raynaud's phenomenon include negative or low-titer ANA, the absence of both clinical features (e.g., sclerodactyly, calcinosis, ischemic tissue injury) and history of underlying connective tissue disease, and normal nailfold capillaries. Nailfold capillaries are readily visible with dermoscopy; abnormalities observed in SSc and related disorders may include enlarged or disorganized capillaries, hemorrhages, and capillary drop-out. These changes are a marker for risk of progression to SSc or other autoimmune connective tissue disease in patients presenting with Raynaud's phenomenon.

Treatment for Raynaud's phenomenon includes lifestyle modification (staying warm, moderating caffeine, and smoking cessation) for all patients. In treating patients with SSc, dihydropyridine-type calcium channel blockers (e.g., nifedipine) are considered first-line. Consideration can be given to adding or switching to a phosphodiesterase 5 inhibitor (e.g., sildenafil) if response is inadequate. Prostanoids, such as intravenous iloprost, can be employed as a temporizing measure in cases of critical ischemia, e.g., while awaiting surgical intervention such as digital sympathectomy. Fluoxetine 20 to 40 mg/day may be an alternative or adjunctive agent in the setting of low blood pressure. Other agents occasionally employed include angiotensin receptor blockers, alpha-blockers, pentoxifylline, and botulinum toxin.

Digital ulcers and/or pitting scars in patients with Raynaud's phenomenon are indicative of ischemic injury (Fig. 3-10) and herald the presence of an underlying connective tissue disease such as SSc. Digital ulcers in patients with SSc are frequently multifactorial with contributions from ischemia, sclerosis, trauma, poor healing, calcinosis, and/or infection. Workup includes Doppler exam for pulses, evaluation for hypercoagulability and vasculitis, swab cultures, radiographs, and vascular imaging and/or consult, as appropriate. Wound care may include hydrocolloid and other occlusive dressings. The therapeutic ladder for the prevention and treatment of digital ulcers is otherwise similar to that for Raynaud's phenomenon.

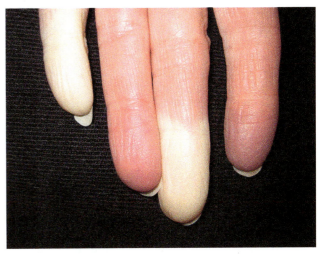

FIGURE 3-10 ■ Raynaud's phenomenon.

MIXED CONNECTIVE TISSUE DISEASE

Patients with mixed connective tissue disease (MCTD) demonstrate overlapping features of two or more autoimmune connective tissue diseases and high titers of pathogenic autoantibodies against the U1 small nuclear ribonucleoprotein autoantigen. Frequent clinical manifestations in this group of patients include puffy fingers, Raynaud's phenomenon, polyarthritis, esophageal dysmotility, and ILD. While initial reports had suggested a milder disease course in these patients, more recent data suggest that severe internal organ involvement, including PAH, may be a late manifestation with a negative prognostic impact. Some patients may also evolve to more clear-cut SSc. Importantly, MCTD is distinct from undifferentiated connective tissue disease. In the latter, patients have some features highly suggestive of an underlying autoimmune connective tissue disease, but do not presently fulfill criteria for a specific entity.

NEPHROGENIC SYSTEMIC FIBROSIS (SEE ALSO CHAPTER 38)

Nephrogenic systemic fibrosis (NSF) is a systemic fibrosing disease occurring in patients exposed to gadolinium-based contrast agents (GBCAs) in the setting of severe acute or chronic renal impairment. Patients often have a concurrent proinflammatory event (e.g., sepsis). All three factors (GBCA exposure, severe renal disease, concurrent major illness) are often required for disease expression. First described as a novel disease under the term "nephrogenic fibrosing dermopathy" in 2000, NSF was linked to GBCAs in 2006. Over the past several years, new guidelines restricting the use and limiting the dose of GBCAs in at-risk patients with renal dysfunction have resulted in a dramatic reduction if not complete elimination of new incident cases. The exact pathogenesis of NSF remains unclear but may be related to release of free toxic gadolinium from less stable linear chelates such as gadodiamide. The sudden appearance of multiple cases of NSF followed by dramatically reduced incidence after identification of the relevant exposure is reminiscent of earlier epidemics of sclerosing disease related to other historic toxins (e.g., toxic oil syndrome, eosinophilia myalgia syndrome).

Clinical features of NSF include a relatively acute onset of irregularly shaped, intensely painful or pruritic indurated plaques, most commonly involving the extremities with a peau d'orange or papulonodular appearance, and associated debilitating joint contractures. In contrast to scleromyxedema, the face is spared. Skin biopsy demonstrates features of fibrosis with increased CD34+ spindle cells and variable increase in mucin. There is no reliably effective treatment for NSF, though considerations might include photopheresis, phototherapy, sodium thiosulfate, intravenous immunoglobulin, and renal transplantation. The most effective approach to managing NSF is prevention, through screening and identification of at-risk patients prior to administration of GBCAs, dialysis within hours of administration, and using only GBCAs with macrocyclic chelation.

SUGGESTED READINGS

Chiu YE, Vora S, Kwon E-KM, Maheshwari M. A significant portion of children with morphea en coup de sabre and Parry-Romberg syndrome have neuroimaging findings. Pediatr Dermatol 2012;29(6): 738–48.

Daftari Besheli L, Aran S, Shaqdan K, Kay J, Abujudeh H. Current status of nephrogenic systemic fibrosis. Clin Radiol 2014;69(7): 661–8.

Fett N. Scleroderma: nomenclature, etiology, pathogenesis, prognosis, and treatments: facts and controversies. Clin Dermatol 2013;31(4):432–7.

Fett N, Werth VP. Update on morphea: part I. Epidemiology, clinical presentation, and pathogenesis. J Am Acad Dermatol 2011a;64(2):217–28.

Fett N, Werth VP. Update on morphea: part II. Outcome measures and treatment. J Am Acad Dermatol 2011b;64(2):231–42.

Frech TM, Shanmugam VK, Shah AA, Assassi S, Gordon JK, Hant FN, et al. Treatment of early diffuse systemic sclerosis skin disease. Clin Exp Rheumatol 2013;31(2 Suppl 76):166–71.

Kim A, Marinkovich N, Vasquez R, Jacobe HT. Clinical features of patients with morphea and the pansclerotic subtype: a cross-sectional study from the morphea in adults and children cohort. J Rheumatol 2014;41(1):106–12.

Lebeaux D, Francès C, Barete S, Wechsler B, Dubourg O, Renoux J, et al. Eosinophilic fasciitis (Shulman disease): new insights into the therapeutic management from a series of 34 patients. Rheumatology 2012;51(3):557–61.

Maverakis E, Patel F, Kronenberg DG, Chung L, Fiorentino D, Allanore Y, et al. International consensus criteria for the diagnosis of Raynaud's phenomenon. J Autoimmun 2014;48–49:60–5.

Nihtyanova SI, Brough GM, Black CM, Denton CP. Mycophenolate mofetil in diffuse cutaneous systemic sclerosis—a retrospective analysis. Rheumatology 2007;46(3):442–5.

Schlosser BJ. Missing genital lichen sclerosus in patients with morphea: don't ask? don't tell?: comment on "high frequency of genital lichen sclerosus in a prospective series of 76 patients with morphea". Arch Dermatol 2012;148(1):28–9.

Tani C, Carli L, Vagnani S, Talarico R, Baldini C, Mosca M, et al. The diagnosis and classification of mixed connective tissue disease. J Autoimmun 2014;48–49:46–9.

van den Hoogen F, Khanna D, Fransen J, Johnson SR, Baron M, Tyndall A, et al. 2013 Classification criteria for systemic sclerosis: an American College of Rheumatology/European League Against Rheumatism collaborative initiative. Ann Rheum Dis 2013;72(11):1747–55.

Yaqub A, Chung L, Rieger KE, Fiorentino DF. Localized cutaneous fibrosing disorders. Rheum Dis Clin N Am 2013;39(2):347–64.

Zulian F, Martini G, Vallongo C, Vittadello F, Falcini F, Patrizi A, et al. Methotrexate treatment in juvenile localized scleroderma: a randomized, double-blind, placebo-controlled trial. Arthritis Rheum 2011;63(7):1998–2006.

Zwischenberger BA, Jacobe HT. A systematic review of morphea treatments and therapeutic algorithm. J Am Acad Dermatol 2011;65(5):925–41.

CHAPTER 4

VASCULITIS

Miguel A. González-Gay • Trinitario Pina

KEY POINTS

- Vasculitic processes may be idiopathic or associated with infections, drugs, malignancies, or connective tissue diseases.
- Drugs and infections are the most common underlying etiologies in adults with cutaneous vasculitis (CV).
- IgA vasculitis (Henoch-Schönlein purpura) is the most frequent vasculitic condition associated with CV in children.
- Clinical manifestations depend on the localization and size of the involved vessel.
- Although the Chapel Hill Consensus Conference has established nomenclature that might be useful for the classification of vasculitis, there exists controversy on the definitions and manifestations of cutaneous disease in this classification system.

INTRODUCTION

The term vasculitis refers to a wide spectrum of diseases characterized by blood vessel inflammation and necrosis. Vasculitic processes may be associated with infections, drugs, malignancies, or connective tissue diseases (CTDs). In the absence of an underlying disease we refer to them as primary or idiopathic systemic vasculitides. These conditions exhibit a wide spectrum of manifestations depending on the localization and size of the involved vessels, and often have overlapping clinical and pathologic manifestations. When skin vessels are affected we talk about cutaneous vasculitis (CV). CV may be a process confined exclusively to the skin, or a manifestation of a more widespread entity associated with a variable grade of visceral involvement.

NOMENCLATURE AND CLASSIFICATION CRITERIA

Classification of vasculitis has been a challenging problem for decades. A widely accepted set of diagnostic criteria for the vasculitides has never been established. To fill this void classification criteria were developed to create homogeneous cohorts for clinical research. There are two classification schemes that have been proposed. One developed in 1990 by the American College of Rheumatology (ACR) and one developed by a consensus conference of multiple specialists held in Chapel Hill, North Carolina, known as the Chapel Hill Consensus Conference (CHCC). The CHCC classification was initially published in 1994 and a 2012 revision was published in January 2013 (Table 4-1). Dermatologists were not involved in the development of any of these classifications systems and thus there are some entities seen on the skin that are not included and there are some nuances regarding cutaneous involvement that might be seen differently by the dermatologic community. The CHCC deals with and tries to define noninfectious vasculitides.

In view of different classification and definition schemes, vasculitis of the skin has been referred to over time by using a number of terms, namely, hypersensitivity vasculitis, leukocytoclastic angiitis, and more recently single-organ cutaneous small-vessel vasculitis (SoCSVV). SoCSVV refers to a vasculitis confined to the skin with no features suggesting a limited expression of a systemic vasculitis.

Nevertheless, three major groups of systemic vasculitides could be identified in all classification schemes: large-vessel vasculitis (giant cell arteritis and Takayasu), medium-sized vessel vasculitis (polyarteritis nodosa [PAN] and Kawasaki), and small-sized vessel vasculitis. Within this latter group we can identify disorders associated with antineutrophil cytoplasmic antibody (ANCA), disorders associated with immune complex deposition, and Henoch-Schönlein purpura characterized by IgA dominant immune deposits, among others.

EPIDEMIOLOGY

In Norwich, UK, the reported annual incidence of biopsy-proven CV in a population 16 years of age and older was 38.6 per million. In northwestern Spain, in a population 21 years of age and older it was 55.2 per million. In Olmsted County, Minnesota, USA, the incidence rate was 45 per million considering all age groups.

In reports from the United States, Malaysia, and Kuwait, men and women were affected almost equally. In series reported from the United Kingdom and Singapore, females outnumbered males in a ratio of approximately 2:1. In contrast, in series reported from northwestern Spain and Australia males outnumbered females in a ratio of approximately 2:1.

In series of adult patients reported from Spain and Kuwait, CV as an idiopathic process limited to the skin accounted for 32% and 36.8% of cases, respectively. In these series, CV was a manifestation of a primary systemic vasculitis (PSV), other than hypersensitivity vasculitis, in 22% of patients from Spain and 12.2% from Kuwait. In both series, Henoch-Schönlein purpura was the commonest underlying PSV, accounting for 15% and 8.8% of cases, respectively.

TABLE 4-1 Nomenclature for Vasculitides Adopted by the 2012 Chapel Hill Consensus Conference

Primary Vasculitis
Large-vessel vasculitis
    Takayasu arteritis
    Giant cell arteritis
Medium-vessel vasculitis
    Polyarteritis nodosa
    Kawasaki disease
Small-vessel vasculitis
    Antineutrophil cytoplasmic antibody (ANCA)-associated vasculitis
        Microscopic polyangiitis
        Granulomatosis with polyangiitis
        Eosinophilic granulomatosis with polyangiitis
        Single-organ ANCA-associated vasculitis
    Immune complex small-vessel vasculitis
        IgA vasculitis
        Cryoglobulinemic vasculitis
        Hypocomplementemic urticarial vasculitis
        Antiglomerular basement membrane disease
Variable-vessel vasculitis
    Behçet's disease
    Cogan's syndrome
Single-organ vasculitis
    Cutaneous leukocytoclastic angiitis
    Cutaneous arteritis
    Primary central nervous system vasculitis
    Isolated aortitis
    Others

Secondary Vasculitis
Vasculitis associated with systemic disease
    Lupus vasculitis
    Rheumatoid vasculitis
    Sarcoid vasculitis
    Others
Vasculitis associated with probable etiology
    Cancer-associated vasculitis
    Hepatitis C virus-associated cryoglobulinemic vasculitis
    Hepatitis B virus-associated vasculitis
    Syphilis-associated aortitis
    Drug-associated ANCA-associated vasculitis
    Drug-associated immune complex vasculitis
    Others

Modified from Jennette et al. (2013).

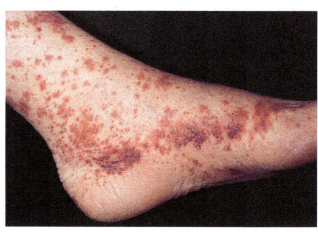

FIGURE 4-1 ■ Typical palpable purpuric lesions seen in a patient with hypersensitivity vasculitis/small-vessel vasculitis.

Among the patients with secondary CV, CTDs were the most frequently reported conditions in Spanish series (30%). This percentage was lower in series from Malaysia (16.5%), Belgium (15.8%), Kuwait (12.1%), and Australia (8.6%). Rheumatoid arthritis constituted the most common CTD associated with CV.

Taken on the whole, drugs and infections are the most common underlying etiologies. In most series Gram-positive cocci (*Streptococcus* and *Staphylococcus*) and *Neisseria* species were the most common bacteria implicated. However, Gram-negative bacteria, anaerobes, mycobacteria, and *Brucella* have also been implicated in the development of CV. In series reported from Australia and Malaysia, infection accounted for 25.8% and 20.2% of cases, respectively. In Kuwait and Spain these percentages were lower (14% and 11%, respectively). Drugs have been reported as the causative agent in 8.7% to 28.2% of patients with CV. Among the drugs, antibiotics and nonsteroidal anti-inflammatory drugs were the most commonly implicated.

Malignancy associated with CV is uncommon. Reported frequencies from Kuwaiti, Australian, Malaysian, and Spanish series were 1.7%, 2.2%, 2.4%, and 4%, respectively. Hematologic disorders are the most common group of neoplasms associated with CV.

CV may affect all age groups. Noteworthy, the clinical spectrum is broader in adults. Blanco et al. (1998) retrospectively reviewed 303 consecutive patients with CV: 172 adults and 131 children (≤20 years). Fourteen children were classified as having hypersensitivity vasculitis (10.7%), and 116 as having Henoch-Schönlein purpura (88.5%), representing the most frequent vasculitic condition associated with CV in this age group. Therefore, almost 100% of children with CV had one of these two conditions.

CLINICAL MANIFESTATIONS

General Concepts

Cutaneous lesions seen in CV are correlated with the size of the affected vessel. Small-sized blood vessels generally include capillaries, post-capillary venules, and nonmuscular arterioles (diameter <50 μm). These are mainly localized within the superficial papillary dermis. The pattern of skin involvement when cutaneous small vessels are affected is usually a maculopapular rash followed by palpable purpura (Fig. 4-1), resulting from extravasation of erythrocytes through damaged blood vessel walls into the dermis. These lesions, in contrast to simple purpura, do not blanch when pressure is applied to the skin. Other skin lesions such as nonpalpable macules and patches, urticaria, bullous lesions, vesicles, pustules, splinter hemorrhages, and ulcerations may also be seen (Fig. 4-2). Moreover, a combination of different lesions is common. Because of increased hydrostatic pressure, skin lesions are commonest on the legs and buttocks. Medium-sized blood vessels (diameter between 50 and 150 μm) have muscular walls and are located principally in the deep reticular dermis, near the junction of the dermis and subcutaneous tissues. Vasculitis involving cutaneous medium-sized blood vessels manifests as subcutaneous nodules, ulcers, livedo reticularis, digital infarctions, and papulonecrotic lesions (Figs 4-3 and 4-4). Larger vessels are not found within

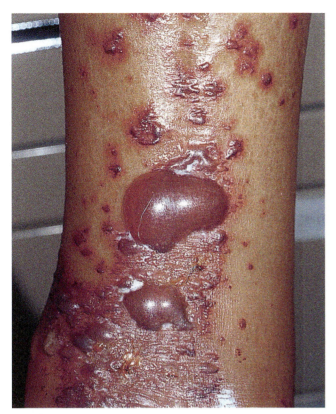

FIGURE 4-2 ■ Bullous lesions exist within typical areas of palpable purpura in this patient with cutaneous small-vessel vasculitis.

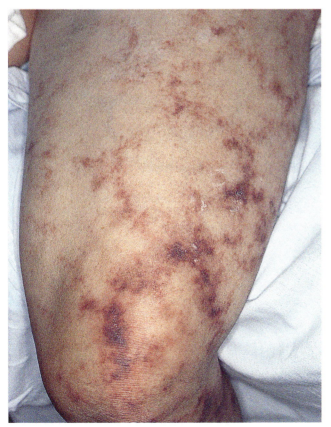

FIGURE 4-3 ■ Cutaneous polyarteritis nodosa as manifested by a livedo pattern with purpuric and necrotic lesions.

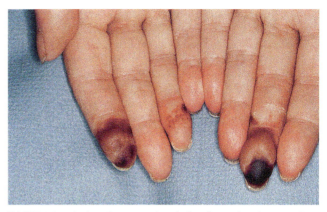

FIGURE 4-4 ■ Ischemic necrosis of the fingertips in a patient with polyarteritis nodosa secondary to hepatitis B antigenemia. (Courtesy of Dr. Neil A. Fenske, Tampa, FL, USA.)

the skin. CV may also be the presenting manifestation of an overlap of small and medium-sized blood vessel involvement. Furthermore, other conditions like pigmented purpuric eruptions, severe thrombocytopenic purpura, or scurvy may mimic CV. This is why a skin biopsy is always required to confirm the presence of vasculitis.

Palpable purpura is the most common type of cutaneous lesion seen in patients with CV. It is observed in up to 70% of cases. Nodules, ulcers, and nonpalpable purpura are probably the more common lesions observed. Lower extremities are affected in up to 100% of cases, with isolated lower-limb involvement occurring in 50% to 68% of patients. Localized lesions above the waist and with a generalized distribution may also be seen.

Extracutaneous involvement is present in 39.8% to 56.1% of patients with CV. The main extracutaneous manifestations are arthralgia/arthritis (21% to 50%), kidney (15% to 38%), and gastrointestinal involvement (7% to 14%). Lung involvement is usually found in less than 10% of cases, and eye and nervous system in less than 5%.

Spectrum of CV in Systemic Vasculitides with Predominant Organ Involvement Different from the Skin

Takayasu Arteritis

Takayasu arteritis, while being a predominantly large-vessel vasculitis, could affect smaller arteries. Skin lesions have been reported in 2.8% to 28% of cases. Cutaneous manifestations include Raynaud's phenomenon, pyoderma gangrenosum-like ulcers, erythema nodosum-like lesions, necrotic or ulcerated nodules, livedo reticularis, and purpura. Erythema nodosum-like lesions are the most commonly reported lesions in Europe and North America.

Polyarteritis Nodosa

There are two variants of PAN. One that is a systemic disease and one that is known as benign cutaneous PAN (BC-PAN) (see below under "Vasculitis variants"). Systemic PAN is defined as a necrotizing arteritis of medium or small arteries including arterioles. Systemic PAN is not associated with the presence of ANCA. Cutaneous involvement in patients with systemic PAN is a controversial subject. In studies from France, up to 50% of patients have had cutaneous disease. In addition, it appears that in these populations, cutaneous involvement is more commonly associated with nonhepatitis B virus-related systemic PAN (57.8% vs 35%). In addition, these studies report that the most common skin lesions are purpura, followed by nodules and livedo reticularis. Nodules usually measure between 0.5 cm and 2 cm in diameter and are usually located on the legs or feet. The presence of cutaneous lesions at the time of diagnosis might be associated with a higher risk of relapse.

ANCA-Associated Vasculitis

The ANCA-associated vasculitis (AAV) is defined as pauci-immune necrotizing vasculitis predominantly affecting small to medium vessels. The AAV comprises three different entities, namely, microscopic polyangiitis (MPA), granulomatosis with polyangiitis (GPA), and eosinophilic granulomatosis with polyangiitis (EGPA). Patients with AAV exhibit vasculitic and nonvasculitic skin lesions, with a complex clinical and histopathological spectrum. Cutaneous vasculitic lesions usually present as palpable purpura in the lower extremities. Less commonly, cutaneous lesions such as livedo racemosa, nodular erythema, or subcutaneous nodules may be observed.

Unlike GPA, MPA does not have granulomatous inflammation. In MPA necrotizing glomerulonephritis is very common and lung capillaritis often occurs. Skin involvement is common (60%). Palpable purpura constitutes the main cutaneous manifestation (40%), followed by livedo and nodules (13% each), and urticaria (3.5%).

GPA, formerly called Wegener's granulomatosis, is characterized by granulomatous inflammation usually involving the upper and lower respiratory tract. Extravascular inflammation (granulomatous and nongranulomatous) and necrotizing glomerulonephritis are common in GPA. Lung capillaritis may also be observed. The proportion of patients reported to have skin and mucosal involvement varies between less than 15% and 46%. Cutaneous lesions are the presenting manifestations in 10% to 21% of cases. Some authors have suggested that vasculitic cutaneous lesions could be correlated with the activity and course of the disease. In this regard patients with cutaneous leukocytoclastic vasculitis (LCV) seem to have an earlier debut of GPA with a more rapidly progressive and widespread disease.

EGPA, also called Churg-Strauss vasculitis, is characterized by an eosinophil-rich necrotizing granulomatous inflammation often involving the respiratory tract. It is associated with asthma and eosinophilia, and nasal polyps are common. Between 40% and 81% of patients have cutaneous lesions, being the presenting sign of the disease in about 14% of cases. Palpable purpura of the lower extremities is the most common manifestation accounting for up to 50% of patients with skin involvement. Urticarial lesions are not uncommon (12% to 31%). Other less frequent manifestations are papular/nodular lesions, livedo reticularis, ulcerations, bullous lesions, cutaneous infarcts, Raynaud's phenomenon, vesicles, and sterile pustules.

Neutrophilic vasculitis (LCV characterized by a predominant infiltrate of neutrophils mixed with nuclear dust) is the commonest histopathologic finding in skin lesions of patients with MPA and GPA. In patients with EGPA, the most common pathologic finding is extravascular necrotizing granuloma, follow by LCV. In addition, vasculitic skin lesions of patients with EGPA show neutrophilic or eosinophilic vasculitis, with most cases involving a mixed infiltrate of both neutrophils and eosinophils. Furthermore, EGPA patients with neutrophilic vasculitis have positive myeloperoxidase (MPO)-ANCA and renal involvement more often than patients with eosinophilic vasculitis, who usually are negative for MPO-ANCA and do not have renal involvement.

Immune Complex Small Vessel Vasculitis

IgA vasculitis (IgAV), more commonly known as Henoch-Schönlein purpura, is a vasculitis affecting small vessels with IgA1-dominant immune deposits. It is the most common vasculitis in children and typically involves skin, gut, and joints, with renal involvement constituting its more serious manifestation. The pediatric form of the disease is generally considered a benign, self-limited condition. In adults, however, it is an infrequent condition with a worse outcome. Skin involvement is present in 100% of cases and it is characterized by a rash of symmetric erythematous papules of the buttocks and lower extremities, which progresses to palpable purpura. Other skin lesions, generally macular, papular, or more rarely urticarial or vesicular, are observed in up to 44% of children. Histological analysis of purpuric lesions shows a small-vessel LCV with direct immunofluorescence revealing an IgA-1 predominant immune deposit. Several studies have evaluated predictive factors of renal involvement and relapse in IgAV. In this regard, recurrent purpura lasting more than 1 month seems to be an important independent predictive factor in the development of nephritis and relapse in children. In adults, relapsing disease has been related to purpura lasting for at least 1 month, and with the presence of severe LCV with a significant deposition of IgA with no IgM on direct immunofluorescence. Notably, patients without relapse tend to have deposition of both IgM and IgA. Also in adults, an inverse association of eosinophils on skin biopsy with renal involvement has been reported, suggesting that adult patients with LCV and absence of eosinophils on histopathology are more likely to have renal involvement. Furthermore, patients with LCV and absence of histiocytes on histopathology seem to have more gastrointestinal involvement.

Cryoglobulinemic vasculitis is a small-vessel vasculitis with cryoglobulin immune deposits, and associated with cryoglobulins in serum. Three basic types of cryoglobulins can be distinguished according to the clonality and type of immunoglobulins. Type I (monoclonal), type II (monoclonal and polyclonal), and type III (polyclonal). Types II and III are referred to as mixed cryoglobulinemias because they consist of both IgG and IgM components. Cryoglobulinemia type I accounts for 10% to 15% of patients with cryoglobulinemia and is found in patients with B-cell lymphoproliferative disorders. Types II and III are commonly associated with infectious (60% to 90% infected with hepatitis C virus), autoimmune (mainly primary Sjögren syndrome and systemic lupus erythematosus [SLE]), or neoplastic diseases. Nearly 10% of cases

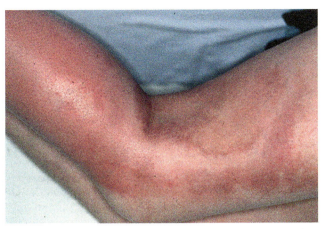

FIGURE 4-5 ■ Hypocomplementemic urticarial vasculitis, presenting with urticarial-like pink plaques. (Courtesy of Dr. Pujol RM. Head of the dermatology division. Department of Dermatology; Hospital del Mar-Parc de Salut Mar, Barcelona, Spain.)

of mixed cryoglobulinemia are idiopathic (essential). The percentage of patients with circulating cryoglobulins who develop symptoms varies from 2% to 50%. Among those who develop symptoms, cutaneous manifestations are the most common at onset (24%), with palpable purpura being the most frequent cutaneous manifestation (54% to 82%). The typical presentation consists of intermittent episodes of small petechial palpable lesions predominantly localized in lower extremities. Those patients with a cryocrit >5%, low C4, and positive rheumatoid factor, are at a higher risk of palpable purpura. In patients with noninfectious mixed cryoglobulinemic vasculitis, cutaneous involvement is observed in up to 83% of cases. Compared with patients with type III cryoglobulins, patients with type II cryoglobulins have more frequent purpura, lower C3 and C4 complement fractions, and higher cryoglobulin levels. Patients with type I cryoglobulinemia were supposed to have a less frequent cutaneous involvement, mainly due to a hyperviscosity-related vasculopathy. However, Terrier et al. (2013) reported a series of 64 patients with type I cryoglobulinemic vasculitis, showing a two-fold increase in frequency of severe cutaneous involvement in comparison with mixed cryoglobulinemic vasculitis. Cutaneous manifestations at diagnosis included purpura in 69%, acrocyanosis in 30%, skin necrosis in 28%, and skin ulcers in 27%.

Hypocomplementemic urticarial vasculitis (HUV) represents an uncommon systemic vasculitis with various clinical manifestations. This is included within the spectrum of urticarial vasculitis (UV), which is a clinicopathological entity characterized by an inflammatory injury of dermal capillaries and postcapillary venules. Although the cutaneous presentation may resemble urticaria, lesions of UV are often painful more than pruritic, typically persist for 24 hours, and resolve with faint residual pigmentation (Fig. 4-5).

The mean age at diagnosis of HUV is 40 years with a predominance in women. Clinically, angioedema, arthralgias, and ocular inflammation are described in at least 50% of patients with HUV, with systemic presentation in two-thirds of cases. Patients with HUV typically present low C1q complement level and normal C1 inhibitor level, in association with anti-C1q antibodies in approximately 50% of cases.

Spectrum of Cutaneous Vasculitis Associated with Autoimmune Systemic Diseases

Vasculitis may occur in many autoimmune diseases, usually affecting small-sized vessels. Rheumatoid arthritis (RA) is a chronic systemic inflammatory disease affecting primarily the synovial joints, but may also be associated with heterogeneous extra-articular manifestations. Skin is the most commonly involved extra-articular site in RA, rheumatoid nodules being the most frequent lesions. Autopsy data have reported systemic vasculitis in 15% to 31% of patients with RA. However, clinically apparent vasculitis in patients with RA is much less frequent. Rheumatoid vasculitis typically affects middle-aged patients with severe RA with an average of 14 years after the onset of the disease. Involved vessels range from small skin vessels to the aortic root. Skin blood vessels are involved in approximately 90% of cases, followed by vasa nervorum of peripheral nerves in approximately 40%. CV is an uncommon finding in patients with RA. European series yielded a prevalence of CV in patients with RA of 5.4% in Belgium, 4.5% in Spain, 3.7% in Italy, and 3.6% in Sweden. Similar results have been reported from Japan (3.8%). A lower prevalence was found in Turkey, accounting for 0.9% of patients with RA. Palpable purpura in the lower extremities is the most common cutaneous presentation. Other manifestations include deep skin ulcers found in unusual locations of the lower extremities, mainly in the dorsum of the foot or the upper calf, ischemic focal digital lesions, maculopapular erythema, hemorrhagic blisters, erythema elevatum diutinum, livedo reticularis, subcutaneous nodules, and atrophie blanche. Three different histological patterns of CV may be seen in RA: (1) a necrotizing LCV of dermal venules, (2) an arteritis resembling PNA, and (3) a mixed arteritis and venulitis in the same sample.

SLE is an often severe, systemic autoimmune disease, with protean clinical and serological manifestations. Approximately 10% of patients with SLE develop vasculitis, with CV as its main clinical presentation (up to 90%). Cutaneous manifestations, in decreasing frequency, are erythematous punctate lesions of the fingertips and palms (36%), palpable purpura (25%), ischemic/ulcerated lesions (14%), erythematous papules/macules (14%), urticarial lesions (11%), and nodular lesions (5%). A combination of lesions is seen in up to 30% of patients. The most common histopathologic finding in SLE patients with CV is LCV. Medium-sized vessel vasculitis may also be seen. Those SLE patients with anti-Ro antibodies have higher risk of developing CV.

Primary Sjögren syndrome (PSS) is an inflammatory autoimmune disease primarily affecting the exocrine glands but with frequent systemic manifestations. CV occurs in 4% to 10% of patients with PSS. The most common histopathologic finding, as described in SLE, is a small-vessel LCV, with occasional medium-sized vessel involvement (5%).

VASCULITIS VARIANTS

An unusual cutaneous vasculitic syndrome, known as erythema elevatum diutinum, is worthy of special

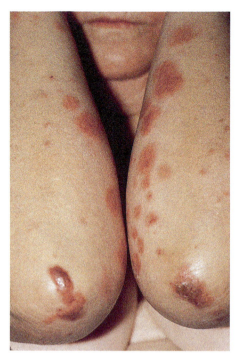

FIGURE 4-6 ■ Erythema elevatum diutinum. These violaceous nodular lesions on the extensor surfaces and over bony prominences represent a localized leukocytoclastic vasculitis. (Courtesy of Dr. Neil A. Fenske, Tampa, FL, USA.)

mention. It is rare, but its major manifestation is cutaneous disease. The lesions begin as red-purple papules that coalesce to form red-yellow plaques (Fig. 4-6). The lesions are most prominent over points of trauma, such as the elbows, knees, dorsum of the hands, and buttocks. Systemic disease is rare. Erythema elevatum diutinum is said to be responsive to the antileprosy agent dapsone, whereas most cases of the other cutaneous vasculitides may be less responsive to this drug. The entity known as BCPAN can present variably in the skin, but most often presents as nodules or ulcers that may be surrounded by livedo reticularis. Although there are some authorities who believe that this disease has the potential to progress to classic systemic PAN, the majority of dermatologists who have encountered this disorder have found it not to progress. These patients may have an accompanying neuropathy, fever, and/or malaise, but BCPAN never involves kidneys, lungs, or gastrointestinal tract. Biopsy of these lesions reveals involvement of arterioles often found in subcutaneous fat. Treatment for BCPAN often includes prednisone early in the course, which is followed by the use of dapsone, mycophenolate mofetil, azathioprine, or methotrexate as steroid-sparing agents.

DIAGNOSTIC APPROACH

Skin biopsy is the gold standard for the diagnosis of CV, and the first step to be carried out. Accurate histological classification is the cornerstone upon which our diagnostic process will be built. For that reason, some important considerations about the biopsy process should be taken into account.

A punch or excisional biopsy extending to the subcutis should be taken from the most tender, reddish or purpuric, lesional skin. In ulcerative lesions, the yield of detecting the affected vessel may be increased by including the center of the ulcer in the biopsy specimen. When biopsing livedo reticularis, the white center of the circular livedo segment should be the focus, as the erythema is due to venous congestion caused by the involved artery.

The optimal time for skin biopsy is less than 48 hours after the appearance of a vasculitic lesion. After 24 hours neutrophilic infiltration of wall vessels is progressively replaced by lymphocytes and macrophages. In consequence, lesions older than 48 hours may show a predominant lymphocyte infiltrate regardless of the underlying form of vasculitis. A direct immunofluorescence analysis is also mandatory, since it does not confirm the diagnosis but may guide us in the appropriate direction. Here timing is also important. The older the biopsied lesion is, the fewer immunoglobulins are found. After 72 hours only C3 is detected.

A histopathological diagnosis of vasculitis must be correlated with clinical history (recent drug exposure, infections, etc.), physical examination, and laboratory and radiological findings in order to establish the presence or absence of systemic involvement. Routine complementary examinations should include chest X-ray, complete blood cell count, erythrocyte sedimentation rate, C-reactive protein, liver and kidney function test, urinalysis, rheumatoid factor, antinuclear antibodies, ANCA, serum IgA, cryoglobulins, complement levels (C3, C4), and determinations for hepatitis B and C virus.

In those patients in whom a suspected well-defined entity may explain the presence of CV, specific studies should be considered (HIV and other viral determinations, blood cultures, echocardiography, colonoscopy, renal biopsy, lumbar puncture, etc.). Figure 4-7 shows a work-up in a patient with CV.

TREATMENT

Treatment of SoCSVV is empiric, as large, well-controlled studies are lacking. Nevertheless, SoCSVV is remarkably predictable in its rapid and sometimes complete improvement after bed-rest, and in some cases with low-dose prednisone therapy. Any factor causing or exacerbating vasculitis should be treated or removed. Patients should also be informed that tight-fitting clothing, cold exposure, and extended periods of standing can all exacerbate the disease. Nonsteroidal anti-inflammatory agents have been suggested for treatment of milder disease, but definitive evidence is lacking. If moderate to severe cutaneous disease develops, particularly if this is persistent, recurrent, or necrotic/ulcerative, the use of colchicine or dapsone as alternatives to corticosteroid therapy is supported by many case series and case reports, though large, well-controlled trials are lacking for almost all suggested therapies for CV. If patients with more severe or persistent disease continue to require corticosteroid therapy, or only partially respond, the addition of methotrexate, azathioprine, or mycophenolate mofetil are some of the more frequently recommended steroid-sparing agents.

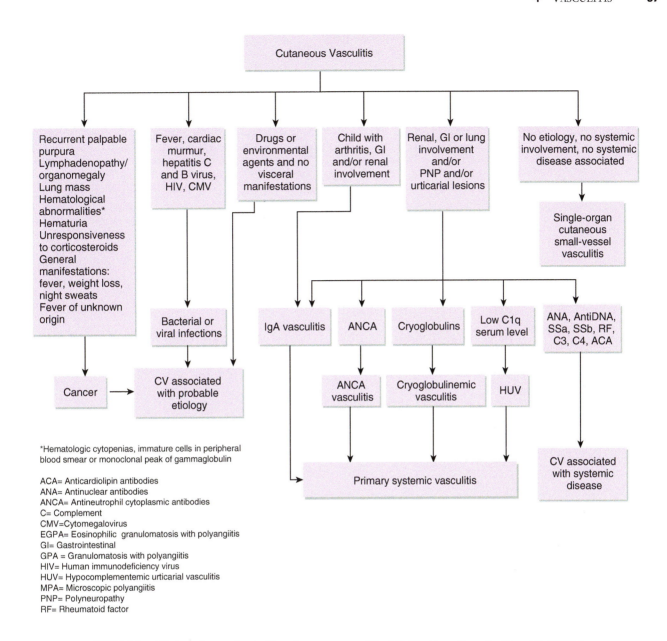

FIGURE 4-7 ■ Work-up in a patient with cutaneous vasculitis. (Modified from Gonzalez-Gay et al. (2005).)

In those patients in whom CV is a manifestation of a systemic vasculitis or a connective tissue disease, therapy must be individualized and must be focused on the management of the systemic disease. In some of these cases, immunosuppressive drugs such as methotrexate, azathioprine, mycophenolate mofetil, cyclophosphamide or rituximab, among others, may be considered. Also, when CV occurs in the setting of a malignancy or an infection, treatment of the underlying disease often leads to improvement of the cutaneous manifestations.

SUGGESTED READINGS

Arora A, Wetter DA, Gonzalez-Santiago TM, Davis MDP, Lohse CM. Incidence of leukocytoclastic vasculitis, 1996 to 2010: a population based study in Olmsted County, Minnesota. Mayo Clin Proc 2014;89(11):1515–24.

Blanco R, Martinez-Taboada VM, Rodriguez-Valverde V, Garcia-Fuentes M. Cutaneous vasculitis in children and adults. Associated diseases and etiologic factors in 303 patients. Medicine 1998;77:403–18.

Bloch DA, Michel BA, Hunder GG, McShane DJ, Arend WP, Calabrese LH, et al. The American College of Rheumatology 1990 criteria for the classification of vasculitis. Patients and methods. Arthritis Rheum 1990;33:1068–73.

Callen JP. Cutaneous vasculitis: what we have learned in the past 20 years? Arch Dermatol 1998;134:355–7.

Carlson JA. The histological assessment of cutaneous vasculitis. Histopathology 2010;56:3–23.

Chen KR, Carlson JA. Clinical approach to cutaneous vasculitis. Am J Clin Dermatol 2008;9(2):71–92.

Gonzalez-Gay MA, García-Porrua C, Pujol RM. Clinical approach to cutaneous vasculitis. Curr Opin Rheumatol 2005;17:56–61.

Gonzalez-Gay MA, Garcia-Porrua C. Epidemiology of the vasculitides. Rheum Dis Clin North Am 2001;27(4):729–49.

Hodge SJ, Callen JP, Ekenstam E. Cutaneous leukocytoclastic vasculitis: correlation of histopathological changes with clinical severity and course. J Cutan Pathol 1987;14:279–84.

Jachiet M, Flageul B, Deroux A, Le Quellec A, Maurier F, Cordoliani F, et al. The clinical spectrum and therapeutic management of hypocomplementemic urticarial vasculitis: data from a French nationwide study of fifty-seven patients. Arthritis Rheumatol February 2015;67(2):527–34.

Jennette JC, Falk RJ, Bacon PA, Basu N, Cid MC, Ferrario F, et al. 2012 Revised International Chapel Hill consensus conference nomenclature of vasculitides. Arthritis Rheum 2013;65(1):1–11.

Kinney MA, Jorizzo JL. Small-vessel vasculitis. Dermatol Therapy 2012;25(2):148–57.

Pina T, Gonzalez-Gay MA. Cutaneous vasculitis: a rheumatologist perspective. Curr Allergy Asthma Rep 2013;13:545–54.

Rocha LK, Romitti R, Shinjo S, Neto ML, Carvalho J, Criado PR. Cutaneous manifestations and comorbidities in 60 cases of Takayasu arteritis. J Rheumatol May 2013;40(5):734–8.

Stone JH, Nousari HC. "Essential" cutaneous vasculitis: what every rheumatologist should know about vasculitis of the skin. Curr Opin Rheumatol 2001;13:23–34.

Terrier B, Karras A, Kahn JE, Le Guenno G, Marie I, Benarous L, et al. The spectrum of type I cryoglobulinemia vasculitis. New insights based on 64 cases. Medicine (Baltimore) 2013;92(2):61–8.

Watts RA, Jolliffe VA, Grattan CE, Elliott J, Lockwood M, Scott DG. Cutaneous vasculitis in a defined population. Clinical and epidemiological associations. J Rheumatol 1998;25:920–4.

CHAPTER 5

NEUTROPHILIC DERMATOSES

Joanna Harp • Joseph L. Jorizzo

KEY POINTS

- Neutrophilic dermatoses encompass a spectrum of diseases marked by cutaneous lesions that on histopathologic examination show intense inflammation composed primarily of mature neutrophils.
- Behçet's disease is a neutrophilic dermatosis characterized by an immune-mediated occlusive vasculitis of small, medium, and large blood vessels that is associated with a wide range of cutaneous and systemic findings.
- Sweet's syndrome is typified by a cutaneous infiltrate of dermal or subcutaneous neutrophils often with fever that has been associated with a variety of underlying diseases and medications.
- Pyoderma gangrenosum is a neutrophilic dermatosis marked by ulcerating skin lesions. It is a diagnosis of exclusion and other etiologies of cutaneous ulceration must be ruled out.
- Bowel bypass syndrome, later known as Bowel-associated dermatosis–arthritis syndrome, is a neutrophilic dermatosis characterized by typical skin lesions in the setting of bowel surgery or inflammatory bowel disease.

BEHÇET'S DISEASE

Clinical Manifestations

Behçet's disease is a complex multisystem vasculitis first described by the Turkish dermatologist Hulusi Behçet in the late 1930s. It is characterized by recurrent oral and genital ulcers, as well as ocular, articular, vascular, intestinal, and nervous system manifestations. Although relatively common in the Middle East and Asia, it is uncommon in northern Europe, Great Britain, and the United States. Behçet's occurs in both genders and is primarily a disease of young adults.

Because there is no pathognomonic laboratory test, the diagnosis is based on clinical criteria (Table 5-1). The oral aphthae experienced by these patients are like those seen in patients with simple aphthosis (i.e., canker sores). They are usually multiple, painful, and occur in crops (Fig. 5-1). The genital aphthae are similar, except that they occur less frequently (Figs 5-2 and 5-3). Pathergy—the development of cutaneous papulopustular lesions 24 hours after cutaneous trauma (e.g., by needle prick or intradermal injection)—is a characteristic feature seen in many patients with Behçet's disease. Various skin manifestations including vesiculopustular lesions, palpable purpura, Sweet's syndrome-like edematous papules and PG-like ulcerations may be seen. Deeper subcutaneous lesions that mimic erythema nodosum can also occur.

Behçet's disease is a multisystem disorder. Posterior uveitis (i.e., retinal vasculitis) is the most classic ocular lesion seen, though various other ocular findings can occur. The arthritis seen in patients with Behçet's disease is nonerosive and inflammatory, and affects both large and small joints. Neurologic manifestations have a late onset in patients with Behçet's disease and are remarkably variable in their presentation. A vasculitis of the vasa vasorum, with a propensity to affect large arteries and veins, can be a cause of death in patients with Behçet's. Vessel thrombosis and aneurysms likely due to chronic endovascular damage are reported typically as a late manifestation of disease. The kidneys are relatively spared in Behçet's patients compared to other systemic vasculitides.

Pathogenesis

Behçet's disease is considered an autoinflammatory disorder typified by an immune-mediated occlusive vasculitis of small, medium, and large blood vessels affecting both the arterial and venous circulation. The etiology of Behçet's disease remains unknown, but various studies have implicated genetic factors, environmental pollution, viral and bacterial agents, and immunologic factors. Behçet's has been associated with certain human leukocyte antigens (HLAs) including HLA-B51. A genetic predisposition that triggers immunologic disease in response to viral or other infection is one theory of disease pathogenesis and studies have implicated various antigens including streptococcal antigens, *Helicobacter pylori*, herpes simplex virus, and parvovirus B19. Dysregulation of innate and adaptive immunity, including increased activation of neutrophils, has also been demonstrated in patients with Behçet's.

TABLE 5-1	Clinical Criteria for Behçet's Disease

Recurrent oral aphthosis (at least three times in 1 year)
AND
At least two of the following:
    Recurrent genital aphthosis
    Eye lesions (uveitis, cells in vitreous on slit lamp, or retinal vasculitis)
    Skin lesions (erythema nodosum, pseudovasculitis, papulopustular lesions or acneiform nodules consistent with Behçet's)
    Positive pathergy test

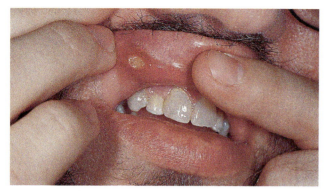

FIGURE 5-1 ■ Oral aphthous lesions in a patient with Behçet's disease.

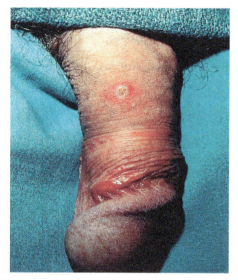

FIGURE 5-2 ■ Aphthae on the penis in a patient with Behçet's disease.

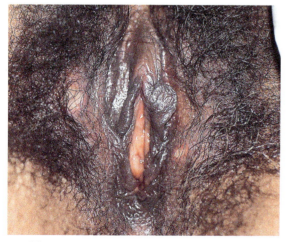

FIGURE 5-3 ■ Vulvar aphthae in Behçet's disease.

Histopathology

Early mucocutaneous lesions typically show a neutrophilic vascular reaction or true leukocytoclastic vasculitis on histopathology. Tissue from late or chronic mucocutaneous lesions shows a more lymphocyte-dominant infiltrate. Similar histopathologic findings of a lymphocytic "perivasculitis" are reported from autopsy specimens of internal organs in Behçet's patients.

Treatment

Therapy for mucosal lesions includes topical viscous lidocaine, potent topical corticosteroids, or intralesional corticosteroid injections. Oral colchicine therapy may be associated with a reduced severity and frequency of aphthae. Oral thalidomide therapy is extremely effective for mucocutaneous involvement. Low-dose weekly methotrexate therapy may be beneficial in selected patients. Oral dapsone may be substituted or added.

Systemic corticosteroid therapy, alone or with azathioprine, is a mainstay of treatment for more severe ocular and systemic disease. Cyclophosphamide and cyclosporine may be considered for patients with resistant ocular or neurologic disease. There is also increasing evidence for the efficacy of biologics including infliximab, etanercept, adalimumab, and rituximab, especially in patients with uveitis. In most case reports where biologics were initiated, the extraocular manifestations also improved, but tended to recur if the drug was withdrawn. Early reports suggest possible benefit with agents directed against interleukin-1 (IL-1) or interleukin-6, especially in severe or refractory disease.

SWEET'S SYNDROME (ACUTE FEBRILE NEUTROPHILIC DERMATOSIS)

Clinical Manifestations

Sweet described a group of patients with one or more attacks of painful, erythematous plaques accompanied by fever, arthralgias, and leukocytosis. This syndrome is more frequent in women (female:male, 4:1) between the ages of 30 and 60 years. The characteristic lesion is a well-defined erythematous plaque often with a pseudovesicular, vesicular, or pustular surface (Fig. 5-4). Lesions can occur at any location though they predominantly affect the face, trunk, and proximal extremities, and may develop at sites of trauma (pathergy). In some cases, lesions may present as deeper subcutaneous nodules with mild overlying erythema termed subcutaneous Sweet's. Though ulceration is generally considered rare in classic Sweet's, a new necrotizing variant with soft tissue necrosis has been reported. The lesions are accompanied by fever in most patients, and by myalgias and/or arthralgias in about half. Untreated lesions resolve over 6 to 8 weeks though recurrence may occur, especially in the setting of malignancy. Sites of extracutaneous organ involvement include bone (sterile osteomyelitis) and ocular (conjunctivitis, ulcerative keratitis) involvement as well as neutrophilic infiltration of the lungs, heart, nervous system, kidney, and gastrointestinal system.

Pathogenesis

The pathogenesis of Sweet's syndrome is not well understood but is thought to result from the interplay of genetic susceptibility, exogenous triggers, and immune

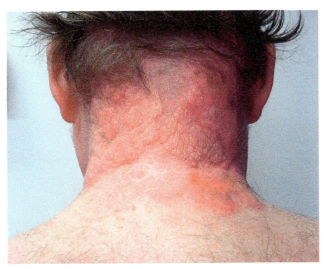

FIGURE 5-4 ■ Pseudovesiculated, mammillated plaques of acute febrile neutrophilic dermatosis.

dysregulation. Some evidence suggests that infections, neoplasms, and other triggers lead to Sweet's through the activation of proneutrophil and proinflammatory cytokines such as IL-1 and IL-8 and granulocyte-colony stimulating factor (G-CSF). G-CSF has been shown to be elevated in some patients with Sweet's and is postulated to be produced directly by tumor cells in certain cases of malignancy-associated Sweet's. In addition, exogenous G-CSF is a known trigger for drug-induced Sweet's syndrome.

Histopathology and Laboratory Findings

Histopathologically there is a dense dermal infiltrate composed of mature neutrophils and dermal edema. In subcutaneous Sweet's, neutrophils are localized to the subcutis. Though the infiltrate may be more pronounced in perivascular areas, vasculitis is classically absent. Given the predominance of neutrophils, infection must be ruled out. "Histiocytoid" Sweet's refers to a histological variant of Sweet's syndrome most commonly reported in patients with hematologic malignancies characterized by tissue infiltration of immature myeloid cells that resemble histiocytes. Laboratory findings include increased erythrocyte sedimentation rate and C-reactive protein as well as leukocytosis often with neutrophilia. Clinicians should be aware, however, that Sweet's can develop in neutropenic patients, typically in the setting of acute myelogenous leukemia.

Associated Conditions

Sweet's syndrome has been described with a variety of diseases including malignancy (most commonly acute myelogenous leukemia and myelodysplastic syndrome, but also lymphomas and solid organ tumors), autoimmune disease, sarcoid, inflammatory bowel disease (IBD), and infection (*Streptococcus*, *Mycobacterium tuberculosis*, viral hepatitis). Sweet's has also been reported with pregnancy and after vaccination. Many medications have been implicated in cases of Sweet's including G-CSF, trimethoprim–sulfamethoxazole, azathioprine, oral contraceptives, hydralazine, and minocycline, among others.

Treatment

Sweet's syndrome is usually an acute, steroid-responsive disease. Oral prednisone (generally 40 to 60 mg/day) typically leads to a dramatic response, with resolution of fever and improvement of skin lesions. Steroids are generally tapered over 2 to 6 weeks. Pulse dosing of methylprednisolone may be required for severe or refractory disease. Colchicine and potassium iodide are also considered first-line treatment, with dapsone, cyclosporine, clofazimine, and indomethacin considered second line. Individual cases and small case series have reported success with thalidomide, chlorambucil, cyclophosphamide, retinoids, and, more recently, tumor necrosis factor-alpha (TNF-α) inhibitors and IL-1 antagonists. In patients with underlying disease the onset of Sweet's lesions often occurs in the setting of poor control of the underlying disease, which should be a primary consideration in therapeutic decisions.

PYODERMA GANGRENOSUM

Clinical Manifestations

Pyoderma gangrenosum (PG) is an uncommon neutrophilic dermatosis typically presenting with rapidly expanding cutaneous ulcerations. The diagnostic evaluation of a patient presumed to have PG has two objectives: (1) to exclude other causes of cutaneous ulceration, as this is a diagnosis of exclusion; and (2) to determine whether there is an associated treatable systemic disorder.

The ulceration(s) of classic PG are often clinically characteristic. The border is well defined with a deep erythematous to violaceous color (Fig. 5-5). The lesion extends peripherally, and often the border overhangs the ulceration (undermined). Pain is a prominent feature. As the lesion heals, scar formation occurs that may be in a cribriform pattern. Lesions may display pathergy and aggressive debridement of PG lesions should be avoided especially during the active, expanding disease phase. Several variants of PG have been described.

Pyostomatitis Vegetans

This process is one in which chronic, pustular, and eventually vegetative erosions develop on the mucous membranes, most notably in the mouth.

Atypical or Bullous Pyoderma Gangrenosum

In this variant, the ulcerations are more superficial than in classic PG. There is often a bullous, blue-gray margin, and the upper extremities and face are the most commonly affected sites (Fig. 5-6). This variant has been reported in patients with hematologic disease, specifically, myelodysplastic syndrome or acute myelogenous leukemia.

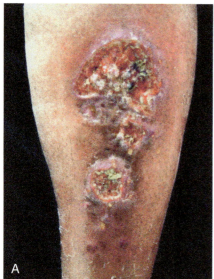

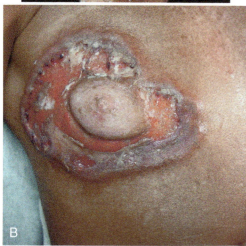

FIGURE 5-5 ■ **A,** Classic pyoderma gangrenosum in a patient with partially controlled Crohn's disease. **B,** Pyoderma gangrenosum developed following a breast biopsy performed at the same time as abdominal surgery in this patient with Crohn's disease.

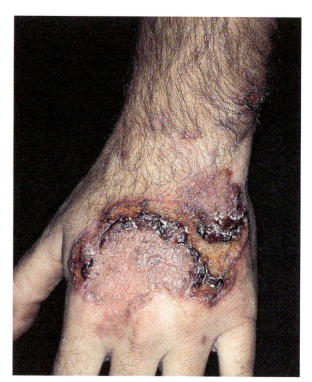

FIGURE 5-6 ■ Atypical pyoderma gangrenosum.

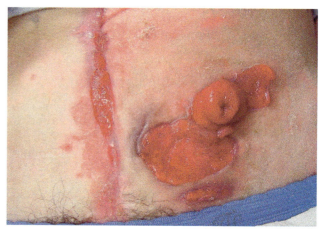

FIGURE 5-7 ■ Several peristomal ulcerations developed following colectomy in this young woman with Crohn's disease. Also of note is the ulceration in the midline incision created during surgery.

Peristomal Pyoderma Gangrenosum

These patients often have a stoma created after surgery for IBD or cancer (Fig. 5-7). Some patients have no evidence of active bowel disease, whereas in others careful study reveals active disease, in particular Crohn's disease. These patients are often thought to have an infection, and surgeons may debride the ulcer or relocate the stoma—approaches that often result in worsening or recurrence of the disease.

Pathogenesis

The pathogenesis of PG is poorly understood but increasing evidence points toward immune dysregulation and altered neutrophil chemotaxis. Some consider PG on the spectrum of autoinflammatory disorders, which may explain the association between PG and other autoinflammatory diseases such as Crohn's disease. Genetics factors can play a role in some cases and may help elucidate the pathogenesis of idiopathic cases. PAPA syndrome (pyogenic sterile arthritis, PG, and acne) is characterized by an autosomal dominant mutation in proline/serine/threonine phosphatase-interacting protein 1 (PSTPIP1), which is thought to result in dysregulation of the cryopyrin inflammasome and activation of IL-1β leading to inflammation. This pathway may be central to many autoinflammatory conditions.

Histopathology

The histopathologic features of PG are nonspecific, but histology is often useful in ruling out other causes

TABLE 5-2 Diseases Associated with Pyoderma Gangrenosum

Common Associations
Inflammatory bowel disease
   Chronic ulcerative colitis
   Regional enteritis, granulomatous colitis (Crohn's disease)
Arthritis
   Seronegative with inflammatory bowel disease
   Seronegative without inflammatory bowel disease
   Rheumatoid arthritis
   Spondylitis
   Osteoarthritis
Hematologic diseases
   Myelocytic leukemias
   Hairy cell leukemia
   Myelofibrosis, agnogenic myeloid metaplasia
   Monoclonal gammopathy (IgA)

Rarely Reported Associations
Chronic active hepatitis
Myeloma
Polycythemia rubra vera
Paroxysmal nocturnal hemoglobinuria
Takayasu's arteritis
Primary biliary cirrhosis
Systemic lupus erythematosus
Hidradenitis suppurativa
Acne conglobata
Malignancy
Thyroid disease
Pulmonary disease
Sarcoidosis
Diabetes mellitus
Other pustular dermatoses

---

of cutaneous ulceration including infection, vasculitis/vasculopathy, and neoplasm. New lesions in untreated patients have been reported to show a neutrophilic histology with endothelial swelling. Classically there is extensive neutrophilic infiltration with resultant necrosis and hemorrhage. Focal vasculitis may be seen but should not be prominent.

Associated Conditions

There is an associated systemic disease in roughly 50% of patients with PG (Table 5-2). The most common associated conditions are IBD, arthritis, paraproteinemia, and hematologic malignancy. Work-up for an associated disease is an important part of the evaluation for a patient diagnosed with PG.

Arthritis is a frequent finding in patients with PG. In general, the arthritis associated with PG is a symmetrical polyarthritis, which may be seronegative or seropositive. As described with Sweet's syndrome, patients with PG may also have neutrophilic infiltration of internal organs, including the lung, liver, heart, and bone.

Treatment

Treatment for PG must be directed at optimization of wound healing and control of inflammation. Wound care includes selecting appropriate dressings, monitoring for and treating infection, and minimizing exacerbating factors. Strategies for controlling inflammation are varied and depend on the number and size of lesions, rate of progression, and presence of associated underlying disorders.

In mild cases, local measures such as topical agents including corticosteroids, calcineurin inhibitors, or topical dapsone, or intralesional injections may be sufficient to control disease. In patients with severe or rapidly progressive disease, systemic corticosteroids and cyclosporine are generally considered first-line therapies. For patients with PG associated with IBD, corticosteroid-sparing strategies are generally preferred and biologics are becoming the treatment of choice to control both the skin and gut disease. Infliximab and adalimumab have shown efficacy in patients with PG and IBD, the former in a randomized placebo-controlled trial. Other agents including azathioprine, mycophenolate mofetil, intravenous immunoglobulin, anakinra, canakinumab, and cyclophosphamide have been used for refractory disease or in patients who develop side effects to other therapies. Finally, agents such as dapsone and minocycline may be considered as adjunctive or maintenance treatments.

BOWEL-ASSOCIATED DERMATOSIS–ARTHRITIS SYNDROME

Clinical Manifestations

Bowel-associated dermatosis–arthritis syndrome is characterized by recurrent crops of cutaneous pustular vasculitis, synovitis, fever, and flu-like symptoms that develop subsequent to a variety of bariatric procedures or with IBD. The incidence of this syndrome was initially reported to be as high as 20% after jejunoileal bypass surgery, though it is generally considered to be less common with more modern bariatric procedures. Patients experience the onset of the serum sickness-like illness typically 2 to 3 months, but ranging from several days to years, after the gastrointestinal procedure. An increased frequency of diarrhea and gastrointestinal disturbance accompanies the systemic disease. Polyarticular arthralgias, myalgias, and a nonerosive arthritis are frequent findings. Cutaneous pustular vasculitis is frequently seen, though erythema nodosum-like lesions may also occur (Fig. 5-8). Bouts may occur every 4 to 6 weeks.

Pathogenesis

The proposed pathophysiology of bowel bypass–bowel-associated dermatosis–arthritis syndrome is bacterial overgrowth with subsequent immune complex formation in areas of altered gastrointestinal tract. Circulating immune complexes then deposit in target tissues, such as the skin and synovium, producing the clinical features of this syndrome.

Histopathology

Early lesions are characterized by papillary edema and subepidermal vesiculation, while later lesions display a

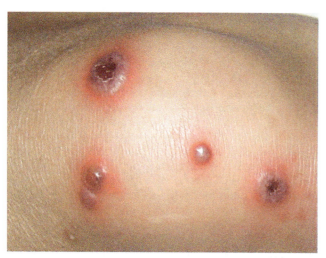

FIGURE 5-8 ■ Pustular vasculitis in a patient with uncontrolled ulcerative colitis.

dense neutrophilic dermal infiltrate. True leukocytoclastic vasculitis is rare. Findings are very similar histopathologically to lesions of Behçet's disease.

Treatment

Systemic corticosteroid therapy is typically effective for controlling the signs and symptoms of bowel-associated dermatosis–arthritis syndrome. Bowel bypass patients may be cured by restoration of normal bowel anatomy. Systemic antibiotics (e.g., tetracycline, metronidazole, and erythromycin) are efficacious, perhaps because of their effect on the reduction of bowel bacterial overgrowth. Efficacy has also been demonstrated with TNF-α inhibitors. Thalidomide, colchicine, and dapsone have been successfully used in individual patients. Patients with inflammatory bowel disease require better control of their underlying disease.

SUGGESTED READINGS

Agarwal A, Andrews J. Systemic review: IBD-associated pyoderma gangrenosum in the biologic era, the response to therapy. Aliment Pharmacol Ther 2013;38:563–72.

Ahronowitz I, Harp J, Shinkai K. Etiology and management of pyoderma gangrenosum: a comprehensive review. Am J Clin Dermatol June 1, 2012;13(3):191–211.

Alavi A, Sajic D, Cerci FB, Ghazarian D, Rosenbach M, Jorizzo J. Neutrophilic dermatoses: an update. Am J Clin Dermatol October 2014;15(5):413–23.

Anzalone C, Cohen P. Acute febrile neutrophilic dermatosis (Sweet's syndrome). Curr Opin Hematol January 2013;20(1):26–35.

Butler D, Shinkai K. What do autoinflammatory syndromes teach about common cutaneous diseases such as pyoderma gangrenosum? A commentary. Dermatol Clin 2013;31:427–35.

Mazzoccoli, et al. Behçet syndrome: from pathogenesis to novel therapies. Clin Exp Med December 2, 2014. Epub ahead of print.

Yazici H, Ben-Chetrit E, Bang D, et al. Behçet's disease and other autoinflammatory conditions. Clin Exp Rheumatol 2007;25: S1–119.

CHAPTER 6

PSORIASIS AND SYSTEMIC DISEASE

Jashin J. Wu • Johann E. Gudjonsson

KEY POINTS

- Psoriasis is common, affecting over 125 million worldwide.
- Comorbidities include diabetes, hypertension, dyslipidemia, obesity, myocardial infarction, stroke, cardiovascular death, lymphoma, autoimmune disorders, and renal disease.
- TNF signaling and the IL-23/Th17 pathways are critical in the pathogenesis of psoriasis, and effective therapies interfere with these pathways.
- Treatment with systemic therapy may improve risk for cardiovascular disease.
- About one-third of psoriasis patients may develop psoriatic arthritis, on average 10 years after the onset of skin disease.
- Psoriatic arthritis can be differentiated from other arthritides with the CASPAR diagnostic criteria.

EPIDEMIOLOGY

Psoriasis is a chronic immune-mediated skin condition that affects 2% to 3% of the US population. Psoriasis is found worldwide, and over 125 million people are thought to be afflicted. The lowest prevalence rates are reported in Asia with less than 0.5%, and the highest in Norway at 4.82% and France at 5.20%.

Psoriasis is more than just a skin disease. Several comorbidities are associated with psoriasis. About one-third of patients may develop psoriatic arthritis, on average 10 years after psoriasis appears. It has been shown that those with psoriasis are also at higher risk for cardiometabolic conditions such as diabetes, hypertension, dyslipidemia, obesity, and metabolic syndrome. These patients are at higher risk for myocardial infarction, stroke, and cardiovascular death. They are more likely to develop lymphoma, autoimmune disorders, and renal disease. Furthermore, patients with psoriasis are more likely to have psychiatric conditions such as depression and anxiety, and are more likely to smoke and drink alcohol.

PATHOGENESIS

The most striking feature of psoriasis is the silvery scaling and redness that sharply demarcates the plaques from the surrounding normal skin. Histologically it is characterized by marked hyperproliferation of keratinocytes, altered epidermal differentiation, and proliferation of endothelial cells accompanied by an influx of various inflammatory cells. Substantial evidence implicates activated T-cells in the pathogenesis of psoriasis. Both CD4+ and CD8+ T-cells are found in psoriatic skin lesions, with CD4+ T-cells being primarily located in the upper dermis and CD8+ T-cells within the epidermis. CD8+ T cells in the epidermis are required for the development of psoriasis lesions. The CD8+ T-cells are oligoclonal, suggesting that they are responding to a restricted set of antigens, likely in the psoriatic epidermis. Multiple other cell types participate in this process including keratinocytes, dendritic cells, macrophages, mast cells, endothelial cells, and neutrophils. Cytokines initiate and sustain inflammation through pathways that involve cells of both the innate and acquired immune systems. These pathways, including tumor necrosis factor (TNF) signaling and the IL-23/Th17 (interleukin-23/T helper 17) pathways, are critical, as blockade of either one is highly effective for treatment. Interestingly, the mechanism of action for TNF inhibitors, such as etanercept, appears to be due to suppression of IL-17 signaling rather than a direct response to TNF. Besides IL-17 and TNF-α, multiple other cytokines and growth factors participate in this process, and the interaction is incompletely understood.

It has been known for over 100 years that psoriasis has a strong genetic component. However, it is only in the past few years that major strides have been made in identifying the specific genetic risk factors, mostly through genome-wide association studies. To date over 40 independent genetic signals have been identified. One of the most prominent genetic signals identified in psoriasis is HLA-Cw6. Several other risk loci are close to genes involved in antigen processing and presentation, including the *ERAP1* and *ERAP2* genes, which may tie in with the role of CD8+ T-cell function, as those cells respond to antigens in the context of major histocompatibility complex class I. Several of the risk loci are close to genes that play key roles in IL-23/IL-17 responses and others map to regions involved in epidermal barrier formation, inflammatory dendritic cell function, nuclear factor kappa beta, interferon signaling, and Th1/Th2 polarization. These genetic findings, along with progress in our understanding of the immunology, highlight the key pathogenic circuits and increase our ability to more effectively treat this disease.

CLINICAL MANIFESTATIONS

Chronic plaque psoriasis/psoriasis vulgaris is the most common clinical form of psoriasis, and is found in approximately 90% of patients. The skin manifestations are

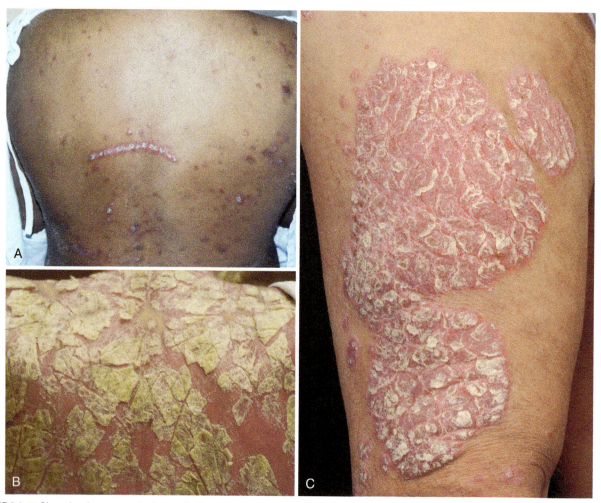

FIGURE 6-1 ■ Chronic plaque psoriasis/psoriasis vulgaris. **A,** Photo on upper left shows Koebner response after scratching. **B,** Photo on lower left shows extensive chronic plaque psoriasis involving the entire back. **C,** Typical psoriasis plaques with overlying silvery white scale on an erythematous background sharply demarcated from normal skin.

characterized by well-demarcated, raised, erythematous plaques with a white scaly surface (Fig. 6-1). Lesions can vary in size from a few millimeters up to plaques that cover an entire extremity or large areas of the trunk. Under the scale, the skin has a homogeneous shiny appearance, and small bleeding points can appear when the scale is removed (Auspitz's sign). Symmetrical distribution of lesions is a helpful feature in establishing a diagnosis. The lesions in chronic plaque psoriasis are characteristically located on the extensor aspects of the extremities, including elbows and knees. Other sites of predilection include the scalp. When the lesions are predominantly located in the umbilicus, axillary or intergluteal clefts, the term inverse psoriasis is commonly used. Signs of nail psoriasis are listed in Table 6-1. Lesions themselves may have variable presentation and may be geographic, resulting from merging of many individual lesions, annular, and less commonly verrucous or hyperkeratotic. A ring of hypopigmentation may sometimes be seen around individual plaques (Woronoff's rings). This phenomenon is usually associated with treatment response during active treatment, most commonly UV phototherapy.

Guttate psoriasis is a common form of psoriasis during childhood and early adolescence that classically arises concomitant with and shortly after streptococcal throat infection. It is characterized by eruption of small scaly plaques and papules, 5 to 10 mm in size, over the trunk and proximal extremities (Fig. 6-2). These eruptions are usually self-limited and resolve over 3 to 4 months. About a third of patients may develop repeated episodes of guttate psoriasis and about a third go on to develop chronic plaque psoriasis. This subtype of psoriasis has the strongest association with HLA-Cw6. Patients with chronic plaque psoriasis may experience guttate flares following streptococcal throat infections.

Erythrodermic psoriasis is a severe form that involves most if not all of the skin surface. Diffuse erythema is the most prominent sign, and in contrast to the thick adherent scale seen in chronic plaque psoriasis, erythrodermic

TABLE 6-1 Manifestations of Nail Psoriasis

Psoriasis of the Nail Matrix	Psoriasis of the Nail Bed
• Pitting	• Onycholysis
• Leukonychia	• Splinter hemorrhages
• Red spots in the lunula	• Subungual hyperkeratosis
• Crumbling	• "Oil drop" (salmon patch)

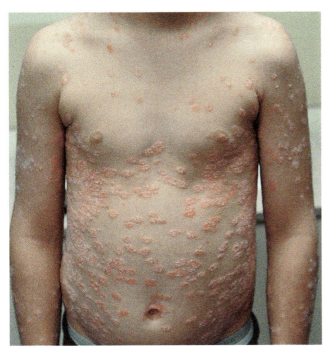

FIGURE 6-2 ■ Guttate psoriasis in a young child following a strep infection.

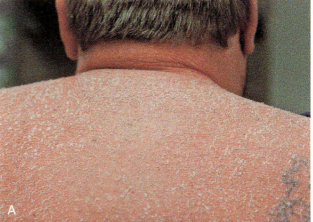

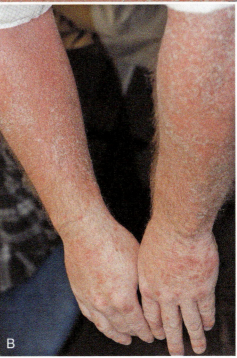

FIGURE 6-3 ■ Erythrodermic psoriasis. **A,** Extensive erythema is the most prominent sign as can be seen in this photo from the upper back of an erythrodermic patient, and scaling is typically much finer than what is seen in plaque psoriasis. **B,** Erythrodermic psoriasis is more diffuse in nature and characteristically lacks the sharp demarcation from normal skin as can be seen in this photograph of the arms from the same case as in (**A**).

psoriasis is characterized by fine delicate scale that easily flakes off (Fig. 6-3). Patients with this form of psoriasis generally feel unwell. They have difficulties maintaining thermoregulation, and are often hypohidrotic due to occlusion of the sweat ducts. High-output cardiac failure may occur given the increased blood flow to the skin surface.

Pustular psoriasis is an uncommon presentation of psoriasis. Several variants exist, including generalized pustular psoriasis, acrodermatitis continua of Hallopeau, annular pustular psoriasis, and palmoplantar pustulosis (Fig. 6-4). Generalized pustular psoriasis is the most severe form. This is an acute form characterized by fevers that last several days followed by a sudden eruption of sterile pustules 3 to 4 mm in size. The pustules arise on erythematous skin that may become confluent. Characteristically this form occurs in waves of fevers and pustules. It may resolve spontaneously, although treatment is usually required given the severe nature of this eruption. Generalized pustular psoriasis can occur on the background of chronic plaque psoriasis, is commonly triggered by withdrawal of treatments especially systemic steroids, and has been shown to be associated with CARD14 mutations. Whereas spontaneous pustular psoriasis is associated with mutations in the IL-36 receptor antagonist (*IL36RN*), suggesting that it belongs within the spectrum of autoinflammatory diseases.

DIFFERENTIAL DIAGNOSIS

Differential diagnosis depends on the specific subtype of psoriasis (Table 6-2). A large number of conditions can have manifestations that resemble psoriasis but often can be distinguished on clinical grounds alone. Where diagnosis is questionable clinically, a biopsy is indicated.

TREATMENT

A discussion of the full spectrum of therapies for psoriasis is beyond the scope of this chapter. We will pass over discussion of topical therapies and phototherapy and focus on the basics of systemic therapy and the potential effect on systemic disease.

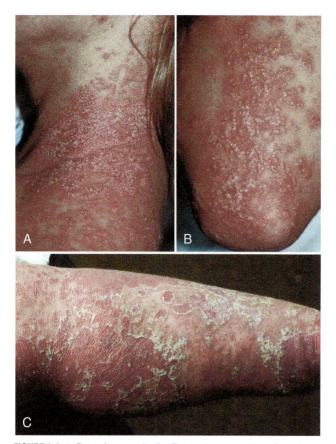

FIGURE 6-4 ■ Pustular psoriasis. Extensive eruption of pustular psoriasis of the neck (**A**) and elbow (**B**) in a young female. When pustular psoriasis resolves it typically leaves behind erythematous background and peeling scale (**C**).

TABLE 6-2 Differential Diagnoses

Chronic plaque psoriasis/psoriasis vulgaris
    Chronic eczema/nummular eczema
    Tinea
    Cutaneous T-cell lymphoma
    Subacute cutaneous lupus erythematosus
    Chronic cutaneous lupus
    Lichen simplex chronicus
    Contact dermatitis
    Pityriasis rubra pilaris
    Fixed plaques of keratoderma variabilis and/or progressive symmetric erythrokeratoderma
Guttate psoriasis
    Pityriasis lichenoides chronica
    Pityriasis rosea
    Syphilis
    Lichen planus
    Small plaque parapsoriasis
    Drug eruption
Erythrodermic psoriasis
    Eczema
    Cutaneous T-cell lymphoma/Sezary syndrome
    Pityriasis rubra pilaris
    Drug-induced erythroderma
Pustular psoriasis
    Reactive arthritis syndrome
    Superficial folliculitis
    Superficial candidiasis
    Impetigo
    Pemphigus foliaceus
    IgA pemphigus
    Sneddon–Wilkinson's disease
    Migratory necrolytic erythema
    Acute generalized exanthematous pustulosis

Methotrexate was the first oral systemic therapy approved by the Food and Drug Administration for psoriasis. It may be used first-line for psoriasis as well as psoriatic arthritis. It works well in combination with a biologic and reduces the risk of antidrug antibodies, which can over time decrease the effectiveness of the biologic. There is some evidence that methotrexate may lower cardiovascular disease in psoriasis.

Cyclosporine is indicated for the treatment of adult, nonimmunocompromised patients with severe (i.e., extensive and/or disabling), recalcitrant, plaque psoriasis who have failed to respond to at least one systemic therapy, or in patients for whom other systemic therapies are contraindicated, or cannot be tolerated. Of the systemic agents, it is the authors' opinion that cyclosporine has the quickest onset of action, which makes it a preferred therapy for patients with a severe psoriasis flare, erythrodermic psoriasis, or pustular psoriasis. Cyclosporine may increase blood pressure and lipids, which is a consideration for this patient population already at risk for cardiovascular disease.

When taking acitretin, patients may experience intolerable side effects such as chapped skin, hair loss, and peeling skin on the palms and soles. Acitretin may increase triglycerides and less commonly blood glucose. The authors consider acitretin as a second-line oral therapy for psoriasis.

Apremilast was approved in September 2014 for plaque psoriasis and in March 2014 for psoriatic arthritis. In two pivotal phase 3 trials, 33.1% and 28.8% of patients reached PASI75 at week 16. We consider apremilast as third-line due to the low effectiveness and high rate of gastrointestinal adverse events.

Etanercept was approved in April 2004 for plaque psoriasis and in January 2002 for psoriatic arthritis. Two pivotal phase 3 trials showed that 49% of patients reached PASI75 at week 12.

Adalimumab was approved in January 2008 for plaque psoriasis and in October 2005 for psoriatic arthritis. In a pivotal phase 3 trial, 71% of patients reached PASI75 at week 16.

Infliximab was approved in September 2006 for plaque psoriasis and in August 2006 for psoriatic arthritis. The pivotal phase 3 EXPRESS trial showed that 80% of patients reached PASI75 at week 10, 82% at week 24, and 61% at week 50.

Ustekinumab was approved in September 2009 for plaque psoriasis and in September 2013 for psoriatic arthritis. The pivotal phase 3 PHOENIX 1 trial showed that 66% on the 45 mg dose and 67% on the 90 mg dose reached PASI75 at week 12. The pivotal phase 3 PHOENIX 2 trial showed that 67% on the 45 mg dose and 76% on the 90 mg dose reached PASI75 at week 12.

Secukinumab was approved in January 2015 for plaque psoriasis. In two pivotal phase 3 trials at the 300 mg dose, 82% and 76% of patients reached PASI75 at week 12.

Secukinumab should not be given to patients with active Crohn's disease as exacerbations may then result.

It is the opinion of the authors that of the biologics, adalimumab should be considered first-line due to its efficacy for both psoriasis and psoriatic arthritis, safety profile, and its dosing schedule. Although etanercept has a lower effectiveness compared to the other biologics, it should be considered a first-line biologic due to its long safety record and lower level of immunosuppression compared to the other biologics. Although it has a comparable effectiveness to adalimumab in psoriasis, ustekinumab may be considered a second-line biologic due to a lower effectiveness and slower onset of action in psoriatic arthritis. However, it may be a better option than a TNF inhibitor if the patient has latent hepatitis B, is at higher risk for serious infections, and has a first-degree relative with multiple sclerosis. Secukinumab should be considered a second-line therapy since there are no long-term safety data that exist yet. It has particular utility in patients who have failed TNF inhibitors. Although it has the fastest onset and is the most effective initially, infliximab should be considered a third-line biologic due to the nature of its intravenous administration and typical loss of efficacy within 1 to 2 years.

There is some literature that suggests that treating patients with systemic therapy (biologic therapy in particular) may improve their risk for cardiovascular disease. Etanercept and adalimumab therapy reduce C-reactive protein (CRP) levels in patients with psoriasis, which correlates with improvement in psoriasis. Among patients with psoriasis, the adjusted risk of diabetes was lower for individuals starting a TNF inhibitor compared with initiation of other nonbiologic disease-modifying antirheumatic drugs such as methotrexate. Another study showed that use of TNF inhibitors for psoriasis was associated with a significant reduction in myocardial infarction risk and incident rate compared with treatment with topical agents, and that use of TNF inhibitors for psoriasis was associated with a nonstatistically significant lower myocardial infarction incident rate compared with treatment with oral agents or phototherapy. A Danish nationwide cohort showed that TNF inhibitors were associated with reduced event rates of cardiovascular death, myocardial infarction, and stroke when compared to cyclosporine, retinoids, and other therapies.

Currently under way is a National Institutes of Health-funded clinical trial to prospectively study the effect of therapy on biomarkers and on [18F]-fluorodeoxyglucose positron emission tomography-computed tomography (FDG-PET/CT). Patients are enrolled into one of three groups: adalimumab, UVB phototherapy, and placebo. Every 4 weeks for 52 weeks, biomarkers such as CRP and lipids will be checked. An FDG-PET/CT scan will be performed at weeks 0, 12, and 52. The theory is that adalimumab will improve biomarkers and reduce vascular inflammation as measured by the FDG-PET/CT scan. It is also believed that UVB phototherapy will not improve biomarkers and not reduce vascular inflammation. This study could show that aggressive systemic therapy may alter the natural history of the cardiovascular disease in psoriasis.

On the horizon, there are therapies in the pipeline targeting IL-17, IL-23, and Janus kinase for both psoriasis and psoriatic arthritis. In addition, there are clinical trials under way for biosimilars of the TNF inhibitors approved for psoriasis.

PSORIATIC ARTHRITIS

Epidemiology

Psoriatic arthritis is an erosive inflammatory joint disease with variable clinical manifestations. The prevalence is believed to be 0.5%, with studies ranging from 0.02% to 1.4%. It is estimated that up to 42% of patients with psoriasis have concomitant psoriatic arthritis. The great majority of patients develop arthritis about 10 years after the onset of their skin disease, but about 15% of patients develop arthritis before the appearance of psoriasis. There is no direct correlation between the severity of joint and skin manifestations. Males and females are affected equally. The peak age of onset is between 35 and 45 years.

Pathogenesis

Psoriatic arthritis can involve the synovium of the peripheral, the spine and sacroiliac joints, as well as the entheses, which are the attachment sites of ligaments, tendons, and joint capsules to bone. The pathogenesis of psoriatic arthritis is poorly understood. However, one of the features characterizing psoriatic arthritis is extensive bone resorption, unlike what is seen in most other arthritic conditions. Patients with psoriatic arthritis have increased numbers of circulating osteoclast precursors, and osteoclasts arise spontaneously in cultures of peripheral blood mononuclear cells from patients with psoriatic arthritis suggesting that osteoclasts have a major role in its pathogenesis. What drives the activation of the osteoclasts and the cytokine involved is not clear, but there is abundant overexpression of proinflammatory cytokine in the inflamed synovium including TNF-α, IL-1β, and IL-6. Recent data from clinical trials have implicated IL-17A as having an important role in the pathogenesis of psoriatic arthritis.

Clinical Manifestations

Psoriatic arthritis has several distinctive clinical features that distinguish it from more common arthritides such as rheumatoid arthritis. Apart from the frequent cutaneous involvement with psoriasis, these features include involvement of the distal interphalangeal joints (DIP); an asymmetric distribution of involved joints; and the presence of dactylitis, enthesitis, and sacroiliitis. Radiologic changes often present as osteolysis with widespread erosive bone lesions, and as periarticular new bone formation. Patients with psoriatic arthritis typically test negative for rheumatoid factor and anticitrullinated peptide antibodies. These features are incorporated into the CASPAR (ClASsification of Psoriatic Arthritis) diagnostic criteria for psoriatic arthritis (Table 6-3). If the patient has three of out six possible points, the CASPAR criteria have a specificity of 98.7% and sensitivity of 91.4% for psoriatic arthritis. However, of note is that despite these distinctive clinical

TABLE 6-3 CASPAR Criteria for Psoriatic Arthritis

To meet the CASPAR (ClASsification criteria for Psoriatic ARthritis) criteria, a patient must have inflammatory articular disease (joint, spine, or entheseal) with three points from the following five categories:
1. Evidence of current psoriasis, a personal history of psoriasis, or a family history of psoriasis. Current psoriasis is defined as psoriatic skin or scalp disease present today as judged by a rheumatologist or dermatologist.* A personal history of psoriasis is defined as a history of psoriasis that may be obtained from a patient, family physician, dermatologist, rheumatologist, or other qualified healthcare provider. A family history of psoriasis is defined as a history of psoriasis in a first- or second-degree relative according to patient report
2. Typical psoriatic nail dystrophy including onycholysis, pitting, and hyperkeratosis observed on current physical examination
3. A negative test result for the presence of rheumatoid factor by any method except latex but preferably by enzyme-linked immunosorbent assay or nephelometry, according to the local laboratory reference range
4. Either current dactylitis, defined as swelling of an entire digit, or a history of dactylitis recorded by a rheumatologist
5. Radiographic evidence of juxta-articular new bone formation, appearing as ill-defined ossification near joint margins (but excluding osteophyte formation) on plain radiographs of the hand or foot

*Current psoriasis is assigned a score of 2; all other features are assigned a score of 1.

TABLE 6-4 Classification of Psoriatic Arthritis

Types	Incidence	Major Characteristics
Asymmetrical oligoarthritis	70	Usually one or a few small joints of the hands and feet
Symmetrical polyarthritis	15	Clinically indistinguishable from rheumatoid arthritis, yet more benign
Primarily distal interphalangeal joints	5	So-called classic pattern; marked nail involvement and "sausage digits"
Arthritis mutilans	5	Severe, rapid development that is destructive, telescoping
Psoriatic spondylitis	5	Not an uncommon accompaniment of other forms (uncommon alone)

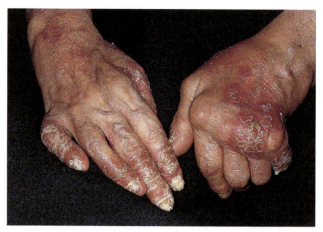

FIGURE 6-5 ■ Severe psoriatic arthritis mutilans.

features of psoriatic arthritis, there is great heterogeneity in clinical presentation (Table 6-4).

Differential Diagnosis

Psoriatic arthritis needs to be mainly differentiated from rheumatoid arthritis, particularly in patients presenting with oligo- and polyarthritis. For spine involvement the main differential is seronegative arthritic conditions, which include reactive arthritis, ankylosing spondylitis, spondylitis associated with inflammatory bowel disease, juvenile rheumatoid arthritis, and undifferentiated spondyloarthropathy. For DIP joint disease, the main differential diagnosis is osteoarthritis. Another less common consideration, particularly for arthritis mutilans, is the arthritis seen with multicentric reticulohistiocytosis (Fig. 6-5).

SUGGESTED READINGS

Elder JT, Bruce AT, Gudjonsson JE, et al. Molecular dissection of psoriasis: integrating genetics and biology. J Invest Dermatol May 2010;130(5):1213–26.
Famenini S, Sako EY, Wu JJ. Effect of treating psoriasis on cardiovascular co-morbidities: focus on TNF inhibitors. Am J Clin Dermatol February 2014;15(1):45–50.
Lowes MA, Suarez-Farinas M, Krueger JG. Immunology of psoriasis. Annu Rev Immunol 2014;32:227–55.
Menter A, Gottlieb A, Feldman SR, et al. Guidelines of care for the management of psoriasis and psoriatic arthritis: Section 1. Overview of psoriasis and guidelines of care for the treatment of psoriasis with biologics. J Am Acad Dermatol May 2008;58(5):826–50.
Menter A, Korman NJ, Elmets CA, et al. Guidelines of care for the management of psoriasis and psoriatic arthritis: section 4. Guidelines of care for the management and treatment of psoriasis with traditional systemic agents. J Am Acad Dermatol September 2009;61(3):451–85.
Nestle FO, Kaplan DH, Barker J. Psoriasis. N Engl J Med July 2009;361(5):496–509.
Robinson A, Van Voorhees AS, Hsu S, et al. Treatment of pustular psoriasis: from the Medical Board of the National Psoriasis Foundation. J Am Acad Dermatol August 2012;67(2):279–88.
Rosenbach M, Hsu S, Korman NJ, et al. Treatment of erythrodermic psoriasis: from the medical board of the National Psoriasis Foundation. J Am Acad Dermatol April 2010;62(4):655–62.
Wu JJ, Nguyen TU, Poon KT, Herrinton LJ. The association of psoriasis with other autoimmune disorders. J Am Acad Dermatol 2012a;67(5):924–30.
Wu JJ, Poon KT, Channual JC, Shen AY. Association between tumor necrosis factor inhibitor therapy and myocardial infarction risk in patients with psoriasis. Arch Dermatol 2012b;148(11):1244–50.

CHAPTER 7

OTHER RHEUMATOLOGIC–DERMATOLOGIC CONDITIONS

Natalie A. Wright • Joseph F. Merola

KEY POINTS

- Rheumatoid arthritis (RA) is a multisystem disorder with many extra-articular manifestations that may affect the skin, including rheumatoid nodules and rheumatoid vasculitis.
- Rheumatoid nodules are the most characteristic cutaneous manifestation of RA. They, along with other extra-articular manifestations, are most common among seropositive RA patients.
- Systemic-onset juvenile idiopathic arthritis and adult-onset Still's disease are diagnoses of exclusion that are characterized by intermittent fevers with an accompanying exanthem, arthritis, hepatosplenomegaly, lymphadenopathy, and nonspecific serologic findings.
- Screening for underlying autoimmune disease and malignancy should be considered in patients with newly diagnosed interstitial granulomatous dermatitis or palisaded neutrophilic granulomatous dermatitis.
- Kawasaki disease is a small-to medium-vessel vasculitis characterized by high fevers and a constellation of clinical findings most notably involving the skin and coronary vessels. Prompt therapy with combination intravenous immunoglobulin and high-dose aspirin is the treatment of choice to prevent coronary artery aneurysms.
- Sjögren's syndrome is an autoimmune condition that affects the secretory glands. Cutaneous manifestations include xerosis, cutaneous small-vessel vasculitis, urticarial vasculitis, cryoglobulinemic vasculitis, and hypergammaglobulinemic purpura. Patients are at increased risk for B-cell lymphomas.
- Gout is caused by persistent elevation of serum uric acid levels leading to acute attacks of crystal-induced arthritis and chronic deposition of monosodium urate in the skin, joints, and surrounding synovium known as tophi.

RHEUMATOID ARTHRITIS

Definition, Diagnosis, and Epidemiologic Data

Rheumatoid arthritis (RA) is a multisystem disease of unknown etiology, which is primarily characterized by synovitis that can lead to erosive joint deformity and significant morbidity. Extra-articular manifestations commonly involve the skin and/or the lungs, but may also involve the hematologic, cardiovascular, and neurologic systems. RA primarily affects females between the fourth and sixth decades of life, but can occur at all ages.

The diagnosis of RA is relatively easy to make in its advanced stages but is challenging early in the disease course. The diagnosis is based on a combination of clinical, radiographic, and laboratory findings, including the serum rheumatoid factor. Criteria have been developed by the American College of Rheumatology for the diagnosis of classic, definite, probable, and possible RA, as well as for determining clinical remission, disease progression, and the functional capacity of patients. Histologic changes in the synovium and the presence of skin nodules are additional criteria. The rheumatoid factor (RF), measured primarily as IgM with specificity against altered IgG, is positive in approximately 75% of patients with RA and in 5% to 10% of normal subjects. The presence of second-generation anticyclic citrullinated peptide is similar in sensitivity to RF, but is more specific at 90% to 95%. High levels of RF are generally associated with more severe, erosive forms of the disease, as well as with the presence of extra-articular manifestations including rheumatoid nodules and other associated skin disorders. HLA-DRB1*04 is the most significant genetic association with seropositive RA. Additional confirmed genetic variants include peptidylarginine deiminase type 4 (PADI4) and protein tyrosine phosphatase nonreceptor type 22 (PTPN22). Interleukin (IL)-4 receptor single-nucleotide polymorphisms have been associated with increased risk of joint destruction and rheumatoid nodules.

Cutaneous Manifestations

A number of cutaneous findings are reported with RA. Few of these are characteristic for the disease, with the notable exception of the rheumatoid nodule. Pyoderma gangrenosum and a wide spectrum of vasculitic lesions may occur in patients with RA, but they occur more frequently in association with other disorders. There also are a wide variety of cutaneous changes associated with therapeutic agents used to treat RA (Table 7-1).

Rheumatoid Nodules

Rheumatoid nodules are firm, nontender, mobile subcutaneous nodules that occur in 20% to 35% of adult patients with RA. The incidence can be as high as 75% in those with Felty's syndrome, a disorder characterized by resistant leg ulcers, granulocytopenia, and splenomegaly

TABLE 7-1 Cutaneous Findings in Rheumatoid Arthritis

Neutrophilic and/or Granulomatous Skin Lesions
Rheumatoid nodules
Palisaded neutrophilic granulomatous dermatitis
Interstitial granulomatous dermatitis
Sweet's syndrome
Rheumatoid neutrophilic dermatitis
Superficial ulcerating rheumatoid necrobiosis

Nail Changes
Onychorrhexis, onychomadesis, onycholysis, clubbing, red lunulae

Vasculopathic/Vasculitic Lesions
Capillaritis
Livedo reticularis
Erythema elevatum diutinum
Petechiae
Purpura
Gangrenous/ulcerating plaques

Leg Ulcers
Felty's syndrome
Pyoderma gangrenosum
Vasculitis

Miscellaneous Associations
Urticaria-like lesions of Still's disease
Amyloidosis
Bullous diseases including epidermolysis bullosa acquisita

Skin Changes Secondary to Medications
Corticosteroids
    Cushingoid features
    Macular purpura and striae
    Atrophy/fragility
Methotrexate
    Accelerated/eruptive nodulosis
Nonsteroidal anti-inflammatory drugs
    Pseudoporphyria
    Toxic epidermal necrolysis
    Fixed drug eruption
Tumor necrosis-α blockers
    Leukocytoclastic vasculitis
    Psoriasiform dermatitis
    Palmoplantar pustulosis
    Urticaria, angioedema, anaphylaxis
    Injection site reaction
    Interstitial granulomatous dermatitis
    Cutaneous lupus erythematosus (subacute > chronic/discoid variants)
    Dermatomyositis
    Accelerated or eruptive nodulosis
    Nonmelanoma skin cancer
Leflunomide
    Toxic epidermal necrolysis
    Accelerated or eruptive nodulosis
Thiol containing compounds (i.e., penicillamine)
    Pemphigus foliaceus and vulgaris
    Lichenoid drug eruption
    Elastosis perforans serpiginosa
    Pseudoxanthoma elasticum-like changes
    Cutis laxa-like changes
Tocilizumab
    Palmoplantar pustulosis
    Halo nevi

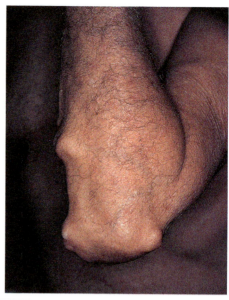

FIGURE 7-1 ■ Rheumatoid nodules on the elbow.

in the setting of seropositive RA. Rheumatoid nodules are the most characteristic cutaneous manifestation of RA, most commonly seen in white males with severe arthritis, high-titer RF seropositivity, and rheumatoid vasculitis. Smokers are more likely to have rheumatoid nodules. Rheumatoid nodules have also been reported in association with other entities including lupus erythematosus/rheumatoid arthritis overlap and antiphospholipid syndrome.

The dome-shaped flesh-colored nodules vary from 0.5 cm to several centimeters in diameter and tend to occur on the extensor extremities, usually overlying bony prominences that are frequently subjected to trauma (Fig. 7-1). Any subcutaneous site can be affected, however, and histologically identical lesions have been found in the sclerae, larynx, heart, lungs, and abdominal wall. Rheumatoid nodules can cause discomfort, be disfiguring, and interfere with activities of daily living. Larger nodules can cause compressive neuropathies and are at risk for ulceration and secondary local infection. Eruptive rheumatoid nodules have been reported with the administration of methotrexate ("methotrexate accelerated nodulosis"), and less commonly with tumor necrosis factor (TNF) antagonists, azathioprine and leflunomide. The clinical differential diagnosis of rheumatoid nodules includes gouty tophi, xanthomas, deep (subcutaneous) or nodular granuloma annulare, subcutaneous sarcoidosis, and ganglion and epidermal inclusion cysts.

Histologically, three distinct zones are observed in well-developed rheumatoid nodules: a central zone of fibrinoid necrosis, a middle zone of palisading histiocytes, and a peripheral zone of highly vascularized granulation tissue with a chronic, mononuclear inflammatory cell infiltrate. Early lesions are composed primarily of granulation tissue but have focal areas of leukocytoclastic vasculitis that are believed to be relevant in the pathogenesis of the nodules. The histopathologic differential diagnosis includes the transient nodules seen in acute rheumatic fever, deep granuloma annulare, and necrobiosis lipoidica diabeticorum.

Rheumatoid Vasculitis

The spectrum of clinical lesions reported to be rheumatoid vasculitis is wide and varies with the size and location of the vessels involved, and with the extent of the disease. Leukocytoclasis occurs most commonly in the small arterioles and venules of the skin, but this same necrotizing process may occur in larger vessels of the mesentery, heart, and central nervous system. Most evidence suggests that the vasculitic lesions are related to circulating immune complexes. Cutaneous lesions include petechiae, capillaritis (pigmented purpuric dermatoses), palpable purpura, digital infarcts, retiform purpura, and large ischemic ulcerations of the lower extremities, especially over the malleoli. Vasculitis develops late in the disease course in patients with high-titer RF, severe erosive disease, and rheumatoid nodules. Although it has been reported to occur in only 2% to 5% of individuals with RA, rheumatoid vasculitis has been noted in up to 30% of patients on autopsy.

The cutaneous lesions of mild rheumatoid vasculitis include small digital infarcts, especially of the nail folds and digital pulp (often called Bywater's lesions), petechiae, and livedo reticularis or livedo racemosa. Palpable purpura of the lower extremities and buttocks is typical in moderate disease, and is clinicopathologically indistinguishable from cutaneous small-vessel vasculitis due to other causes. Severe disease can occur in an explosive fashion, involving both the skin and systemic organs and having a mortality rate approaching 30%. Cutaneous involvement may include the changes seen in mild or moderate rheumatoid vasculitis, in addition to large ulcers from retiform purpura and digital gangrene. It is associated with a high degree of mortality so aggressive work-up with skin biopsy, serologic assessment, rheumatologic consultation, and rapid therapeutic intervention is merited. It is also important to consider the possibility of drug-induced cutaneous vasculitis in patients receiving biologic treatment for RA. Several biologic agents, infliximab in particular, have been associated with the development of cutaneous small-vessel vasculitis.

Miscellaneous Dermatologic Conditions Associated with Rheumatoid Arthritis

Several nonspecific cutaneous lesions and nail changes have been reported in patients with RA (Table 7-1). In addition, there are numerous reports linking RA to pyoderma gangrenosum, as well as rheumatoid neutrophilic dermatitis, Sweet's syndrome, interstitial granulomatous dermatitis, palisaded neutrophilic granulomatous dermatitis, connective tissue-associated panniculitis, erythema nodosum, and blistering diseases, particularly epidermolysis bullosa acquisita.

SYSTEMIC-ONSET JUVENILE IDIOPATHIC ARTHRITIS (STILL'S DISEASE)

Juvenile idiopathic arthritis (JIA), previously termed juvenile rheumatoid arthritis, is characterized by the onset

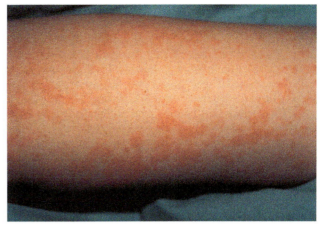

FIGURE 7-2 ■ Transient faint erythema of juvenile idiopathic arthritis. (Courtesy of Kenneth E. Greer, MD, Charlottesville, VA.)

of arthritis in childhood to young adulthood and is classified into seven subtypes. Systemic-onset JIA, or Still's disease, makes up 15% to 20% of JIA cases. Children with systemic-onset JIA display a characteristic evanescent, pink to salmon-colored urticarial or morbilliform eruption of the trunk or extremities associated with high, spiking fevers, which can precede the associated arthritis (Fig. 7-2). The cutaneous eruption is asymptomatic and exhibits a predilection for the axillae and waist. Rarely, koebnerized, linear lesions can occur. The cutaneous eruption and fever are typically transitory and usually peak in the late afternoon to early evening. However, these symptoms may persist for several days. Patients typically have a polyarthritis of the hips, knees, ankles, wrists, and temporomandibular joints, which rarely may become erosive. Lymphadenopathy, serositis, and hepatomegaly can be seen. Laboratory findings are often unhelpful when diagnosing Still's disease as >95% of patients have a negative RF and antinuclear antibody (ANA). However, significant hyperferritinemia (>4000 mg/mL) in addition to elevated acute-phase reactants, leukocytosis, anemia, and thrombophilia have been noted. Mortality has been linked to macrophage activating syndrome (MAS) that is characterized by an unremitting fever, cytopenias, coagulopathies, low sedimentation rate, and evidence of end-organ dysfunction. MAS can be triggered by underlying disease flare, medications or infections, and should be promptly diagnosed to avoid life-threatening multiorgan failure.

ADULT STILL'S DISEASE

Adult Still's disease typically affects females prior to age 30, although cases have been reported in adults up to their 60s. Patients with adult Still's disease exhibit spiking fevers in the afternoon to early evening accompanied by an asymptomatic, evanescent cutaneous eruption most commonly found on truncal pressure points. The presence of a sore throat, either prior to or early in the disease course, is a frequent complaint. The arthritis is typically localized to the ankles, knees, and wrists, and can progress to a symmetric, destructive polyarthritis. Carpal ankylosis, characterized by fusion of the carpometacarpal joints, is a classic finding in the disease that can also be seen in the juvenile form of the disease. Still's remains a diagnosis of exclusion and is often a clinical diagnosis as laboratory findings are nonspecific. Hyperferritinemia, elevated acute-phase reactants, and elevated liver function tests have been noted. The natural progression of the disease can be limited to one or multiple flares of systemic and joint complaints that resolve over the course of months to 2 years. Those with a persistent polyarthritis can have a chronic form of the disease that can result in disability.

Treatment

The mainstay of RA therapy is the early institution of disease-modifying antirheumatic drugs (DMARDs), even in those with early disease. Methotrexate is often the first-line treatment utilized as a monotherapy for those with mild disease, and in combination therapy for those with moderate to severe disease with poor prognostic features. Other frequently used treatments include so-called "triple therapy" consisting of concurrent hydroxychloroquine, sulfasalazine and methotrexate, and inhibitors of pyrimidine synthesis (leflunomide). Systemic corticosteroids are often given for short intervals for control of disease flares, but are also sometimes used chronically in low doses. Biologic therapies include those that inhibit TNF-α (e.g., etanercept, adalimumab, infliximab, golimumab, certolizumab), those that modulate T-cell activation (abatacept), inhibitors of IL-6 (tocilizumab), inhibitors of type I receptors of IL-1 (anakinra), inhibitors of specific JAK kinases (tofacitinib), and agents that affect B-cell activation (rituximab). No controlled studies have been performed to assess the benefit of RA therapies in treating the cutaneous manifestations of the disease. Rheumatoid nodules develop insidiously and are usually persistent, but may regress spontaneously. Larger and/or symptomatic nodules can be treated with excision, but have a high rate of recurrence. Intralesional corticosteroids can decrease the size of the nodules; however, response is often temporary. Eruptive rheumatoid nodules tend to regress with discontinuation of methotrexate. Rheumatoid vasculitis should be viewed as an extra-articular manifestation of RA that dictates more aggressive control of the underlying disease.

Recent guidelines by the American College of Rheumatology recommend treatment with DMARDs for children and adolescents with Still's disease who are not well controlled with nonsteroidal anti-inflammatory drugs or intra-articular corticosteroid injections. Sulfasalazine should be avoided in this population as it can induce macrophage activating syndrome. Skin manifestations of Still's disease often improve with treatment of the underlying disease.

INTERSTITIAL GRANULOMATOUS DERMATITIS

Interstitial granulomatous dermatitis (IGD) is a rare, polymorphous disorder first described by Ackerman in 1993. Some authors believe that it exists along a clinical disease spectrum with palisaded neutrophilic granulomatous dermatitis (PNGD); however, many of the clinical and histologic features are distinctive. The underlying etiology of IGD is unknown, but it is hypothesized to be secondary to immune complex deposition given its well-known association with autoimmune and connective tissue disorders, most notably RA, lupus erythematosus, autoimmune thyroiditis, vitiligo, diabetes mellitus, and autoimmune hepatitis. Malignancies have also been reported to be associated with IGD, including both lymphoproliferative disorders and solid organ tumors. Those affected by IGD are most commonly middle-aged females, and can have arthritis symptoms prior to, concurrent with, or subsequent to development of the cutaneous manifestations.

Clinical Manifestations

IGD typically presents with symmetric erythematous papules and plaques, often with an annular configuration, on the lateral trunk, medial thighs, and buttocks. Occasionally the lesions can be skin-colored or associated with burning or pruritus. The "rope sign," which is characterized by linear cords in the aforementioned sites, is considered pathognomonic for IGD when present, but has only been seen in 9% of reported cases. The associated arthritis is described as a seronegative, nonerosive polyarthritis of both the small and large joints. This association has been labeled the "IGD with arthritis syndrome" by some. The closely related entity, IGD drug reaction, is typically not associated with an underlying arthritis, but can resemble IGD clinically. It has been reported with a number of medications including calcium channel blockers, angiotensin-converting enzyme inhibitors, statins, anti-TNF-α therapy, IL-1 inhibitors, furosemide, and antihistamines.

Histopathologic Features

Given the polymorphous nature of the cutaneous manifestations of IGD, histopathologic analysis is needed to determine the diagnosis. Interstitial palisading histiocytes are noted around degenerated collagen, with a surrounding dense, bottom-heavy dermal infiltrate comprised of neutrophils and eosinophils. There is an absence of associated vasculitis. In IGD drug reaction, a vacuolar interface dermatitis with a prominent infiltrate of eosinophils and minimal degenerated collagen is typical. Interstitial granuloma annulare can be difficult to differentiate from IGD both clinically and histologically, but classically exhibits a "top heavy," focal infiltrate with associated mucin. A detailed histologic description of PNGD is described below.

Treatment

Data regarding treatment of IGD are largely limited to case reports and small series. Successful reports of systemic and topical corticosteroids, thalidomide, hydroxychloroquine, TNF antagonists, intravenous immunoglobulin, and tofacitinib exist. A recent review of the literature revealed that two-thirds of patients with IGD achieved remission between 3 months and 3 years, while the remaining patients exhibited a chronic relapsing course. Therapy did not affect disease course.

PALISADED NEUTROPHILIC AND GRANULOMATOUS DERMATITIS

PNGD is a rare neutrophilic dermatosis with varied cutaneous findings. Previously described clinicopathologic entities that likely represented PNGD were Churg-Strauss granulomas, rheumatoid papules, and cutaneous extravascular necrotizing granuloma of Winkelmann. Usually seen in adult females, with only rare reports in children, PNGD is most frequently associated with an underlying connective tissue disease or systemic vasculitis. RA is the most commonly associated systemic disorder, but PNGD has also been reported in the setting of systemic lupus erythematosus, limited systemic sclerosis, Behçet's disease, and granulomatosis with polyangiitis and autoimmune thyroid disease. It has rarely been reported in the absence of underlying systemic illness. In addition to connective tissue diseases, PNGD is also noted to be associated with underlying malignancy, most commonly lymphoproliferative disorders, and infections such as HIV. Rare reports have described the development of PNGD secondary to medications such as TNF antagonists and allopurinol.

Clinical Manifestations

Although the clinical presentation of PNGD varies, it classically presents as erythematous and skin-colored papules and nodules on the extensor surfaces of the extremities with a predilection for the elbows and fingers (Fig. 7-3). A review of 81 patients with PNGD revealed that 51% of cases involved the upper extremities, 27.7% involved the lower extremities, and 21% had lesions on the head or neck. The lesions of PNGD can be umbilicated or crusted with associated pain. In addition, annular plaques, urticarial lesions, and livedo reticularis patterns have been described.

Histopathologic Features

Palisaded neutrophilic and granulomatous dermatitis is histologically notable for zones of basophilic collagen degeneration with a surrounding infiltrate made up predominantly of histiocytes, neutrophils, and nuclear dust. In comparison to IGD, there is an associated leukocytoclastic vasculitis in PNGD.

Treatment

A diagnosis of PNGD should prompt screening for underlying autoimmune disease and malignancy. Therapeutic strategies are based primarily on data from case reports and small series, including positive responses to systemic corticosteroids, methotrexate, cyclosporine, leflunomide, and dapsone. In addition, a number of severe cases are reported to have improved with cyclophosphamide. Spontaneous resolution has been noted in up to 20% of patients.

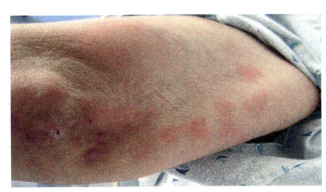

FIGURE 7-3 ■ Erythematous and skin-colored papules and nodules on the elbow of a rheumatoid arthritis patient with palisaded neutrophilic granulomatous dermatitis. (Courtesy of Joseph F. Merola.)

KAWASAKI DISEASE (MUCOCUTANEOUS LYMPH NODE SYNDROME)

Clinical Manifestations

Kawasaki, a Japanese pediatrician, first described an acute febrile mucocutaneous syndrome with striking lymphadenopathy occurring in Japanese children in the late 1960s. This syndrome, which has now been reported worldwide, is a vasculitis affecting small- and medium-sized vessels. Diagnostic criteria detailed by the American Heart Association (AHA) include unexplained fever for greater than 5 days in addition to at least four clinical symptoms (Table 7-2). Incomplete forms of the disease have been described that meet only two to three of the diagnostic criteria. Echocardiograms and coronary angiography can be a helpful adjuvant in diagnosis of these patients.

The cause of Kawasaki disease (KD) remains unknown. Epidemiologic factors suggest an infectious cause, but no bacterial, viral, or toxic agent has been identified. The disease is most common in children between 6 months and 5 years of age. Asian ancestry is a high-risk factor, although the syndrome occurs in all races. While there is no clear human leukocyte antigen association, genetic factors appear to contribute to disease onset and several susceptibility loci have been suggested.

KD is defined by three phases: acute, subacute, and convalescent. The acute phase lasts until fever resolution. High fevers (up to 40.5°C) are typically unresponsive to antipyretics and may last up to 3 weeks. The exanthem, present in 80% to 90% of patients with KD, has been described as a morbilliform, scarlatiniform, or erythema multiforme-like diffuse eruption on the trunk and the extremities (Fig. 7-4). The eruption often begins perineally, which is followed quickly by desquamation in the area. Edema and erythema can be localized to the palms and soles only, or encompass the entire acral surface. Pain often accompanies the changes. Mucosal findings include strawberry tongue, cheilitis, or pharyngitis (Fig. 7-5). Nonpurulent conjunctival injection is seen with sparing of the limbus. There is often concurrent photophobia, and patients are at increased risk for uveitis. The cervical lymphadenopathy may be dramatic and is often unilateral. During the subacute phase, brawny change and desquamation occur acrally (posterythemal desquamation). Several nail findings have been described including Beau's

TABLE 7-2 Diagnostic Criteria and Treatment of Kawasaki Disease

Signs and Symptoms	Treatments

High fever persisting for >5 days, plus at least four of the following five features:
  Peripheral extremity changes: acute stage with erythema or edema of the palms and soles; chronic stage with acral desquamation and Beau's lines
  Polymorphous exanthem, usually generalized but may be limited to groin or lower extremities
  Oropharyngeal changes: strawberry tongue, erythema, fissuring, crusting of the lips or cheilitis, pharyngeal injection
  Painless bilateral bulbar conjunctival injection without exudate
  Acute nonpurulent cervical lymphadenopathy with lymph node diameter greater than 1.5 cm, usually unilateral
	Intravenous immunoglobulin plus high-dose aspirin
	Avoid corticosteroid monotherapy
	Intravenous immunoglobulin (IVIG)-resistant cases:
	  Combination corticosteroids with IVIG and aspirin
	  Cyclosporine
	  Methotrexate
	  Plasmapheresis
	  Tumor necrosis factor antagonists
	  Cyclophosphamide

Note: "Atypical" or "incomplete" Kawasaki disease can be diagnosed when coronary artery disease is present on echocardiography or coronary angiography.
Modified from the 2004 American Heart Association Diagnosis, Treatment, and Long-Term Management Guidelines for Kawasaki Disease.

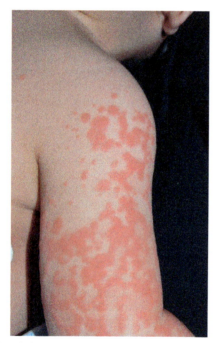

FIGURE 7-4 ■ Polymorphous exanthematous eruption seen in a patient with Kawasaki disease. (Courtesy of Joseph F. Merola.)

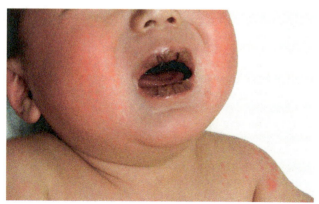

FIGURE 7-5 ■ Cheilitis and oral mucosal involvement observed in a child with Kawasaki disease. (Courtesy of Joseph F. Merola.)

lines, chromonychia (color change of the nails), leukonychia striata (white longitudinal bands), pincer nails, and onychomadesis (shedding of the nails). Periungual desquamation is one of the most common cutaneous findings in KD, but it proves to be unhelpful in diagnosis as it occurs late in the disease course. The arthritis usually presents as a polyarthritis of the small joints evolving to a pauciarthritis of the large joints of the lower extremities. It typically improves rapidly with treatment with no permanent sequelae. The final, convalescent phase of KD begins after all clinical manifestations have resolved and inflammatory markers and platelet counts have returned to normal, typically 4 to 8 weeks from disease onset.

The most important clinical complication of KD is the development of coronary aneurysms, which may result from coronary artery vasculitis, and can produce death from myocardial infarction. Approximately 20% of patients have coronary artery involvement. The mortality rate in KD may be as high as 1% to 2%, and adult coronary artery disease has been recognized as a complication of KD. Cardiac changes in KD are indistinguishable from the changes seen in juvenile polyarteritis nodosa.

Many laboratory abnormalities have been noted in KD, but none are specific. Elevated inflammatory markers, leukocytosis with a neutrophilia, eosinophilia, thrombophilia, normocytic anemia, and transaminitis are common. In children being treated with intravenous immunoglobulin, a continued rise in white blood cells, platelets, and C-reactive protein are associated with a higher risk of coronary artery findings.

A number of other acute syndromes may mimic some features of KD. The differential diagnosis includes Stevens–Johnson syndrome, toxic shock syndrome, scarlet fever, juvenile polyarteritis nodosa, Rocky Mountain spotted fever, leptospirosis, mononucleosis, viral exanthems, the drug reaction with eosinophilia and systemic symptoms syndrome, and collagen–vascular diseases.

Treatment

The current AHA standard of care for KD includes intravenous immunoglobulin (IVIG) in addition to high-dose aspirin. Therapy within the first 10 days of illness reduces the incidence of coronary artery aneurysms by more than

70%. Aspirin as monotherapy is helpful in the treatment of the fever and arthritis associated with KD, but does not decrease the incidence of coronary artery aneurysms. Despite early treatment, 10% to 15% of cases are resistant to IVIG. A variety of adjuvant therapies have been reported in cases refractory to IVIG, including systemic corticosteroids, infliximab, cyclosporine, methotrexate, plasmapheresis, and cyclophosphamide.

Early data suggested an increased cardiovascular risk when systemic corticosteroid monotherapy was employed. However, a more recent study in the Japanese literature found reduction in cardiovascular sequelae when patients were treated with a combination of systemic corticosteroids, IVIG, and aspirin as opposed to IVIG and aspirin alone. It is unclear whether these data can be extrapolated to affected populations in other parts of the world.

SJÖGREN'S SYNDROME

Sjögren's syndrome (SS) is an autoimmune condition that primarily affects the secretory glands leading to xerostomia and xerophthalmia, often with associated arthritis. Other organs can also be affected including the lungs, kidneys, neurologic system, and liver. The pathogenesis is attributed to abnormal B-cell activation and dysfunction within the Th17 pathway.

SS can be seen as a primary disorder or in the setting of other autoimmune conditions. An array of systemic manifestations may occur including B-cell lymphomas and vasculitis. Mucosa-associated lymphoid tissue marginal zone lymphoma is the most common associated malignancy and is seen in approximately 5% of patients. SS is more common in women, particularly presenting in the fourth and fifth decades, although the syndrome has even been reported in the pediatric population. Serologic findings include the presence of ANA, anti-Ro and anti-La antibodies, RF, and hypergammaglobulinemia. To date, the American College of Rheumatology and the American-European Consensus group have differing classifications for the disorder.

Xerosis remains the most frequent skin manifestation of SS. In the setting of xerostomia, perleche and thrush can result from yeast overgrowth. Halitosis and dental caries arise with decreased saliva production. Other cutaneous manifestations include cutaneous small-vessel vasculitis presenting as palpable purpura, urticarial vasculitis of the hypo- and normocomplementemic types, hypergammaglobulinemic purpura that can result in peripheral neuropathy, Raynaud's disease, amyloidosis, Sweet's syndrome, erythema nodosum, and cryoglobulinemic vasculitis (Fig. 7-6). Cryoglobulinemia, vasculitis, hypocomplementemia and parotid swelling are associated with increased lymphoma risk among Sjögren's patients. Annular erythema has been reported primarily in Asian populations and presents with annular plaques with or without scale on sun-exposed areas of the face and extremities that usually occurs in those with seropositivity to Ro autoantibodies. A recent retrospective review detailed 43 cases in non-Asian patients. Some authors suggest that the photodistributed annular scaly plaques seen in annular erythema of Sjögren's strongly resembles subacute cutaneous lupus erythematosus; however, they

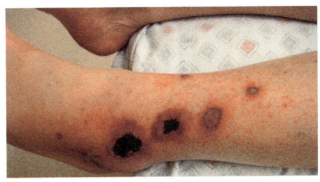

FIGURE 7-6 ■ Multiple ulcerated purpuric plaques in a patient with cryoglobulinemic vasculitis in the setting of Sjögren's syndrome. (Courtesy of Joseph F. Merola.)

differ histologically with annular erythema exhibiting perivascular and periadnexal cuffing of lymphocytes.

Current treatments for SS are largely aimed at managing symptoms. Emollients are beneficial in repairing barrier function and humidifiers are helpful to combat xerosis. Regular ophthalmologic exams are warranted as corneal abrasions can occur in the setting of xerophthalmia. Lubricating drops are the first-line therapy to decrease eyelid friction over the corneal surface. Punctal occlusion, topical cyclosporine, and topical tacrolimus are alternative treatments. Regular professional dental cleanings, home hygiene, salivary stimulants, and diet management can prevent loss of teeth. Annular erythema has been noted to respond to antimalarials, topical or systemic corticosteroids, and low-dose cyclosporine. SS with associated systemic symptoms often requires therapies including systemic corticosteroids, antimalarials, methotrexate, azathioprine, cyclosporine, cyclophosphamide, intravenous immunoglobulin, or rituximab. B-cell-targeted agents such as rituximab, epratuzumab, and belimumab have shown promising, albeit inconsistent, results in treating the signs and symptoms of Sjögren's, and have produced remission in some lymphoma patients. TNF antagonists have failed to show positive therapeutic outcomes in several studies.

GOUT

Gout is an inflammatory arthropathy caused by persistent elevation of serum uric acid levels leading to deposition of monosodium urate in the joints and surrounding synovium. This results in painful episodes of crystal-induced arthritis. Chronic gout can lead to joint damage, erosions, marked disability, uric acid nephrolithiasis, and renal impairment. A detailed discussion of gout is beyond the scope of this chapter, but this entity is predominantly seen in middle-aged to older males with concurrent risk factors including obesity, alcoholism, renal impairment, medication use most notably with diuretics, a history of psoriasis, thyroid disease, malignancy, or disorders of purine metabolism.

Acute gout attacks are characterized by acute joint pain with associated erythema and edema. A single joint is usually affected, but presentations may be polyarticular. Podagra, which is characterized by involvement of the first metatarsophalangeal joint, is seen in 75% of cases.

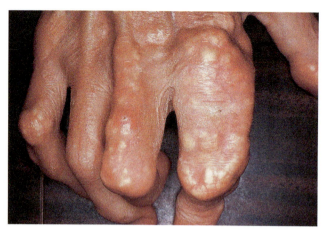

FIGURE 7-7 ■ Multiple yellowish nodules representative of tophi.

Chronic cutaneous deposits of gout are intradermal or subcutaneous nodules called tophi, which preferentially occur in avascular tissue over the ears, olecranon, and prepatellar bursae, or in acral sites, often associated with tendons (Fig. 7-7). Tophi may discharge a chalky material.

Microscopic examination of this material reveals the typical crystals of gout, which have negative birefringence. These crystals may also be seen in biopsy specimens when fixed in alcohol, but not in formaldehyde. Therapy for gout includes oral colchicine and/or allopurinol as a prophylactic measure. Indometacin and occasionally systemic corticosteroids may be used for acute attacks.

SUGGESTED READINGS

Bayers S, Shulman ST, Paller AS. Kawasaki disease. J Amer Acad Dermatol 2013;69(4):501.e1–11, 513.e1–8.

Gerfaud-Valenin MG, Jamilloux Y, Iwaz J, Seve P. Adult-onset Still's disease. Autoimmun Rev 2014;13(7):708–22.

Merola JF, Wu S, Han J, Choi HJ, Qureshi AA. Psoriasis, psoriatic arthritis, and risk of gout in US men and women. Ann Rheum Dis 2015;74(8):1495–500.

Peroni A, Colato C, Schena D, Gisondi P, Girolomoni G. Interstitial granulomatous dermatitis: a distinct entity with characterisitic histological and clinical pattern. Br J Dermatol 2012;166(4):775–83.

Prete M, Racanelli V, Digiglio L, Vacca A, Dammacco F, Perosa F. Extra-articular manifestations of rheumatoid arthritis: an update. Autoimmun Rev 2011;11(2):123–31.

Sada PR, Isenberg D, Ciurtin C. Biologic treatment in SS. Rheumatol (Oxford) 2015;54(2):219–30.

CHAPTER 8

AUTOINFLAMMATORY SYNDROMES

Kieron S. Leslie

KEY POINTS

- Autoinflammatory syndromes are characterized by excessive multisystem inflammation from activation of innate pathways rather than the acquired immune system.
- Autoinflammatory syndromes are mostly rare monogenic disorders that generally first present in childhood.
- Most of these diseases are, at least in part, modulated by the interleukin-1 pathway, which has provided targeted treatment strategies. Tumor necrosis factor-alpha antagonists have also proved useful agents for these diseases.

INTRODUCTION

Inflammation is a highly adapted necessary response to both infection and neoplasia. However, damage to tissues may occur from maladaptive autoimmune processes where self-directed T-cells or antibody-producing B-cells are activated in disorders such as systemic lupus erythematosus. Alternatively, damage may be initiated by various germline-encoded innate immune receptors with the absence of involvement of the adaptive immune system. The term "autoinflammation" has been coined for this process. This chapter will outline the various syndromes where dysregulation of innate immunity is central to their pathogenesis.

MOLECULAR PRIMER

Various molecules that are recognized by cells of the innate immune system mediate the initiation of host response to infection or tissue damage (Fig. 8-1). Chiefly, these are called pathogen-associated molecular patterns (PAMPs), which recognize bacterial and viral components, and danger-associated molecular patterns (DAMPs), which recognize signals related to cell death and toxins. PAMPs and DAMPs interact with pattern recognition receptors such as Toll-like receptors and Nod-like receptors (NLRs), which leads to downstream inflammation. This inflammation is predominantly mediated by the relatively recently described multimeric proteins called inflammasomes. Most autoinflammatory syndromes have genetic mutations in these pathways that lead to increased and inappropriate inflammasome activity (Table 8-1).

CRYOPYRIN-ASSOCIATED PERIODIC SYNDROME

Cryopyrin-associated periodic syndrome (CAPS) is the preferred diagnostic term for three originally separately described syndromes: familial cold autoinflammatory syndrome (FCAS), Muckle-Wells syndrome (MWS), and neonatal onset multisystem inflammatory disorder (NOMID). In practice, the severity of clinical presentation is observed as mild (FCAS), moderate (MWS), and severe phenotypes.

Pathogenesis

CAPS is an autosomal dominant inherited condition. It is caused by "gain-of-function" mutations in *NLRP3*, about half of patients have a family history of CAPS with the remainder representing spontaneous (new) mutations. *NLRP3* encodes cryopyrin, which activates the NLRP3 inflammasome. The downstream effect of this is excessive production of the proinflammatory cytokine interleukin-1 (IL-1), which is responsible for the clinical manifestations of CAPS.

Clinical Features

Characteristically, patients present with an urticarial rash in the neonatal period (Fig. 8-2). This differs from chronic urticaria in a number of ways. The rash is present lifelong, tends not to be pruritic although patients may describe heat or tightness in affected skin, and has a circadian rhythm with little or no rash in the morning with progressive worsening as the day progresses. It is associated with constitutional symptoms, which include fever, arthralgia, headache, myalgia, and conjunctival injection. Most patients will describe these inflammatory episodes on a daily basis and furthermore may be precipitated or worsened by other factors like cold exposure. As the clinical severity advances patients may additionally have high-tone sensorineural hearing loss and systemic amyloidosis. The most severely affected patients may have neurological symptoms from raised intracranial pressure resulting in neurological impairment and rapidly progressive deforming arthropathies.

Evaluation

Skin biopsy is helpful, as it tends to reveal a neutrophilic dermal infiltrate, which is perieccrine and perivascular without evidence of vasculitis. Genetic evaluation may reveal a germ-line mutation in *NLRP3*, although

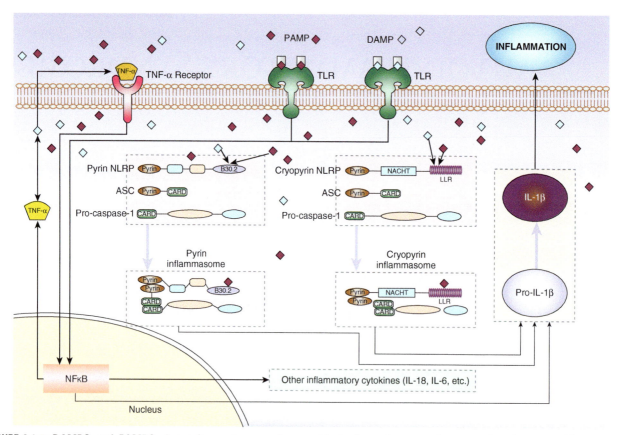

FIGURE 8-1 ■ DAMPS and PAMPS. Autoinflammatory syndromes. Illustration of commonly targeted pathways. *ASC,* apoptosis-associated speck-like protein; *DAMP,* danger-associated molecular pattern; *IL,* interleukin; *NFκB,* nuclear factor kappa beta; *NLRP,* nucleotide-binding domain leucine-rich repeat-containing protein; *PAMP,* pathogen-associated molecular pattern; *TLR,* toll-like receptor; *TNF-α,* tumor necrosis factor alpha. (From Nguyen TV, Cowen EW, Leslie KS. Autoinflammation: from monogenic syndromes to common skin diseases. J Am Acad Dermatol May 2013;68(5):834–53.)

a significant proportion of patients will have negative mutational analysis on conventional genetic testing. It has been shown recently that the majority of these patients are actually mosaic for *NLRP3* mutations. Acute phase reactants such as C-reactive protein (CRP) will be elevated, as will serum amyloid A (SAA) although this lab test is not widely available in clinical practice. Due to prolonged elevation of SAA, patients are susceptible to systemic amyloidosis (AA type). The most serious sequelae of amyloidosis is the development of renal impairment secondary to nephrotic syndrome; therefore, regular urinalysis is required for the monitoring of proteinuria. Audiometry should be performed at initial assessment to identify sensorineural hearing impairment. Referral to rheumatology and neurology may also be considered.

Treatment

Drugs that block the IL-1 pathway are highly efficacious and generally achieve complete clinical remission for patients. There are currently three drugs that the Food and Drug Administration has approved for use in CAPS. Anakinra, which is an IL-1 receptor antagonist; daily dosing is required as its half-life is 4 to 6 hours. Rilonacept is an IL-1 trap molecule with a longer half-life so requires weekly administration. Canakinumab is a fully human monoclonal antibody directed against IL-1β and is dosed every 8 weeks. This class of drugs is generally well tolerated but side effects include rare neutropenia and increased risk of infection.

SCHNITZLER'S SYNDROME

In the 1970s, Liliane Schnitzler, a French dermatologist, reported a syndrome characterized by chronic urticaria, bone pain, fever, and the presence of an IgM paraprotein. Since the original observations about 200 cases have been reported in the literature.

Pathogenesis

Although IgM or rarely IgG gammopathy is the invariable biological characteristic of the disease, it is unclear how this contributes to the pathophysiology. It is evident that the cytokine IL-1β is elevated and contributes to the clinical features of systemic inflammation. The effects of IL-1β on the gammopathy or vice versa are unknown.

Clinical Features

Schnitzler's syndrome (SS) should be suspected in any patient with a chronic recurrent urticarial rash, fever, and arthralgia/myalgia or bone pain. The urticarial lesions are similar to patients with CAPS or adult-onset Still's disease (AOSD) as they are evanescent and rarely itchy.

TABLE 8-1 Autoinflammatory Syndromes: Key Characteristics

	Cryopyrin Associated Periodic Syndrome (CAPS)	Schnitzler's Syndrome (SS)	Deficiency of IL-1 Receptor Antagonist (DIRA)	Tumor Necrosis Factor Receptor Associated Periodic Syndrome (TRAPS)	Familial Mediterranean Fever (FMF)	Hyperimmunoglobulinemia D Syndrome (HIDS)	Pyogenic Arthritis, Pyoderma Gangrenosum and Acne Syndrome (PAPA)	Synovitis, Acne, Pustulosis, Hyperostosis and Osteitis Syndrome (SAPHO)
Cutaneous findings	Daily nonitchy urticarial rash	Urticarial rash	Pustular rash, Ichthyosis	Erythema overlying areas of myalgia, Periorbital edema	Erysipelas-like erythema	Exanthem-like rash, urticarial and purpuric lesions also reported	Acne, pyoderma gangrenosum	Acne, palmoplantar pustulosis
Systemic features	Arthralgia, sensorineural healing loss, neurological impairment, systemic amyloidosis	IgM paraprotein, arthralgia/myalgia, bone pain	Fetal distress, osteolytic lesions, periostitis, epiphyseal ballooning, multiorgan failure	Periodic febrile episodes, myalgia, abdominal cramping and nausea	Febrile episodes, peritonitis, pleuritis, synovitis, systemic amyloidosis	Febrile episodes, abdominal pain, arthralgia, lymphadenopathy, splenomegaly	Monoarthritis typically seen in first decade, cutaneous manifestations present later (puberty)	Synovitis, osteoarticular disease affecting chest wall, sacroileitis
Age of onset	Infancy	>40 years (typically)	Neonatal	3 years (rarely present in adulthood)	<20 years	Infancy	<10 years	Any
Inheritance	AD	N/A	AR	AD	AR	AR	AD	Unknown
Gene	NLR3P	N/A	IL1RN	TNFRSF1A	MEFV	MVK	PSTPIP1	N/A
Protein	Cryopyrin	N/A	IL-1 receptor antagonist	TNFRSF1A	Pyrin	Mevalonate kinase	CD2 binding protein	N/A
Treatments	Anakinra, rilonacept, canakinumab	Colchicine, NSAIDs, anakinra	Anakinra	Corticosteroids during attack, etanercept, anakinra, canakinumab	Colchicine, thalidomide, sulfasalazine, TNF blockers, anakinra	Simvastatin, corticosteroids, etanercept, anakinra	Etanercept, adalimumab, infliximab, anakinra, corticosteroids, retinoids for acne	NSAIDs and intra-articular corticosteroids for joint disease, methotrexate, azathioprine, TNF blockers, anakinra

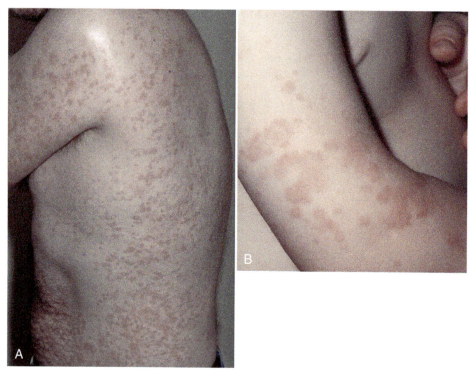

FIGURE 8-2 ■ **CAPS rash.** Cryopyrin-associated periodic syndrome. **A,** Familial cold autoinflammatory syndrome, urticaria-like eruption in adult. **B,** Muckle-Wells syndrome, urticaria-like dermatitis in child. (From Nguyen TV, Cowen EW, Leslie KS. Autoinflammation: from monogenic syndromes to common skin diseases. J Am Acad Dermatol May 2013;68(5):834–53.)

Additionally, patients may have lymphadenopathy and hepatosplenomegaly. Phenotypically there is a broad overlap between SS, CAPS, and AOSD, which is likely explained as they all result in elevated levels of IL-1β. A feature that differentiates them is age of onset; SS tends to present after the age of 40 whereas CAPS is typically lifelong. Still's disease may present initially with a severe pharyngitis.

Evaluation

Serum electrophoresis and/or immunofixation are key to establishing a diagnosis of SS. Other laboratory makers include a leukocytosis and raised inflammatory markers including erythrocyte sedimentation rate (ESR) and CRP. Transaminitis is rarely seen in SS but is common in AOSD, as is a very elevated ferritin level. Skin histology will reveal a neutrophilic infiltrate but no evidence of leukocytoclastic vasculitis as would be evident in urticarial vasculitis. Regular monitoring of the gammopathy is important as approximately 20% of patients will develop a lymphoproliferative disorder, which is similar in proportion to that seen in other patients with monoclonal gammopathy of uncertain significance.

Treatment

In patients with mild disease, a therapeutic trial of colchicine is reasonable. Nonsteroidal anti-inflammatory drugs (NSAIDs), such as ibuprofen, may help with bone or joint pain. There are reports of hydroxychloroquine being helpful for a small number of patients. In patients with significant impairment of quality of life and/or persistent raised inflammatory markers, anakinra can be commenced, which is generally highly effective.

DEFICIENCY OF THE INTERLEUKIN-1 RECEPTOR ANTAGONIST

This is an exceptionally rare autoinflammatory syndrome with fewer than 20 cases reported to date. It is characterized by a rash clinically similar to pustular psoriasis, osteomyelitis, periostitis, and elevated acute phase markers presenting in the perinatal period.

Pathogenesis

Deficiency of interleukin-1 receptor antagonist (DIRA) is an autosomal recessive condition caused by the homozygous loss of function mutations in *IL1RN*. This gene encodes the endogenous IL-1 receptor antagonist. The absence of the IL-1 receptor antagonist leads to unopposed excessive activity of the IL-1 pathway and resultant inflammation.

Clinical Features

DIRA patients present within the first few weeks of life with fetal distress, pustular rash, and joint inflammation. They may be born prematurely. The skin rash manifests from discrete crops of pustules to widespread pustulosis (Fig. 8-3). Ichthyosis and nail changes such as onychomadesis and pitting have also been reported. Bone and joint changes are evident with multiple osteolytic

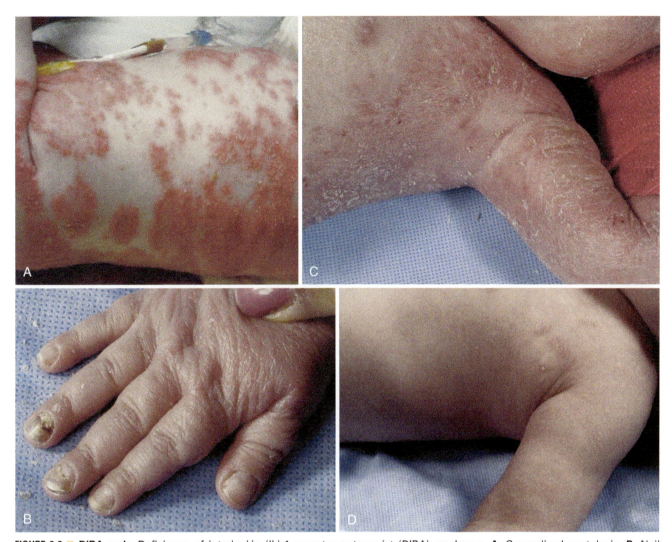

FIGURE 8-3 ■ **DIRA rash.** Deficiency of interleukin (IL)-1 receptor antagonist (DIRA) syndrome. **A,** Generalized pustulosis. **B,** Nail dystrophy. **C,** Patient with DIRA before IL-1 blockade therapy. **D,** Same child after 5-day course of subcutaneous anakinra 100 mg/day. (From Nguyen TV, Cowen EW, Leslie KS. Autoinflammation: from monogenic syndromes to common skin diseases. J Am Acad Dermatol May 2013;68(5):834–53.)

lesions, periostitis, and epiphyseal ballooning of the long bones. This condition, if untreated, is associated with an extremely high mortality secondary to multiorgan failure from uncurbed severe inflammation.

Evaluation

Acute phase reactants such as CRP and ESR will be markedly elevated with a leukocytosis. Skin histology shows neutrophilic infiltration of the epidermis and dermis with pustule formation. Genetic sequencing should be undertaken to confirm homozygous mutations in *IL1RN*.

Treatment

Anakinra should be commenced as soon as possible to prevent irreversible damage and decrease mortality. Rapid clearance of inflammation has been recorded with resolution of skin lesions and reduction in acute phase reactant within a few days of initiating therapy.

TUMOR NECROSIS FACTOR RECEPTOR ASSOCIATED PERIODIC SYNDROME

Tumor necrosis factor receptor associated periodic syndrome (TRAPS) is an autosomal dominant condition characterized by recurrent febrile episodes typically presenting early in childhood. This syndrome was first described in the 1980s when it was reported in a Scottish/Irish family and was called familial Hibernian fever. It became known as TRAPS after its molecular basis was discovered.

Pathogenesis

TRAPS is a monogenic condition with mutations in the *TNFRSF1A* gene (TNF receptor super family1A). This results in increased activity in the TNF pathway. Downstream effects appear to include decreased apoptosis, increased nuclear factor kappa beta (NF-κB), defective receptor trafficking, and increased reactive oxygen species leading to increased mitogen-activated protein kinase activity.

Clinical Features

The median age of onset of febrile episodes is 3 years but occasionally patients may first present later in adolescence or adulthood. The episodes last 1 to 3 weeks and recur every 1 to 2 months. They may occur spontaneously or may be triggered after local injury or minor infections. Myalgia and fever are characteristic features of attacks. Frequently, the sole cutaneous manifestation may be erythema overlying the affected muscles (Fig. 8-4). The erythema may migrate to distal extremities. Other morphologies such as dermal papules, plaques, and reticulated erythema have less commonly been described. The majority of patients will also have abdominal symptoms such as cramping and nausea. Other described signs and symptoms include periorbital edema, conjunctivitis, uveitis, pleuritic, and testicular pain.

Evaluation

Acute phase reactants are elevated in an attack, specifically ESR, CRP, fibrinogen, haptoglobin, and ferritin. A complete blood count may reveal a neutrophil leukocytosis, thrombocytosis, and anemia. Soluble TNF receptor can be measured showing low serum levels (<1 mg/mL). SAA levels are invariably raised so monitoring for amyloidosis is important (urinalysis for proteinuria), which has been reported in about 14% of TRAPS patients. Genetic analysis for the *TNFR1SF1A* gene should be ordered. Histopathology of the skin lesions may show perivascular inflammation with lymphocytes or monocytes but is non-specific.

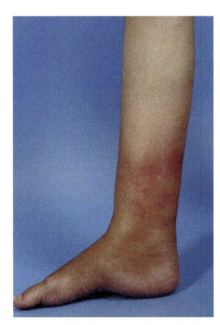

FIGURE 8-4 ■ **Familial Mediterranean fever.** Erysipelas-like erythema above ankle of patient's right leg. (From Radakovic, S., Holzer, G., Tanew, A. Erysipelas-like erythema as a cutaneous sign of familial Mediterranean fever: A case report and review of the histopathologic findings. J Am Acad Dermatol. 2013; 68(2): e61-e63.)

Treatment

Symptomatic control of attacks may be sufficiently achieved with systemic corticosteroids (prednisone >20 mg/day during attack). TNF blockade with etanercept may reduce symptoms and inflammatory markers in some patients. However, there are reports of a paradoxical worsening of inflammation with other TNF-α inhibitors such as adalimumab and infliximab. There are reports that IL-1 inhibition with both anakinra and canakinumab may resolve clinical manifestations and prevent relapses.

FAMILIAL MEDITERRANEAN FEVER

Familial Mediterranean fever (FMF) is the most common monogenic autoinflammatory syndrome. As its name suggests it predominantly affects people of eastern Mediterranean origin, especially Sephardic Jewish, Armenian, Turkish, and Arab individuals. Prevalence of FMF in this region is in the order of 1:400 to 1:1000 although there have been cases reported in Western Europe and the United States.

Pathogenesis

FMF is an autosomal recessive disorder caused by mutations in the marenostrin-encoding fever (*MEFV*) gene. *MEFV* encodes pyrin, which is part of the inflammasome complex and is an inhibitor of the NLRP3 inflammasome. There are five highly conserved missense mutations identified that account for the majority of affected individuals, suggesting a founder effect. It appears that disease expression is related to the amount of mutated pyrin produced, with greater expression leading to increased IL-1β production. This explains why some patients who are heterozygous can have clinical manifestations. There is some degree of genotype predicting phenotype with a poor prognosis associated with M694V mutation.

Clinical Features

Most patients will present with their first attack before the age of 20 years. Fever is typically accompanied with clinical serositis such as peritonitis, pleuritis, and/or synovitis. The sterile peritonitis may be confused with an acute abdomen, as patients will present with pain, distention, and loss of bowel sounds, which may result in unnecessary surgery. Generally, the attacks of FMF will resolve after 48 to 96 hours. The characteristic rash of FMF is called erysipelas-like erythema (ELE) although it affects only 5% to 30% of patients (Fig. 8-5). Typical involvement is unilateral well-demarcated erythematous patches on the lower extremity. More rarely described cutaneous presentations include panniculitis, purpura, and polyarteritis nodosa-like lesions and urticaria.

Evaluation

In the Eastern Mediterranean region, diagnosis of FMF is made clinically. The "Tel Hashomer" Criteria are used to make a diagnosis of FMF fever with one or more major signs and two or more minor signs of fever. Major criteria are abdominal pain, chest pain, skin eruption (ELE), and joint pain, whereas minor criteria include elevated ESR, leukocytosis, and elevated fibrinogen level. Affected individuals with FMF are particularly susceptible to systemic amyloidosis so frequent monitoring of renal function and evaluation of proteinuria are mandatory.

Treatment

Colchicine is highly effective at preventing systemic amyloidosis and is helpful at reducing the frequency and severity of acute attacks. It is also useful in preventing progression in patients who already have established renal amyloidosis. There are reports of thalidomide and sulfasalazine being useful antiflammatories in FMF. Increasingly there are many reports of anti-TNF-α agents such as etanercept, infliximab, and adalimumab being successful. Anakinra has also been reported as useful for FMF.

HYPERIMMUNOGLOBULINEMIA D SYNDROME

Hyperimmunoglobulinemia D syndrome (HIDS) is characterized by recurrent febrile episodes frequently associated with elevated polyclonal IgD levels. It is also known as mevalonate kinase deficiency.

Pathogenesis

HIDS is an autosomal recessive condition caused by mutations to the *MVK* gene. This gene encodes an enzyme involved in the biosynthesis of cholesterol. Most mutations are loss of function with a wide phenotypic expression. Severe disease expression is associated with lower residual enzymatic activity. HIDS patients typically have less than 10% of enzymatic activity. A related condition called mevalonic aciduria (MA), also as a result of *MVK* mutations, presents with a more severe phenotype and less than 1% of enzymatic activity. It is unclear whether inflammation results from either accumulation of products upstream such as mevalonic acid or as a result of reduction of downstream products. It appears that there is activation of both TNF-α and IL-1β pathways.

Clinical Features

Patients present with febrile episodes in infancy typically lasting 3 to 7 days. The frequency of attacks is variable but the median interval is 4 to 6 weeks. As the child ages the attacks may become less frequent and less severe. The febrile episodes are accompanied by abdominal pain, arthralgias, lymphadenopathy, and splenomegaly. The majority of patients (80%) will have some cutaneous manifestations during an attack (Fig. 8-6). Various morphologies have been

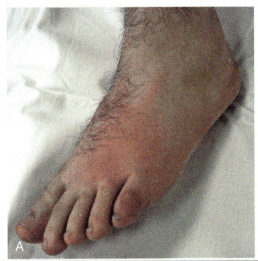

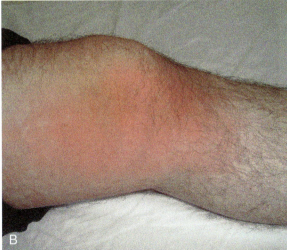

FIGURE 8-5 ■ **FMF rash. A,** Erysipelas-like erythema (ELE) of familial Mediterranean fever (FMF): erythematous plaques on the foot. **B,** ELE of FMF: erythematous plaques on the lower extremity. (Courtesy of Aydin Fatma, MD. Professor in Dermatology. Ondokuz Mayis University, School of Medicine, Department of Dermatology, Samsun, Turkey. From Tripathi SV, Leslie KS. Autoinflammatory diseases in dermatology: CAPS, TRAPS, HIDS, FMF, Blau, CANDLE. Dermatol Clin July 2013;31(3):387–404.)

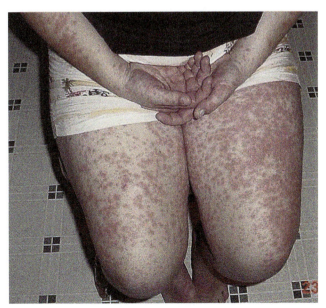

FIGURE 8-6 ■ **HIDS rash.** The rash of hyperimmunoglobulinemia D syndrome (HIDS) may be a diffuse maculopapular eruption, often extending to the palms and soles. (From Nguyen TV, Cowen EW, Leslie KS. Autoinflammation: from monogenic syndromes to common skin diseases. J Am Acad Dermatol May 2013;68(5):834–53.)

described including erythematous macules, papules, urticarial lesions, annular erythema, and purpura. The rash tends to involve the trunk and the extremities for the duration of the febrile episode. For patients with MA, in addition to the febrile episodes, they may have psychomotor retardation, facial dysmorphia, cataracts, and failure to thrive.

Evaluation

During febrile episodes inflammatory markers are elevated such as CRP and SAA. The majority of patients will have an elevated IgD although a low/normal level does not exclude HIDS. They may also have a slightly elevated urinary mevalonic acid level. In between attacks all labs may be normal. The definitive diagnostic test is to look for *MVK* mutations.

Treatment

Simvastatin, an HMG-CoA reductase inhibitor, which reduces mevalonate levels, has been helpful in reducing the duration of febrile episodes. The other treatments where favorable responses have been reported include prednisone, etanercept, and anakinra. Colchicine appears to be ineffective for HIDS.

PYOGENIC ARTHRITIS, PYODERMA GANGRENOSUM AND ACNE SYNDROME

Pyogenic arthritis, pyoderma gangrenosum, and acne (PAPA) syndrome is characterized by joint and skin inflammation. Typically arthritis presents initially in the first decade with variable skin expression as the patient ages.

Pathogenesis

PAPA is a rare autosomal dominant autoinflammatory syndrome. It is caused by mutations in the *PSTPIP1* gene. This encodes CD2 binding protein 1, which interacts with pyrin. The mutated protein exhibits greater affinity with pyrin, which leads to dysregulation of IL-1β production. Genotypic analysis of affected families has demonstrated variable penetrance with some family members without any apparent symptoms.

Clinical Features

The typical presenting sign of the disease is aseptic, recurrent, painful monoarthritis in the first decade. The joints most commonly affected are the elbows, knees, and ankles, which may result in significant joint destruction over time. Severe nodulocystic acne and pyoderma gangrenosum (PG) may develop in puberty (Fig. 8-7). Skin disease may well persist into adulthood. A few cases of concomitant hidradenitis suppurativa have also been reported in PAPA patients.

Evaluation

As with other autoinflammatory syndromes elevated acute phase reactants and leukocytosis may be observed. Histology from PG lesions is identical to PG not related to PAPA and therefore is not diagnostic. Ideally mutational analysis for the *PSTPIP1* gene should be ordered.

Treatment

Satisfactory responses have been described from various TNF-α antagonists including etanercept, adalimumab, and infliximab. Blocking the IL-1 pathway with anakinra has also been helpful although it may be better for joint disease than cutaneous manifestations. Corticosteroids have also been useful for arthritis but their use may exacerbate acne. Topical and systemic retinoids in combination with biological agents have been effective for control of the cystic acne.

Pyoderma Gangrenosum, Acne, and Suppurative Hidradenitis (PASH)

Recent reports have described a PSTPIP1 gene mutation associated syndrome distinct from PAPA. This syndrome includes dramatic hidradenitis suppurativa, along with pyoderma gangrenosum and acne conglobata. This syndrome presents significant therapeutic difficulty. A therapeutic role for tumor necrosis factor antagonists, or interleukin-1 inhibitors including anakinra has been supported by case reports.

SAPHO SYNDROME

SAPHO syndrome presents as osteoarticular and skin inflammation in childhood and young adult life. SAPHO stands for synovitis, acne, pustulosis, hyperostosis, and osteitis. It is likely that chronic multifocal osteomyelitis, a syndrome described predominantly in a pediatric population, lies within the same clinical spectrum as SAPHO as they share numerous characteristics.

Pathogenesis

The genetic basis of SAPHO is unknown although familial cases of SAPHO have been reported where genetic analysis has failed to reveal genetic associations. The presence of *Propionibacterium acnes* and coagulase-negative staphylococci has been found in bone lesions, although it is unclear what role the microorganisms may be playing. It has been postulated that SAPHO syndrome may be the result of abnormal cellular and humoral response to the presence of *P. acnes*.

Clinical Features

The cardinal feature of SAPHO is osteoarticular disease with the chest wall most commonly affected followed by the spine. Sacroileitis may also occur whereas long bone involvement is less common (especially in adults). Distal synovitis may be seen, which is more common in adults than in children. Dermatological manifestations are seen independently of osteoarticular inflammation, so may precede or appear concurrently or after bone and joint disease. The most frequent skin findings are palmoplantar pustulosis followed by acne conglobate and acne fulminans. There

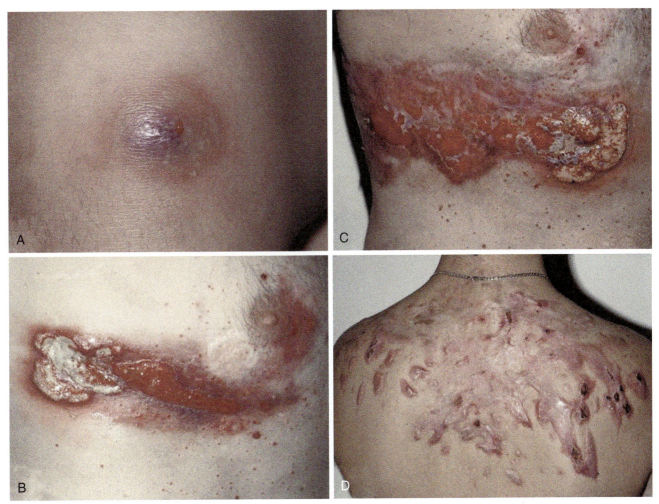

FIGURE 8-7 ■ PAPA rash. Pyogenic arthritis, pyoderma gangrenosum (PG), and acne (PAPA) syndrome. **A,** PG in its early stage. **B,** Developing PG. **C,** Progression and scarring of the same PG. **D,** Extensive hypertrophic scarring at sites of severe acne involvement. (From Nguyen TV, Cowen EW, Leslie KS. Autoinflammation: from monogenic syndromes to common skin diseases. J Am Acad Dermatol May 2013;68(5):834–53.)

have also been reports of hidradenitis suppurativa, folliculitis, pyoderma gangrenosum, and Sweet's syndrome.

Evaluation

Laboratory evaluations tend to be normal so diagnosis tends to be based on clinical features consistent with SAPHO. Radiological studies are helpful in assessing disease activity. Imaging of the sternoclavicular region is important, as this is the region that is most frequently affected. Plain radiographs may reveal ossifications and erosions in the costoclavicular ligament, clavicles, and manubrium sternii. The axial skeleton is affected in one-third of cases so may reveal spondylodiscitis, osteosclerosis, and sacroileitis. Nuclear medicine imaging is the most sensitive imaging modality for SAPHO. The ^{99}Tc scan may show increased uptake in the sternoclavicular region, which is called the "bull's head" sign.

Treatment

NSAIDs and intra-articular corticosteroids are helpful for joint inflammation. Systemic corticosteroids in combination with methotrexate or azathioprine may be beneficial for both bone and skin disease. All the TNF-α antagonists have been used in SAPHO with reports of early reduction of bone pain. Anakinra has also been reported as useful in a small open study for SAPHO.

SUGGESTED READINGS

Aksentijevich I, Masters SL, Ferguson PJ, et al. An autoinflammatory disease with deficiency of the interleukin-1-receptor antagonist. N Engl J Med 2009;360(23):2426–37.

Bauernfeind F, Ablasser A, Bartok E, et al. Inflammasomes: current understanding and open questions. Cell Mol Life Sci 2011;68(5):765–83.

Braun-Falco M, Kovnerystyy O, Lohse P, Ruziaka, T. Pyoderma gangrenosum, acne, and suppurative hidradenitis (PASH): a new autoimflammatory syndrome distinct from PAPA syndrome. J Am Acad Dermatol 2012;66:409–15.

Calderón-Castrat X, Bancalari-Diaz D, Román-Curto C, Romo-Melgar A, Amorós-Cerdán D, Alcaraz-Mas L, et al. PSTPIP1 gene mutation in a pyoderma gangrenosum, acne and suppurative hidradenitis (PASH) syndrome. Br J Dermatol December 29, 2015.

Cantarini L, Lucherini OM, Mucari I, et al. Tumor necrosis factor receptor-associated periodic syndrome (TRAPS): state of the art and future perspectives. Autoimmun Rev 2012;12(1):38–43.

Gattorno M, Federici S, Pelagatti MA, Caorsi R, Brisca G, Malattia C, et al. Diagnosis and management of autoinflammatory diseases in childhood. J Clin Immunol 2008;28(S1):S73–83.

Naik HB, Cowen EW. Autoinflammatory pustular neutrophilic diseases. Dermatol Clin 2013;31(3):405–25.

Nguyen TV, Cowen EW, Leslie KS. Autoinflammation: from monogenic syndromes to common skin diseases. J Am Acad Dermatol 2013; 68(5):834–53.

Savic S, Dickie L, Battelino M. Familial Mediterranean fever and related periodic fever syndromes/autoinflammatory diseases. Curr Opin Rheumatol 2012;24(1):103–12.

Simon A, et al. Schnitzler's syndrome: diagnosis, treatment, and follow-up. Allergy 2013;68(5):562–8.

Ter Haar N, Lachmann H, Özen S, et al. Treatment of autoinflammatory diseases: results from the Eurofever Registry and a literature review. Ann Rheum Dis 2013;72(5):678–85.

van der Hilst J.C., Frenkel J.. Hyperimmunoglobulin D syndrome in childhood. Curr Rheumatol Rep 2010;12(2):101–107.

Yu JR, Leslie KS. Cryopyrin-associated periodic syndrome: an update on diagnosis and treatment response. Curr Allergy Asthma Rep 2011;11(1):12–20.

Zemer D, Revach M, Pras M, et al. A controlled trial of colchicine in preventing attacks of familial Mediterranean fever. N Engl J Med 1974;291:932–4.

Zhao Z, Li Y, Li Y, Zhao H, Li H. Synovitis, acne, pustulosis, hyperostosis and osteitis (SAPHO) syndrome with review of the relevant published work. J Dermatol 2011;38(2):155–9.

CHAPTER 9

EOSINOPHIL-ASSOCIATED DISEASES WITH DERMATOLOGIC MANIFESTATIONS

Kristin M. Leiferman

KEY POINTS

- Peripheral blood eosinophilia provides clues to diagnosis, but it is not a diagnostic marker except when levels of peripheral blood eosinophils are in the "hypereosinophilic" range as found in the hypereosinophilic syndromes.
- Many diseases with increased peripheral blood eosinophils have accompanying tissue eosinophil infiltration, including skin, often with degranulation and loss of morphological identity of infiltrating eosinophils.
- Eosinophils are observed in biopsy specimens of various skin lesions, with and without accompanying peripheral blood eosinophilia, and clinicopathological correlation is needed to arrive at the correct diagnosis; eosinophil-associated dermatoses include drug eruptions, arthropod bite reactions, parasite infestations ("drugs and bugs"), certain autoimmune blistering diseases, Wells syndrome, eosinophilic granulomatosis with polyangiitis (Churg–Strauss syndrome), and IgG4-related diseases.
- Eosinophils commonly disrupt and lose their morphological integrity as they deposit toxic granule proteins and other inflammatory mediators in tissues, prominently in urticarial, eczematous, and pruritic skin lesions; therefore, the presence or absence of intact eosinophils in tissue specimens may not accurately reflect their pathogenic role in disease.
- In patients with *persistent* peripheral blood eosinophilia from any cause, including the hypereosinophilic syndromes, tissue infiltration, and eosinophil-derived effector molecules may cause clinically relevant pathology, including irreversible organ damage.

Eosinophils are leukocytes with cytoplasmic granules that are named for their characteristic staining with the acidic dye, eosin. They circulate in blood as mature cells. Normally, they are not found in human tissues other than blood except in the bone marrow where they develop, in the gastrointestinal tract distal to the esophagus where they likely are eliminated, and in lymphoid tissues where they function in both innate and acquired immunity. Peripheral blood eosinophils are increased in various inflammatory diseases, classically in parasitic infections, allergic diseases and drug reactions, in hematological malignancies, and in some solid tumors. Eosinophils infiltrate tissues in response to certain inflammatory signals, which may or may not be accompanied by peripheral blood eosinophilia. Eosinophils commonly disrupt and lose their morphological identity as they deposit toxic granule proteins, and the presence or absence of intact eosinophils may not accurately reflect a pathogenic role for eosinophils in affected tissues. New therapies that target eosinophils show promise in treating eosinophil-associated diseases.

CLASSIFICATION

Peripheral blood eosinophilia can be transient, episodic, or persistent and can fluctuate between eosinophilia ($0.5-1.5 \times 10^9$/L) and hypereosinophilia (greater than 1.5×10^9/L). Tissue hypereosinophilia can occur in the absence of increased blood eosinophils, although, often, at least episodic eosinophilia is present. Blood hypereosinophilia can be classified as follows:
- Primary hypereosinophilia (clonal/neoplastic) in which eosinophils are neoplastic cells with underlying stem cell, myeloid, or eosinophil neoplasm, as classified by World Health Organization criteria
- Secondary hypereosinophilia (reactive) in which eosinophilia is cytokine-driven in most cases by an underlying condition/disease and eosinophils are nonclonal
- Hereditary hypereosinophilia (familial) in which a familial clustering of individuals with hypereosinophilia is found without hereditary immunodeficiency and no evidence of neoplastic or reactive conditions underlying the eosinophilia
- Hypereosinophilia of undetermined significance in which hypereosinophilia develops with no evidence of underlying cause including no neoplastic or reactive conditions and no family history and with no organ damage; this category may be prodromal to primary or secondary forms.

Various patterns of tissue eosinophil involvement are recognized:
- Eosinophil infiltration of few to many intact cells
- Intact eosinophils with extracellular eosinophil granule protein deposition proportionate to the numbers of infiltrating eosinophils
- Intact eosinophils with extensive extracellular eosinophil granule protein deposition disproportionately greater than the numbers of infiltrating eosinophils
- Extensive extracellular eosinophil granule protein deposition with few or no infiltrating eosinophils (in this pattern, eosinophil involvement may not be recognized on histopathology examination).

Eosinophils likely are activated as they infiltrate tissues resulting in the deposition of their toxic granule proteins in many reaction patterns. Virtually every organ, including skin, is affected by inflammatory conditions accompanied by tissue hypereosinophilia.

PATHOGENESIS

Eosinophils circulate transiently in blood (8 to 18 hours) and are constantly replenished from bone marrow progenitor cells. Major growth factors for eosinophils are interleukin (IL)-5, granulocyte–macrophage colony-stimulating factor (GM-CSF), and IL-3, which are produced and secreted by activated T cells, mast cells, stromal cells, and eosinophils themselves. Eosinophils express cell surface receptors for these cytokines throughout development. These cytokines induce not only proliferation of eosinophil progenitor cells, but migration, adherence, cytokine production, activation, and survival of mature eosinophils. The mobilization of eosinophils from bone marrow into blood is regulated predominantly by IL-5 and eotaxin. Eosinophils derived from inflamed tissues express higher levels of certain cell surface adhesion receptors.

Several lines of investigation indicate that eosinophils are recruited to and activated in tissues by cytokine activity from the Th2 subset of T cells, which produces IL-4, IL-5, IL-10, and IL-13, in addition to cytokines common to Th1 cells, such as GM-CSF and IL-3. Eosinophils themselves elaborate important inflammatory and regulatory cytokines. As a result, eosinophil activation occurs in an autocrine manner. In cytotoxicity assays, eosinophils are maximally activated by GM-CSF, followed by IL-3, IL-5, tumor necrosis factor (TNF)-α, and IL-4, in order of potency.

Upon activation, eosinophils release granule contents into their extracellular spaces via three mechanisms: cytolytic degranulation, piecemeal degranulation, and regulated secretion. Cytolytic degranulation is characterized by cytoplasmic membrane rupture, chromatolysis of nuclei with loss of morphological integrity and identity of eosinophils, and extensive deposition of eosinophil granules and granule products within tissue; this process occurs in many inflammatory disorders, including skin diseases as well as in affected organs in other diseases. The distinctive eosinophil granule proteins, including eosinophil major basic protein (eMBP)1, eMBP2, eosinophil-derived neurotoxin, eosinophil cationic protein, and eosinophil peroxidase, have many biological activities (reviewed in detail in other publications) implicating their roles in pathophysiology with effects on tissues and cells, including basophils, neutrophils, and platelets, as well as infectious organisms including helminths, RNA viruses, and bacteria. Eosinophil granule proteins persist in tissues for long periods of time; eMBP1 up to 6 weeks.

Eosinophils possess receptors for glucocorticoids, which inhibit eosinophil growth and function, and receptor numbers correlate with responses of eosinophils to glucocorticoids. Additionally, glucocorticoids and other anti-inflammatory agents inhibit cytokine-induced expression of adhesion molecules on eosinophils and endothelial cells and, therefore, eosinophil adhesion and transendothelial migration.

Certain specific diseases and syndromes are strongly associated with and/or are defined by peripheral blood and tissue eosinophilia in which cutaneous manifestations are common (Tables 9-1 and 9-2).

Peripheral blood hypereosinophilia and end-organ damage attributable to tissue hypereosinophilia are diagnostic criteria for the hypereosinophilic syndromes (HES). Dermatologic involvement is the most frequent presenting clinical manifestation in HES (Table 9-3).

Patients with primary (neoplastic) HES present with signs and symptoms related to the organ systems affected by eosinophilic infiltrates with mucocutaneous lesions in almost 40% and eventually involving almost 70%. Along with skin lesions, the presenting complex may include fever, weight loss, fatigue, and malaise, in addition

TABLE 9-1 Etiopathogenic Disease Associations with Eosinophils

Common/Strong Etiologies	Less Common/Rare Etiologies
Adrenal insufficiency (Addison's disease)	B- and T-cell lymphomas/leukemias
Allergic reactions	Chronic graft-versus-host disease
Atopic diseases	Chronic inflammatory disorders, including inflammatory bowel disease
Drug reactions	Fibrotic reactions
Hypereosinophilic syndromes	Fungal infections, allergic bronchopulmonary aspergillosis, and others
Immunobullous diseases, particularly pemphigoid	Hodgkin's disease
Parasitosis including ectoparasitic infestations and helminthic infections	Human immunodeficiency virus (HIV) and human T-cell lymphotropic virus (HTLV) I and II
IgG4-related diseases
Indolent systemic mastocytosis
Langerhans cell histiocytosis
Sarcoidosis
Solid tumors/malignancy

Modified from Table E2 in Valent P, Klion AD, Horny HP, Roufosse F, Gotlib J, Weller PF et al. Contemporary consensus proposal on criteria and classification of eosinophilic disorders and related syndromes. J Allergy Clin Immunol 2012;130(3):607–12.e9. Epub March 31, 2012.

to increased serum vitamin B12 levels and increased serum tryptase levels. Skin lesions include pruritic erythematous macules, papules, plaques, or nodules on the trunk and extremities or urticaria and angioedema. Mucosal ulcers of the oropharynx or anogenital region associated with primary HES previously had a grim prognosis. Most afflicted patients died within 2 years of presentation; however, these patients are very responsive to imatinib. Embolic events also occur, particularly during the thrombotic stage, and constitute a medical emergency because of their likely serious sequelae; cutaneous involvement with splinter hemorrhages and/or nail fold infarcts may be present and can provide the initial clues to thromboembolic disease. Other cutaneous manifestations of HES include erythema annulare centrifugum-like lesions, retiform purpura, livedo reticularis, and superficial thrombophlebitis (Table 9-4).

Secondary (reactive) HES are commonly associated with severe pruritus, dermatitis, erythroderma and/or urticaria, and angioedema, in addition to lymphadenopathy. Patients with secondary (reactive) HES have an underlying inflammatory, neoplastic, or other disease known to induce hypereosinophilia. Eosinophils are nonclonal in this variant but abnormal clonal lymphocyte populations, frequently with unique surface phenotypes such as $CD3^+CD4^-CD8^-$ or $CD3^-CD4^+$, may be present or develop. Monoclonality of T cells as demonstrated by rearrangement in the T-cell receptor gene also may be detected. Therefore, patients with such clones should be regarded as having premalignant or malignant T-cell lymphoma and be closely observed.

Formerly, HES was termed "idiopathic" because underlying mechanisms were not understood. Currently, disease presentation that satisfies HES diagnostic criteria

TABLE 9-2 Defined Eosinophil-Associated Syndromes

Eosinophilia myalgia syndrome (EMS) and toxic oil syndrome (TOS)	Severe myalgia with hypereosinophilia, often accompanied by neurological symptoms and skin changes; epidemic cases of EMS have been attributed to contaminated L-tryptophan exposure and of TOS to rapeseed oil denatured with aniline
Eosinophilic granulomatosis with polyangiitis (Churg-Strauss syndrome)	Necrotizing vasculitis with hypereosinophilia (ANCA1 and ANCA2 subvariants)
Gleich's syndrome	Cyclic recurrent angioedema, hypereosinophilia, and increased IgM levels, often with clonal T cells, one of several possible clinical presentations of secondary/reactive HES
Hypereosinophilic syndromes (HES)	Peripheral blood hypereosinophilia, hypereosinophilia-related organ damage; variants classified
Hyper-IgE syndromes	Hereditary immunodeficiency syndrome with hypereosinophilia and increased IgE levels, often with eczema and facial anomalies; autosomal dominant variant has STAT3 mutations and autosomal recessive variant has DOCK8 mutations
IgG4-related diseases	Spectrum of disorders with fibrosis as a major finding, tissue eosinophilia and increased IgG4
Omenn syndrome	Severe combined immunodeficiency with hypereosinophilia, often with erythroderma, hepatosplenomegaly, and lymphadenopathy and autosomal recessive genetic disease (mutations in RAG1 or RAG2)

ANCA, Antineutrophil cytoplasmic antibodies; STAT3, signal transducer and activator of transcription 3; DOCK8, dedicator of cytokinesis 8; RAG, recombination-activating gene.
Modified from Table E3 in Valent P, Klion AD, Horny HP, Roufosse F, Gotlib J, Weller PF et al. Contemporary consensus proposal on criteria and classification of eosinophilic disorders and related syndromes. J Allergy Clin Immunol 2012;130(3):607–12.e9. Epub March 31, 2012.

TABLE 9-3 Clinical Manifestations of Hypereosinophilic Syndromes (HES) on Initial Presentation

Clinical Manifestations on Initial Presentation	Number Affected*	Description
Cardiac	9	Congestive heart failure (4), valvular abnormality (1), cardiomyopathy (1), pericardial effusion (1), myocarditis (2)
Constitutional	10	Fever (3), weight loss (6), malaise (7), fatigue (4), night sweats (3), flu-like illness (2)
Dermatologic	70	Urticaria (6), angioedema (15), pruritus (26), dermatitis (26), erythroderma (1), bullous lesions (1), eosinophilic cellulitis (Wells syndrome) (3), unspecified edema (8), mucosal erosions (3)
Gastrointestinal	26	Abdominal pain (9), vomiting (6), diarrhea (5)
Hematologic	6	Deep venous thrombosis (4), anemia (1), superficial thrombophlebitis (1)
Neurologic	9	Vertigo (2), paresthesia (4), change in mentation (1), aphasia (1), visual disturbances (3)
Pulmonary	47	Asthma (21), sinusitis (9), rhinitis (2), cough (19), dyspnea (11), recurrent upper respiratory infection (2), pulmonary infiltrates (4), pleural effusion (1)
Rheumatologic	14	Arthralgia (3), myalgia (9), arthritis (1), myositis (1)
Routine laboratory test	11	Incidental abnormality found on routine laboratory testing (11)

*Some patients had multiple manifestations, 188 total patients.
Modified from Table E1 in Ogbogu PU, Bochner BS, Butterfield JH, Gleich GJ, Huss-Marp J, Kahn et al. Hypereosinophilic syndrome: a multicenter, retrospective analysis of clinical characteristics and response to therapy. J Allergy Clin Immunol December 2009;124(6):1319–25.e3. doi:10.1016/j.jaci.2009.09.022.

TABLE 9-4	Mucocutaneous Manifestations in Hypereosinophilic Syndromes (HES)

Angioedema
Bullae
Dermographism
Digital gangrene
Eczema
Eosinophilic cellulitis (Wells syndrome)
Erosions
Erythema
Erythema annulare centrifuge
Erythroderma
Excoriation(s)
Livedo reticularis
Lymphomatoid papulosis
Macules
Mucosal ulcer(s) (oropharynx and anogenital)
Nail fold infarction(s)
Necrosis
Nodules (including prurigo nodularis)
Papules
Patches
Pruritus
Purpura
Raynaud's phenomenon
Splinter hemorrhage(s)
Ulcer(s)
Urticaria
Vasculitis
Vesicle(s)

Modified from Leiferman KM, Gleich GJ, Peters MS: Dermatologic manifestations of the hypereosinophilic syndromes, Box 1. Immunol Allergy Clin North Am 2007;27(3):415–41 and Leiferman KM, Peters MS. Eosinophils in cutaneous diseases, Chapter 36, Table 36-3. In: Goldsmith LA, Katz SI, Gilchrest BA, Paller AS, Leffell DJ, Wolff K, editors. Fitzpatrick's Dermatology in General Medicine. 8th ed. San Francisco: McGraw Hill Medical; 2012. p. 386–400.

but does not have an underlying explanation, i.e., not primary (neoplastic) or secondary (reactive), is called "idiopathic." Over time, patients with this "idiopathic" HES variant may evolve to one of the other variants or resolve.

"Eosinophil-associated dermatoses" encompass a wide variety of diseases characterized by the presence of few to many eosinophils and/or evidence of eosinophil degranulation in the skin and/or mucous membranes (Table 9-5). The disorders traditionally associated with eosinophil infiltration include arthropod bite reactions, drug eruptions ("bugs and drugs"), atopic disorders, parasitic infestations (e.g., ectoparasites and helminths), and Wells syndrome. In addition, autoimmune blistering diseases, particularly bullous pemphigoid, demonstrate eosinophil infiltration. The histopathological features of urticaria, urticarial dermatitis, and cutaneous vasculitis, especially eosinophilic granulomatosis with polyangiitis (Churg–Strauss syndrome), often include eosinophils. Mild to moderate eosinophil infiltration is one of the key morphological features of the recently described IgG4-related disease (IgG4-RD) spectrum in which fibrosis is a major finding. IgG4-RD subsequently has been reported to involve any/multiple organs, and many disorders of specific organs are now considered to be variants of IgG4-RD, including certain eosinophil-associated dermatoses (e.g., granuloma faciale, angiolymphoid hyperplasia with eosinophilia, and Kimura's disease). IgG4 is lowest in concentration of the four IgG subclasses and normally constitutes 3% to 6% of total serum IgG; its functions are not well understood but seemingly bridge innate and acquired immunity.

HISTOPATHOLOGY

Histopathological reaction patterns with eosinophils are found in cutaneous compartments throughout the depth of the skin from epidermis into muscle.

Eosinophils are a predominant inflammatory cell observed by histopathology in many diverse dermatological diseases and categorized into various histopathological patterns including those that are defined by eosinophils, others that are characterized by tissue eosinophils, and yet others that are typically associated with tissue eosinophils (Table 9-5). In some of these disorders, eosinophil activation with extracellular deposition of eosinophil granule proteins is known (e.g., urticaria, atopic dermatitis, pemphigoid, Wells syndrome), but, because immunopathological staining for eosinophil granule proteins is not commonly performed, the presence and extent of eosinophil granule protein deposition and, thus, eosinophil involvement may not be known. Flame figures in eosinophilic cellulitis as a dermatopathological feature with prominent deposition of eosinophil granule proteins (Fig. 9-1), in particular, are found in various conditions (Table 9-6). In certain other lesions, recognition of eosinophils in the histopathology is of doubtful or limited benefit in the diagnosis, although they still may be part of the pathophysiology.

DIFFERENTIAL DIAGNOSIS

The differential diagnosis (Table 9-7) depends on the patient's presentation with respect to the type and distribution of skin lesions, pattern of eosinophil infiltration in the skin, other apparent organ involvement, and/or presence and level of peripheral blood eosinophils. The differential diagnoses overlap with various cutaneous manifestations and include the spectrum of eosinophil-associated dermatoses.

TREATMENT

The goal of treatment is to relieve symptoms and improve organ function while keeping peripheral blood eosinophils at or less than 1 to a maximum of $2 \times 10^9/L$ and minimizing treatment side effects. Recent publications have reviewed management of eosinophil-associated diseases including HES specifically. For reactive eosinophilia, management of the underlying disease directs therapy. If blood and/or tissue eosinophilia persists with likely organ-related dysfunction or damage, glucocorticoid therapy is the mainstay of therapy. However, consider screening for *Strongyloides stercoralis* in patients from or traveling in endemic areas because of risk of life-threatening hyperinfection (severe complicated strongyloidiasis) with immunosuppressive therapy.

TABLE 9-5 Eosinophil-Associated Dermatoses

Histopathological patterns defined by eosinophils
- Eosinophilic spongiosis
  - Acute dermatitis
    - Allergic contact dermatitis
    - Atopic dermatitis
  - Arthropod bite and sting
  - Immunobullous diseases
    - Pemphigoid
    - Pemphigus
  - Incontinentia pigmenti
- Eosinophilic cellulitis with flame figures (Fig. 9-1)
  - See Table 9-6
- Eosinophilic panniculitis
  - Arthropod bite
  - Erythema nodosum
  - Gnathostomiasis
  - Injection granuloma
  - Wells syndrome
- Eosinophilic vasculitis
  - Recurrent cutaneous necrotizing vasculitis
  - Connective tissue disease with necrotizing eosinophilic vasculitis
  - Hypocomplementemia associated
  - Eosinophilic granulomatosis with polyangiitis (Churg–Strauss syndrome)

Diseases characterized by tissue eosinophils
- Angiolymphoid hyperplasia with eosinophilia
- Annular erythema of infancy
- Eosinophilic, polymorphic, and pruritic eruption associated with radiotherapy
- Eosinophilic pustular folliculitis
  - Classical (Ofuji disease)
  - Human immunodeficiency virus associated
  - Infantile/neonatal
- Erythema toxicum neonatorum
- Eosinophilic annular erythema
- Eosinophilic dermatosis of hematologic malignancy
- Eosinophilic ulcer of oral mucosa
- Hypereosinophilic dermatitis of Nir–Westfried
- Hypereosinophilic syndromes
- IgG4-related cutaneous diseases
  - Angiolymphoid hyperplasia with eosinophilia
  - Granuloma faciale
  - Kimura's disease
- Pachydermatous eosinophilic dermatitis
- Wells syndrome (eosinophilic cellulitis)

Diseases associated with tissue eosinophils
- Arthropod bites and sting reactions
- Bullous dermatoses
  - Pemphigoid
  - Pemphigus
  - Epidermolysis bullosa acquisita
  - Incontinentia pigmenti
- Dermatoses of pregnancy
  - Pemphigoid gestationis
  - Polymorphic eruption of pregnancy, pruritic urticarial papules, and plaques of pregnancy
- Drug reactions
  - DRESS (drug rash with eosinophilia and systemic symptoms)/drug hypersensitivity syndrome
  - Interstitial granulomatous drug reaction
- Eosinophilic granulomatosis with polyangiitis (Churg–Strauss syndrome)
- Fungal infections
  - Coccidioidomycosis, paracoccidioidomycosis, basidiobolomycosis, histoplasmosis, cryptococcosis
- Histiocytic diseases
  - Langerhans cell histiocytosis
  - Juvenile xanthogranuloma
- Itchy, red bump disease (papular dermatitis)
- Juvenile temporal arteritis
- Oid-oid disease (exudative discoid and lichenoid chronic dermatosis of Sulzberger and Garbe)
- Papuloerythroderma of Ofuji
- Parasitic diseases/infestations
  - Cysticercosis, dirofilariasis, fascioliasis, gnathostomiasis, larva migrans, loiasis, myiasis (Fig. 9-2), onchocerciasis, paragonimiasis, schistosomiasis, strongyloidiasis, tungiasis
  - Scabies, bed bugs
  - Swimmer's itch (cercarial dermatitis) and seabather's itch
- Pruritic papular eruption of human immunodeficiency virus (HIV) disease
- Sclerodermoid disorders
  - Eosinophilic fasciitis (Shulman's syndrome)
  - Eosinophilia myalgia syndrome and toxic oil syndrome
  - Drugs including statins
  - Iron infusion
  - Lymphoma and leukemia
  - Graft versus host, stem cell, and bone marrow transplantation
- Urticaria and angioedema
- Vasculitis

Eosinophils pathophysiologically present but of doubtful, limited, or no value in histopathological diagnosis
- Drug reaction versus graft-versus-host disease
- Granuloma annulare
- Interstitial granulomatous dermatitis
- Lymphoproliferative disorders (except hypereosinophilic syndromes [HES] variants)
  - Mycosis fungoides
  - Anaplastic large cell lymphoma
  - Lymphomatoid papulosis
- Mastocytosis
- Neoplasms
  - Keratoacanthoma
  - Squamous cell carcinoma

Modified from Leiferman KM, Peters MS. Eosinophils in cutaneous diseases, Chapter 36, Table 36-1. In: Goldsmith LA, Katz SI, Gilchrest BA, Paller AS, Leffell DJ, Wolff K, editors. Fitzpatrick's Dermatology in General Medicine, 8th ed. San Francisco: McGraw Hill Medical; 2012.p. 386–400.

If glucocorticoid side effects become limiting, if patients have poor tolerance or otherwise do not respond well, steroid-sparing agents are used, most commonly hydroxyurea and interferon (IFN)-α. New steroid-sparing therapies that target IL-5 are becoming available. Mepolizumab, a humanized IL-5 monoclonal antibody, has been shown to be safe and effective as a steroid-sparing therapy in patients with secondary and idiopathic HES, as well as asthma, eosinophilic granulomatosis with polyangiitis, and nasal polyposis, and has recently received

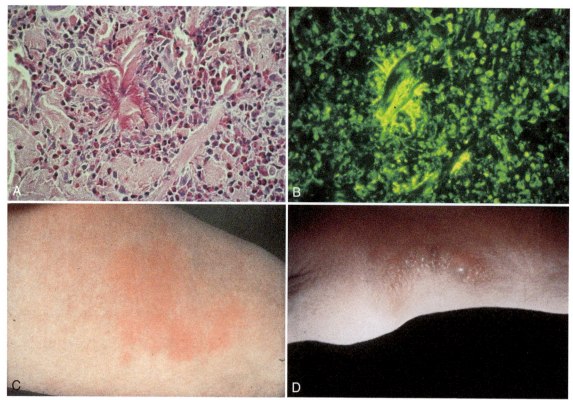

FIGURE 9-1 ■ Flame figure (**A**) by hematoxylin and eosin stain (H&E) and (**B**) by immunostaining for eosinophil major basic protein 1 (eMBP1) showing extensive extracellular eosinophil granule protein deposition on the degenerating collagen fibers characteristically found in (**C**) Wells syndrome and (**D**) bullous eosinophilic cellulitis lesions and in multiple other inflammatory conditions (Table 9-6). (Figures A, B and D are from Davis MDP, Brown AC, Blackston RD, Gaughf C, Peterson EA, Gleich GJ, Leiferman KM. Familial Eosinophilic Cellulitis, Dysmorphic Habitus and Mental Retardation. J Am Acad Dermatol, 38:919-928, 1998; figure C is from Leiferman KM, Peters MS. Eosinophils in Cutaneous Diseases, Chapter 36. In: Goldsmith LA, Katz SI, Gilchrest BA, Paller AS, Leffell DJ, Wolff K, editors. Fitzpatrick's Dermatology in General Medicine. 8th ed. San Francisco: McGraw Hill Medical; 2012. p. 386–400.)

TABLE 9-6 Associations with Flame Figures

Arthropod bite reaction
Bronchogenic carcinoma
Colonic adenocarcinoma
Dental abscess
Dermographism
Drug reaction
Eczema
Eosinophilic fasciitis
Eosinophilic granulomatosis with polyangiitis (Churg–Strauss syndrome)
Eosinophilic pustular folliculitis
Herpes simplex infection
Human immunodeficiency virus infection
Hymenoptera sting
Hypereosinophilic syndromes
Immunobullous diseases
Mastocytoma
Molluscum contagiosum
Myeloproliferative disorders
Parasite infestation (ascariasis, onchocerciasis, toxocariasis)
Pemphigoid gestationis
Tinea
Urticaria
Ulcerative colitis
Vaccinations
Varicella

Modified from Leiferman KM, Peters MS. Eosinophils in cutaneous diseases, Chapter 36, Table 36-5. In: Goldsmith LA, Katz SI, Gilchrest BA, Paller AS, Leffell DJ, Wolff K, editors. Fitzpatrick's Dermatology in General Medicine, 8th ed. San Francisco: McGraw Hill Medical; 2012.p. 386–400.

FDA approval for treating asthma. Another humanized IL-5 monoclonal antibody, reslizumab, and a humanized monoclonal antibody to the IL-5 alpha receptor (present on eosinophils) are in clinical trials and have had reported steroid-sparing activities in eosinophilic asthma. In patients with primary HES with the mutant gene *FIP1L1-PDGFRA* and other *PDGFRA* and *PDGFRB* mutations, administration of imatinib mesylate (Gleevec®) is indicated and induces hematologic remission.

In the absence of the gene mutation, after *Strongyloides* infection has been excluded, first-line therapy is prednisone. Approximately 70% of patients will respond, with peripheral eosinophil counts returning to normal. Patients for whom glucocorticoid monotherapy fails have a worse prognosis generally; in such cases or when long-term side effects become problematic, alternative treatments should be used. Extracorporeal photopheresis alone or in combination with IFN-α or other therapies represent additional therapeutic options. Other treatments for HES with reported benefit include hydroxyurea, dapsone, vincristine sulfate, cyclophosphamide, methotrexate, 6-thioguanine, 2-chlorodeoxyadenosine and cytarabine combination therapy, pulsed chlorambucil, etoposide, cyclosporine, intravenous immunoglobulin, and psoralen plus ultraviolet A phototherapy. Refractory disease may respond to infliximab (anti-TNF-α) or alemtuzumab (anti-CD52), as well as to bone marrow and peripheral blood stem cell allogeneic transplantation.

TABLE 9-7	Differential Diagnosis of Eosinophil-Associated Diseases with Cutaneous Manifestations
Angioedema/ dermographism/ edema/urticaria	Cellulitis Drug reaction Eosinophilia myalgia and toxic oil syndromes Eosinophilic cellulitis (Wells syndrome) Erysipelas Hereditary angioedema Hypereosinophilic syndromes Mast cell disease Parasitic infection Urticaria Urticarial vasculitis
Blisters and/or ulceration	Aphthous stomatitis Behçet's syndrome Drug reaction Erythema multiforme Herpes simplex infection Hypereosinophilic syndromes Incontinentia pigmenti Immunobullous disease Lichen planus Lesions in diseases listed above (angioedema/dermographism/edema/urticaria) may blister
Dermatitis/ eczema/pruritus	Atopic dermatitis Contact dermatitis Drug reaction Ectoparasite infestation Fungal infection Hypereosinophilic syndromes Parasitic infection
Erythema/pruritus	Drug reaction Ectoparasite infestation Hypereosinophilic syndromes Sézary syndrome Seborrheic dermatitis
Fibrosis	IgG4-related diseases Morphea Eosinophilia myalgia and toxic oil syndromes
Hyperpigmentation	Adrenal insufficiency (Addison's disease) Drug reaction Hemochromatosis Hyperthyroidism

Nodules/papules/ plaques/pustules	Acne, including acne neonatorum
	Acropustulosis
	Epithelioid angiosarcoma
	Epithelioid hemangioendothelioma
	Erythema toxicum neonatorum
	Folliculitis
	Follicular mucinosis
	Fungal infection
	Hypereosinophilic syndromes
	IgG4-related diseases
	  Angiolymphoid hyperplasia with eosinophilia
	    Granuloma faciale
	    Kimura's disease
	Kaposi's sarcoma
	Lichen planus
	Lupus erythematosus
	Mast cell disease
	Morphea
	Mycosis fungoides
	Nodules, eosinophilia, rheumatism, dermatitis and swelling (NERDS)
	Palmar–plantar pustular psoriasis
	Pityriasis lichenoides chronica
	Pyogenic granuloma
	T-cell lymphoma
	Vasculitis

TABLE 9-7	Differential Diagnosis of Eosinophil-Associated Diseases with Cutaneous Manifestations—cont'd
Various, miscellaneous disease associated	Asthma Crohn's disease Erythema multiforme Fungal infection including allergic bronchopulmonary aspergillosis Hyper IgE syndromes Immunodeficiencies Reiter's syndrome Sarcoidosis Syphilis Ulcerative colitis

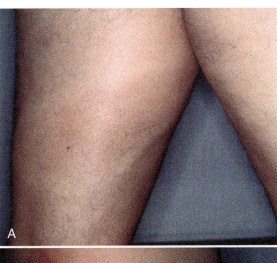
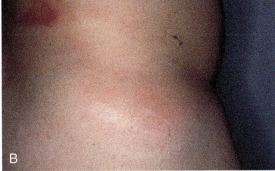
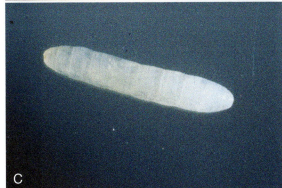

FIGURE 9-2 ■ Myiasis with indurated, erythematous pruritic plaques on (**A**) backs of legs and (**B**) lateral trunk, recurrent lasting 4 to 7 days, associated with protracted multisystem disease and hypereosinophilia in peripheral blood and tissue caused by (**C**) *Hypoderma lineatum*. (From Starr J, Pruett JH, Yunginger JW, Gleich GJ. Myiasis due to *Hypoderma lineatum* infection mimicking the hypereosinophilic syndrome. Mayo Clin Proc July 2000;75(7):755–9.)

Treatments targeting IL-5 have provided new insights into understanding eosinophil-associated disease. Furthermore, several of the wide variety of surface molecules, including cytokine receptors, adhesion receptors, peptide (chemokine) receptors, and Siglec molecules, that regulate eosinophil growth, differentiation, homing, and activation, are being considered as potential therapeutic targets in eosinophil-related disorders; their utility for treatment remains to be determined in preclinical studies and future clinical trials. Importantly concerning these targeted therapies that deplete eosinophils, several lines of investigation indicate that deficiency of eosinophils is not associated with health consequences.

SUGGESTED READINGS

Fulkerson PC, Rothenberg ME. Targeting eosinophils in allergy, inflammation and beyond. Nat Rev Drug Discov 2013;12(2):117–29.

Gleich GJ, Klion AD, Lee JJ, Weller PF. The consequences of not having eosinophils. Allergy 2013;68(7):829–35.

Khoury P, Grayson PC, Klion AD. Eosinophils in vasculitis: characteristics and roles in pathogenesis. Nat Rev Rheumatol 2014;10(8): 474–83.

Lee J, Rosenberg HF. Eosinophils in Health and Disease. 1st ed. London; Waltham, MA: Elsevier/Academic Press; 2013. xxiii, 654 pp.

Radonjic-Hoesli S, Valent P, Klion AD, Wechsler ME, Simon HU. Novel targeted therapies for eosinophil-associated diseases and allergy. Annu Rev Pharmacol Toxicol 2015;55:633–56.

Valent P, Klion AD, Horny HP, Roufosse F, Gotlib J, Weller PF, et al. Contemporary consensuroposal on criteria and classification of eosinophilic disorders and related syndromes. J Allergy Clin Immunol 2012;130(3):607–612.e9.

Valent P, Gleich GJ, Reiter A, Roufosse F, Weller PF, Hellmann A, et al. Pathogenesis and classification of eosinophil disorders: a review of recent developments in the field. Expert Rev Hematol 2012;5(2):157–76.

Wagelie-Steffen A, Aceves SS. Eosinophilic disorders in children. Curr allergy asthma Rep 2006;6(6):475–82.

CHAPTER 10

URTICARIA

Julie B. Zang • Joseph L. Jorizzo

KEY POINTS

- Urticaria is characterized by development of wheals and/or angioedema of the skin or mucosa. Individual lesions have a transient nature lasting less than 24 hours.
- Infection, drugs, chemicals, foods, inhalants, contactants, and physical stimuli are several recognizable triggers of urticaria. Urticaria can also be associated with endocrinopathies, autoimmune connective tissue diseases, and malignancies. However, in many cases, the cause of urticaria can remain unexplained despite extensive work-up, especially in chronic urticaria.
- Lesions that last longer than 24 hours are urticarial. On cursory clinical examinations, a few diseases, such as urticarial vasculitis, bradykinin-mediated angioedema, and mast cell disorders, can be mistaken as urticaria.
- Treatments of urticaria aim at eliminating the triggers as well as symptomatic control. Antihistamines, anti-inflammatory and immunosuppressive agents have demonstrated efficacy.

Urticaria is characterized by wheals (hives) and/or angioedema. It affects up to 20% of the population at some point and occurs across the age spectrum. Wheals are well-demarcated swelling of the superficial dermis surrounded by a reflex erythema (Fig. 10-1, A). The size and number of the lesions vary. It is associated with an itching or burning sensation. Lesions typically come and go within 24 hours, although the overall condition may persist with fresh crops of wheals occurring in other areas. Angioedema is characterized by sudden pronounced swelling in the deeper dermis, subcutaneous or submucosal tissue. It appears as brawny nonpitting edema. It is less well demarcated than wheals and often painful rather than pruritic. It lasts for 2 to 3 days. Lips, tongues, eyelids, genitalia, and rarely bowels are affected (Fig. 10-1, B).

Acute urticaria is defined as occurrence of spontaneous wheals, angioedema, or both for less than 6 weeks. If an allergic cause is suggested by the patient's history, such as medications or food, occasionally skin testing or immunoassays to identify the triggers for acute urticaria can be useful. It is important to exclude anaphylaxis in patients presenting with acute urticaria, as they may have common triggers. Involvement of respiratory (wheezing and cough), gastrointestinal (diarrhea and vomiting), neurologic (dizziness and loss of consciousness), or cardiac (change in heart rate and blood pressure) systems are concerning and could progress to anaphylaxis.

Episodes of urticaria and/or angioedema lasting longer than 6 weeks are designated as chronic. Duration can vary from months to many years. In 90% to 97% of patients with chronic urticaria, the cause is found. Fifty percent of patients with chronic urticaria for 6 months will have active disease 10 years later.

PATHOGENESIS

Urticaria and angioedema may be a final common pathway for a number of immunologic or nonimmunologic reactions that lead to cutaneous vasodilatation with extravasation of edema fluid in response to perivascular inflammation. It is believed that the vascular reaction in most patients with urticaria results from the release of proinflammatory mediators from mast cells and basophils. The most important mediator is histamine. Others include heparin, tryptase, platelet-activating factor, prostaglandins, leukotrienes, eosinophil chemotactic factor of anaphylaxis, neutrophil chemotactic factor, serotonin, and cytokines, such as tumor necrosis factor-alpha (TNF-α). Mediators produce vascular permeability with extravasation of plasma into the dermis or subcutaneous tissue. The delayed reaction produces tissue infiltration with eosinophils, neutrophils, and monocytes.

IgE-mediated immediate hypersensitivity reaction is a classical mechanism of mast cell activation. IgE antibody is produced in response to an antigen. IgE binds to mast cell or basophil Fc receptors. Exposure to the antigen results in Fab binding and crosslinking of IgE molecules, initiating a cascade of calcium-dependent processes that leads to release of proinflammatory mediators. Categories of antigen that may produce urticaria by a presumed IgE-dependent mechanism are listed in Table 10-1. Physical stimuli may produce antigens that react with IgE and lead to the release of mast cell-derived mediators, giving rise to a subtype of urticaria, physical urticaria.

Immunologically mediated urticaria may also occur via anti-IgE and anti-FcεRI antibodies. IgG anti-IgE antibody crosslinks IgE molecules, which in turn bind to two adjacent Fc receptors on mast cells. IgG anti-FcεRI antibody crosslinks two adjacent Fc receptors directly and triggers the cascade of mast cell degranulation without allergen exposure. These autoantibodies are present in a large number of patients with chronic idiopathic urticaria, termed chronic autoimmune urticaria.

Urticaria or a distinct disease, urticarial vasculitis, may occur in diseases with circulating immune complexes, such as systemic lupus erythematosus and hepatitis B. Immune complexes activate the complement cascade,

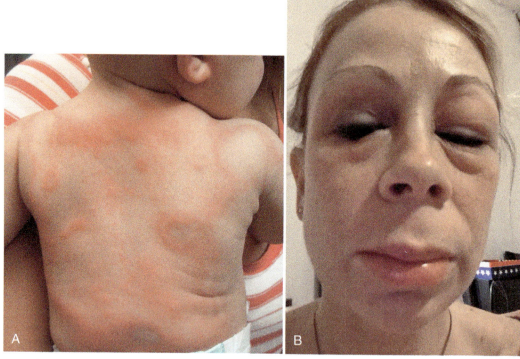

FIGURE 10-1 ■ **A,** Urticaria. **B,** Angioedema.

generating C3a and C5a, potent anaphylotoxins capable of causing mast cell degranulation.

Nonimmunologic mechanisms independent of IgE can also cause release of mast cell mediators. Radiocontrast media, opiates, some neuropeptides (e.g., substance P), and some foods, including eggs, strawberries, and shellfish, are some examples. They bind to specific receptors on mast cells and produce mast cell degranulation. Nonsteroidal anti-inflammatory drugs (NSAIDs), including aspirin, induce the lipoxygenase pathway and increase the synthesis of arachidonic acid metabolites such as leukotrienes, which are potent vasodilators formerly called slow-reacting substances of anaphylaxis.

CLASSIFICATION

There is a wide spectrum of clinical manifestations of urticaria subtypes. Two or more types of urticaria can sometimes coexist in the same patient. Table 10-2 presents the EAACI/GA²LEN/EDF/WAO, an international multispecialty panel consensus on classification of chronic urticaria updated in 2013.

Physical urticarias are an important subgroup of the chronic urticarias, where wheals and/or angioedema are induced by environmental stimuli such as heat, cold, pressure, exercise, water, vibration, and sunlight (Table 10-3). Symptomatic dermatographism (Fig. 10-2) is the most common of all physical urticarias. It manifests as a prompt wheal-and-flare response to stroking pressure applied to the skin. Cold contact urticaria refers to pruritus and swelling with exposure of the skin to contact with a cold stimulus. The diagnosis can be confirmed by applying an ice cube to the forearm skin and observing the wheal-and-flare reaction during rewarming of the skin. Systemic symptoms, such as flushing, headache, syncope, and abdominal pain, can develop if the patient is widely exposed to cold, e.g., cold baths and swimming. A less common and potentially life-threatening form of cold urticaria occurs with cold air exposure. Delayed pressure urticaria is swelling with onset 3 to 12 hours after a pressure stimulus is applied to the skin. Solar urticaria happens when the skin is exposed to various wavelengths of ultraviolet and visible light. Its diagnosis can be confirmed with phototesting. Heat urticaria is one of the rarest forms of urticaria. Within minutes of contact with heat, itching and whealing occur at the site of contact. Vibratory angioedema refers to pruritus and localized swelling within minutes of skin exposure to a vibratory stimulus, with lesions lasting for approximately 1 hour. Cholinergic urticaria occurs 15 minutes after an increase in the core body temperature. Triggers include physical exertion, sudden emotional stress, drinking alcohol, eating spicy food, etc. It presents as multiple pinpointed (1 to 3 mm) papules surrounded by large flares with a predilection for the upper body. Aquagenic urticaria is rare. It is characterized by 1 to 3 mm papules, which occur after direct contact of the skin with any source of water independent of the temperature. Interestingly, patients have no problem consuming water. IgE-mediated immediate hypersensitivity mechanisms are involved in several physical urticarias, supported by passive and reverse passive transfer experiments.

Physical urticarias may last for many years. In most patients, it is caused by a specific physical stimulus; in rare cases, multiple physical stimuli can trigger urticaria in the same patient. Sometimes patients with physical urticaria may also have concomitant chronic idiopathic urticaria, in which case they are less likely to respond to conventional pharmacotherapy.

TABLE 10-1 Some Causes of Urticaria*

Infections
Bacterial infections
    Dental abscess
    Sinusitis
    Otitis
    Pneumonitis
    Gastritis
    Hepatitis
    Cholecystitis
    Cystitis
    Vaginitis
Fungal infections
    Dermatophytes
    Candida
Other infections/infestations
    Scabies
    Helminth
    Protozoa
    Trichomonas

Drugs and Chemicals
Salicylates
Indometacin and other, newer nonsteroidal anti-inflammatory agents[†]
Opiates[†]
Radiocontrast material[†]
Penicillin (medication, milk, blue cheese)
Sulfonamides
Sodium benzoate
Douches
Ear drops or eye drops
Insulin
Menthol (cigarettes, toothpaste, iced tea, hand cream, lozenges, candy)
Tartrazine (vitamins, birth control pills, antibiotics, FDC yellow #5)

Foods
Nuts
Berries[†]
Fish
Seafood
Shellfish[†]
Bananas
Grapes
Tomatoes
Eggs[†]
Cheese

Inhalants
Animal danders
Pollen

Contactants
Wool
Silk
Occupational exposure
Potatoes
Antibiotics
Cosmetics
    Dyes
    Hairspray
    Nail polish
    Mouthwash
    Toothpaste
    Perfumes
    Hand cream
    Soap
Insect repellent

Physical Stimuli
Light
Pressure
Heat
Cold
Water
Vibration

Endocrinopathies
Thyroid disease
Diabetes mellitus
Pregnancy
Menstruation
Menopause

Systemic Diseases
Rheumatic fever
Connective tissue diseases (lupus erythematosus, Sjögren's syndrome, rheumatoid arthritis, Still's disease, dermatomyositis, polymyositis, other)
Leukemia
Lymphoma
Acquired immunodeficiency disease
Ovarian tumors

*Partial list of most frequently described causes in each category.
[†]May be mediated by nonimmunologic mechanisms independent of IgE.

The term contact urticaria describes urticaria after contact with eliciting substances. It occurs within 30 to 60 minutes and resolves within 24 hours. More commonly, it is a nonimmunologic response to chemicals that cause direct release of vasoactive substances. Acetylcholine and serotonin in nettle stings is an example. Contact urticaria can also be an immediate hypersensitivity reaction mediated by IgE antibodies specific to the eliciting allergen. Patients with atopic dermatitis are predisposed to this immunologic type of contact urticaria. Repeated exposure can produce anaphylaxis.

Diseases Related to Urticaria

Table 10-2 lists diseases that may be confused with urticaria.

Individual urticarial lesions of serum sickness-like reactions last for more than 24 hours. These reactions may be circulating immune complex mediated and occur 1 to 2 weeks after exposure to antigens, such as heterologous serum (classical reaction) or certain infectious agents or drugs. Systemic signs and symptoms may include fever, arthralgias, arthritis, myalgias, lymphadenopathy, elevated liver function tests, and proteinuria.

In urticarial vasculitis, lesions resemble urticaria (Fig. 10-3) but are often burning and painful, last for 24 to 72 hours, and leave residual purpura. The diagnosis should be confirmed by biopsy, demonstrating leukocytoclastic vasculitis. Angioedema may occur in 40% of patients. Urticarial vasculitis is reported to be associated with autoimmune connective tissue diseases (especially systemic lupus erythematous and Sjögren's syndrome),

TABLE 10-2	Classification of Chronic Urticaria Subtypes and Diseases Related to Urticaria	
Chronic urticaria subtypes	Chronic spontaneous urticaria	Spontaneous appearance of wheals, angioedema or both ≥6 weeks due to known or unknown causes
	Inducible urticaria	• Symptomatic dermatographism* • Cold urticaria[†] • Delayed pressure urticaria[‡] • Solar urticaria • Heat urticaria[§] • Vibratory angioedema • Cholinergic urticaria • Aquagenic urticaria • Contact urticaria
Diseases related to urticaria		• Serum sickness-like reaction; urticarial vasculitis • Bradykinin-mediated angioedema (e.g., hereditary angioedema) • Mast cell disorders (e.g., urticaria pigmentosa) • Exercise-induced anaphylaxis

Syndromes that present with wheals and/or angioedema		• Cryopyrin-associated periodic syndromes (CAPS)
		  • Familial cold autoinflammatory syndrome (FCAS)
		  • Muckle–Wells syndrome (MWS)
		  • Neonatal onset multisystem inflammatory disease (NOMID)
		• Schnitzler syndrome
		• Gleich's syndrome

*Also called *urticaria factitia* dermatographic urticaria.
[†]Also called cold contact urticaria.
[‡]Also called pressure urticaria.
[§]Also called heat contact urticaria.

cryoglobulinemia, paraproteinemia, and infections, such as hepatitis B and C. Urticarial vasculitis can have either low or normal complement levels (C4, C3, and C1q). Patients with normal complement levels often have skin-limited diseases. When complement levels are decreased, the disease course tends to be more severe and persistent. In some cases this may be due to IgG antibodies to C1q.

When recurrent angioedema occurs without wheals or pruritus, it is important to consider the possibility of C1 esterase inhibitor deficiency. C1 esterase deficiency is usually hereditary, but may be acquired. Hereditary angioedema (HAE) occurs as an autosomal dominant genodermatosis caused by mutation in one copy of the C1 esterase inhibitor gene. It results in reduced levels of C1 inhibitor (type I HAE, 85% of cases) or reduced C1 inhibitor function (type II HAE, 15% of cases). Acquired angioedema (AAE) is due to the formation of inhibitory autoantibodies against C1 inhibitor, often in the setting of lymphoproliferative diseases, paraproteinemia, or systemic lupus erythematosus. The subsequent consumption of complements leads to low levels of C4, which is a diagnostic feature between and during attacks in untreated patients. Type III hereditary angioedema is a newly reported type of familial angioedema with a female preponderance, where patients have normal C1 esterase inhibitor levels and activity. Skin is the most commonly affected organ, showing painful and disfiguring swelling. Gastrointestinal colic, nausea, vomiting, and diarrhea occur in one-quarter of the attacks and are experienced at some point by most HAE patients. The least common (<1%) but potentially life-threatening complication of upper airway attacks may even result in asphyxiation. Attacks usually last 48 to 72 hours and are followed by a refractory period. Angiotensin-converting enzyme (ACE) inhibitor can induce angioedema without urticaria. It is believed to be mediated by bradykinin as well.

Mastocytosis is frequently associated with urticarial lesions (Chapter 42).

Urticaria can be a manifestation of exercise-induced anaphylaxis (EIAn). There are two subgroups of patients with EIAn. One group experiences anaphylaxis provoked by exercise alone. The second group experiences anaphylaxis when exercise happens in temporal proximity to ingestion of food such as gluten. Cholinergic urticaria, a type of physical urticaria, can be associated with exercise as well. However, EIAn differs from cholinergic urticaria in that it can happen in temperature-controlled environments, whereas cholinergic urticaria is associated with sweating/increased core body temperature. Diagnostically, cholinergic urticaria but not EIAn can be triggered by a hot bath.

Distinctive Urticarial Syndromes

Urticaria is also a feature of several syndromes (Table 10-2). Cryopyrin-associated periodic syndromes (CAPS) are a group of autoinflammatory syndromes generally caused by autosomal-dominant mutation of the *NLRP3* gene (formerly the *CIAS1* gene), which encodes for the cryopyrin protein. The mutation causes a complex cascade that results in increased IL-1β, activating the inflammation seen in CAPS. There are three subtypes—familial cold autoinflammatory syndrome (FCAS), Muckle–Wells syndrome (MWS), and neonatal-onset multisystem inflammatory disease (NOMID)/chronic infantile neurologic, cutaneous, and articular syndrome (CINCA). FCAS

TABLE 10-3 Comparison of the Physical Urticarias

Urticaria	Relative Frequency	Precipitant	Time of Onset	Duration	Local Symptoms	Systemic Symptoms	Tests	Mechanism	Treatment
Symptomatic dermatographism	Most frequent	Stroking skin	Minutes	2–3 hours	Irregular pruritic attacks	None	Scratch skin	Passive transfer, IgE, histamine, possible role of adenosine triphosphate, substance P, possible direct pharmacologic mechanism	Continual antihistamines
Delayed dermatographism	Rare	Stroking skin	30 minutes to 8 hours	<48 hours	Burning, deep swelling	None	Scratch skin, observe early and late	Unknown	Avoidance of precipitants
Primary cold contact urticaria	Frequent	Cold contact	2–5 minutes	1–2 hours	Pruritic wheals	Wheezing, syncope, drowning	Apply ice-filled copper beaker to arm, immerse	Passive transfer, reverse passive transfer, IgE (IgM), histamine, vasculitis can be induced	Cyproheptadine hydrochloride, other antihistamines; desensitization; avoidance of precipitants
Familial cold urticaria	Rare	Change in skin temperature	30 minutes to 3 hours	<48 hours	Burning wheals	Tremor; headache; arthralgia; fever	Expose skin to cold air	Unknown	Avoidance of precipitants
Delayed pressure urticaria	Frequent	Pressure	3–12 hours	8–24 hours	Diffuse, tender swelling	Flu-like symptoms	Apply weight	Unknown	Avoidance of precipitants; if severe, low doses of corticosteroids given for systemic effects
Solar urticaria	Frequent	Various wavelengths of light	2–5 minutes	15 minutes to 3 hours	Pruritic wheals	Wheezing, dizziness, syncope	Phototest	Passive transfer, reverse passive transfer, IgE, possibly histamine	Avoidance of precipitants; antihistamines, sunscreens, antimalarials
Heat urticaria	Rare	Heat contact	2–5 minutes (rarely delayed)	1 hour	Pruritic wheals	None	Apply hot water-filled cylinder to arm	Possibly histamine; possibly complement	Antihistamines; desensitization; avoidance of precipitants
Vibratory angioedema	Very rare	Vibrating against skin	2–5 minutes	1 hour	Angioedema	None reported	Apply vibration to forearm	Unknown	Avoidance of precipitants
Cholingeric urticaria	Very frequent	General overheating of body	2–20 minutes	30 minutes to 1 hour	Papular, pruritic wheals	Syncope; diarrhea; vomiting, salivation; headaches	Bathe in hot water; exercise until perspiring, inject methacholine chloride	Passive transfer; possible immuno-globulin; product of sweat gland stimulation; histamine, reduced protease	Application of cold water or ice to skin; hydroxyzine regimen; refractory period; anticholinergics
Aquagenic urticaria	Rare	Water contact	Several minutes	30–45 minutes	Papular, pruritic wheals	None reported	Apply water compresses to skin	Unknown	Avoidance of precipitants; antihistamines; application of inert oil

From Jorizzo JL, Smith EG. The physical urticarias. Arch Dermatol 1982;118:194–201, with permission.

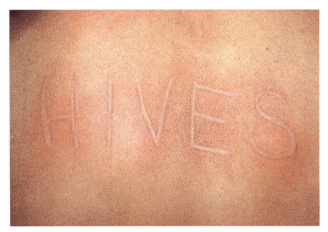

FIGURE 10-2 ■ Dermatographism. Stroking of the skin leads to the urticarial reaction.

patients develop a systemic inflammatory response a few hours following exposure to even mild cold. Symptoms include burning papular urticaria-like lesions, fever, chills, arthralgias, myalgias, headaches, and conjunctivitis. Duration of most flares lasts less than 1 day. MWS is similar to FCAS, but is more chronic and has random unknown triggers. NOMID/CINCA is the most severe form of CAPS with onset within the first 6 weeks after birth. Patients not only have urticaria, fever/chills, and other symptoms of CAPS, but also develop significant disabilities including bony overgrowth (especially knees and elbows), mental retardation, optic nerve malformation (papilledema), and chronic aseptic meningitis. Anti-IL-1 therapies, such as anakinra, rilonacept, and canakinumab, are beneficial for the treatment of CAPS.

Schnitzler syndrome patients develop chronic recurrent nonpruritic urticaria accompanied with recurrent fevers, a monoclonal IgM gammopathy, and bone and joint pain. NSAIDs, systemic corticosteroids, immunosuppressive agents, and IL-1 receptor antagonists have been reported to be beneficial.

Gleich's syndrome is characterized by episodic angioedema and fever lasting usually less than a week, associated with hypereosinophilia and elevated immunoglobulin M. It is benign with no internal organ involvement; however, recurrent episodic angioedema can be incapacitating. Severe attacks may be controlled by systemic corticosteroids.

DIAGNOSIS AND DIFFERENTIAL DIAGNOSIS

The diagnosis of a cutaneous eruption as urticaria is not usually difficult, because of the characteristic appearance and short duration of the individual lesions. During the cutaneous examination, clinicians can assess for dermatographism by firmly stroking the skin on the patient's back. Clinicians may draw a circle with a pen around a new lesion and ask the patient to report later on the duration of that individual lesion. Lesions that last for more than 24 hours are urticarial, not urticaria.

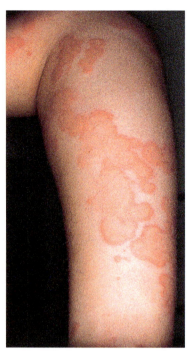

FIGURE 10-3 ■ Urticarial lesions in a patient with urticarial vasculitis. These lesions may take several days to resolve.

The presence of purpura after the wheal resolves may aid to distinguish urticarial vasculitis from urticaria, especially if purpura is present on nonexcoriated truncal skin. Histopathologic examination is not required for routine urticaria; however, if circled individual lesions last longer than 24 hours, then these urticarial lesions must be biopsied. Urticarial vasculitis is characterized by fibrinoid necrosis of blood vessel walls, infiltration with neutrophils showing karyorrhexis, extravasation of red blood cells, and endothelial swelling. The histopathology of urticaria is characterized by dermal edema and a scant mixed perivascular infiltrate of lymphocytes, neutrophils, and eosinophils.

Other dermatologic diseases may have diagnostic lesions that occur in association with or are superimposed on urticarial eruptions, such as bullous pemphigoid with an urticarial eruption and subsequent tense blisters, and erythema multiforme with target-like urticarial lesions. Insect bites often appear urticarial but last for several days, and close examination usually discloses a central punctum.

The lesions of urticaria result from infiltration of the dermis with fluid, giving the tissue an orange-peel appearance like that produced by intradermal injections (e.g., intradermal skin tests). Other dermal infiltrative diseases can occasionally be confused with urticaria on cursory cutaneous examination. These longstanding infiltrative conditions include granulomatous infiltrates (e.g., sarcoidosis, leprosy, and cutaneous tuberculosis), malignant infiltrates (e.g., cutaneous T-cell lymphoma, and metastatic disease), fibrous processes (e.g., morphea), metabolic deposits (e.g., amyloidosis and mucinosis), and nonurticarial inflammatory infiltrates (e.g., tumid lesions of lupus erythematosus, and lymphocytoma cutis).

When only angioedema is present, without wheals and pruritus, bradykinin-dependent angioedema must be considered.

PATIENT EVALUATION

Evaluation of the patient with urticaria begins with a thorough history. The patient must understand that urticaria may result from a newly developed allergy to a medication or other substance to which they have been exposed for years. The patient may be encouraged to keep a personal diary of possible exposures associated with meals, work, medication, environmental exposures, etc., during 12 to 24 hours prior to the onset of each outbreak of urticaria. The clinician should inquire specifically about certain exposures typically associated with urticaria (Table 10-1).

A specific trigger is much more likely to be identified in acute urticaria than in chronic urticaria. A comprehensive physical examination is important for all patients with chronic urticaria. Not only might systemic signs associated with the urticaria be revealed, but also clues as to etiologic systemic disease might be unveiled.

Laboratory testing should be ordered when suggested by the history and physical examination. A complete blood count with differential, Westergren sedimentation rate, urinalysis, and chemistry profile might be a screening approach for the patient with urticaria of unknown cause that lasts for more than 1 to 2 weeks. These tests might provide leads for obtaining supplemental information from the history and physical examination, and suggest additional evaluation (Table 10-4).

A number of chronic infectious processes have been reported to cause urticaria, including viral infections, such as hepatitis B and C, Epstein–Barr virus, and herpes simplex virus; *Helicobacter pylori* infections; and helminthic parasitic infections. For example, a patient with urticaria who has intermittent diarrhea and peripheral blood eosinophilia should undergo multiple stool evaluations for ova and parasites. Urticaria is associated with numerous autoimmune connective tissue diseases (Table 10-1). It can sometimes be a presenting symptom. Serology is warranted if there are any additional features to suggest a concomitant autoimmune disease. Screening for thyroid-stimulating hormone and thyroid antibodies in a patient with weight gain and other thyroid-related symptoms is recommended. However, without any symptoms or history, laboratory screening tests have a low yield. A significant number of urticaria patients with thyroid antibodies are euthyroid. It is unclear whether treatment of the euthyroid patients with thyroxine can lead to improvement of urticaria. Lymphoproliferative malignancies and endocrine tumors, such as ovarian tumors, although rare, may also present with urticaria.

Lastly, autologous serum skin test (ASST) and autologous plasma skin test (APST) are assays developed to measure autoantibodies, such as anti-IgE and anti-FcεRI antibodies, present in a large number of chronic idiopathic urticaria patients. However, positive ASSTs have been seen in patients with allergic rhinitis and healthy individuals without urticaria. Moreover, patients with a positive ASST do not appear to respond to treatments differently compared with patients with a negative ASST. Thus, routine performance of an ASST or APST in chronic urticaria patients is not recommended.

TABLE 10-4 Laboratory Tests that May Be Helpful in the Evaluation of Urticaria

Complete blood count
Liver function tests
Renal function tests
Thyroid function tests
Erythrocyte sedimentation rate/C-reactive protein
Antinuclear antibody test
C3, C4, CH50, and C1q
Hepatitis B and C serology
Herpes simplex virus and Epstein-Barr virus serology or culture
Urinalysis
Stool specimen examination for ova and parasites
Helicobacter pylori serology or breath test
Herpes simplex virus and Epstein-Barr virus serology or culture
Anti-DNase B or the streptococcal serology
Mononucleosis serology
Syphilis serology
Sinus radiographs
Dental radiographs
Chest radiograph
Vaginal smear
Pulmonary function tests
Serum and urine protein electrophoresis and immunofixation
Skin biopsy
Autologous serum skin test (ASST) and autologous plasma skin test (APST)
Basophil and mast cell histamine release assays
Other specific tests as directed by history and physical examination

TREATMENT

The treatment of acute or chronic urticaria consists of removal of the cause when and if possible, and treatment of the signs and symptoms. Acute urticaria is, by definition, self-limiting. An evaluation aimed at uncovering the cause of acute urticaria is warranted to permit avoidance of the offending precipitant to prevent future attacks. Therapy of urticaria is aimed at controlling signs and symptoms (Fig. 10-4).

As part of the treatment approach, many clinicians advocate empiric trials with elimination diets, even if a careful history excludes the common precipitants listed in Table 10-1 One approach is to use a very restrictive diet, such as rice and water, for 3 to 4 days. If the patient has urticaria while eating only rice and water, the urticaria is almost certainly not food related. However, if the urticaria resolves on this diet, foods can be reintroduced gradually until the urticaria recurs. In this way, the offending substance may be identified. Other general points of therapy include the avoidance of dairy products in penicillin-sensitive individuals (dairy products from penicillin-treated cattle may contain traces of penicillin) and the avoidance of

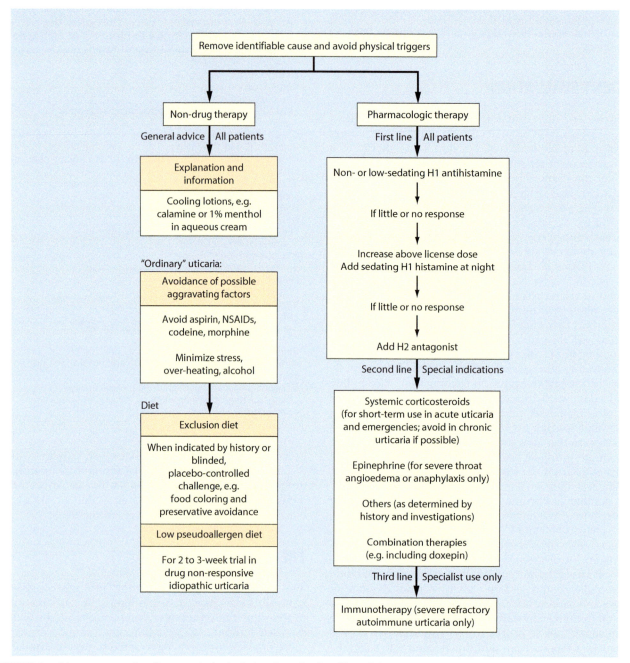

FIGURE 10-4 ■ Management of ordinary and physical chronic urticarias. (From Bolognia JL, Jorizzo JL, Schaffer, JV, Dermatology. 3rd ed. vol 1; © 2012, Elsevier Limited.)

NSAIDs, opiate derivatives, or ACE inhibitors that may exacerbate urticaria of any cause by nonimmunologic mechanisms.

Emergency measures include the administration of epinephrine (adrenaline) (1:1000, 0.3 to 0.5 mL subcutaneously), which reduces the release of histamine from mast cells by increasing cyclic adenosine monophosphate levels within the cells, and also directly affects respiratory smooth muscle. Tracheostomy may rarely be required. Patients prone to develop laryngeal edema, such as those with hereditary angioedema, should be given commercially available kits containing preloaded epinephrine (adrenaline) syringes with instructions for intramuscular injection.

Antihistamines with a specificity for H_1 receptors are the treatment of choice for almost all types of urticaria. These agents competitively inhibit histamine at the H_1 receptor of blood vessels. Antihistamines do not prevent the release of histamine from mast cells; therefore, they must be given to the patient around the clock. Simply taking the antihistamine "when I get hives" is practically useless because the histamine will have already bound to H_1 receptors and have induced its pathologic effects. In most studies, hydroxyzine is the most effective traditional antihistamine. The dosage can be low initially (10 mg orally every 6 hours, with 20 to 30 mg at bedtime), with a relatively prompt increase to the maximal dosage to control lesions (50 to 100 mg four times daily).

TABLE 10-5 Antihistamines for Urticaria

Class	Examples	Half-life (hours)	Daily Adult Dose*
Classic (sedating) H_1 antihistamines	Chlorpheniramine (1)	12–15	4 mg three times daily (up to 12 mg at night)
	Hydroxyzine (1)	20	10–25 mg three times daily (up to 75 mg at night)
	Diphenhydramine (2)	4	10–25 mg at night
	Doxepin† (1)	17	10–50 mg at night
Second-generation H_1 antihistamines	Acrivastine‡ (1)	2–4	8 mg three times daily
	Cetirizine§ (1)	7–11	10 mg once daily
	Loratadine (1)	8–11	10 mg once daily
	Mizolastine‖ (1)	13	10 mg once daily
Newer second-generation H_1 antihistamines	Desloratadine (1)	19–35	5 mg once daily
	Fexofenadine (1)	17	180 mg once daily
	Levocetirizine (1)	7–10	5 mg once daily
	Rupatadine (1)	6	10 mg once daily
H_2 antagonists¶	Cimetidine (1)	2	400 mg twice daily
	Ranitidine (2)	2–3	150 mg twice daily

A short-acting classic antihistamine may be added at night to a daily second-generation antihistamine, with or without the addition of an H_2 antagonist for maximal antihistamine blockade. Key to evidence-based support: (1) prospective controlled trial; (2) retrospective study or large case series; (3) small case series or individual case reports.
*Current prescribing manuals should be consulted for details on doses in children.
†Possesses potent H_1 and H_2 antihistamine properties.
‡Only available in the United States as a combination product with pseudoephedrine for seasonal allergic rhinitis.
§The active metabolite of hydroxyzine.
‖Not available in the United States.
¶Used in combination with H_1 antagonist.
From Bolognia JL, Jorizzo JL, Schaffer, JV. Dermatology. 3rd ed. vol. 1, Table 18.5. Elsevier Limited.

The major side effects are sedation and anticholinergic effects, such as dry mouth, tachycardia, double vision, urinary retention, and constipation. If hydroxyzine is ineffective, an H_1 antihistamine from another class may be added (Table 10-5).

Controlling signs and symptoms of chronic urticaria can be much more challenging. First-line therapy includes the second-generation H_1 antihistamines such as loratadine and fexofenadine. These antihistamines are safe, effective, and associated with less sedation than the classic antihistamines. Newer nonsedating antihistamines, such as desloratadine and levocetirizine, may offer greater clinical improvement. If symptomatic improvement is not fully achieved with initial licensed doses, additional benefit may be obtained from increasing to 2 to 3 times the daily dose. Caution is advised with high doses of fexofenadine, as it is an active metabolite of terfenadine, an antihistamine associated with arrhythmias and no longer available. Adding a sedating H_1 antihistamine to the regimen at bedtime can be helpful if symptoms interfere with sleep.

Doxepin is a potent agent with H_1 and H_2 antihistaminic effects that is commonly used to treat urticaria. Side effects including agranulocytosis, hallucinations, ataxia, cardiac effects, and photosensitization are generally controllable with lower dosing. Reports of synergistic therapeutic benefits from combining H_1 antihistamines and H_2 antagonists, such as cimetidine or ranitidine, have been balanced by reports showing no added benefit (Table 10-5). Some, but not all, studies have found leukotriene receptor antagonists, such as montelukast or zafirlukast to have efficacy in chronic urticaria. Given that these agents are generally well tolerated, they can be considered in patients with unsatisfactory responses with H_1 antihistamines (Table 10-6).

Patients with hereditary angioedema may have a dramatic reduction in the frequency and severity of attacks and may benefit during acute attacks from systemic treatment with attenuated androgens, such as danazol or stanozolol. These agents stimulate the synthesis of the deficient C1 esterase inhibitor.

Systemic corticosteroids are not recommended in the routine therapy of chronic urticaria, although they may be useful for urticarial vasculitis, urticarial lesions of bullous pemphigoid, and drug-induced hypersensitivity syndrome (DIHS, also called DRESS). High doses are required to benefit patients with chronic urticaria, but these doses cannot be maintained for the many years that numerous patients with chronic urticaria would require them.

Anti-inflammatory agents, such as hydroxychloroquine, dapsone, sulfasalazine, and colchicine have been demonstrated to have some efficacy and can be considered for treatment of patients with antihistamine-refractory chronic urticaria (Table 10-6). Newer data showing the presence of autoantibodies in many patients with chronic idiopathic urticaria have led to trials of immunosuppressive therapies, including cyclosporine (3 to 5 mg/kg/day), intravenous immunoglobulin (2 g/kg in total over 5 days), and plasmapheresis. Phototherapy with psoralens and ultraviolet A light has been reported to be beneficial. Ultimately, the cost and potential morbidities of these therapies and their inability to deliver the desired long-term remissions limit their value in patients with chronic idiopathic urticaria. Mycophenolate has been shown in a number of studies to be effective to treat antihistamine-refractory chronic urticaria. Methotrexate has been demonstrated to be a useful treatment for steroid-dependent, recalcitrant

TABLE 10-6 Alternative Therapies for Chronic or Physical Urticaria

Generic Name	Drug Class	Route	Dose	Special Indication/Associated Diseases
Prednisone (2)	Corticosteroid	Oral	0.5 mg/kg daily	Severe exacerbations (days only)
Epinephrine (2)	Sympathomimetic	Subcutaneous, intramuscular (self-administered)	300–500 mcg	Idiopathic or allergic angioedema of throat/anaphylaxis
Montelukast (3)	Leukotriene receptor antagonist	Oral	10 mg daily	Aspirin-sensitive urticaria, ? delayed pressure urticaria
Thyroxine (2)	Thyroid hormone	Oral	50–150 mcg daily	Autoimmune thyroid disease
Colchicine (3)	Neutrophil inhibitor	Oral	0.5/0.6–1.5/1.8 mg* daily	Neutrophilic infiltrates in lesional biopsy specimens or urticarial vasculitis
Sulfasalazine (3)	Aminosalicylates	Oral	2–4 g daily	Delayed pressure urticaria
Hydroxychloroquine (3)	Antimalarial	Oral	200 mg twice daily	Urticarial vasculitis and connective tissue diseases
Dapsone (3)	Myeloperoxidase inhibitor	Oral	25–50 mg daily	Angioedema, delayed pressure urticaria, and urticarial vasculitis
Cyclosporine (1)	Immunosuppressant	Oral	3–4 mg/kg/day	Chronic idiopathic and autoimmune urticaria
Mycophenolate (2)	Immunosuppressant	Oral	1000 mg twice daily	Chronic idiopathic and autoimmune urticaria
Methotrexate (2)	Antimetabolite	Oral	10–15 mg weekly	Steroid-dependent chronic urticaria
Omalizumab (1)	Monoclonal antibody	Subcutaneous (physician's office)	150–300 mg every 4 weeks	Asthma

Current prescribing manuals should be consulted for details on dose, drug interactions, and contraindications for individual patients. The stated doses represent guidelines only. Key to evidence-based support: (1) prospective controlled trial; (2) retrospective study or large case series; (3) small case series or individual case reports.
*Available in doses of 0.5 mg or 0.6 mg depending upon the country.
Adapted from Bolognia JL, Jorizzo JL, Schaffer. Dermatology, 3rd ed. vol. 1, Table 18.6. Elsevier Limited.

chronic urticaria (Table 10-6). The newest treatment is omalizumab (Xolair), a recombinant monoclonal antibody that binds to free IgE and inhibits binding of IgE to FcεRI on the mast cells. A number of large randomized trials have demonstrated its efficacy in the treatment of refractory chronic urticaria at a dose of 150 mg or 300 mg every month (Table 10-6). In 2014, omalizumab was Food and Drug Administration-approved for chronic idiopathic urticaria in patients 12 years of age and older.

SUGGESTED READINGS

Abajian M, Mlynek A, Maurer M. Physical urticaria. Curr Allergy Asthma Rep 2012;4:281–7.
Berstein JA, Lang DM, Khan DA. The diagnosis and management of acute and chronic urticaria: 2014 update. J Allergy Clin Immunol 2014;1270–1277.e66.
Brown NA, Carter JD. Urticarial vasculitis. Curr Rheumatol Rep 2007;9:312–9.
Frigas E, Park MA. Acute urticaria and angioedema: diagnostic and treatment considerations. Am J Clin Dermatol 2009;10:239–50.
Greenberger PA. Chronic urticaria: new management options. World Allergy Organ J 2014;7:31.
Sharman M, Bennett C, Cohen SN, Carter B. H1-antihistamines for chronic spontaneous urticaria. Cochrane Database Syst Rev 2014;11:CD006137.
Zuberbier T, Aberer W, Asero R, et al. The EAACI/GA²/EDF/WAO guideline for the definition, classification, diagnosis, and management of urticaria: the 2013 revision and update. Allergy 2014:868–87.

CHAPTER 11

Erythema Multiforme, Stevens–Johnson Syndrome, and Toxic Epidermal Necrolysis

Andrew Avarbock • Joseph L. Jorizzo

KEY POINTS

- Herpes simplex virus infection is a frequent cause of erythema multiforme, while drugs most often cause Stevens–Johnson syndrome and toxic epidermal necrolysis.
- Erythema multiforme is often self-limited, skin lesions often target-appearing, and mucosal lesions can occur in the absence of skin lesions.
- Stevens–Johnson syndrome patients have systemic illness with prominent mucosal involvement and may have skin sloughing.
- Toxic epidermal necrolysis patients have systemic illness and present with painful red skin that progresses to extensive skin sloughing.
- Survival for patients with Stevens–Johnson syndrome and toxic epidermal necrolysis improves with early intervention, and the benefit of immunomodulatory therapies is inconclusive.

Erythema multiforme (EM), Stevens–Johnson syndrome (SJS), and toxic epidermal necrolysis (TEN) are immunologically mediated, mucocutaneous reactions triggered by medications and infections. Disease can be self-limited as in EM or potentially fatal as in TEN. The current clinical classification of EM, SJS, and TEN is based on pattern and distribution of skin lesions and maximum extent of skin detachment. However, the clinical classification of these diseases is often debated, and although there is a better understanding of the molecular events leading to the disease state, there remains no standard of care for treatment.

EM is the least severe of the mucocutaneous reactions. It is self-limited, characterized by classic true target lesions—with three zones of inflammation—in the absence of widespread skin sloughing; there is variable mucous membrane involvement, and causality frequently from herpes simplex virus (HSV) or less often other causes. When systemic symptoms or extensive skin sloughing is present, with or without targetoid lesions or mucosal involvement, the diagnoses of SJS and TEN are considered.

PATHOGENESIS

Immune-mediated pathogenesis has long been suspected for EM, SJS, and TEN. Current concepts center on host immune response to various specific antigenic stimuli from drugs and infections. In EM patients, cutaneous lesions often result from cytotoxic reactions against HSV antigens expressed in epidermal keratinocytes. For the vast majority of patients with SJS and TEN, a cytotoxic reaction results from immunoreactivity against keratinocytes expressing drug-related antigens. Evidence supports a theory that patients are immunogenetically predisposed to developing their disease.

Multiple etiologic agents have been implicated as causes of EM, SJS, and TEN (Table 11-1). The best-documented causes of EM include HSV and *Mycoplasma pneumoniae*. Fragments of HSV DNA can be found in the cutaneous lesions of EM in more than 80% of cases. While many drugs have been reported to cause EM, such cases may lack classic target lesions and are currently often labeled as mild SJS. Other associations include mononucleosis, other viral infections (e.g., mumps, poliomyelitis, milker's nodule, and vaccinia), granuloma inguinale, psittacosis, histoplasmosis, syphilis, streptococcal infection, radiation therapy of tumors, sarcoidosis, pregnancy, carcinomas, reticuloses, leukemias, systemic lupus erythematosus (Rowell's syndrome), and other collagen–vascular diseases. A significant percentage of cases remain idiopathic.

Although there is a complex interplay between host immune cells, CD8+ cytotoxic T lymphocytes and natural killer cells appear mainly responsible for the keratinocyte apoptosis seen in the mucocutaneous reactions. The mechanism of immune cell activation is theorized to be secondary to the pro-hapten concept, p-i concept, or both. In the pro-hapten concept drug metabolites bind to cellular peptides creating a highly immunogenic molecule capable of immune system activation. In the p-i concept the drug or drug metabolite can bind directly to MHC or T-cell receptors and stimulate an immune response.

Several MHC I allotypes have been associated with increased incidence of SJS and TEN. Han Chinese, Thai, Malaysian, and South Indian populations with MHC I allotype (HLA)-B*1502 have increased risk of

TABLE 11-1	Possible Causes of Erythema Multiforme, Stevens–Johnson Syndrome, and Toxic Epidermal Necrolysis

Infectious agents
    Herpes simplex
    Mycoplasma pneumoniae
    Epstein–Barr virus
    Mumps
    Polio
    Calymmatobacterium
    Streptococcus
    Vaccinia
    Yersinia
    Tuberculosis
    Treponema pallidum
    Chlamydia
    Deep mycoses (e.g., histoplasmosis)
    Dengue virus
    Cytomegalovirus
Medications
    Sulfonamides
    Sulfasalazine
    NSAIDs
    Carbamazepine
    Phenytoin
    Lamotrigine
    Barbiturates
    Allopurinol
    Penicillins
    Cephalosporins
    Quinolones
    Tetracyclines
    Contrast agents
    Nevirapine
Other conditions
    Irradiation of tumors
    Immunizations
    Connective tissue disease (e.g., systemic lupus erythematosus)
    Sarcoidosis
    Inflammatory bowel disease
    Pregnancy

SJS/TEN from aromatic antiepileptic agents such as phenytoin, carbamazepine, lamotrigine, and oxcarbazepine. Likewise, populations of European descent with allotype HLA-B*5801 have increased incidence of allopurinol-induced SJS/TEN. These allotypes may be genetic markers or could be involved in the pathogenesis of the mucocutaneous syndromes. The US Food and Drug Administration recommends that patients of East Asian descent have testing for the HLA-B*1502 genotype prior to receiving carbamazepine.

The crucial mediator of keratinocyte apoptosis in the mucocutaneous reactions appears to be granulysin, a molecule found in the cytotoxic granules of CD8+, NK, and NK/T cells, which is capable of causing membrane instability and destruction resulting in cell death. Increased levels of granulysin are found in TEN blisters as well as serum and correlate with disease severity. Multiple other factors are implicated in the disease pathogenesis of SJS and TEN as well, including death receptor Fas (CD95), soluble Fas ligand (FasL) produced by peripheral blood mononuclear cells, and FasL on epidermal keratinocytes, cytotoxic T cells, and NK cells. Interaction of Fas and FasL induces signaling, which rapidly leads to apoptosis. Antibodies present in pooled human intravenous immunoglobulins (IVIg) may block Fas-mediated keratinocyte death, and use of IVIg for treatment of TEN rests on this theory. Markers of oxidative stress are also elevated in TEN patients, and may result from TNF-α- and IFN-γ-induced production of nitric oxide within inflammatory cells and keratinocytes. Other inflammatory mediators found elevated in TEN patients include alarmins, TRAIL (TNF-related apoptosis-inducing ligand), TWEAK (TNF-related weak apoptosis inducer), alpha-defensins, and granzyme B and perforin released by cytolytic T cells.

CLINICAL MANIFESTATIONS

The current classification of EM, SJS, and TEN is based on consensus definitions published in 1993. An international group reviewed hundreds of historical cases and agreed upon clinical definitions based on pattern and distribution of skin lesions and maximum extent of skin detachment. The consensus group determined that EM differed significantly enough from SJS and TEN that it represented its own clinical group, and SJS and TEN were variants of a single disease. However, while there is general agreement that EM represents a different disease, many believe that within the SJS and TEN spectrum exist two distinct diseases with different clinical presentations. Additionally, a mycoplasma-induced rash and mucositis syndrome may exist, distinct from EM/SJS and characterized by a mild disease course. Thus, the diagnosis of EM, SJS, and TEN is often debated and different clinical classifications exist.

Erythema Multiforme

EM begins with either a mild prodrome of malaise and low-grade fever or no systemic involvement at all. Skin lesions are often target-appearing (Fig. 11-1) with three concentric zones, most commonly: (1) a central dusky area, (2) a middle pink or edematous zone, and (3) an outer red ring. Although target lesions are characteristic of EM, lesions need only be monomorphic for an EM diagnosis, and target lesions themselves are not diagnostic for EM. Target lesions can be seen in viral-induced eruptions and may not show the characteristic histology necessary to confirm a diagnosis of EM. Lesions may be asymptomatic to burning or pruritic, last from 1 to 2 weeks, and tend to evolve to have a dusky appearance. Mucosal surfaces may be involved in EM (Fig. 11-2), and mucosal involvement can occur in the absence of skin lesions. Within EM, two variants have been observed and studied: HSV-associated cases with target lesions predominantly on the extremities and drug-associated cases with target lesions in a diffuse or central pattern. The distinct clinical presentations of EM appear to have different molecular mechanisms, as HSV-associated EM lesions express IFN-γ and drug-induced EM lesions express TNF-α. Recurrent EM is not uncommon, and is often due to HSV reactivation.

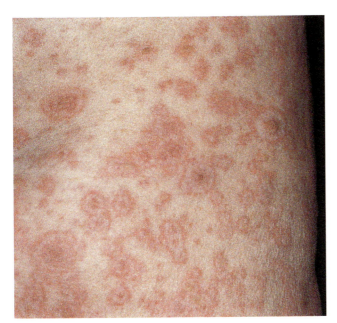

FIGURE 11-1 ■ Erythema multiforme with typical target lesions.

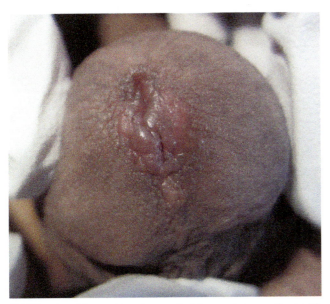

FIGURE 11-2 ■ Mucosal involvement of the penis in a patient with erythema multiforme.

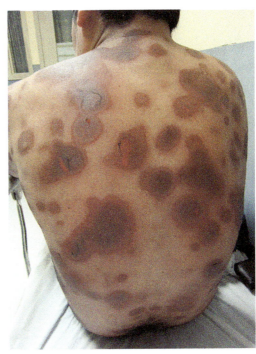

FIGURE 11-3 ■ Stevens–Johnson syndrome. Targetoid lesions as well as multiple bullae.

erythema), or other monomorphic lesions that may progress to skin denudation that is indistinguishable from TEN (Fig. 11-3). This definition emphasizes presenting symptoms and mucosal involvement and is similar to the original case descriptions of Stevens and Johnson in 1922 and Thomas in 1950 where patients had prodromal symptoms, mucosal involvement that was often ocular and oral, and a generalized skin eruption. Mucosal lesions of SJS may affect the ocular conjunctivae (Fig. 11-4), oral cavity (Fig. 11-5), vaginal mucosa or penis meatus, anal mucosa, and esophagus. Mucosal complications may include keratitis, conjunctival scarring, uveitis, scleral perforation, urethral stricture, vaginal scarring, and esophageal stricture. Patients may experience fevers, arthralgias, arthritis, myalgias, hepatitis, bronchopulmonary disease, glomerulonephritis, or acute renal tubular necrosis.

Stevens–Johnson Syndrome

The consensus group in 1993 suggested that SJS is a less severe variant of TEN, only differing by percent of skin involvement and not on clinical presentation. SJS was defined to involve less than 10% denudation of the total body surface area. Although this is a widely accepted definition, other opinion suggests SJS diagnostic criteria based on clinical disease presentation rather than resulting percent of skin sloughing. The classification we favor suggests that SJS presents with (1) a prodrome of fever and malaise for 1 day to 2 weeks, (2) two or more sites of mucous membrane involvement, and (3) skin involvement that may include characteristic true target lesions, targetoid lesions (with two zones of inflammation, such as central nonblanching redness surrounded by blanching

Toxic Epidermal Necrolysis

Lyell coined the term toxic epidermal necrolysis in the mid-1950s to refer to a severe illness characterized by a generalized scalded appearance of the skin and life-threatening serum-sickness-like features. The most common cause of TEN is hypersensitivity to a systemically administered medication. TEN is currently described to: (1) be preceded by a prodrome including fever, cough, and malaise, followed by a painful macular exanthem in a symmetrical distribution on the face and trunk, which spreads to the extremities, (2) develop the Nikolsky sign, where gentle lateral pressure causes skin separation, (3) blister with large sheets of epidermis sloughing off, and (4) feature gastrointestinal, respiratory, and genitourinary mucosal denudation. The 1993 consensus group defined TEN to involve more than 30% denudation of

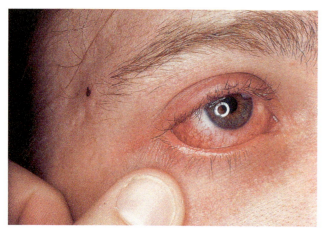

FIGURE 11-4 ■ Stevens–Johnson syndrome: conjunctivitis.

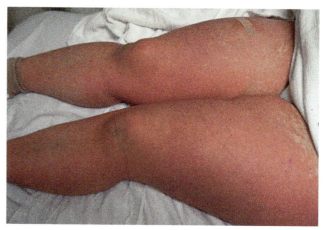

FIGURE 11-6 ■ Toxic epidermal necrolysis. This patient presented with painful erythematous skin.

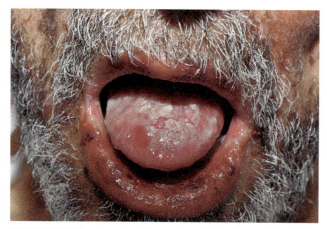

FIGURE 11-5 ■ Erosive glossitis and erosive lesions on the lips in this patient with Stevens–Johnson syndrome.

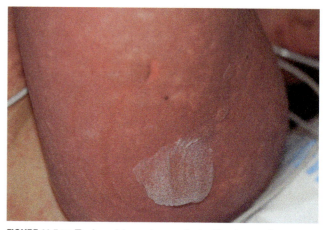

FIGURE 11-7 ■ Toxic epidermal necrolysis. Tender erythematous eruption with bullae formation and positive Nikolsky sign.

the total body surface area. For cases of epidermal detachment between 10% and 30%, an "SJS-TEN overlap" category was created. An important feature of TEN is the presentation of painful erythematous skin (Fig. 11-6) that progresses to denudation (Fig. 11-7).

Recovery from skin sloughing is slow, but it may be complete without scarring if excellent care is administered early in the disease course. Mortality is mainly from multiorgan failure secondary to sepsis. TEN mortality is predicted from the verified SCORTEN tool. One point is given for each clinical or biochemical risk factor, which includes: age >40 years, heart rate >120 beats per minute, comorbid malignancy, affected body surface area >10%, blood urea nitrogen >28 mg/dL, glucose >252 mg/dL, and bicarbonate <20 mEq/L. Mortality increases with points; 3.2% prediction for 0 or 1 point, 35.3% for 3 points, and up to 90% with 5 points or more.

Differential Diagnosis

The differential diagnosis of EM, SJS, and TEN must be divided into two categories: a differential for the cutaneous eruption and one for the mucosal lesions, which may occur alone. Erosive mucosal diseases include pemphigus vulgaris (histopathology showing acantholysis, with confirmatory direct and indirect immunohistochemistry), paraneoplastic pemphigus (diagnostic immunohistochemistry), herpetic gingivostomatitis (histopathology showing multinucleated giant cells, a diagnostic culture), recurrent aphthous stomatitis (morphology and time course of lesions suggesting diagnosis), cicatricial pemphigoid (histopathology showing dermoepidermal junction blister and confirmatory direct immunofluorescence), erosive lichen planus (diagnostic histopathology), graft-versus-host disease (GVHD) (suggestive if history includes transplantation, but indistinguishable on histopathology).

The differential diagnosis of the cutaneous lesions of EM is extensive, particularly if the skin lesions are not typical targets. Patients with typical EM with target lesions may have other cutaneous lesions that are clinicopathologically similar to those of simple erythema, urticaria, annular erythemas, viral exanthemas, secondary syphilis, toxic shock, or the following vasculitides: cutaneous small-vessel (leukocytoclastic) vasculitis, pustular vasculitis (disseminated gonococcemia or meningococcemia, or lesions of Behçet's or bowel bypass syndromes), or vasculitis associated with collagen–vascular diseases. Rowell's syndrome, characterized by EM-like lesions in a patient with lupus erythematosus, is also in the differential diagnosis. Detection of the classic target lesions together with typical histology confirm an EM diagnosis.

In typical cases the explosive presentation and dramatic physical findings leave little confusion about the diagnosis of TEN. However, other blistering conditions may resemble TEN, including drug-induced linear IgA bullous dermatosis, paraneoplastic pemphigus, and pemphigus vulgaris. Consideration must also be given for GVHD, AGEP, staphylococcal scalded skin syndrome, and initially a toxic erythroderma. GVHD can show similar clinical and histologic features to TEN, so distinguishing TEN from GVHD in a transplant patient may be difficult. AGEP may have confluent lakes of pus which can blister, but there is persistent intact epidermis. Staphylococcal scalded skin syndrome is excluded by histopathologic confirmation of a more superficial blister than that seen in TEN. There are many causes of acute erythroderma, but other than the blistering disorders, they do not progress to skin sloughing.

Histopathologic Findings

Although the classic target lesions of EM have a reproducible, typical histopathologic appearance, the clinician must be aware that individual lesions evolve over several days, and that the histopathologic findings in an individual lesion will vary depending on when in a lesion's lifespan it is biopsied and if therapy has been initiated. Also, if the clinician samples a lesion with the clinical characteristics of erythema or urticaria rather than with those of a target lesion, the histopathologic appearance may mimic that of those conditions. Biopsy specimens should be taken from the periphery of target lesions, not from the center, to have the best chance of showing keratinocyte changes.

Typical EM lesions show focal keratinocyte necrosis and spongiosis associated with vacuolar alterations of basal epidermal cells that may progress to a dermoepidermal junction zone blister. Nonspecific dermal changes include endothelial swelling, a superficial perivascular mononuclear cell infiltrate, and papillary dermal edema. The basement membrane remains intact and the lesions do not produce scarring. Extravasation of erythrocytes does occur in the dermis, but leukocytoclasia (infiltration of neutrophils with nuclear fragmentation) and fibrinoid necrosis of blood vessel walls never occurs. Oral lesions show similar histopathologic changes.

Direct immunofluorescence microscopy from lesions of EM is not diagnostic; however, a biopsy for immunofluorescence microscopy should be considered especially for mucosal lesions in the absence of skin lesions to exclude autoimmune bullous diseases such as paraneoplastic pemphigus. In early lesions of EM, immunoreactants such as C_3 and IgM may be detected in a granular pattern in the dermal blood vessels.

The histopathologic appearance of lesions of SJS and TEN may be identical to that of EM with extreme epidermal necrosis. The severity of the histologic findings in SJS and TEN is not associated with increased mortality. The cutaneous basement membrane remains at the base of the blister in TEN. Therefore, if secondary infection is prevented, it is believed that scarring will not occur; however, clinically, results vary widely. Scarring may occur on mucosal surfaces, the scalp, the fingernails, and the skin, probably as a result of secondary infection. A biopsy for routine processing should always be done, frozen sections for rapid diagnosis, and immunofluorescence should be considered in diagnostically uncertain cases.

Evaluation

The evaluation of a patient with mucocutaneous disease must address both confirmation of the diagnosis and exclusion of significant underlying disease as a cause. There is no specific laboratory abnormality associated with EM; therefore, the diagnosis is based on clinical parameters with histopathologic confirmation. Patients with EM may have leukocytosis, an elevated erythrocyte sedimentation rate, elevated liver function test results, proteinuria, and occasionally hematuria.

In addition to the routine histopathologic examination, a bedside evaluation of oral mucosal blisters may involve a Tzanck smear. In this preparation, a blister is unroofed, the base of the blister is scraped firmly, and the material obtained is placed on a glass slide and stained with Wright, Giemsa, or other suitable stain. EM blisters show only mixed inflammatory cells, but the acantholytic cells of pemphigus vulgaris or the multinucleate giant cells of herpes simplex infections can be excluded.

A thorough history and physical examination should be a prerequisite for the laboratory evaluation of the underlying causes of mucocutaneous disease. A careful drug history is particularly important. Obviously, suspected drugs should not be readministered, because of the risk of even more severe reactions. The signs and symptoms of infection must be sought. The history may suggest recent vaccination or hyposensitization as a precipitant.

A high index of suspicion for HSV infection is particularly relevant in recurrent EM. The diagnosis of HSV can be confirmed by Tzanck's preparation of an active vesicle, biopsy of a herpetic lesion, or culture of the virus from a herpetic lesion. Immunoperoxidase-labeled monoclonal antibodies and polymerase chain reaction are sensitive techniques that can substantiate the diagnosis of HSV infection. It is often difficult to distinguish the herpetic lesion from the EM lesion on mucosal surfaces, and it can be difficult to confirm HSV infection because of the time lag between HSV infection and onset of EM.

If other infections are suspected, appropriate imaging and laboratory studies can be ordered for confirmation. In particular, *M. pneumoniae* should be considered in cases of EM and SJS. A complete blood count, erythrocyte sedimentation rate, urinalysis, and liver function tests may be useful screening procedures in patients with EM, SJS, and TEN. Specialized tests (hepatitis serology; cultures for bacteria, fungi, and viral agents; syphilis serology; tuberculin skin testing; antinuclear antibody profile; rheumatoid factor; pregnancy test; imaging for infection or occult malignancies) can be ordered as suggested by the history, physical examination, and screening tests.

Treatment

Patients with drug-induced SJS and TEN should wear a bracelet carrying a warning of their drug allergy because a second exposure may result in even more severe illness; given potential genetic risk factors, some advocate counseling first-degree relatives to practice avoidance if feasible. However, there are also rare patients who have been inadvertently reexposed to putative agents that caused their disease and have had no further reactions. Treatment options have focused on suppressing an exaggerated immune response, but no treatment has been demonstrated in a double-blind study to consistently shorten disease course or reduce mortality.

EM may be an uncomplicated, self-limited condition that requires no treatment. Recurrent EM that is caused by HSV infection may be prevented by reducing the frequency of herpes infections (e.g., sunscreen use on the lips to reduce the frequency of sun-exacerbated herpes labialis). Oral acyclovir (200 mg twice daily), valacyclovir (500 mg once or twice daily), or famciclovir (250 mg twice daily) can reduce the incidence of herpes infection recurrences. Higher doses may be needed for HIV patients or other immunocompromised states. Oral prednisone may be utilized to decrease the mucocutaneous inflammation in EM and should be considered for patients with severe oral disease who cannot tolerate oral intake or require hospitalization.

The mortality rate in SJS may approach 5% and overall mortality in TEN may approach 30%. Mortality is reduced by withdrawal of the causative agent within 24 hours and early intervention with supportive care in an ICU or burn unit. An underlying drug allergy or infection must be diagnosed and corrected quickly. Supportive care may include maintaining the patient's fluid balance, temperature control, skin and mucosal barrier protection with aggressive emollient use, and recognition and treatment of infections. Ophthalmologic consultation should be obtained early to prevent corneal scarring from secondary bacterial infections. Oral care should include compresses and oral rinses. Urethral stricture must be prevented in male patients with penile involvement, and gynecologic supportive care is essential in cases of vaginal mucosal sloughing. These patients should also be monitored to exclude urinary retention.

Systemic pharmacologic therapy is controversial and there remains no consensus. Corticosteroid therapy is a controversial treatment in SJS and TEN. Several studies have found conflicting conclusions about the efficacy of corticosteroids compared to supportive therapy. In fact, some studies have found an association with increased infections, duration of hospital stay, and mortality. Several reports, as well as our own observations, suggest that SJS can respond rapidly to high-dose intravenous corticosteroids (1 to 2 mg/kg) given early and short term (7 to 10 days). As for TEN, we may briefly use high-dose intravenous corticosteroids, but small studies and expert consensus opinion favor the use of IVIg or cyclosporine for treatment.

IVIg has been of interest in the treatment of TEN because of its potential to inhibit Fas-FasL-mediated keratinocyte apoptosis. Although the use of IVIg is controversial because some reports suggest a lack of benefit, examination of the literature notes, variations in timing of treatment, dosing, IVIg batch preparations, and most of the case series have variable numbers of patients with comorbid conditions that might affect the outcome. Our experience and several reports suggest that the use of early (especially when the Nikolsky sign is still positive), high-dose IVIg can reduce mortality. Therapy must be given early in the course of the disease over several days, usually 3, in order to deliver a total of 3 to 4 g/kg.

More recently there has been interest in therapy for TEN with cyclosporine, a calcineurin inhibitor that reduces lymphokine production and interleukin release resulting in reduced function of effector T cells. In a few recent studies it has been found to improve mortality. The dose of cyclosporine used varies between 3 and 5 mg/kg/day for an average of 7 days. TNF-α inhibitors have also been suggested, but cautious use is recommended because of the detrimental effects seen with thalidomide. Plasmapheresis has been shown in several reports to provide rapid improvement, possibly from the removal of proinflammatory cytokines. Supportive therapy is otherwise the standard of care for TEN and usually requires an ICU or burns unit. Maintenance of fluid and electrolyte balance and prevention of infection require constant vigilance. Artificial dressings (e.g., Duoderm, Vigilon, or keratinocyte culture grafts) that are designed for the care of burned patients may be life-saving.

SUGGESTED READINGS

Bastuji-Garin S, Rzany B, Stern RS, et al. Clinical classification of cases of toxic epidermal necrolysis, Stevens-Johnson syndrome, and erythema multiforme. Arch Dermatol 1993;129:92–6.

Cartotto R, Mayich M, Nickerson D, Gomez M. SCORTEN accurately predicts mortality among toxic epidermal necrolysis patients treated in a burn center. J Burn Care Res 2008;29:141–6.

Chung WH, Hung SI, Yang JY, et al. Granulysin is a key mediator for disseminated keratinocyte death in Stevens-Johnson syndrome and toxic epidermal necrolysis. Nat Med 2008;14(12):1343–50.

Kirchhof MG, Miliszewski MA, Sikora S, et al. Retrospective review of Stevens-Johnson syndrome/toxic epidermal necrolysis treatment comparing intravenous immunoglobulin with cyclosporine. J Am Acad Dermatol 2014;71(5):941–7.

Lee HY, Dunant A, Sekula P, et al. The role of prior corticosteroid use on the clinical course of Stevens-Johnson syndrome and toxic epidermal necrolysis: a case-control analysis of patients selected from the multinational EuroSCAR and RegiSCAR studies. Br J Dermatol 2012;167(3):555–62.

Schneck J, Fagot JP, Sekula P, et al. Effects of treatments on the mortality of Stevens-Johnson syndrome and toxic epidermal necrolysis: a retrospective study on patients included in the prospective EuroSCAR study. J Am Acad Dermatol 2008;58:33–40.

Schwartz RA, McDonough PH, Lee BW. Toxic epidermal necrolysis: Part I. Introduction, history, classification, clinical features, systemic manifestations, etiology, and immunopathogenesis. J Am Acad Dermatol August 2013;69(2):173.e1–3.

Schwartz RA, McDonough PH, Lee BW. Toxic epidermal necrolysis: Part II. Prognosis, sequelae, diagnosis, differential diagnosis, prevention, and treatment. J Am Acad Dermatol 2013;69(2):187.e1–6.

Sekula P, Dunant A, Mockenhaupt M, et al. Comprehensive survival analysis of a cohort of patients with Stevens-Johnson syndrome and toxic epidermal necrolysis. J Invest Dermatol 2013;133:1197–204.

Viard-Leveugle I, Gaide O, Jankovic D, et al. TNF-alpha and IFN-gamma are potential inducers of Fas-mediated keratinocyte apoptosis through activation of inducible nitric oxide synthase in toxic epidermal necrolysis. J Invest Dermatol 2013;133:489–98.

CHAPTER 12

PANNICULITIS

Ana M. Molina-Ruiz • Luis Requena

KEY POINTS

- The panniculitides comprise a heterogeneous group of inflammatory diseases that involve the subcutaneous fat.
- Various panniculitides may show the same clinical appearance, consisting of erythematous nodules, which frequently makes histopathologic study necessary in order to obtain the specific diagnosis.
- In patients presenting with panniculitis, performing an excisional biopsy that incorporates at least a fat lobule and its surrounding connective tissue septa is crucial in making the correct diagnosis.
- From a histopathologic point of view, most panniculitides are somewhat mixed because the inflammatory infiltrate tends to involve both the septa and the lobules. However, differentiating between a predominantly septal and a predominantly lobular panniculitis is often straightforward at scanning magnification on the basis of identifying the subcutaneous structures more intensely involved by the inflammatory infiltrate.
- Erythema nodosum, a predominantly septal panniculitis, is the most common form of panniculitis.
- Erythema induratum and nodular vasculitis have generally been considered to be synonyms referring to a clinicopathologic entity with several possible causes, one of which is tuberculosis.

INTRODUCTION

Panniculitis refers to inflammation within the subcutis. As for most inflammatory skin disorders, it is especially true for panniculitis that a combined assessment of all available clinical, laboratory, and histopathologic features may be required in order to establish a correct diagnosis. From a clinical point of view, different types of panniculitis with diverse etiologies can closely resemble one another clinically. There is usually deep induration or inflammation of the skin, accompanied by erythema, warmth, pain, and occasionally ulceration or drainage. Sometimes, panniculitis may represent the dermatologic manifestation of a systemic disease, with erythema nodosum (EN) being a classic example. Moreover, histopathologic differences among the various forms of panniculitis may be very subtle, as the subcutaneous fat responds in a limited number of ways to different stimuli. Therefore, when performing a biopsy in a patient with panniculitis, it is crucial to include an entire fat lobule and its surrounding connective tissue septa. Excisional biopsies are preferable to punch biopsies. Furthermore, panniculitis, like other inflammatory diseases of the skin, constitutes a dynamic process in which both the composition and the distribution of the inflammatory infiltrate may change within the course of a few days, making the achievement of the correct diagnosis challenging. Finally, management of patients with panniculitis may also be difficult, particularly given that treatment of both the specific panniculitis and the underlying illness is often necessary.

Table 12-1 provides a pattern-based histologic classification of the multiple forms of panniculitis. The categories have been determined based on histopathologic features, as *septal* versus *lobular* panniculitis, according to the location in which the inflammatory infiltrate is more abundant. Although there is no purely septal or purely lobular panniculitis, certain forms of panniculitis can be characterized as having predominantly septal or lobular involvement, and this finding can provide a useful clue to diagnosis when combined with other histopathologic features, such as the presence or absence of vasculitis and the nature of the cells present in the inflammatory infiltrate. Not all of the disease entities in Table 12-1 are presented in detail in this chapter, and the reader is referred to other chapters of this publication or to the suggested reading material for a comprehensive review of this subject.

PREDOMINANTLY SEPTAL PANNICULITIS

Erythema Nodosum

Erythema nodosum (EN) is the best known of the various forms of panniculitis, as well as the most common. It can occur at any age, in both sexes, and in all racial groups, although it is more common among women during the second through fourth decades of life. It is widely regarded as a delayed hypersensitivity response to a variety of antigenic stimuli, including bacteria, viruses, and chemical agents, although the mechanisms of its development are complex. The relative ranking of underlying causes may vary according to geographic location, and a summarized list of the most common etiologies is outlined in Table 12-2. However, more than one-third of cases of EN have no known disease association, even when followed over a long period of time. Moreover, although the exact pathogenesis of EN remains unknown, some evidence supports

TABLE 12-1 Proposed Classification of Panniculitides

Predominantly septal	Without vasculitis	Erythema nodosum Subacute nodular migratory panniculitis Necrobiotic xanthogranuloma Rheumatoid nodule Subcutaneous granuloma annulare Morphea profunda Necrobiosis lipoidica		
	With vasculitis	Superficial migratory thrombophlebitis Cutaneous polyarteritis nodosa Leukocytoclastic vasculitis		
Predominantly lobular	Without vasculitis	Noninflammatory Sclerosing panniculitis Calciphylaxis Oxalosis Sclerema neonatorum	Pancreatic panniculitis Alpha-1 antitrypsin deficiency Cold panniculitis Lupus panniculitis (and other connective tissue disease-associated panniculitis) Pancreatic panniculitis Infective panniculitis Factitial panniculitis Cytophagic histiocytic panniculitis Traumatic panniculitis	Inflammatory Lipoatrophy Fat necrosis of the newborn Gout panniculitis Crystal storing panniculitus Poststeroid panniculitis Postirradiation panniculitis Sclerosing panniculitis (lipodermatosclerosis)
	With vasculitis	Erythema induratum of Bazin (nodular vasculitis) Erythema nodosum leprosum Lucio phenomenon Neutrophilic lobular panniculitis		

TABLE 12-2 Etiology of Erythema Nodosum and Patient Evaluation

CAUSES	Common	Idiopathic Common infectious associations: streptococcal infections, bacterial gastroenteritis (*Yersinia, Salmonella, Campylobacter*), viral upper respiratory tract infections, coccidioidomycosis
	Uncommon	Drugs (especially estrogens and oral contraceptive pills; also sulfonamides, penicillin, bromides, iodides; occasionally TNF inhibitors) Sarcoidosis Inflammatory bowel disease (Crohn's disease > ulcerative colitis) Neutrophilic dermatoses (Behçet's disease, Sweet's syndrome) Pregnancy Uncommon infectious associations (brucellosis, *Chlamydophila pneumoniae, C. trachomatis, Mycoplasma pneumoniae*, tuberculosis, hepatitis B, histoplasmosis)
	Rare	Pernicious anemia, diverticulitis, malignancy (acute myelogenous leukemia, Hodgkin's disease) Rare infectious associations: gonorrhea, meningococcemia, *Escherichia coli*, pertussis, syphilis, cat scratch disease, HIV infection, blastomycosis, giardiasis, multiple amebic abscesses
PATIENT EVALUATION	History	Drugs Exposure to infectious agents Symptoms of an infection Symptoms of bowel disease
	Physical examination Laboratory studies	Blood cell count, erythrocyte sedimentation rate, γ-globulin levels, urinalysis Skin test for tuberculosis Throat culture Anti-DNase B titer (for *Streptococcus*) Pregnancy test (in women of childbearing age)
	Other studies	Chest X-ray (to exclude tuberculosis, sarcoidosis, or deep fungal infection)

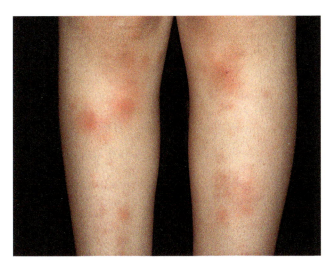

FIGURE 12-1 ■ Erythema nodosum demonstrating erythematous nodules on the anterior aspects of the lower legs.

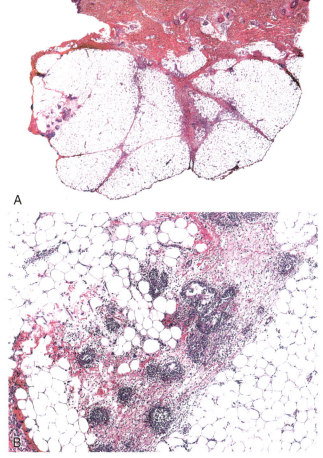

FIGURE 12-2 ■ Histopathologic features of erythema nodosum. **A,** Scanning power magnification showing a predominantly septal panniculitis. **B,** Higher magnification demonstrating numerous Miescher's radial granulomas within the thickened septum.

a circulating immune-complex-mediated pathogenesis. Clinically, patients often have serum-sickness-like signs and symptoms, such as fever, malaise, arthralgias, arthritis, and myalgias, features often associated with circulating immune-complex-mediated disease. EN usually presents as an acute eruption of tender, erythematous subcutaneous nodules over the bilateral pretibial areas (Fig. 12-1), with other locations being occasionally involved, particularly the thighs and forearms. Unlike other forms of panniculitis, ulceration is not a feature of EN. The lesions usually last for a few days or weeks and then slowly involute, changing in color like an ecchymosis, and healing without scar formation. More chronic forms do occur, some of which show a tendency toward migration or centrifugal spread, referred to as *subacute nodular migratory panniculitis* or *erythema nodosum migrans*. This entity is believed by many authors to represent a variant of EN; however, others consider it to be a separate disorder. Untreated, subacute nodular migratory panniculitis can last for months to years.

Histopathologically, EN is the prototype of a predominantly septal panniculitis; however, changes are not entirely confined to the connective septa of the subcutis. Biopsy specimens of early lesions usually show edematous septa and mild lymphocytic infiltrates, although sometimes neutrophils may predominate. True vasculitis is not demonstrable; however, "secondary" vasculitis may occasionally be observed in lesions with heavy, mixed, or neutrophil-rich inflammatory infiltrates. Miescher's radial granulomas, which are small collections of macrophages surrounding small cleft-like spaces, usually found within septa (Fig. 12-2), can also be observed in the early stages of EN. As lesions progress, the septa become widened and contain a mixed, partly granulomatous infiltrate that invades the periphery of the adjacent fat lobules in a lace-like configuration. The extent of lobular involvement may vary, and in some cases can be prominent, especially at the periphery of the fat lobule. Finally, in later stages, the septa become fibrotic, partly replacing the fat lobules, with residual granulomas and lipophages.

The basic evaluation of a patient with EN is summarized in Table 12-2. Further evaluation can be performed in a cost-effective manner if it is guided by the history, physical examination, and laboratory screening test results, always taking into account the most important etiologic considerations depending on geographical location. Finally, identification and treatment of the underlying disorder, if found, is of primary importance, but therapy directed toward the lesions themselves is also an option. In this context, treatments most often recommended for uncomplicated EN include bed rest, salicylates, and nonsteroidal anti-inflammatory drugs. Potassium iodide has been used with success, with adult dosages ranging from 300 to 1500 mg/day, and improvement is typically seen within 2 weeks. In cases of EN associated with underlying conditions, the treatment of the associated disease is usually effective in managing coexistent EN. For example, colchicine is frequently used to treat EN that accompanies Behçet's disease, and various therapies aimed at treating inflammatory bowel disease may also help associated EN lesions. For more severe cases of EN, systemic corticosteroids are occasionally utilized in the absence of an underlying infection.

Superficial Migratory Thrombophlebitis

Superficial migratory thrombophlebitis (SMT) usually presents with painful, erythematous subcutaneous nodules arranged in a linear fashion, with a cord-like thickening along the inflamed vein. Frequently, these nodules are located on the lower limbs, although involvement on the arms and trunk may be also seen. Acute superficial thrombophlebitis of the superficial veins of the anterolateral thoraco-abdominal wall is known as Mondor's disease. The term migratory is applied to describe this disorder because some lesions regress at the same time that new foci of thrombosis develop along the involved vein. Although a hypercoagulable stage, either primary or secondary, should be investigated, venous insufficiency of the lower extremities is the only precipitating factor in most cases. Classically, emphasis is placed on the paraneoplastic character of SMT; however, an internal malignancy is seldom associated. Patients with Behçet's syndrome may also present with SMT of the lower extremities.

Histopathologically, cutaneous lesions of SMT involve large veins of the septa in the upper subcutaneous tissue, with luminal thrombosis and inflammatory infiltrates within the vessel wall. In early lesions, the inflammatory cell infiltrate is mostly composed of neutrophils, whereas in later stages lymphocytes, histiocytes, and occasional multinucleated giant cells are present. Granulomatous inflammation contributes to recanalization of the thrombus. A striking feature is that, despite the intense damage of the involved vein, there is little or no involvement of the adjacent fat lobule, and the process is more vasculitic than panniculitic in nature.

Once malignancy has been ruled out and identification and correction of any underlying hypercoagulable state has been performed, treatment of SMT is conservative, with bed rest, analgesics, and the use of a compression stocking or bandage on the involved leg. In chronic or recurrent cases, especially those associated with malignancy, heparin and fibrinolytic therapies may be used.

PREDOMINANTLY LOBULAR PANNICULITIS

Erythema Induratum of Bazin/Nodular Vasculitis

Erythema induratum (EI) and nodular vasculitis have generally been considered to be synonyms referring to a clinicopathologic entity with several possible causes, one of which is tuberculosis. In some geographic areas, recent polymerase chain reaction investigations have demonstrated that *Mycobacterium tuberculosis* DNA is present in most cutaneous biopsy specimens of patients with EI, supporting the notion that tuberculosis is the most important etiologic factor for this type of panniculitis. However, there are some clinicians who prefer to use the term nodular vasculitis when referring to individuals with a nontuberculous etiology. Nontuberculous cases have been reported to be related to other infectious agents (e.g., *Nocardia*) or to drugs (e.g., propylthiouracil).

EI shows an overwhelming female predominance, with a mean age of presentation between 30 and 40 years. Clinically, EI is characterized by tender, erythematous to violaceous nodules and plaques that most often develop on the lower legs, especially the calves. Lesions are persistent, tend to ulcerate, heal with scarring, and are prone to recurrence.

On histopathology, EI is generally described as a predominantly lobular or mixed septal/lobular panniculitis. Inflammation is mixed, and can include neutrophils, lymphocytes, macrophages, and multinucleated giant cells. Vasculitis is identifiable in the vast majority of cases, and most frequently involves small venules of the fat lobules and, less frequently, veins or arteries of the connective tissue septa. Necrosis, with a coagulative or caseous appearance, has been described in both tuberculous and nontuberculous cases, but the incidence and degree of necrosis are greater in cases related to *M. tuberculosis*.

Spontaneous regression may occur in a large percentage of cases of EI, making evaluation of response to therapy challenging. In most patients, simple measures such as avoidance of physical exercise, bed rest, and compression stockings result in complete remission of the lesions in weeks. In more severe cases, nonsteroidal anti-inflammatory drugs, potassium iodide, dapsone, colchicine, antimalarials, tetracycline, gold salts, mycophenolate mofetil, and prednisone have been administered with favorable response. In those patients with a strong positive reaction to the Mantoux test or when *M. tuberculosis* DNA is demonstrated in the cutaneous biopsy specimen, a full course of 9 months of antituberculous drugs is recommended.

Pancreatic Panniculitis

Pancreatic panniculitis (PP) is an uncommonly reported complication of pancreatic disorders (approximately 2% of patients), and its chief importance is as a sign of a systemic disorder, particularly because the panniculitis may be recognized prior to detection of the underlying pancreatic disease. There is considerable evidence that the enzymes lipase, amylase, and trypsin are involved in producing the lesions of PP, with lipase having the clearest relationship with the panniculitis. However, elevated enzyme levels are not the complete explanation for the changes of PP, and immunologic factors may also play a role. Clinically, subcutaneous, erythematous, and often painful nodules develop, frequently on the extremities (Fig. 12-3), but also on the abdomen, chest, arms, and scalp, and even in the visceral fat. The lesions may become fluctuant and ulcerate, discharging an oily material, and usually involute within a period of weeks, leaving hyperpigmented scars. Associated findings include fever, abdominal pain, inflammatory polyarthritis, ascites, and pleural effusions. The combination of subcutaneous nodules, polyarthritis, and eosinophilia is known as Schmid's triad and is associated with a poor prognosis. Some patients have radiographic evidence of multiple lytic areas involving the cortical bone near large joints.

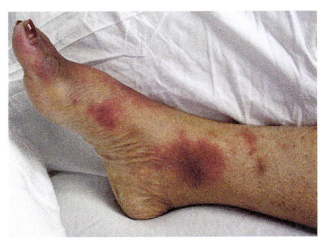

FIGURE 12-3 ■ Pancreatic panniculitis: Multiple erythematous tender nodules were present in this patient with pancreatitis. (Courtesy of J. Callen.)

Histopathologically, PP is a predominantly lobular panniculitis, with intense necrosis of the adipocytes at the center of the fat lobule. A characteristic feature is ghost adipocytes, which are necrotic adipocytes that have lost their nuclei and show a finely granular and basophilic material within their cytoplasm due to calcification. Ghost adipocytes result from the hydrolytic action of pancreatic enzymes on fat, followed by calcium deposition, a process known as saponification. Although characteristic of PP, ghost adipocytes have also been recently found as a histopathologic feature in lesions of subcutaneous mucormycosis. Finally, in late-stage lesions of PP, the fat lobule is replaced by a granulomatous inflammatory infiltrate composed of foamy histiocytes and multinucleated giant cells.

Treatment of PP is primarily directed toward managing the underlying pancreatic disease; however, supportive measures such as compression and elevation can also be helpful.

Alpha-1 Antitrypsin Deficiency Panniculitis

Alpha-1 antitrypsin (A1AT) deficiency is an uncommon cause of panniculitis. In this genetic disorder, defective production of A1AT, a serine protease inhibitor protein produced in the liver, allows for accumulation of abnormal A1AT in hepatocytes as well as decreased A1AT activity in the lungs, where the protein typically protects the pulmonary tissue from neutrophil elastase. Systemic manifestations may include chronic liver disease with cirrhosis, emphysema, pancreatitis, membranoproliferative glomerulonephritis, rheumatoid arthritis, antineutrophil cytoplasmic antibody-positive vasculitis, other cutaneous vasculitides, and angioedema. In this genetic disorder, the most severe manifestations arise in patients with profound proteinase inhibitor deficiency, although the panniculitis can also occur in heterozygotes. The initiating event in individuals who develop panniculitis is not always clear; trauma-related and postpartum flares of the disease have been reported in genetically susceptible individuals. Clinically, large, erythematous to purpuric, tender nodules or plaques appear in a variety of sites, especially the lower trunk and proximal extremities. Frequently, ulcers develop and may be deep and necrotic, accompanied by an oily discharge. Healing is accompanied by scarring and subcutaneous atrophy. The clinical course is often prolonged, and lesions are usually resistant to therapy.

On histopathology, early stages show a neutrophilic panniculitis, followed rapidly by necrosis and destruction of fat lobules. Splaying of neutrophils between collagen bundles in the deeper reticular dermis has been described as an early clue to the diagnosis. Dissolution of dermal collagen, with resultant liquefactive necrosis and separation of fat lobules from adjacent septa, is a key feature in most cases. Another characteristic finding is the presence of "skip areas" of normal fat adjacent to foci of severe necrotizing panniculitis.

The most effective therapeutic measure is replacement of A1AT via intravenous infusions. Dosages are generally 60 mg/kg per week, administered over a period of 3 to 7 weeks. Improvement is relatively rapid, and clearing of the panniculitis can occur after only a few weekly doses. Recurrences are possible when A1AT levels fall below 50 mg/dL, but these typically respond to further replacement therapy. Other successful therapies include plasma exchange, carbamazepine, doxycycline, dapsone, and liver transplantation. Reduction of alcohol intake has also been recommended, since ethanol (as a hepatotoxin) may precipitate A1AT-associated hepatitis. Cigarette smoking must also be strictly avoided in patients with A1AT deficiency.

Lipoatrophy

Lipoatrophy and lipodystrophy are often used as synonyms; however, even though both disorders lead to a loss of subcutaneous fat, they are pathogenically different entities. Lipoatrophy refers to loss of subcutaneous fat due to a previous inflammatory process involving the subcutis, while lipodystrophy is applied to an absence of subcutaneous fat with no evidence of inflammation.

Several forms of localized lipoatrophy have been described according to their clinical appearance and location, such as annular lipoatrophy, abdominal lipoatrophy, semicircular lipoatrophy, and postinjection localized lipoatrophy. Localized lipoatrophy has even been described secondary to compression by tight-fitting clothes. However, the most common localized lipoatrophy is the one that appears as the final stage of different types of panniculitis.

On the other hand, lipodystrophy may be either localized or generalized, as well as either congenital or acquired. This loss of subcutaneous tissue may appear in the context of genetic syndromes or in patients with HIV infection treated with protease inhibitors.

In most cases of lipoatrophy, the histopathologic findings are those of a lipophagic granuloma surrounding a small-sized fat lobule, with perilobular fibrosis. In fully developed lesions of lipodystrophy, there is an absence of subcutaneous fat with deposition of new collagen and no evidence of inflammation. Recently, two histopathologic variants of lipodystrophy have been proposed, a first type showing prominent involutional changes of the fat lobule, and a second type with inflammation. However, lipoatrophy and lipodystrophy are controversial terms that some authors use as synonymous terms. In our opinion, lipoatrophy should be used when the process is accompanied by inflammatory response and lipodystrophy when inflammation is absent. But it is also possible that lipodystrophy is a late and residual stage of lipoatrophy.

Treatments of localized lipoatrophy include soft tissue augmentation using fillers, fat transplantation, or reconstructive surgery, while partial lipodystrophy has been treated with troglitazone.

SUGGESTED READINGS

Ackerman AB. Panniculitis. In: Ackerman AB, editor. Histopathologic diagnosis of inflammatory skin diseases. Philadelphia: Lea & Febiger; 1978. p. 779–825.

Craig AJ, Cualing H, Thomas G, et al. Cytophagic histiocytic panniculitis – a syndrome associated with benign and malignant panniculitis: case comparison and review of the literature. J Am Acad Dermatol 1998;39:721–36.

Pincus LB, LeBoit PE, McCalmont TH, et al. Subcutaneous panniculitis-like T-cell lymphoma with overlapping clinicopathologic features of lupus erythematosus: coexistence of 2 entities? Am J Dermatopathol 2009;31:520–6.

Requena L, Sanchez Yus E. Panniculitis. Part I. Mostly septal panniculitis. J Am Acad Dermatol 2001;45:163–83.

Requena L, Sanchez Yus E. Panniculitis. Part II. Mostly lobular panniculitis. J Am Acad Dermatol 2001;45:325–61.

Requena L, Sanchez Yus E. Erythema nodosum. Semin Cutan Med Surg 2007;26:114–25.

Requena L, Sitthinamsuwan P, Santonja C, et al. Cutaneous and mucosal mucormycosis mimicking pancreatic panniculitis and gouty panniculitis. J Am Acad Dermatol 2012;66:975–84.

Segura S, Pujol RM, Trindade F, Requena L. Vasculitis in erythema induratum of Bazin: a histopathologic study of 101 biopsy specimens from 86 patients. J Am Acad Dermatol 2008;59:839–51.

Walsh SN, Santa Cruz DJ. Lipodermatosclerosis: a clinicopathologic study of 25 cases. J Am Acad Dermatol 2010;62:1005–12.

CHAPTER 13

PRURITUS

Gil Yosipovitch

> **KEY POINTS**
>
> - Chronic itch can occur without primary skin rash associated with underlying systemic diseases.
> - Itch can be the presenting symptom of lymphoma and hepatic diseases.
> - Chronic systemic itch is associated with imbalance of μ versus κ opioids.
> - Topical antipruritic treatments include local anesthetics, coolants, emollients, and topical immunomodulators.
> - Systemic antipruritic treatments include drugs that are used for neuropathic pain, such as gabapentin, pregabalin, selective serotonin reuptake inhibitors, and κ opioids.

Pruritus is a complex symptom that is very similar to pain and affects all humans in the course of their lives. Chronic pruritus is defined as an itch that lasts more than 6 weeks. It has a significant impact on patients' quality of life, very similar to chronic pain. It is the primary symptom in a diverse range of inflammatory skin diseases, such as atopic eczema, psoriasis, dry skin, and chronic urticaria (Table 13-1). It can occur without any primary skin eruption associated with underlying systemic diseases (Table 13-2), and can be the presenting symptom of lymphoma, hepatic diseases such as biliary cirrhosis and hepatitis C, and HIV viral infections. It can occur in relation to primary damage to nerve fibers, such as postherpetic neuropathy, as well as spinal nerve root injuries such as brachioradial pruritus and notalgia paresthetica, and in afferent nerves in the central nervous system post stroke. Pruritus is a common symptom in psychiatric diseases such as obsessive compulsive disorders, depression, and in delusions of parasitosis.

SKIN SIGNS OF CHRONIC PRURITUS

There are common skin lesions that develop in pruritus as a result of repetitive scratching and rubbing of the skin. These lesions are not considered a primary skin eruption. They include excoriations such as prurigo nodules (excoriated papules that lead to nodule formation). These are usually distributed on the extensor side of the limbs and upper back. Lichenification is a thickened plaque with marked accentuation of the skin creases, which develops as a result of continuous rubbing and scratching, generally in areas that the patient can easily scratch and rub, such as the nape of the neck, below the elbow, the ankle, the buttocks, and the genitalia. Changes in skin pigmentation—both hyper- and hypopigmentation—can occur because of repeated scratching. Excoriated lesions resulting from repetitive scratching, as well as primary eczematous lesions, can become infected, particularly in patients with atopic dermatitis.

The middle of the back, which cannot be easily reached, may show normal skin or relative hypopigmentation, in contrast to the hyperpigmentation of the areas subjected to persistent scratching, thereby resulting in a butterfly pattern. The finger nails may be shiny because of prolonged rubbing.

COMMON COMPLICATIONS IN PATIENTS WITH GENERALIZED PRURITUS

Patients with chronic pruritus often have difficulty sleeping, are agitated, and suffer from depression, and decreased sexual desire and sexual function, suggestive of a significant impairment of quality of life.

DIAGNOSIS

When no diagnosis of a primarily dermatological disorder can be made, a history, review of systems, physical examination, and screening laboratory examination are needed.

A detailed history is important. One should investigate whether the patient suffers from generalized or localized itching. A localized itch may be associated with a burning sensation and pain in peripheral neuropathy, such as damage to cervical spinal nerve roots in brachioradial pruritus or thoracic nerve roots in notalgia paresthetica. Careful history also includes a drug history, as drugs such as opiates, aspirin, and the new targeted cancer therapies such as estimated glomerular filtration rate inhibitors can induce itch with and without a cutaneous eruption. A simple question, such as whether pruritus occurs in other family members, can indicate the possibility of scabies and prevent unnecessary investigation. Recent travel to endemic areas of parasitic infection and gastrointestinal complaints may be suggestive of parasitic infection. A positive review of systems, especially in relation to general health, such as weight loss, night sweats, and tremor, could point to a systemic cause.

Some pruritic states have specific clinical patterns. Despite severe pruritus, chronic urticaria does not usually show secondary skin lesions associated with scratching. Patients with cholestatic itch initially present with itch

TABLE 13-1	Common Skin Diseases and Infectious Skin Diseases that Cause Pruritus

Atopic eczema
Psoriasis
Contact dermatitis
Urticaria
Dry skin
Elderly idiopathic itch
Seborrheic dermatitis
Lichen planus
Cutaneous T-cell lymphoma
Scars and post burns
Pityriasis rosea
Bullous pemphigoid (including the prebullous phase)
Dermatitis herpetiformis
Pregnancy-associated cutaneous eruptions
Superficial fungal diseases
Folliculitis
Scabies
HIV
Varicella
Onchocerciasis

TABLE 13-2	Systemic Diseases that Cause Itch

End-stage chronic renal disease
Cholestasis
    Primary biliary cirrhosis
    Hepatitis C viral infection
    Cholestasis of pregnancy
Hematopoietic
    Hodgkin's lymphoma
    Non-Hodgkin's lymphoma
    Mastocytosis
    Multiple myeloma
    Polycythemia vera
    Iron deficiency anemia
    Myeloid and lymphocytic leukemias
    Myelodysplastic disorders
Solid malignant tumors (paraneoplastic manifestation)
Endocrine
    Hyperthyroidism
    Diabetes
    Mastocytosis
    Anorexia nervosa
Drugs (such as opioids, hydroxyethyl starch, chloroquine, epidermal growth factor inhibitors, and ipilimumab)
Connective tissue diseases
    Dermatomyositis
    Scleroderma
    Sjögren's syndrome
Itch in post-transplant patients
Peripheral neuropathy
    Postherpetic neuralgia
    Brachioradial pruritus
    Notalgia paresthetica
    Diabetic neuropathy
Central nervous system neuropathy
    Multiple sclerosis
    Brain tumors
    Cerebrovascular events
    Creutzfeldt–Jakob disease
Psychogenic itch
    Depression
    Obsessive compulsive disorder
    Fibromyalgia
    Delusional state of parasitophobia disorder

in an acral distribution in the palms and soles, whereas patients with other chronic types of itch rarely do so. Neuropathic itch in disease entities such as postherpetic neuralgia, brachioradial pruritus, and notalgia paresthetica involves itch in the relevant nerve distributions.

EXAMINATION

A thorough physical examination with particular attention to lymph nodes (lymphoreticular malignancy) and organomegaly of liver and spleen (lymphoreticular malignancy and paraneoplastic manifestations) is essential. Fine tremor may suggest underlying hyperthyroidism. Examination of the genital area, finger webs, the ulnar border of palms, wrists, elbows, axilla, and nipples is carried out to exclude scabies.

INVESTIGATIONS

Based on the initial findings, further laboratory evaluation and imaging studies may be necessary. Although the appropriate tests will vary with the individual circumstances, one suggested approach is to obtain the studies indicated in Table 13-3. Most patients with pruritus will not need further tests. A detailed history and examination will reveal the cause. Investigations in patients with pruritus with an eruption include a skin biopsy (sometimes including a biopsy for direct immunofluorescence) and appropriate laboratory investigations. Figure 13-1 provides an algorithm for the diagnosis and investigation of pruritus.

PATHOPHYSIOLOGY OF GENERALIZED PRURITUS

In many cases, pruritus originates in the upper layers of the skin, although damage to nerve fibers along the peripheral and central nervous system can induce itch. There are histamine and nonhistaminergic C nerve fibers that transmit itch. These C nerve fibers represent only 5% to 10% of the C nerve fibers and have slow conduction velocity.

There are many mediators and receptors involved in pruritus, both peripherally and centrally. Important

TABLE 13-3	Initial Laboratory Studies in Patients with Generalized Pruritus

  I. Complete blood count and differential
 II. Chemistry profile
    A. Hepatic enzymes
    B. Urea nitrogen and creatinine levels
III. Thyroid function (e.g., thyroid-stimulating hormone)
IV. Chest radiography
 V. Optional
    A. Stool examination for parasites
    B. HIV testing
    C. Abdominal and chest imaging
    D. Skin biopsy for routine and immunofluorescence microscopy

mediators include proteinases such as tryptase and cathepsins, histamines, substance P, cytokines such as interleukin 31, nerve growth factor, and central mediators including μ opiates and gastrin-releasing peptide. Important receptors are G-protein-coupled receptors including histamine receptor 1 and 4, proteinase 2 receptors, heat-sensing receptors TRPV1, TRPA1, and TRPV3, chloroquine receptor Mrgprs, tyrosine kinase receptors TrkA, opioid receptors, and interleukin 31 receptor oncostatin.

For the most part, "itch factors," or pruritogens, in the various systemic diseases in which itching occurs have not yet been identified. In the last decade there has been accumulating evidence suggesting that generalized pruritus is induced by an imbalance between the μ- and the κ-opioid systems. Activation of μ-opioid receptors stimulates itch perception, whereas κ-opioid receptor stimulation inhibits μ-receptor effects both centrally and peripherally.

END-STAGE RENAL DISEASE PRURITUS

Pruritus is a frequently disabling and distressing symptom of end-stage renal disease (ESRD). It affects more than 50% of patients, especially those on dialysis, and has a significant impact on sleep and mental and physical function. In the International Dialysis Outcomes and Practice Patterns study, which evaluated more than 18,000 patients on hemodialysis, pruritus was associated with a 17% higher mortality risk, an effect that was no longer significant after adjustment for measures of sleep quality. This observation suggests that sleep disturbances may have an important role in the greater mortality risk associated with ESRD pruritus. The pathophysiology of ESRD pruritus is poorly understood. Current data point toward a role for the immune system, central neuropathy, and imbalance in the opioidergic system. Early hypotheses of the pathogenesis of pruritus caused by renal failure related pruritus to secondary hyperparathyroidism, but other factors such as calcium and phosphate levels may have a role in itch. Subtotal parathyroidectomy was occasionally associated with the control of ESRD pruritus. It has been postulated that ESRD itch is associated with a proinflammatory state with elevated C reactive protein and recent data suggest that interleukin 31, a pruritic TH-2 cytokine, is elevated in ESRD itch. In concordance with this theory, immunomodulators such as ultraviolet light (UVB), thalidomide, and topical immunomodulators such as tacrolimus reduced pruritus. The pruritus can be so intense that excoriations lead to cutaneous nodules (prurigo nodularis). Kyrle's disease and other perforating disorders may be present as well, as either a sign of or cause of pruritus in some patients. The most prevalent body site is the back, but the arms, head, and abdomen are also commonly affected. The symptom tends to be more severe at night.

PRURITUS OF CHOLESTASIS

Cholestatic pruritus is highly distressing. It often begins in an acral distribution but later becomes generalized. Clinicians are familiar with the causes of cholestasis, including intrahepatic (e.g., hepatitis of all causes and intrahepatic cholestasis of pregnancy), extrahepatic (e.g., bile duct

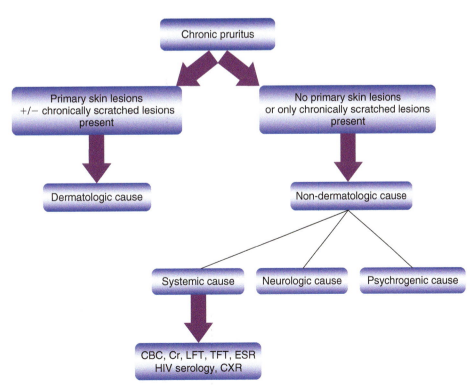

FIGURE 13-1 ■ An algorithm for the diagnosis and investigation of pruritus. (Adapted from Yosipovitch G, Bernhard JD. Clinical practice. Chronic pruritus. N Engl J Med April 25, 2013;368(17):1625–34.)

stricture, cholelithiasis, or malignant bile duct or pancreatic tumors), and drug-induced (e.g., chlorpromazine, testosterone, norethindrone, phenothiazines, tolbutamide, erythromycin estolate, and estrogens). The pathogenesis of pruritus of cholestasis is unknown. It has been associated with accumulation of bile salts and increased opioidergic tone, and recent studies suggest an important role of elevated lysophosphatidic acid (LPA). LPA is a phospholipid that is formed by autotaxin. Both LPA and elevated autotaxin have been found to be correlated with cholestatic itch of different types. Therapy with bile acid sequestrants such as cholestyramine and ursodeoxycholic acid may provide some relief. As patients also have high plasma levels of opioids, opioid antagonists (such as naltrexone) have been shown to reduce cholestatic itch. Hepatitis C can be associated with severe generalized itching, and in severe cases itch is considered an indication for liver transplantation, although with novel hepatitis C antiviral treatments and their high response rates this may no longer be necessary in the future.

LYMPHOMAS, LEUKEMIA, AND HEMATOLOGIC DISEASE

Pruritus is an important sign that may have prognostic significance in several of the malignant lymphomas. It could be the presenting symptom of lymphoma. Widespread cutaneous T-cell lymphoma and erythrodermic forms, including Sézary syndrome (T-cell leukemia), cause an intractable severe itch that is difficult to treat. Thirty percent of patients with Hodgkin's lymphoma experience generalized pruritus at some time during the course of their disease. The pruritus of Hodgkin's lymphoma is usually related to the disease's activity. Pruritus may be experienced more intensely at night. Pruritus is an infrequent accompanying symptom of multiple myeloma. The mechanism of pruritus in these conditions remains unknown. Recent studies have shown that increased serum and mRNA levels of interleukin 31, a TH2 pruritic cytokine, correlate with the severity of cutaneous T-cell lymphoma pruritus. Reduced serum levels of this cytokine post treatment with oral corticosteroids and histone deacetylase inhibitors correlated with significant reduction in itch in these patients.

Approximately 50% of patients with polycythemia vera develop pruritus that usually occurs after exposure to water (bath itch). This short-lasting pruritus is most probably mediated by increased histamine release from mast cells. Iron deficiency is associated with pruritus. This is reversible with iron supplementation. The mechanism of pruritus in iron deficiency is unknown.

ENDOCRINE DISEASE

Pruritus is an important symptom of hyperthyroidism and could be a presenting symptom. The underlying mechanism of this itch is unknown. Hypothyroidism less frequently causes itch related to the associated asteatosis (dry skin).

Secondary hyperparathyroidism associated with renal disease is often associated with generalized pruritus.

Diabetes mellitus is now believed to be a cause of localized, not generalized, pruritus. Recent studies suggest that scalp and truncal itch in diabetics is associated with diabetic neuropathy.

PRURITUS OF HUMAN IMMUNODEFICIENCY VIRUS INFECTION

Itch is the most common skin manifestation of HIV disease and has a significant impact on patients' quality of life. It may be associated with skin diseases that are more prevalent or aggravated by HIV, such as psoriasis and seborrheic dermatitis, as well as skin dryness. It may occur as a primary symptom of HIV, such as in eosinophilic folliculitis, insect bite hypersensitivity reaction, and pruritic papules of HIV. These papular pruritic eruptions cause severe itch. It continues to be a common symptom of HIV in the era of highly active antiretroviral therapy.

NEUROPATHIC ITCH

Neuropathic itch has been defined as an itch initiated or caused by a primary lesion or dysfunction at any point along the afferent pathway of the nervous system. Characteristics of neuropathic itch that differentiate it from other forms of itch include associations with other sensory symptoms in a dermatomal distribution and the presence of other neural damage, including motor damage or autonomic damage.

Neuropathic itch can coincide with pain, as is seen in 30% to 40% of patients with postherpetic neuralgia. Characteristic sensory complaints associated with neuropathic itch are burning, paresthesia, tingling, and stinging. Localized itching can follow dermatomes at the level of C5–C8, such as the dorsolateral aspect of the arms in brachioradial pruritus, and unilateral itch midback in dermatomes at the level of T2–T6 in notalgia paresthetica.

PREGNANCY

Pregnant women may experience generalized pruritus as a result of cholestasis, which is common in pregnancy; in addition, several dermatoses of pregnancy, which are extremely itchy, have been described, such as polymorphic eruption of pregnancy and pemphigoid (herpes) gestationis (see Chapter 41).

TREATMENT OF PRURITUS

There are no specific antipruritic drugs that benefit all forms of pruritus. Treatment depends on identifying and removing the cause, whether systemic or cutaneous. If treatment of the cause is not possible there are a number of preventive and therapeutic treatment options. Treatments are divided into topical and systemic.

Topical treatments to relieve itch are particularly helpful for pruritus resulting from skin inflammation. These include emollients and moisturizers, especially when the skin is dry, such as in old age, atopic eczema, and ESRD itch. Although they are capable of relieving pruritus due to inflammatory skin disease, corticosteroids are not intrinsically antipruritic. Topical immunomodulators such as tacrolimus or pimecrolimus have a role in itch associated with eczema.

Coolants and counterirritants such as menthol activate nerve fibers for cold and inhibit C nerve fibers that transmit warmth and itch. Other topical agents include local anesthetics such as pramoxine and topical capsaicin, which have a role in the treatment of localized itch, in particular that associated with neuropathic itch.

Systemic corticosteroids are not indicated, except when the diagnosis of a specific steroid-responsive disease (such as bullous pemphigoid) has been established.

Systemic antipruritic treatments include drugs that are used for neuropathic pain, such as gabapentin, pregabalin, and mirtazapine and paroxetine. As mentioned, opioids have a role in systemic generalized itch. Therefore, opiate antagonists such as naltrexone have been used for the treatment of pruritus, in particular itch associated with cholestasis, but owing to their significant side effects they are not commonly used. There are currently new κ agonists in development that seem a promising avenue for treating severe pruritus. Butorphanol is a κ agonist and μ antagonist that is a commercially available analgesic and has fewer side effects than the μ antagonists. It has been reported to be effective for different types of severe generalized pruritus.

Antihistamines are only antipruritic if the pruritus is caused by histamine, as in urticarial or drug eruptions. They only benefit nonhistamine-mediated itch through their sedating/tranquilizing properties. First-generation H_1 antihistamines such as hydroxyzine have marked sedative and anticholinergic actions and are useful in severe chronic urticaria, enabling patients with chronic itch to sleep. Second-generation antihistamines such as loratadine, desloratadine, cetirizine, and levocetirizine are suitable in the daytime for relief of pruritus due to urticaria. The role of these nonsedating antihistamines in other pruritic disorders is limited. Thalidomide was found to have a role in treating chronic itch in particular prurigo nodularis, but because of the high cost and monitoring requirements is rarely used.

Phototherapy has been used for more than a decade to treat different types of itch. UVB therapy, both broadband and narrowband, seems to be the most effective. The treatment is safe and can be repeated as necessary. It is beneficial for itch associated with atopic dermatitis, psoriasis, and chronic renal failure. Remissions may last for as long as 18 months.

Several studies have shown that behavioral modification therapy reduces the intensity and perception of itch. Other possible behavioral interventions include stress reduction and biofeedback. These treatments are especially effective in chronic pruritus associated with psychogenic cofactors.

SUGGESTED READINGS

Patel T, Yosipovitch G. Therapy of pruritus. Expert Opin Pharmacother 2010;11(10):1673–82.

Wang H, Yosipovitch G. New insights into the pathophysiology and treatment of chronic itch in patients with end-stage renal disease, chronic liver disease, and lymphoma. Int J Dermatol 2010;49(1):1–11.

Yosipovitch G, Bernhard JD. Clinical practice. Chronic pruritus. N Engl J Med 2013;368(17):1625–34.

Yosipovitch G, Greaves M, Fleischer A, McGlone F, editors. Itch: basic mechanisms and therapy. New York: Marcel Dekker; 2004.

Yosipovitch G, Patel TJ. Pathophysiology and clinical aspects of pruritus. In: Goldsmith KS, Wolff K, Gilchrest B, et al., editors. Fitzpatrick's dermatology in general medicine. 8th ed. New York: McGraw Hill; 2012. p. 902–11.

Yosipovitch G, Papoui A. Cutaneous neurophysiology. In: Bolognia JL, Jorizzo JL, Rapini RP, et al., editors. Dermatology. 3rd ed. London: Mosby; 2012. p. 81–90.

CHAPTER 14

ERYTHRODERMA

Megan H. Noe • Karolyn A. Wanat

KEY POINTS

- Erythroderma is erythema, with or without scaling, involving more than 90% of the cutaneous surface.
- Many cases of erythroderma are idiopathic, but the most common causes are exacerbation of an underlying skin disease, a drug hypersensitivity reaction, and cutaneous T-cell lymphoma.
- Although pathology can be nonspecific, a biopsy should typically be performed because it may give clues to the underlying diagnosis.
- Hospitalization may be required for appropriate monitoring of fluid–electrolyte balance, nutrition, and thermoregulation, as well as for diligent skin care.
- Treatment should be focused on the underlying disease, if known, in addition to skin-directed therapy with topical corticosteroids applied twice daily under moist occlusion.
- Prognosis depends on the underlying condition but tends to be worse for those with malignancy-related erythroderma and for those who develop high-output cardiac failure or sepsis.

INTRODUCTION

Erythroderma is the clinical finding of erythema, with or without scaling, on more than 90% of an individual's body surface area. The term "exfoliative dermatitis" is used in some contexts and is often considered to be the same entity, but erythroderma is a more encompassing and often favored term. Numerous conditions can result in erythroderma, and identifying the exact inciting cause or underlying pathology may be challenging. Extreme disruption in the barrier function of the skin can lead to systemic manifestations such as fluid and electrolyte abnormalities, tachycardia, and problems with thermoregulation. Management of erythroderma should be focused on treatment of the underlying cause, if possible, in addition to supportive care for the skin and systemic manifestations.

The incidence of erythroderma is difficult to determine given lack of standardized reporting, and the incidence likely varies depending on location. In the United States and Europe, the incidence has been estimated to be between 1 and 2 cases per 100,000 individuals/year, but some reports from India have reported an incidence as high as 35 cases per 100,000 dermatologic outpatients. Erythroderma is more commonly seen in patients older than 45 years, with an average age of 55 years, which may be related to an increase in conditions that result in erythroderma in older individuals. There also appears to be a male predominance, with males being affected 2 to 3 times more often than females.

CAUSE AND PATHOGENESIS

Erythroderma represents a final clinical endpoint for many dermatological and systemic disease states (Table 14-1). The most common causes are exacerbation of an underlying skin disease such as psoriasis or atopic dermatitis, a drug hypersensitivity reaction, and cutaneous T-cell lymphoma; however, many cases are considered idiopathic, as an inciting cause is not identified. Erythroderma is likely secondary to a complex interaction of cytokines and cellular adhesion molecules affecting T-cells within the skin. Keratinocytes and Langerhans cells both produce IL-1, which increases vascular permeability, acts as a chemotactic factor for T-cells, and upregulates ICAM-1. ICAM-1 is found on venous endothelial cells and plays an important role in T-cell binding to both endothelial cells and keratinocytes. This complex interaction of T-cells and cytokines leads to the erythema and desquamation seen clinically. Increased cell turnover in the epidermis occurs secondary to an increase in both the number of proliferative cells and the mitotic rate. These rapidly shed epidermal cells contain amino acids and proteins normally retained by the skin, leading to significantly higher than normal levels of protein loss.

Exacerbation of an underlying skin disease is a common cause of erythroderma. Psoriasis, atopic dermatitis, contact dermatitis, stasis dermatitis, and seborrheic dermatitis can all lead to erythroderma. Psoriatic erythroderma can be triggered by abrupt withdrawal of a systemic medication, including oral corticosteroids, addition of a new medication, topical irritants such as tar or phototherapy burns, pregnancy, or systemic illness. Erythrodermic psoriasis can present with extensive involvement of characteristic psoriatic plaques (Fig. 14-1) or with diffuse erythroderma, often with small pustules or coalescing "lakes" of pus. Erythroderma from atopic dermatitis tends to present as part of a chronic course with extensive lichenification following an uncontrolled flare, but may also present with a more acute erythroderma. New-onset pityriasis rubra pilaris (PRP) is another important consideration in the differential diagnosis of erythroderma. Lesions in PRP tend to have an orange-red hue and are classically separated by islands of sparing (Fig. 14-2). The eruption typically starts on the face or scalp and spreads downwards, with an associated palmoplantar keratoderma. Photosensitivity is a common feature. Follicularly

TABLE 14-1	Causes of Erythroderma	
Primary Skin Diseases	**Malignancy**	**Other**
Psoriasis	Cutaneous T-cell	Drug
Atopic dermatitis	lymphoma	hypersensitivity
Pityriasis rubra	Systemic	reaction
pilaris	lymphoma	Dermatomyositis
Contact dermatitis	Leukemia	Hepatitis
Chronic actinic	Myelodysplastic	HIV
dermatitis	syndrome	Graft-versus-host
Bullous	Solid organ	disease
pemphigoid	malignancy	Omenn syndrome
Pemphigus	Paraneoplastic	Dermatophyte
foliaceus	reaction	infection
Ichthyoses		Crusted scabies
Seborrheic dermatitis (rare)		
Stasis dermatitis		

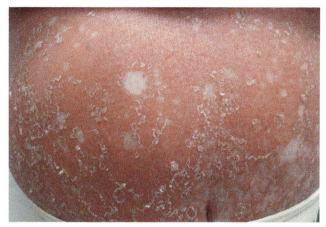

FIGURE 14-2 ■ Pityriasis rubra pilaris causing erythroderma. Pink-orange erythema, with islands of sparing and overlying desquamation.

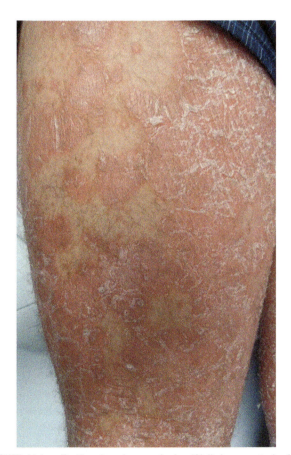

FIGURE 14-1 ■ Erythrodermic psoriasis. Well-demarcated pink plaques with overlying silvery scale, covering more than 90% of body surface area.

based, hyperkeratotic papules on the fingers, wrists, and elbows may be another clue to the diagnosis.

Drug eruptions that start as morbilliform, lichenoid, or urticarial reactions can all progress to generalized erythema. Onset and resolution tend to be more rapid than in erythroderma caused by other etiologies. Common medications implicated in inducing erythroderma are sulfas, allopurinol, gold, penicillin, carbamazepine, phenytoin, and barbiturates, but many others have been reported. At presentation, serious drug reactions such as drug reaction with eosinophilia and systemic symptoms, acute generalized exanthematous pustulosis (Fig. 14-3), and Stevens–Johnson syndrome/toxic epidermolytic necrolysis can present with erythroderma, and clinicians should have a high index of suspicion with close clinical monitoring for progression when evaluating patients with erythroderma. Patients with these more serious drug reactions will often have fever, additional laboratory abnormalities, mucous membrane involvement, skin pain, or will show clinical progression to pustules or bullae with subsequent desquamation.

Malignancy is another common cause of erythroderma. Cutaneous T-cell lymphoma (CTCL), including mycosis fungoides and Sézary syndrome, is the most common cause of malignancy-related erythroderma (Fig. 14-4). Patients with erythroderma from CTCL often have more pruritus than is seen with other types of erythroderma. Hodgkin's disease, non-Hodgkin's lymphoma, leukemia, and myeloplastic syndrome have also been reported to cause erythroderma, along with other solid-organ malignancies including prostate, thyroid, esophageal, liver, melanoma, ovarian, rectal, and breast. Chronic, subacute erythroderma can be a clue to an underlying malignancy.

Other systemic illnesses have also been reported to present with generalized erythroderma, including dermatomyositis, hepatitis, seroconversion in HIV-positive individuals, graft-versus-host disease, and Omenn syndrome, among others. Extensive dermatophyte infections and crusted scabies can also present with generalized erythema. Less commonly, bullous pemphigoid, pemphigus foliaceus, and chronic actinic dermatitis can also present as erythroderma. Preceding history and clinical morphology can help identify underlying etiologies, although clinicians should reconsider inciting causes if patients do not respond to therapy as expected.

CLINICAL MANIFESTATIONS

Patients present with erythema, with or without scaling, involving greater than 90% of the skin. The erythema usually develops over weeks to months and is followed by prominent desquamation. Lymphadenopathy is common

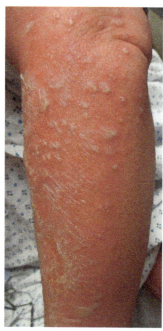

FIGURE 14-3 ■ Acute generalized exanthematous pustulosis (AGEP): a pustular drug eruption causing erythroderma. The presence of pustules on a diffusely erythematous base helps narrow the differential diagnosis in this setting.

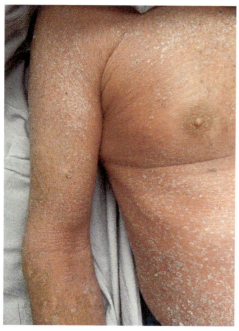

FIGURE 14-4 ■ Paraneoplastic erythroderma. Diffuse erythema of the trunk and upper extremities with overlying fine scale in the setting of new-onset malignancy.

and can be reactive or secondary to an underlying malignancy. Edema is also a common finding and can result from or lead to large fluid shifts in a patient. Pruritus can be a notable complaint in most patients, and severity is often based on the underlying pathology. Skin can become lichenified when the pruritus is persistent, which is seen more often in patients with chronic skin conditions that subsequently worsen, such as atopic dermatitis or CTCL. In general, there is sparing of the palms, soles, and mucous membranes, although keratoderma of the palms and soles can suggest CTCL or pityriasis rubra pilaris. Alopecia, nail dystrophy, and ectropion can be associated with chronic erythroderma, and the presence of these should prompt clinicians to perform further evaluation.

EVALUATION

A careful and detailed history should be obtained, focusing on a history of preexisting skin diseases, prior biopsies performed, new medications, increases or decreases in doses of medications, exposure to chemicals or other allergens, sun exposure, and other systemic symptoms such as fatigue, night sweats, or unintentional weight loss. In early erythroderma, the skin findings may be characteristic of the underlying skin disease, such as typical psoriatic or eczematous plaques (Fig. 14-1) or orange-red plaques with islands of sparing (Fig. 14-2). Although pathology may sometimes be nonspecific, a biopsy should be performed in all patients when the diagnosis is unclear as it may give clues to the underlying diagnosis. If lymphadenopathy is present, lymph node sampling should be considered if the history, physical examination, and histopathology do not provide clues to an underlying etiology, the lymphadenopathy does not resolve with treatment, or the patient does not respond to treatment as expected. Evaluation for systemic associations should be performed including a complete blood count, comprehensive metabolic panel, and blood cultures. In cases in which the etiology remains unclear, additional workup including imaging, HIV testing, and repeat skin biopsy can also be considered. A potential algorithm for evaluation is presented in Figure 14-5.

HISTOPATHOLOGIC FINDINGS

Although histopathology can be nonspecific, a biopsy or multiple biopsies should be performed in patients with new-onset erythroderma or rapidly evolving erythema as they may provide clues to an underlying etiology. Histopathologic features of erythroderma depend on the underlying etiology as well as the duration of the eruption. Acute cases of erythroderma are more likely to demonstrate spongiosis, papillary dermal edema, and a superficial perivascular infiltrate, whereas chronic cases display more hyperkeratosis, psoriasiform hyperplasia, and a thickened papillary dermis.

Additional features may provide clues to the underlying pathology. Patients with psoriatic erythroderma often have psoriasiform hyperplasia of the epidermis, a reduced or absent granular layer, and focal areas of parakeratosis. Patients with underlying atopic dermatitis often demonstrate spongiosis and mixed perivascular inflammation including eosinophils. An infiltrate of atypical lymphocytes with cerebriform nuclei can be seen in erythrodermic CTCL; the presence of epidermotropism or Pautrier's microabscesses are also helpful clues. Unfortunately, with Sezary syndrome or blood involvement of CTCL, histopathology can be very nonspecific in the skin. Alternating ortho- and parakeratosis in combination with psoriasiform hyperplasia can suggest a diagnosis of PRP.

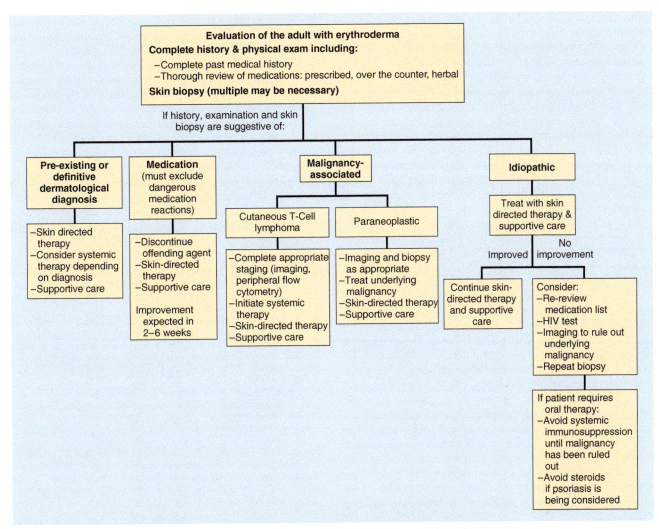

FIGURE 14-5 ■ Algorithm for the evaluation of a patient with erythroderma.

Finally, the presence of eosinophilia can be suggestive of drug-induced erythroderma; however, eosinophilia can be seen in other disease states as well, including atopic dermatitis and CTCL, among others.

COURSE AND TREATMENT

Management of erythroderma should be aimed at treating the underlying cause and any associated complications. For most patients, initial hospitalization is required for appropriate monitoring of fluid–electrolyte balance, nutrition, and thermoregulation, as well as for appropriate skin care. Patients should be kept in a warm, humidified environment, with daily laboratory monitoring including a complete blood count, comprehensive metabolic panel, and electrolyte evaluation. Laboratory abnormalities frequently encountered can include leukocytosis, anemia, electrolyte abnormalities associated with fluid shifts, hypoalbuminemia, hyperuricemia, and elevated inflammatory markers such as erythrocyte sedimentation rate and C-reactive protein. Unnecessary medications should be discontinued. Attention should be paid to ensure the patient has appropriate nutrition, because protein loss through excessive desquamation can cause hypoalbuminemia, edema, and muscle wasting. Patients can also lose a significant amount of heat through the interrupted cutaneous barrier and dilation of the cutaneous vasculature. Increased perfusion of inflamed skin may lead to temperature dysregulation and high-output cardiac failure, which can potentially be life threatening. Bacterial colonization leading to sepsis can also have life-threatening complications, especially in immunocompromised patients.

All patients, regardless of the etiology, should be started on skin-directed therapy, typically topical corticosteroids applied twice daily in conjunction with liberal use of a thick emollient, such as white petrolatum, throughout the day as needed. Consensus is lacking on the appropriate strength of topical corticosteroids. Higher-potency topical steroids may result in systemic absorption due to enhanced permeability of the skin, yet they may also be more efficacious at the outset of treatment. Application of topical corticosteroids under moist gauze wraps can help to increase penetration into the skin. If application under moist dressings is not an option, the "soak and smear" application method can also help to achieve more rapid results. In this method, topical corticosteroids or emollients are applied immediately after a warm bath, while the skin is still damp, followed by tight-fitting cotton garments. Topical corticosteroids and emollients followed by a sauna suit, or nonbreathable clothing, can also achieve similar results.

Given the extensive disruption of their natural skin barrier, patients with erythroderma are at high risk for the development of secondary infections, particularly those of staphylococcal origin. To help prevent infection, acetic-acid-soaked gauze or chlorinated baths can be used. Gauze soaked in 0.25% acetic acid can be applied to the skin and left in place for 10 to 15 minutes daily to reduce bacterial colonization. Alternatively, the patient can soak in a bath with one-quarter cup of household bleach added. Clinicians should have a low threshold for performing blood cultures in patients with a fever and for culturing skin that becomes eroded or yellow-crusted, with subsequent addition of an oral antibiotic if there are concerns for a secondary infection. Coexistent herpetic infection should also be considered in areas of erosion or in those with an acute onset of pain in a previously pruritic eruption.

Oral therapy with antihistamines can help to relieve pruritus. Widespread edema may require oral diuresis, which should be used with caution while focusing on the patient's overall fluid–electrolyte balance. Depending on the underlying disease state, oral corticosteroids may be helpful; however, caution should be utilized as they can worsen erythrodermic psoriasis as well as an infectious process including sepsis. Empiric therapy with a systemic immunosuppressive agent can be considered, but only after CTCL or other malignancy has been ruled out. If the exact etiology of erythroderma is not well understood and systemic therapy is necessary, oral methotrexate or oral retinoids such as acitretin are reasonable options, and therapies such as tumor necrosis factor inhibitors should be avoided to prevent exacerbation of a potential smoldering malignancy. After initial erythroderma is under control, phototherapy also can be considered, but often burns and can worsen skin disease in acute erythroderma.

The prognosis of erythroderma depends on the underlying cause. Erythroderma secondary to a drug reaction can resolve within several weeks, given that the offending agent has been removed. Psoriasis and atopic dermatitis can improve with proper treatment over weeks to months. Erythroderma secondary to CTCL or other malignancy tends to be refractory to standard treatment and can progress quickly with a higher morbidity and mortality. The mortality rate in erythroderma has been reported to be between 11% and 64%, depending on the underlying etiology, but is highest in patients with malignancy-related erythroderma, in individuals who develop high-output cardiac failure, or in those with sepsis.

SUGGESTED READINGS

Callen JP, Bernardi DM, Clark RA, Weber DA. Adult-onset recalcitrant eczema: a marker of noncutaneous lymphoma or leukemia. J Am Acad Dermatol 2000;43:207–10.

Karakayli G, Beckham G, Orengo I, Rosen T. Exfoliative dermatitis. Am Fam Physician 1999;59(3):625–30.

Levine N. Exfoliative erythroderma: skin biopsy is required to determine the cause of this pruritic eruption. Geriatrics 2000;55:25.

Rothe MJ, Bialy TL, Grant-Kels JM. Erythroderma. Dermatol Clin 2000;18(3):405–15.

Rym BM, Mourad M, Bechir Z, Dalenda E, Faika C, Iadh AM, et al. Erythroderma in adults: a report of 80 cases. Int J Dermatol 2005;44(9):731–5.

Sehgal VN, Srivastava G, Sardana K. Erythroderma/exfoliative dermatitis: a synopsis. Int J Dermatol 2004;43(1):39–47.

Sigurdsson V, Toonstra J, Hezemans-Boer M, van Vloten WA. Erythroderma. A clinical and follow-up study of 102 patients, with special emphasis on survival. J Am Acad Dermatol 1996;35(1):53–7.

Wilson DC, Jester JD, King Jr LE. Erythroderma and exfoliative dermatitis. Clin Dermatol 1993;11(1):67–72.

CHAPTER 15

PURPURA

Warren W. Piette

KEY POINTS

- Purpura has an extended and complex differential diagnosis, but can be sorted into three main pathophysiologies: simple hemorrhage, inflammatory (vessel-directed) hemorrhage, and microvascular occlusion.
- Recognition of patterns of morphology, number and distribution can rapidly narrow the diagnostic possibilities enabling a focused and efficient work-up to confirm the diagnosis.
- The differential diagnosis of cutaneous microvascular occlusion only minimally overlaps with traditional differential diagnosis of deep venous thrombosis or pulmonary emboli.
- Distinguishing inflammatory hemorrhage from microvascular occlusion can be difficult because of the clinical and histologic evolution of lesions, but is critical to proper treatment.

PURPURA

The clinical finding of purpura is associated not only with some of the most rapidly life-threatening illnesses known, but also with some of the most common and benign conditions of daily life. Although the evaluation of a patient with purpura can occasionally be complicated, in many cases a good history and physical examination in conjunction with simple tests may be all that is required.

Purpura is a generic term for visible hemorrhage in the skin and mucous membranes. More specific terms describe particular types of purpura, and subtyping purpura is essential for an efficient diagnosis. The term petechia generally implies an area of hemorrhage 4mm or less in diameter (Fig. 15-1). An ecchymosis is a deep reddish-blue, purplish, or blue-black macule, usually at least 1 to 1.5 cm in its greatest dimension. As used in this chapter, the terms petechiae and ecchymoses are also restricted to lesions that are macular (nonpalpable) and without a blanchable component, consistent with simple hemorrhage. A contusion is a major trauma-induced lesion that may be purpuric, and frequently has trauma-related soft-tissue swelling and tenderness. The traditional term palpable purpura is best applied to a lesion that is partially but not completely blanchable, implying a component of early inflammation. Retiform or branching purpura is a term that describes hemorrhage, which may be inflammatory or noninflammatory, but is characterized by a distinctive shape, with branching or reticulate patterning of the whole lesion or of its edges. Noninflammatory retiform purpura most characteristically is due to microvascular occlusive disease in the skin.

PATHOGENESIS

Cutaneous hemorrhage may result from intravascular, vascular, and extravascular causes, and many differential diagnoses use this approach. It may be more helpful to approach the bedside diagnosis of purpura from a morphologic perspective, using the distinctive morphology of purpura to decide between three possible broad pathogenic mechanisms: simple hemorrhage, inflammatory hemorrhage (vessel-directed inflammation), or occlusive hemorrhage with minimal inflammation. This differential applies to lesions of purpura that are primary, meaning that the mechanism of the lesion is also the sole cause of the hemorrhage. Clinical judgment is needed to distinguish primary hemorrhage from hemorrhage secondary to scratching lesions or associated with inflammation such as cellulitis or stasis dermatitis.

Simple Hemorrhage

Simple hemorrhage can be divided into findings with two separate sets of differential diagnoses: petechial or ecchymotic lesions.

Petechial Simple Hemorrhage

Thrombocytopenia or Platelet Dysfunction. Platelet counts above 50,000/mm^3 are usually not accompanied by purpura unless an abnormality of platelet function exists or there is a separate injury. Therefore, thrombocytopenia that might result in hemorrhage occurs at platelet counts of 50,000/mm^3 or less, and typically is not seen until the platelet count is 10,000/mm^3 or below. This is due largely to the role of platelets in releasing a variety of molecules necessary for endothelial cell health, including preserving the cadherin-mediated tight junctions between endothelial cells. Severe thrombocytopenia results in a degradation of endothelial cell health, and an increase in vascular permeability with red cell extravasation, particularly in areas of increased hydrostatic pressure. A variety of disorders can at times produce this degree of thrombocytopenia (Table 15-1). Although severe thrombocytopenia may result in ecchymotic hemorrhage, usually the predominant morphology in any given patient is petechial. Conversely, platelet function defects may result in petechial hemorrhage and must be considered in this differential, but more often

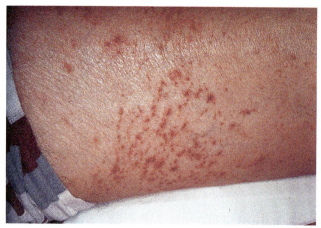

FIGURE 15-1 ■ Small petechiae in an individual with thrombocytopenia.

lead to scattered minor trauma-related ecchymoses. Although thrombocytopenic hemorrhage may occur anywhere, typically it is increased in dependent areas or at sites of minor trauma.

Intravascular Pressure Spikes. Petechial hemorrhage may also result from strong or repetitive localized increases in intravascular pressure. For example, straining during childbirth may produce petechial hemorrhage above the clavicles, solely from the vigorous Valsalva-like pressure effects. This can also occur with vigorous repetitive coughing or retching. In children, vigorous crying may produce a similar supraclavicular distribution of petechial hemorrhage. Ligature placement or strangulation may also produce distinctive patterns of petechial hemorrhage.

Minimally Inflammatory Microvascular Syndromes. There are a variety of minimally inflammatory syndromes affecting the very smallest dermal vessels, which may result in petechial hemorrhage, most included within the syndromes of the chronic pigmented purpuras and benign hypergammaglobulinemic purpura of Waldenström (see Vascular Causes, below).

Platelet function is also important. Intravascular hemorrhage associated with normal platelet counts may result from congenital or hereditary platelet function defects. More commonly encountered are acquired platelet function defects, especially those caused by drugs or metabolic abnormalities, such as severe renal or hepatic impairment. Another type of acquired platelet function defect occurs in patients with monoclonal gammopathies in which there may be interference with normal platelet function by the protein. Finally, patients with myeloproliferative disease and thrombocytosis in the range of 1,000,000/mm^3 will often have platelet dysfunction, and such patients may have problems with both hemorrhage and thrombosis.

Coagulation Cascade Problems in Hemostasis. The ability to form a normal platelet plug is the most important factor for normal hemostasis in the small vessels that supply the skin. The coagulation cascade system becomes important as the diameter of the vessel increases, and increasing forces of pressure and flow require reinforcement of the platelet plug by fibrin clots. This explains why patients with hemophilia or other procoagulant deficiencies of the coagulation cascade system usually do not present with spontaneous petechial hemorrhage. Instead, they present with relatively minor trauma-related injury of larger vessels in skin, fat, joint, or muscle, with the development of an overlying ecchymosis.

Other Intravascular Causes of Hemorrhage. Petechiae may develop in nondependent areas as a result of abrupt increases in capillary and postcapillary venule pressure. Forceful and repetitive Valsalva-like maneuvers, such as paroxysmal vomiting, violent coughing, or straining during childbirth, can cause petechial hemorrhage in supraclavicular areas even in patients whose platelet number and function are normal.

The Gardner–Diamond syndrome, or psychogenic purpura, is sometimes included in discussions of intravascular causes of hemorrhage. Whether this syndrome results from more than factitious disease remains suspect.

Vascular Causes

Vascular causes of hemorrhage include both inflammatory and noninflammatory disorders.

Inflammatory Causes. Inflammatory hemorrhage should include only those disorders in which vessel-directed inflammation is evident. Perivascular inflammation that is not vessel-directed should not be considered vasculitis, and it does not result in palpable purpura, the hallmark but not universal lesion of inflammatory hemorrhage. Lesions of palpable purpura are characterized by a port-wine color, incomplete blanching on pressure or diascopy, and palpability (Fig. 15-2). Partial blanching of an early lesion is an important physical finding, with erythema correlating with inflammation and purpura with hemorrhage. Such lesions, when due to immune complex deposition, usually develop first in dependent areas, which in a bedridden patient may be the back and buttocks. An important cause of palpable purpura is small-vessel leukocytoclastic vasculitis, which has a variety of causes, including idiopathic, postinfectious, and drug-related; IgA-predominant vasculitis (Henoch–Schönlein purpura); mixed cryoglobulinemia; connective tissue disease, such as systemic lupus erythematosus and rheumatoid arthritis; and granulomatosis with polyangiitis (GPA), formerly Wegener's granulomatosis, or allergic granulomatous polyangiitis (AGA) of Churg–Strauss s with or without granulomatous changes. However, the physical findings of palpable purpura may occasionally result from disorders in which vessel-directed inflammation is caused by a predominantly mononuclear cell infiltrate, as in erythema multiforme, and the pityriasis lichenoides group (especially PLEVA [pityriasis lichenoides et varioliformis acuta] syndrome). Patients with the aforementioned conditions who have leukocytoclastic vasculitis demonstrable in young cutaneous lesions may have biopsy specimens from older or treated lesions that show only perivascular lymphocytes.

TABLE 15-1 Partial Differential Diagnosis for Purpura

I. Petechial (nonpalpable)
   A. Hemostatically relevant thrombocytopenia (platelet count <50,000/mm^3, usually <10,000/mm^3)
      1. Idiopathic thrombocytopenic purpura
      2. Thrombotic thrombocytopenic purpura (some cases)
      3. Disseminated intravascular coagulation
      4. Drug-related thrombocytopenia
         a. Peripheral destruction: quinidine, quinine
         b. Marrow: idiosyncratic or dose related
      5. Marrow infiltration, fibrosis, or failure
   B. Abnormal platelet function
      1. Congenital or hereditary platelet function defects
      2. Acquired platelet function defects (e.g., aspirin, renal or hepatic insufficiency, monoclonal gammopathy)
      3. Thrombocytosis in myeloproliferative disease (>1,000,000/mm^3)
   C. Elevated intravascular pressure (Valsalva maneuver-like causes)
   D. Chronic pigmented purpura (occasionally palpable, caused by minimal small-vessel inflammation)
II. Ecchymotic
   A. Procoagulant defect (often localized to sites of minor trauma)
      1. Hemophilia (simple ecchymosis very rare, usually develops over subcutaneous hematoma)
      2. Anticoagulants
      3. Disseminated intravascular coagulation
      4. Vitamin K deficiency
      5. Hepatic insufficiency with poor procoagulant synthesis
   B. Poor dermal support of vessels (usually localized to sites of minor trauma)
      1. Actinic (senile) purpura
      2. Corticosteroid therapy, topical or systemic
      3. Scurvy
      4. Systemic amyloidosis (light chain related)
      5. Ehlers–Danlos syndrome, some types
      6. Pseudoxanthoma elasticum
   C. Abnormal platelet function (see above)
   D. Other
      1. Benign hypergammaglobulinemic purpura of Waldenström (as a result of mild vessel inflammation, usually causes macular hemorrhage, but can produce palpable purpura)
III. Palpable purpura
   A. Classic palpable purpura
      1. Small-vessel leukocytoclastic vasculitis syndromes
         a. Postinfectious, drug-induced, malignancy-associated or idiopathic IgG, IgM immune complex vasculitis
         b. Postinfectious, drug-induced, malignancy-associated or idiopathic IgA-predominant vasculitis (Henoch–Schönlein purpura)
         c. Mixed cryoglobulinemia
         d. Associated with lupus, rheumatoid arthritis, Sjögren's syndrome
         e. Small-vessel lesions of granulomatosis with polyangiitis (GPA—formerly Wegener), allergic granulomatous angiitis (AGA) (of Churg–Strauss), microscopic polyangiitis (MPA)
      2. Pityriasis lichenoides et varioliformis acuta (PLEVA) syndrome
      3. Erythema multiforme (some variants)
   B. Target lesions
      1. Erythema multiforme
   C. Inflammatory retiform purpura (usually vasculitic, both retiform morphology and prominent early erythema)
      1. IgA-predominant small-vessel leukocytoclastic vasculitis (some)
      2. Syndromes of small- and medium-vessel leukocytoclastic vasculitis, such as rheumatic vasculitides, MPA, GPA, AGA
      3. Some early lesions of warfarin- or heparin-induced necrosis demonstrate erythema, but this tends to be at the margin of large, confluent areas of necrosis
IV. Noninflammatory retiform purpura (occlusion syndromes, usually retiform morphology without early erythema)
   A. Disorders of platelet-related thrombopathy: myeloproliferative thrombocytosis, heparin necrosis, paroxysmal nocturnal hemoglobinuria
   B. Disorders of cold-related precipitation or agglutination
   C. Disorders of vessel invasive organisms: ecthyma gangrenosum, aspergillus and other opportunistic fungi, disseminated strongyloidiasis
   D. Disorders of local or systemic control of coagulation: inherited or acquired severe protein C or S deficiency (acquired includes some sepsis/disseminated intravascular coagulation, factor V Leiden thrombophilia, coumadin necrosis, post-varicella/strep purpura fulminans, some antiphospholipid antibody syndromes), antiphospholipid antibody syndrome (APLS), livedoid vasculopathy. Cocaine-levamisole syndrome mostly induces occlusive disease with secondary vasculitic changes, presumable related to induced APLS.
   E. Disorders of embolization: cholesterol or oxalate emboli, atrial myxoma, crystalglobulins
   F. Miscellaneous disorders: cutaneous calciphylaxis, malignant atrophic papulosis (Degos disease), sickle cell ulcerations

The finding of primary palpable purpura indicates only inflammatory hemorrhage, and a biopsy of an early lesion (less than 24 to 48 hours old) is necessary to demonstrate the composition of the initial inflammatory infiltrate and the presence of relevant immune complexes. This has important clinical implications because a patient with cutaneous small-vessel vasculitis may have associated visceral or renal involvement, whereas a patient with palpable purpura as a result of variants of erythema multiforme does not have vasculitis and is instead at risk for

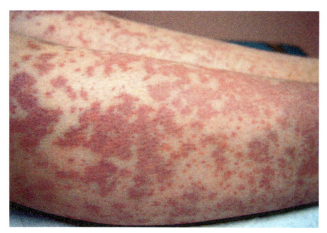

FIGURE 15-2 ■ Typical lesions of palpable purpura in a patient with cutaneous small-vessel vasculitis.

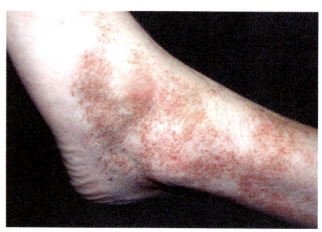

FIGURE 15-3 ■ Clustered petechial hemorrhage with background hyperpigmentation typical of chronic pigmented purpura.

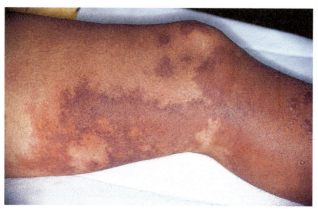

FIGURE 15-4 ■ Noninflammatory retiform purpura in a patient with disseminated intravascular coagulation, Gram-negative sepsis, and diffuse small-dermal-vessel thrombosis and perivascular hemorrhage. These lesions demonstrate little or no erythema (blanching component). (Courtesy of Dr Neil A. Fenske, Tampa, FL.)

the development of mucosal injury, which can be severe. Importantly, not all vasculitic lesions demonstrate early blanching or palpability; this is probably most commonly seen in instances of IgA-predominant vasculitis in adults or children where histologically proven leukocytoclastic vasculitis can manifest at nonblanching purpuric macules, usually 3 to 6 mm in diameter, increasing in number down the legs.

Mild inflammatory conditions that may result in purpura, and occasionally in palpable purpura, include the syndromes of chronic pigmented purpura and benign hypergammaglobulinemic purpura of Waldenström. Chronic pigmented purpura includes several subsets, but patients with this problem usually have areas of recurring hemorrhage, often petechial, with surrounding erythema and brown or "cayenne pepper" hyperpigmentation as a result of hemosiderin deposition in the dermis (Fig. 15-3). Because petechial hemorrhage is common in this syndrome, often the patient or the physician is concerned that there is a serious underlying disorder, such as leukemia. However, chronic pigmented purpura is not associated with internal disease.

Waldenström's hypergammaglobulinemic purpura is usually characterized by macular hemorrhage in either dependent areas or areas covered by restrictive clothing. This condition may be idiopathic or may occur in association with Sjögren's syndrome, sarcoidosis, or other diseases having a polyclonal gammopathy. These lesions may be associated with a burning sensation and may show little or no inflammation on biopsy. This disorder is best characterized by the presence of an IgG or IgA (not IgM) rheumatoid factor, which is demonstrable using analytic ultracentrifugation of serum or plasma. Unfortunately, because this technology is no longer widely used, only those cases with a typical clinical picture and a polyclonal hypergammaglobulinemia will tend to be included in this diagnosis.

Noninflammatory Causes. Bland occlusion syndromes typically present as noninflammatory (and usually retiform) palpable purpura. In these syndromes, fibrin clot, cryoglobulin precipitate, or other material occludes multiple vessels, and this initial occlusion is followed by propagation of a thrombus within the retiform (livedoid) network of superficial dermal venules (Figs 15-4 and 15-5). The list of causes is extensive; these are categorized in Table 15-1. It is important to recognize this subset of purpura as distinct from inflammatory hemorrhage

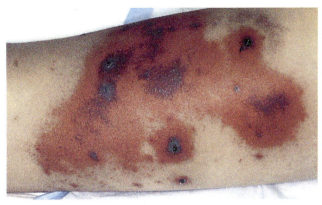

FIGURE 15-5 ■ Purpura fulminans following a varicella infection. Note the retiform extensions at the margins of palpable purpura. Little or no erythema is present.

because, although the therapy differs according to the syndrome, all are treated differently from the syndromes of inflammatory hemorrhage.

Occasionally, lesions of inflammatory retiform purpura will occur. Usually, these result from vasculitides that affect both medium-sized and small vessels, such as GPA, lupus, or rheumatoid vasculitis, and some types of polyarteritis nodosa. However, when such a clinical picture is caused by small-vessel involvement alone, it strongly suggests an IgA-predominant leukocytoclastic vasculitis or cryoglobulin-immune complex vasculitis. Many such patients have multisystem disease, and prolonged or recurrent courses and ulcerations may be more likely in adults. In this setting, the early lesions tend to be classic palpable purpura, with a strong tendency toward the linking of lesions in a livedoid pattern, creating some confluent areas of epidermal or dermal necrosis.

Noninflammatory vascular hemorrhage can occasionally occur as a result of defects in the vascular wall, but such hemorrhage is typically ecchymotic and nonpalpable. The purpura resulting from vessel infiltration in light chain-related systemic amyloidosis is a good example. Because the collagen and elastin content of very small blood vessels is minimal, cutaneous hemorrhage in association with the Ehlers–Danlos syndrome or pseudoxanthoma elasticum is usually not the result of a vessel wall abnormality, but rather of poor vessel wall support by the surrounding connective tissue. The Kasabach–Merritt syndrome, usually seen in infants, occurs with cutaneous or visceral vascular growths of either tufted angioma or Kaposiform hemangioendothelioma. These trigger platelet consumption and thrombosis; a clinical picture mimicking disseminated intravascular coagulation may result.

Extravascular Causes

Extravascular causes of hemorrhage may include either major trauma or minor trauma to the skin. Major trauma results in hemorrhage even in normal skin, is associated with remembered injury, significant tissue swelling, tenderness, or obvious abrasions, and is seldom a diagnostic problem. Purpura related to minor trauma may occur in the absence of obvious tissue

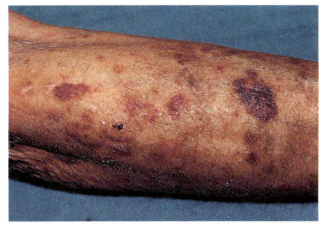

FIGURE 15-6 ■ Ecchymosis as a result of corticosteroid application. Also, note the cutaneous atrophy produced by topical steroids. (Courtesy of Dr Neil A. Fenske, Tampa, FL.)

swelling and often without the patient's recollection of trauma. Such hemorrhage is usually the result of poor support of the small blood vessels by surrounding abnormal connective tissue. The areas of skin most likely to be traumatized include the extensor surface of the forearms, the anterior lower legs, and the dorsum of the hands. Purpura that is caused in part by external trauma tends to be distributed in a geometric pattern, e.g., linearly on the forearm in a scraping injury, or linearly across a periarticular flexural crease. Perhaps the most common type of minor trauma-related purpura is actinic purpura. Most senile purpura should be classified as actinic or solar, because it occurs only in chronically sun-exposed areas with actinic degeneration of the dermis. Corticosteroid excess (endogenous or iatrogenic) is another common cause of poor dermal tissue vascular support (Fig. 15-6).

The presence of perifollicular hemorrhage should suggest the diagnosis of scurvy and requires a nutrition-directed history to exclude scurvy as a cause (Fig. 15-7). The reason for the initial perifollicular localization of vitamin C deficiency is not known. The hemorrhage is probably caused by a collagen defect, because ascorbic acid is a necessary factor for the formation of normal collagen. Light chain-related systemic amyloidosis is a rare but important cause of dramatic minor trauma-related hemorrhage,

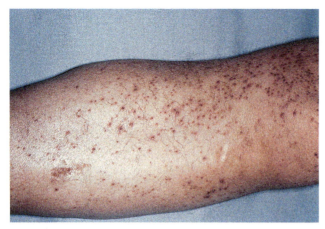

FIGURE 15-7 ■ Perifollicular purpura in a patient with vitamin C deficiency. (Courtesy of Dr Kenneth E. Greer, Charlottesville, VA.)

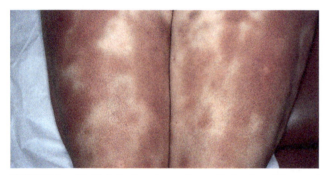

FIGURE 15-8 ■ Multiple bruises in a patient with Gardner–Diamond syndrome.

caused by infiltration of vessel walls and replacement of normal connective tissue by infiltration. Waxy-appearing papules and plaques, or purpura easily induced by light stroking or pinching of the skin, strongly suggest the diagnosis of light chain-related systemic amyloidosis. Cutaneous hemorrhage as a result of Ehlers–Danlos syndrome and pseudoxanthoma elasticum is usually caused by poor dermal tissue support.

The autoerythrocyte sensitization (Gardner–Diamond) syndrome is most likely factitious in its pathogenesis. The disorder occurs primarily in young women who often have significant emotional problems, and is manifested by the rapid development of unexplained noninflammatory purpura (Fig. 15-8). Laboratory studies of immune function and coagulation are within normal limits. It is said that the injection of autologous erythrocytes will reproduce the lesions. Manipulation of injection sites by the patient has been demonstrated in some individuals with this diagnosis.

CLINICAL MANIFESTATIONS

Purpuric Lesion

The first task in unraveling the cause of purpura is to prove that the lesion is purpuric. The color of the lesion should be the result of hemoglobin, i.e., bright red for fully oxygenated; reddish-blue, blue-black, or purple for less-saturated hemoglobin; and blue-black to black for hemorrhage associated with hemorrhagic tissue necrosis. The brown pigmentation of hemosiderin (resulting from the breakdown of hemoglobin) can be impossible to distinguish from melanin pigment, and it is therefore less reliable in establishing past hemorrhage.

Diascopy

Next, at least some of this color must be proved to reside extravascularly. This is done by diascopy, applying direct pressure to a lesion. This is generally done best by using the thicker glass of a pocket hand lens rather than thinner fragile glass slides. Direct lesional compression moves blood within the vessels away from the area, with at lease partial blanching. Blood in the dermis or clotted within the vessels cannot move. A critical assessment is whether a color appropriate for hemorrhage remains within the area being compressed.

Three types of lesions can yield misleading information on diascopy. A tangled mat of small vessels may develop kinks or occluded sections while compressed, thereby trapping blood within vessel segments. A lesion may be too firm, or may develop over soft areas of the skin and simply be pushed into the skin without sufficient compression. For example, cherry (senile) angiomas may be firm, or if they overlie a prominent panniculus (such as on the abdomen) they may be impossible to compress. Finally, any cutaneous eruption may become hemorrhagic when sufficiently traumatized or if it develops in an area of high hydrostatic pressure, e.g., a pruritic area traumatized by scratching, or an active dermatitis occurring near the ankle in an ambulatory patient. By contrast, the presence of symmetrical hemorrhage, especially in dependent areas, or hemorrhage in lesions that the patient cannot easily scratch, and the absence of excoriations suggests that the hemorrhage is primary rather than secondary.

Inflammation

Having established a lesion as primary purpura, the next task to assess is the degree of inflammation using diascopy (see above). Nonpalpable petechiae and simple ecchymoses typically show little or no color change on diascopy, and these represent lesions of simple hemorrhage. Many lesions of vasculitis contain elements of both inflammation (erythema) and hemorrhage (purpura), depending on the pathogenesis of the vessel injury and the age of the lesion. Typical lesions of small-vessel leukocytoclastic vasculitis most commonly present as port-wine papules 5 to 10 mm in diameter (classic palpable purpura), but a subset of vasculitides may present as inflammatory retiform purpura. When due to immune complex deposition, these lesions are concentrated in dependent areas (areas of the highest hydrostatic pressure), whereas clinically identical lesions associated with antineutrophil cytoplasmic antibody (ANCA)-positive syndromes (e.g., GPA, microscopic polyangiitis [MPA]) are much more likely to occur in a random pattern of distribution. Such vasculitic lesions initially have a prominent component of erythema, which becomes less intense and finally disappears as the individual lesion evolves, leaving hemorrhage, vesicles, or ulceration in its place. As previously discussed, some vasculitic lesions present simply as dependent non-blanching macules.

Other forms of inflammatory hemorrhage exist. For example, the lesion most characteristic of erythema multiforme is a target lesion consisting of a central region of intense inflammation with epidermal necrosis or vesicle formation, often associated with an element of purpura. This central area is surrounded by an area of flesh-colored to slightly pale skin, representing relative ischemia, and then by a zone of erythema, thought to represent reactive hyperemia. Erythema multiforme is often idiopathic; the known causes are most frequently medications (including "health foods," vitamins, and other nonprescription items) and herpes simplex infections, especially in recurrent cases.

Bland Occlusion

A third variant of palpable purpura is that which begins as a simple occlusion or thrombosis, usually of multiple dermal vessels, in the absence of significant early inflammation. Such lesions are often palpable but not erythematous, and tend to develop in a livedoid or retiform pattern. Hemorrhage occurs in a perivascular distribution during the early ischemic phase of a lesion as endothelial junctions break down. Inflammation is usually absent initially, but may ultimately develop as a response to ischemic necrosis. Such bland occlusion occurs in a variety of clinical settings, including some types of disseminated intravascular coagulation, or with cold-induced but not immune complex-mediated cryoglobulinemia syndromes.

HISTORY AND PHYSICAL FINDINGS

Because purpura has many different causes, the associated history and physical findings vary greatly. For instance, arthralgias, arthritis, fever, and visceral lesions may accompany cutaneous small-vessel vasculitis. Monoclonal cryoglobulinemia results from benign or malignant lymphoproliferative disease, which may have other manifestations. Hepatitis C infection is now recognized as the most common cause of what was formerly termed essential cryoglobulinemia. Syndromes of disseminated intravascular coagulation usually occur in association with sepsis, malignancy, or other serious underlying disorders. Although many clinicians now seem to use the term purpura fulminans to imply extensive purpuric lesions of any type, the term was originally coined to describe the findings in patients whose dermatologic lesions resulted from extensive noninflammatory thrombosis, presenting clinically as noninflammatory retiform purpura.

The number and pattern of palpable purpura can be very helpful in suggesting the likely etiology of cutaneous hemorrhage. Simple petechial hemorrhage from platelet problems or chronic pigmented purpura often clusters on the lower legs. Immune complex vasculitis also typically produces many lesions on the legs, increasing in number with dependency, but the presence of palpable or partially blanchable lesions favors the diagnosis of vasculitis.

The ANCA-associated vasculitides, along with microvascular occlusion syndromes most often presented with few and scattered lesions. Acral purpura may be cold-localized from cold occlusion syndromes, may be part of the sock–glove purpura syndrome from a virus, usually parvovirus B19, or may be an early localization of disseminated intravascular coagulation/purpura fulminans-related occlusion in hypotensive patients, particularly if on vasopressive agents.

HISTOPATHOLOGIC FINDINGS

Both petechiae and ecchymoses show simple extravasation of red blood cells into the dermis on biopsy, the difference being the total volume of extravasation. Patients with inflammatory hemorrhage may show leukocytoclastic vasculitis, characterized by the presence of at least some neutrophils in and around vessel walls, the presence of perivascular nuclear dust (representing degenerated neutrophil nuclei), and fibrinoid necrosis of the vessel wall. This is the histologic correlate of most forms of necrotizing vasculitis. Other types of inflammatory hemorrhage, such as erythema multiforme, may have relatively few neutrophils in an infiltrate composed largely of mononuclear cells. Syndromes of bland occlusion or thrombus typically include multiple dermal vessels occluded by pink to hyaline material with intermingled red cells, perivascular extravasation of red cells, and often little to no inflammation in early lesions.

Understanding the differences in lesional evolution between these processes is essential in the correct interpretation of clinical and biopsy findings. The earliest lesions of leukocytoclastic vasculitis might have much more erythema than hemorrhage, with early signs of neutrophil-rich inflammation, and significant remaining components of the immune complexes that triggered the lesion. A later stage of the lesion might have comparable degrees of purpura and erythema, a full-blown fibrinoid necrosis on biopsy, but total destruction or removal of the inciting immune complexes in the vessel wall. A resolving lesion would have little or no erythema and a nonspecific inflammatory infiltrate.

By contrast, bland occlusion syndromes typically begin with little inflammation, prominent hemorrhage, and propagation of a clot within vessels; significant necrosis may develop later, followed by a wound-healing response of nonspecific inflammation. Ulcers from any cause may have features of secondary leukocytoclastic vasculitis at their margins. Choosing an appropriate lesion to biopsy is essential for a proper diagnosis. Fundamental to this appropriate selection is recognizing the distinct clinical evolution of lesions that result from different pathogenic processes.

DIFFERENTIAL DIAGNOSIS

The differential diagnosis of purpura is extensive, sometimes confusing, and usually challenging. Table 15-1 lists a partial differential diagnosis that uses morphologic features to separate groups by their likely pathogenesis.

EVALUATION

The history provides much useful information in the assessment of purpuric syndromes, e.g., a family history of a bleeding or thrombotic disorder, the use of drugs that might affect platelet function or coagulation, the presence of underlying metabolic disease that might affect clotting parameters, or a constellation of symptoms that might suggest a particular disease or syndrome.

The bedside correlation of morphology with pathogenesis allows a much more thoughtful and focused approach to aspects of the history and physical examination relevant to the pathogenesis of hemorrhage. This is important in both choosing and interpreting appropriate tests. Abnormal values are not always indicative of important disease, or they can be misleading. For example, a prolonged partial thromboplastin time (PTT) usually implies a coagulation factor deficiency and would correlate with a tendency to develop ecchymotic hemorrhage. The finding of lupus anticoagulant can also prolong the PTT, but if it causes disease will result not in simple ecchymosis but instead in atrophie blanche-like lesions or noninflammatory necrosis or retiform purpura as a result of dermal vessel thrombosis.

A complete blood cell count and differential can be used to assess the number and morphology of platelets, to screen for schistocytes (which suggest a microangiopathic anemia, as may be seen in disseminated intravascular coagulation), and to explore the likelihood of myeloproliferative disease. A bleeding time is a useful screen of abnormal platelet function, but a history is usually adequate for diagnosing the most frequent cause of platelet dysfunction, i.e., aspirin use. Reasonable screens for defects in the coagulation cascade system include the PTT and the prothrombin time. More specialized clotting studies, such as protein C and protein S levels, are important in cases of bland occlusion syndromes, but can be falsely low or high in the months following significant occlusive episodes. Screens for the antiphospholipid antibody syndrome might include a PTT or dilute Russell viper venom test to look for lupus anticoagulant activity, occasionally a venereal disease research laboratory test to look for false positives, and anticardiolipin or antiphospholipid antibody tests. Most studies suggest that elevated IgG anticardiolipin antibodies are more likely to be predictive of or explain thrombosis, but IgM antibodies can occasionally be responsible for thrombotic disease. Unfortunately, IgG or IgM anticardiolipin antibodies have a high rate of false positivity in predicting thrombosis, and may be negative in patients whose thrombosis is due to lupus anticoagulant/antiphospholipid disease. Serum and plasma tubes drawn and spun down at body temperature are essential for excluding cryoglobulin- or cryofibrinogen-related disease. When the clinical picture is appropriate, an antinuclear antibody titer, SS-A and SS-B levels, rheumatoid factor titer, serum protein electrophoresis, or immunoelectrophoresis might be indicated. A biopsy of an appropriate lesion early in its evolution is important for the proper diagnosis of palpable purpura, and immunofluorescence studies of early lesions for immune complexes are useful if leukocytoclastic vasculitis is suspected. Direct immunofluorescence may be negative, especially if older lesions (greater than 48 to 72 hours old) are biopsied. Some lesions of leukocytoclastic vasculitis are negative for direct immunofluorescence in all stages and the pathogenesis of such lesions is unclear. Urinalysis to look for blood, cells, or crystals and testing the stool for occult blood are important to exclude associated or underlying disease, especially in vasculitic syndromes.

TREATMENT

Treatment in purpuric syndromes is directed at the specific cause of the hemorrhage, so the correct diagnosis is critical to proper care. The treatment of cutaneous vasculitis is discussed in Chapter 4.

SUGGESTED READINGS

Carlson JA, Cavaliere LF, Grant-Kels JM. Cutaneous vaculitis: diagnosis and management. Clin Dermatol 2006;24:4414–29.
Nachman RL, Rafii S. Platelets, petechiae, and preservation of the vascular wall. N Engl J Med 2008;359:1261–70.
Piette WW, Stone MS. A cutaneous sign of IgA-associated small dermal vessel leukocytoclastic vasculitis in adults (Henoch–Schönlein purpura). Arch Dermatol 1989;125:53–6.
Piette WW. The differential diagnosis of purpura from a morphologic perspective. Adv Dermatol 1994;9:3–24.
Thornsberry LA, LoSicco KI, English III JC. The skin and hypercoaguable states. J Am Acad Dermatol 2013;69:450–62.
Weinstein S, Piette WW. Cutaneous manifestations of antiphospholipid antibody syndrome. Hematol Oncol Clin North Am 2008;22:67–77.
Wysong A, Venkatesab P. An approach to the patient with retiform purpura. Dermatologic Therapy 2011;24:151–72.

CHAPTER 16

BULLOUS DISEASES

Anneli R. Bowen • John J. Zone

> **KEY POINTS**
>
> - Immunobullous diseases are a complicated multisystem management challenge requiring advanced immunosuppressive regimens.
> - Pathogenesis has been linked to disease-specific autoantibodies to structural antigens within the epidermis and basement membrane zone.
> - The location of blistering, risk of subsequent scarring, and degree of systemic involvement depend upon the type and distribution of antigen targeted.
> - Clinical presentation, histologic findings, and immunofluorescence studies (both indirect and direct) are the cornerstone of diagnosis.
> - Treatment of pemphigus and pemphigoid includes systemic steroids, azathioprine, mycophenolate mofetil, and rituximab, as well as IVIg or plasmapheresis for refractory cases.
> - Epidermolysis bullosa acquisita is notoriously refractory to treatment, but may respond to management similar to that of bullous pemphigoid.
> - Drug-induced and paraneoplastic variants of pemphigoid, pemphigus, and linear IgA bullous dermatosis occur that tend to improve following cessation of the offending drug or treatment of the underlying malignancy.
> - Dermatitis herpetiformis is a manifestation of celiac disease and responds to a strict gluten-free diet.
> - Because dermatitis herpetiformis and linear IgA bullous dermatosis are both neutrophil-mediated processes, dapsone is the most effective immunomodulating agent.

Immunobullous diseases can precipitate extreme stress to multiple organ systems. Severe cases can have extensive mucocutaneous involvement, and have the potential for secondary infection and fluid loss. These diseases are also associated with a variety of systemic disorders, both directly and indirectly. Furthermore, the requirement for systemic corticosteroid and immunosuppressive therapy may produce myriad systemic complications.

Comprehension of the biology of keratinocyte interactions with other keratinocytes and with the extracellular matrix is essential for understanding the autoimmune blistering diseases. Keratinocytes attach to each other by desmosomes, whereas they attach to the underlying basement membrane by hemidesmosomes (Fig. 16-1). Desmosomes consist of an intracellular cytoplasmic plaque made up of the molecules desmoplakin, plakophilin, and plakoglobin. This cytoplasmic plaque interacts with the intracellular scaffolding of tonofilaments and anchors the keratin intermediate filaments to the hemidesmosome. The extracellular portion of the desmosome is comprised of desmogleins and desmocollins, which project onto the cell surface of the keratinocyte and contact desmosomal proteins of neighboring keratinocytes. Disruption of desmosomal interactions leads to acantholysis.

Hemidesmosomes attach basal keratinocytes to the underlying basement membrane. Together with the basement membrane zone (BMZ), hemidesmosomes form the dermoepidermal junction. Proteins that comprise the hemidesmosome are the bullous pemphigoid antigens 1 (BP230) and 2 (BP180), plectin, and α6β4 integrin. BPAG1 is a 230-kDa intracellular molecule, whereas the 180-kDa BPAG2 is an anchoring filament that spans the keratinocyte extracellular membrane, extending into the BMZ. Disruption of hemidesmosomal interactions is implicated in bullous pemphigoid, pemphigoid (herpes) gestationis (discussed in Chapter 35), and linear IgA bullous dermatosis. The BMZ is divided into the lamina lucida and lamina densa, named according to their transmission electron microscopic appearance. Anchoring filaments extend from the hemidesmosome through the lamina lucida to the lamina densa, where they interact with collagen IV and laminin 332. The papillary dermis attaches to the BMZ by anchoring fibrils, which either extend from the lamina densa down to dermal anchoring plaques, or loop back up to reattach to the lamina densa. Anchoring fibrils are composed of collagen VII. The blistering in the epidermolysis bullosa acquisita is thought to be due to disruption of molecular interactions in this region. Important structural proteins in the dermis include types I and II collagen and elastin.

PEMPHIGUS

Pemphigus is characterized by detachment of adhesions between keratinocytes (acantholysis). This process results in vesicles, bullae, and subsequent erosions of both cutaneous and mucosal surfaces. Affected skin in pemphigus vulgaris reveals flaccid blisters that generally develop on

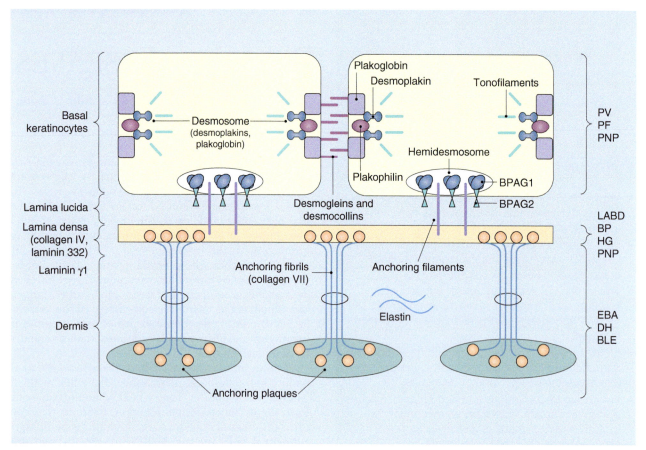

FIGURE 16-1 ■ The dermal–epidermal junction consists of the basal keratinocytes, the basement membrane and the papillary dermis with their structural and attachment molecules. Diseases are listed on the right by the location of their target antigen(s). PV, pemphigus vulgaris; PF, pemphigus foliaceus; PNP, paraneoplastic pemphigus; LABD, linear IgA bullous dermatosis; BP, bullous pemphigoid; HG, herpes gestationis; EBA, epidermolysis bullosa acquisita; DH, dermatitis herpetiformis; BLE, bullous lupus erythematosus; BPAG1 and 2, bullous pemphigoid antigens 1 and 2.

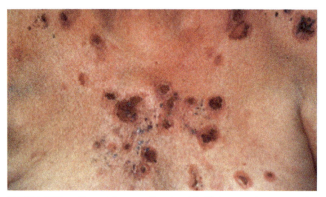

FIGURE 16-2 ■ Pemphigus vulgaris. Multiple erosions on the trunk of this patient were preceded by blisters.

Pathogenesis

The pathogenetic process in pemphigus is that of an organ-specific autoimmune disease. Lesional skin and usually serum demonstrate the presence of an IgG class autoantibody directed against desmoglein antigens present in normal squamous epithelium. The exact mechanism for this loss of self-tolerance is unknown, but CD4+ T cells recognize distinct epitopes of the extracellular portions of desmoglein 1 and 3, and preferentially produce T-helper type 2 (Th2) cytokines. Autoantibody production in pemphigus vulgaris and pemphigus foliaceus is polyclonal, and most antibodies in active disease are of the IgG_4 subclass. Patients in remission who have persistent pemphigus antibodies in their serum have mainly the IgG_1 subtype.

Several lines of evidence support the critical role of antibodies to desmogleins in the clinical acantholytic process. First, the antibody is consistently present in lesional skin and the patient's serum. The serum autoantibody titers correlate with disease activity and there is a therapeutic response to plasmapheresis. Passive transfer of pemphigus from mothers to neonates occurs. Pemphigus antibody produces acantholysis when added to normal human skin in organ culture, and results in detachment when added to epidermal cell cultures. Further

noninflamed skin, are readily broken, and progress to large, weeping, denuded areas (Fig. 16-2). Oropharyngeal erosions are common and may be the presenting sign (Fig. 16-3). The pemphigus group of diseases is divided into pemphigus vulgaris (with its variant pemphigus vegetans), pemphigus foliaceus (with its variants pemphigus erythematosus and fogo selvagem), IgA pemphigus, and paraneoplastic pemphigus.

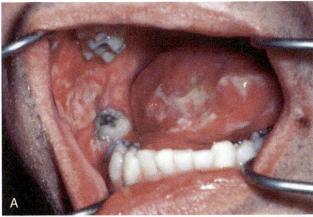

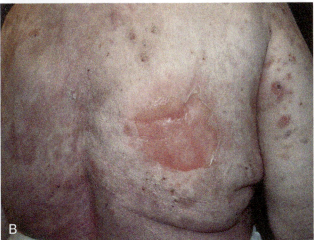

FIGURE 16-3 ■ **A,** Oral erosions of pemphigus are often the earliest lesions, as in this patient. (Courtesy of Mark Bernstein, MD, Louisville, KY.) **B,** Pemphigus foliaceus in this elderly woman was initially misdiagnosed as impetigo.

convincing evidence of the pathogenetic role of pemphigus antibody has been provided by the demonstration that IgG fraction purified from the serum of patients with pemphigus can induce a disease in neonatal mice that reproduces the clinical, histologic, and immunologic features of human pemphigus.

There are two alternative hypotheses to explain the autoantibody-mediated acantholysis: the desmoglein compensation hypothesis and the intracellular signaling hypothesis. In the desmoglein compensation hypothesis, binding of IgG to desmoglein molecules structurally disrupts epidermal cell adhesion. Desmoglein 1 (Dsg 1) expression is very low in mucosa, but it is expressed throughout the skin and increases in the more superficial layers. Desmoglein 3 (Dsg 3), by contrast, is expressed in all levels of mucosa, but only in and near the basal layer of the skin. Therefore, pemphigus foliaceus with Dsg 1 antibodies leads to superficial blistering in the skin, but no oral involvement. Pemphigus vulgaris with only Dsg 3 antibodies (mucosal-dominant pemphigus vulgaris) leads to oral erosions but minimal skin blisters. Amagai has proposed the "desmoglein compensation theory" as an explanation of this phenomenon, suggesting that Dsg 1 in the skin can "compensate" for the loss of Dsg 3 adhesion in this form of the disease. Finally, there can be no desmoglein compensation in pemphigus with both Dsg 1 and 3 antibodies (mucocutaneous pemphigus vulgaris), so acantholysis results in both skin and mucosa. Complement activation is not thought to play a role in acantholysis. The second hypothesis involves binding of IgG to the desmoglein cell surface antigen. This triggers transmembrane signaling and a series of intracellular pathways that lead to separation of the epidermal cells. These pathways are complex, but the validity of the process has been documented in vitro.

Although the stimulus for pemphigus antibody formation is unknown, the endemic nature of pemphigus foliaceus in Brazil suggests the involvement of an environmental factor, possibly an infectious agent. Most of the cases in Brazil occur in populations residing near rivers, and an insect vector for a microorganism has been proposed. Whether pemphigus in other geographic areas is precipitated by similar events is unknown. D-Penicillamine may produce pemphigus (predominantly pemphigus foliaceus) in patients being treated for rheumatoid arthritis, Wilson's disease, scleroderma, or other penicillamine-responsive disorders. Consequently, it is likely that a variety of stimuli may give rise to epidermal antigen intolerance.

There is a strong association of pemphigus vulgaris with the HLA class II alleles HLA DRB*0402, DRB*0401, and DQB1*0503. These HLA alleles may restrict autoreactive responses to desmoglein 3.

Classification

There are two histopathologically distinct forms of pemphigus. Pemphigus vulgaris is the most severe type and is characterized histopathologically by suprabasilar cleft formation, whereas pemphigus foliaceus is less severe and is distinguished by blister formation within or just beneath the granular layer. In pemphigus vulgaris and, to a lesser extent, pemphigus foliaceus, the blister may extend into surrounding nonblistered skin by applying shearing pressure to perilesional tissue (Nikolsky's sign).

Pemphigus vulgaris is the most common form of pemphigus and is generally seen in the fourth to sixth decades of life. It has, however, been described both in children and in the elderly. Prior to the use of corticosteroids, 50% of patients with the disease died within the first 12 months, most frequently from secondary cachexia, sepsis, and/or electrolyte imbalance. Now, with the broad utilization of immunosuppressants, the mortality is 5%.

Pemphigus vegetans is a rare variant of pemphigus vulgaris. Proliferative and verrucous lesions with surrounding pustules gradually develop from denuded bullae on intertriginous cutaneous surfaces. Such lesions were more common in the era before corticosteroid use and may represent a host response to the blistering process. Spontaneous remission is somewhat more likely in the vegetans form. Histopathologically one sees epidermal proliferation with hyperkeratosis, papillomatosis, and acantholysis with intraepidermal abscesses containing eosinophils.

Pemphigus foliaceus is generally less severe than pemphigus vulgaris. The superficial vesicles rupture easily, producing shallow erosions and crusting that clinically resemble impetigo. Clinical blistering may be totally absent. Lesions occur on the chest, back, and scalp, and may produce a seborrhea-like scaling with eventual spread to acral areas after a prolonged period. Clinically visible mucosal lesions are absent, even in advanced cases. Autoantibodies in pemphigus foliaceus are directed predominantly against desmoglein 1. Pemphigus herpetiformis is a morphologic variant of pemphigus vulgaris or pemphigus foliaceus that occurs as grouped vesicles.

Fogo selvagem is an endemic form of pemphigus foliaceus seen in Brazil. It occurs predominantly in children and young adults from poor rural areas. It is characterized by desquamation, erythroderma, and an intense burning in the sun-exposed skin, giving rise to the term fogo selvagem ("wild fire" in Portuguese). Histopathologically and immunopathologically it is indistinguishable from pemphigus foliaceus. Unlike other pemphigus variants, this condition can be seen in multiple members of a single family. There is an increased frequency of HLA-DRB1 haplotypes, DRB1*0404, 1402, 1406, and 1401. An environmental "second hit" is suspected but not identified. Because of the clustering of cases near rivers, *Simulium* black flies have been suggested as a possible vector. IgM-anti-Dsg 1 is found in a majority of fogo selvagem patients in their native environment, but is uncommon in patients with other pemphigus phenotypes and in fogo selvagem patients who move to more urban settings, further supporting a recurrent environmental antigenic exposure in the pathogenesis of this disease.

Pemphigus erythematosus (Senear–Usher's syndrome) represents a localized variant of pemphigus foliaceus characterized by erythematous lupus-like malar dermatitis. Patients frequently manifest an abnormal antinuclear antibody test as well as the presence of pemphigus antibody. Direct immunofluorescence microscopy may show immunoglobulin and complement components along the basement membrane, as well as characteristic intercellular pemphigus antibody deposition. This disorder is believed to represent the coexistence of lupus erythematosus and pemphigus foliaceus.

IgA pemphigus comprises a recently characterized group of IgA-mediated immunobullous diseases. This entity presents as vesicopustules with neutrophils and acantholysis, most commonly affecting the axillae and groin. Oral involvement is rare. IgA pemphigus is subdivided into two histologic types: the subcorneal pustular dermatosis type with blister formation subcorneally, and the intraepidermal neutrophilic type where blisters form throughout the epidermis. The IgA pemphigus antibodies in the subcorneal pustular dermatosis type recognize desmocollin 1, whereas rare IgA pemphigus sera recognize desmoglein 1 and 3. The antigen in the intraepidermal neutrophilic form remains uncharacterized. Only 50% of patients have circulating autoantibody on indirect immunofluorescence. The subcorneal pustular dermatosis form is clinically indistinguishable from Snedden–Wilkinson's disease and must be differentiated by immunofluorescence studies. Rarely, either form of IgA pemphigus may exhibit concomitant expression of IgG autoantibodies—so-called IgA/IgG pemphigus.

Penicillamine and angiotensin-converting enzyme (ACE) inhibitor therapies have been associated with a variety of autoimmune disorders, including pemphigus vulgaris and pemphigus foliaceus. Pemphigus foliaceus accounts for 70% of the penicillamine-induced cases, and pemphigus vulgaris composes the remainder. The development of pemphigus may occur with a wide range of dosages and is often a late complication of therapy. After discontinuation of penicillamine therapy approximately half the patients resolve in 4 months, whereas the other half require suppressive corticosteroid therapy over a longer period. Autoantibodies from drug-induced patients have the same antigenic specificity on a molecular level as do those from idiopathic forms of pemphigus.

Pemphigus has occurred in association with thymoma and myasthenia gravis. Pemphigus vulgaris, pemphigus foliaceus, and pemphigus erythematosus have all been noted associations. There is little, if any, concordance between the clinical activities of the coexistent disorders. The concurrence is believed to involve an underlying failure of thymic-dependent lymphocytes in suppressing autoimmune disease.

The description of paraneoplastic pemphigus (PNP) as a distinct disorder by Anhalt et al. focuses this issue in a small subgroup of patients who had a clear-cut association of pemphigus with a tumor. The patients are clinically heterogeneous and somewhat atypical. Clinical descriptions partially resemble Stevens–Johnson's syndrome, with target lesions and painful oral lesions seen on occasion. Some patients have been described as having a papulosquamous eruption, whereas others have tense bullae. The most common associations, in descending order, are non-Hodgkin's lymphoma, chronic lymphocytic leukemia, Castleman's disease, and solid tumors including carcinomas, sarcomas, and melanoma. Histologically, suprabasilar acantholysis has been described in some cases, whereas keratinocyte necrosis, basal cell vacuolization, interface inflammation, and even basement membrane blisters have been described in others.

The immunofluorescent pattern in paraneoplastic pemphigus is one of intercellular IgG deposition, which may be patchy and focal, and basement membrane zone IgG and complement deposition. Circulating autoantibodies bind to different tissue sources than standard pemphigus antibodies, including urinary bladder, respiratory epithelium, and desmosomal areas of myocardium and skeletal muscle. Indirect immunofluorescence to rat bladder is the most specific diagnostic tool. PNP sera react to a unique complex of antigens, which includes the plakin protein family, including desmoplakin, bullous pemphigoid antigen 1 (BPAG1), envoplakin and periplakin, and desmogleins 1 and 3. Patients with paraneoplastic pemphigus may have antibodies to one or all of these antigens, or may start with a few and with time develop antibodies to other paraneoplastic pemphigus antigens. This observed progression may represent epitope spreading.

Unique to paraneoplastic pemphigus is a large proportion of patients who develop bronchiolitis obliterans, a lethal pulmonary condition characterized by severe hypoxia, a relatively clear chest X-ray, and an association in at least one patient with IgG deposition in bronchial epithelium intracellular spaces. Because desmoplakins are present in bronchial epithelium it is possible that this pulmonary finding is autoimmune-mediated. In summary, it appears that this is an unusual mucocutaneous disorder with myriad clinicopathologic findings, some of which are not a part of any of the forms of pemphigus.

Other sporadic and poorly understood associations with pemphigus include pernicious anemia, red blood cell aplasia, rheumatoid arthritis, and lymphomatoid granulomatosis.

Differential Diagnosis

The differential diagnosis of blistering disorders of the skin ranges from a wide variety of banal dermatoses to more serious and progressive disorders such as pemphigus, bullous pemphigoid (Fig. 16-4), and epidermolysis bullosa acquisita. These disorders require clinical, histopathologic, and immunopathologic evaluation for definite diagnosis. When the etiology of blistering disorders cannot be recognized, biopsy is warranted. Subsequent decisions are made on the basis of these findings. Histopathologic characteristics of potential blistering disorders that will not be discussed here in detail are listed in Table 16-1.

Many patients with oral ulcerations of pemphigus are misdiagnosed as having aphthous stomatitis. After months to years, however, such patients typically progress to have extramucosal involvement.

Acantholysis is the hallmark of immunologically mediated pemphigus, but it may also be seen in Grover's disease (transient acantholytic dermatosis), Darier's disease (keratosis follicularis), and Hailey–Hailey's disease (benign familial pemphigus). In Grover's disease there is involvement of the trunk with pruritic papulovesicles, but no oral involvement. It is frequently precipitated by sun exposure or heat and lasts for weeks to months, although chronic cases are not uncommon.

Darier's disease is an autosomal dominant disorder characterized by yellowish-brown crusted papules on the scalp, intertriginous areas, and seborrheic areas of the face and trunk. The disease is slowly progressive and seldom overtly bullous. Lesions are frequently perifollicular. Although acantholysis is suprabasilar, as in pemphigus vulgaris, characteristic dyskeratotic changes (corps ronds and grains) occur within the epidermis.

Hailey–Hailey's disease (benign familial pemphigus) is an autosomal dominant disorder characterized by multiple grouped erythematous vesicles in intertriginous areas. Mucosal surfaces are usually spared. There is extensive loss of intercellular bridges, with partial coherence of cells throughout all levels of the epidermis.

The clinical pattern of these acantholytic disorders is usually distinctive from that of pemphigus. If confusion exists, direct immunofluorescence of perilesional skin is negative for IgG deposition in these disorders, whereas pemphigus patients demonstrate characteristic intercellular IgG deposition in stratified squamous epithelial tissues.

Patient Evaluation

Close examination of all mucous membranes is indicated. Oral involvement is the rule in pemphigus vulgaris, but esophageal as well as vulvar involvement may occur.

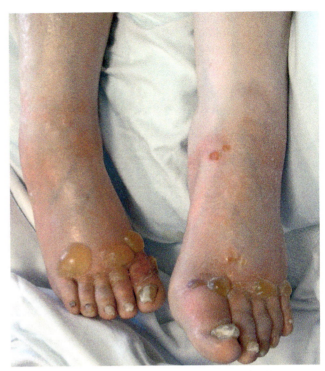

FIGURE 16-4 ■ Tense bullae are representative of bullous pemphigoid.

TABLE 16-1   Blistering dermatoses

1. Subcorneal vesicles
   a. Bullous impetigo
   b. Staphylococcal scalded skin syndrome
   c. Miliaria
   d. Subcorneal pustular dermatosis
   e. Candidiasis
2. Spongiotic blisters
   a. Eczematous disorders, including allergic contact dermatitis, stasis dermatitis, irritant dermatitis, fungal dermatitis, etc.
   b. Incontinentia pigmenti
3. Ballooning degeneration of epidermal cells
   a. Herpes simplex
   b. Herpes zoster and varicella

Significant esophageal symptoms and even stricture may develop. Consequently, esophageal symptoms mandate endoscopy and possible biopsy. Patients presenting with blistering skin disorders that cannot be easily explained (e.g., friction blisters and contact dermatitis) require biopsy. If there is histopathologic acantholysis, biopsy of perilesional skin for direct immunofluorescence should be performed. Indirect immunofluorescence microscopy demonstrating pemphigus antibodies in the serum further confirms the diagnosis, and antibody titers typically correlate with disease activity. Disappearance of antibody from the serum frequently precedes remission.

Chest X-ray to rule out an associated thymoma and a search for clinical symptoms of myasthenia gravis is part of good clinical care, but a low yield of positive findings is to be expected. Culture of potentially infected lesions and close attention to protein loss and malnutrition are necessary in severe cases. Chest X-ray, tuberculosis skin test, complete blood count (CBC), and blood glucose determination should be undertaken prior to initiating corticosteroid or immunosuppressive therapy.

Treatment

Initial therapy of pemphigus involves complete suppression of blistering with oral prednisone (usually 1 to 2 mg/kg daily). Initial control with 3 to 4 mg/kg daily has been suggested, but in the authors' estimation is associated with unnecessarily severe side effects. Because therapy may need to be continued for years, corticosteroid side effects become a major clinical problem. Corticosteroid sparing may be accomplished by the addition of an immunosuppressive agent, as discussed below. Immunosuppression is continued in sufficient doses to suppress blistering until serum antibody titers become negative, at which time tapering of therapy should be attempted. Follow-up biopsy for direct immunofluorescence once clinical manifestations have cleared for >6 months on treatment can predict the likelihood of remission once medications are stopped. Ratnam and Pang showed that three-quarters of patients with negative direct immunofluorescence at this stage remain in remission, and those with negative direct immunofluorescence who do recur have mild disease. In contrast, all patients with a positive follow-up direct immunofluorescence tend to relapse within 3 months of discontinuing therapy.

Systemic methotrexate (oral, intravenous, or intramuscular) can be used in dosages of 20 to 50 mg per week, but may aggravate oral ulcers. Cyclophosphamide is effective in oral dosages of 1 to 3 mg/kg/day, and oral azathioprine may be used in dosages of 1 to 3 mg/kg/day. Mycophenolate mofetil is effective alone or in combination with steroids in doses of 1 to 3 g/day. Close attention should be paid to a variety of potential side effects, including leukopenia, hepatotoxicity, teratogenesis, sterility, oral ulcers, and cystitis, depending on the specific agent used. Patients with excessive toxicity from oral corticosteroids or cyclophosphamide may have reduced side effects with monthly pulse doses.

Plasmapheresis may be useful in pemphigus patients poorly controlled on conventional therapy. Six-liter exchanges on three separate occasions over a 3-week period are necessary to lower the antibody titer significantly. Immunosuppressants such as cyclophosphamide are then necessary to maintain the improvement and prevent the rebound of antibody levels that usually follows plasmapheresis.

Intravenous immunoglobulin (IVIg) therapy is emerging as a promising treatment for many immune-mediated diseases. It works rapidly, and selectively lowers serum levels of pemphigus antibody. The clinical response in individual patients is variable. The concurrent administration of an immunosuppressive agent to prevent the synthesis of new antibody improves the efficacy. The dose is usually 2 g/kg/cycle, administered over 2 to 5 days. It is traditionally given in monthly cycles, but the optimal frequency of cycles is unknown. Caution needs to be taken to avoid fluid overload in elderly patients, and venous thrombosis may occur with administration.

Rituximab is a murine–human chimeric monoclonal antibody to CD20, an antigen present on B cells but not plasma cells. It is approved for use in B-cell lymphoma and is being used off-label for pemphigus and pemphigoid. Administration in a dose of 375 mg/m^2 once weekly for 4 weeks rapidly reduces the peripheral B-cell count to zero and sustains this level for 6 to 12 months. Rituximab has also been used in a dosing schedule similar to its rheumatologic use or 1000 mg initially, followed by a second infusion at 2 weeks. It seems that either dosing schedule results in a similar chance of response. Clinical improvement usually occurs within days to weeks, indicating that mechanisms other than B-cell depletion may be active. Pemphigus antibodies decrease in response to therapy and complete remission may occur. The risk of fatal infection is increased, and at present it is recommended that it be reserved for severe disease unresponsive to conventional therapy.

Because of its neutrophil-mediated pathogenesis, the drug of choice for IgA pemphigus is dapsone. Doses of 100 mg/day are usually sufficient. For patients unable to tolerate dapsone, etretinate is an alternative, providing immunosuppression by interfering with neutrophil and monocyte chemotaxis.

BULLOUS PEMPHIGOID

Bullous pemphigoid (BP) is the most common subepidermal blistering disorder. It is characterized by subepidermal vesicles and bullae that, unlike the lesions of pemphigus vulgaris, do not rupture easily and rarely produce large areas of denuded skin. Oropharyngeal lesions occur commonly, and may be the only manifestation of the disease (mucous membrane pemphigoid). Cutaneous blisters generally arise from erythematous or urticarial plaques (Fig. 16-5). BP is often self-limited, and in contrast to pemphigus vulgaris the mortality is low even in the absence of corticosteroid therapy. However, BP is a potentially serious disease because it typically occurs in older individuals whose compromised status predisposes them to infection and the complications of corticosteroid therapy. BP is characterized by deposition of IgG

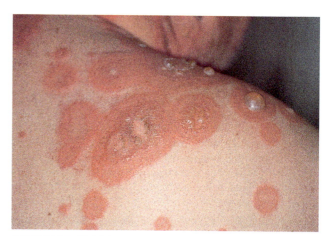

FIGURE 16-5 ■ Multiple tense bullae arising on an urticarial base in a patient with bullous pemphigoid. (Reprinted with permission from Callen JP, Greer KE, Paller A, Swinyer L, editors. Color atlas of dermatology: a morphological approach. 2nd ed. Philadelphia: WB Saunders; 2000.)

antibodies that react with basement membrane antigens in the lamina lucida, stimulating loss of dermoepidermal adherence.

Pathogenesis

Although the specific mechanisms responsible for blister formation in BP are not as well established as those in pemphigus, there is good evidence that IgG antibodies directed against antigens of the hemidesmosome of stratified squamous epithelium are pivotal. Perilesional skin and frequently serum from BP patients demonstrate the presence of IgG autoantibody directed against two distinct hemidesmosomal antigens: a 230-kDa glycoprotein bullous pemphigoid antigen 1 (BPAG1 or BP230) that reacts with circulating antibodies in 50% to 70% of cases, and the 180-kDa bullous pemphigoid antigen 2 (BPAG2 or BP180) with extracellular collagen-like domains that is reactive in 30% to 50% of cases. The BP antigens are normal components of the basement membrane zone, but, as is the case in pemphigus, patients become intolerant to these antigens. The HLA DQB1*0301 allele may be important in initial antigen processing. Autoreactive T lymphocytes producing Th1 and particularly Th2 cytokines are critically involved in the initiation of production of pathogenic autoantibodies in BP.

Antibodies to BPAG2, also known as collagen XVII, bind to a noncollagenous region of the molecule outside the cell membrane in the lamina lucida. Several points support the pathogenic role of anti-BPAG2 antibodies in BP. Firstly, passive transfer experiments in mice have resulted in blister formation when rabbit-derived antibodies to murine BPAG2 are injected. Secondly, sensitive enzyme-linked immunosorbent assay (ELISA) testing shows that BP180 antibody titers correlate with disease severity. Finally, IgG antibodies to BPAG2 in the related condition pemphigoid gestationis can cross the placenta and cause blisters in the fetuses of mothers with this disease. Passive transfer experiments in mice have produced inflammation and subepidermal blistering. Because BPAG1 is an intracytoplasmic molecule it has been suggested that anti-BPAG1 antibodies may develop secondarily after initial skin injury by anti-BPAG2 antibodies.

BPAG2 IgG antibodies are thought to cause blistering by complement and neutrophil activation. Several pieces of information support a role for complement in the pathogenesis of BP lesions. Complement deposits have been detected in vivo in the lamina lucida, and the complement membrane attack complex has been identified in involved skin. The stimulus for leukocyte attachment is activated complement components released by immune complex activation. Neutrophils are recruited by C5a-dependent pathways. Their pathogenicity is inferred by the finding that mice deficient in gelatinase-B (a neutrophil enzyme) were protected from blistering in passive transfer experiments. When neutrophils from normal mice were injected into the gelatinase-deficient mice they developed blisters.

Degranulation of mast cells mediated by complement-derived anaphylatoxins, eosinophil activation, or a direct effect of IgG antibody is responsible for the release of chemotactic factors, proteolytic enzymes, and vasoactive amines, which subsequently mediate dermoepidermal separation. IgE is emerging as an important pathogenic factor in BP. IgE antibodies against BPAG1 and BPAG2 have been detected in a high percentage of BP patients, with anti-BPAG1 IgE levels correlating with local eosinophil recruitment. SCID mice injected with an IgE-producing hybridoma directed toward the shed ectodomain of BPAG2 developed histologically evident subepidermal blisters in human skin grafts. Finally, IgE anti-BPAG2 is related to disease activity and severity.

Several reports have indicated that patients with BP may develop further blistering on exposure to ultraviolet light. The mechanism for this may be related to ultraviolet light activation of mast cells.

Classification

The term BP is generally reserved for patients demonstrating a chronic, vesiculobullous eruption involving predominantly nonmucosal surfaces. The distribution is usually widespread, with sites of predilection including the lower abdomen, inner thighs, groin, axilla, and flexural aspects of the arms and legs. BP antigen may vary in the amount distributed regionally, accounting for this classic distribution. However, 15% to 30% of patients demonstrate tense bullae limited to the pretibial area. Such cases are immunopathologically and histologically identical to BP, and no definite reason for the localized nature has been established. BP has been described in prepubertal children, but it is most common in the seventh and eighth decades of life. In the precorticosteroid era many cases resolved without treatment, although occasional patients developed aggressive and severe disease.

Some patients' biopsy specimens demonstrate a heavy inflammatory infiltrate around dermal blood vessels, with an admixture of neutrophils, eosinophils, and mononuclear cells. The prominence of the eosinophil infiltration serves to differentiate this disorder from dermatitis herpetiformis histopathologically. The second histopathologic type is characterized by a sparse inflammatory infiltrate of mononuclear cells around superficial dermal blood vessels in the presence of prominent vesiculation in the basement membrane zone. Immunopathologic diagnosis is essential to separate this from other immunobullous diseases.

The term cicatricial pemphigoid is reserved for those forms of the disease characterized by blistering and scarring. Classically this is a disease of the elderly, involving erosions of mucosal surfaces, especially the conjunctiva (Fig. 16-6), but also including the nasopharynx, oropharynx, esophagus, larynx, urethra, and anal mucosa. The morbidity and mortality of the disorder are related to the scarring produced by the recurrent lesions. Associated skin lesions occur in a minority of cases. Eye involvement may result in conjunctival symblepharon with obliteration of the conjunctival sulcus. Subsequent scarring of the cornea may produce blindness. The gingivae are commonly involved, and the disease may present only as "desquamative gingivitis." Esophageal lesions begin as smooth-bordered erosions, but stricture may occur and require repeated dilatation. Direct immunofluorescence microscopy of mucous membrane

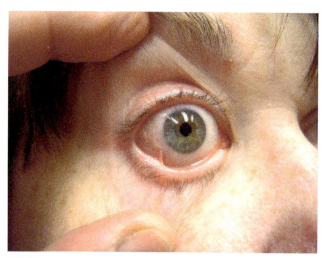

FIGURE 16-6 ■ Scarring ocular disease in a patient with cicatricial pemphigoid.

tissue reveals IgG and/or IgA anti-BMZ antibody in more than 80% of cases. Immunofluorescent-negative cases may represent a technical problem with obtaining adequate tissue from mucosal surfaces such as the eye. However, it is important to obtain positive direct immunofluorescence results, even if multiple biopsies are required, in order to separate the disorder from pemphigus, lichen planus, and cicatrizing conjunctivitis secondary to irritants and allergens. Indirect immunofluorescence studies reveal circulating anti-BMZ antibodies of IgG or IgA class in less than 50% of cases. Antibodies in cicatricial pemphigoid recognize several BMZ molecules, including BPAG1 and -2, laminin 332, α6β4 integrin, and type VII collagen. The scarring nature of this disease may be explained by the fact that the BPAG2 antibodies in cicatricial pemphigoid recognize the distal extracellular domain (carboxy terminus) of this molecule, which ends in the lamina densa, in contrast to classic BP patients where the more proximal NC16A domain of BPAG2 is targeted.

A specific localized scarring variant of cicatricial pemphigoid has been termed the Brunsting–Perry type. In this variant, scarring and blister formation occur on the head and neck without concomitant oral involvement. The pathogenesis of cicatricial pemphigoid is believed to be similar to that of BP, although the reason for localized disease and scarring is not understood.

There have been numerous evaluations of the association between BP and internal malignancy. BP has been reported in association with malignancies of the lymphoreticular system, skin, lung, breast, pancreas, kidney, and gastrointestinal tract. However, rarely have concurrent onset or a parallel course been documented. Ahmed and coworkers, as well as Stone and Schroeter, were able to find no increased rate of malignancy in their BP patients, but a study by Chorzelski et al. did claim a 10% association. Most authors have concluded that there is no increased incidence of malignancy in BP patients compared to age-matched controls. Thus, BP is best considered not to be a cutaneous marker of internal malignancy. However, recent evaluation of a subset of 35 cicatricial pemphigoid patients who had IgG serum antibodies directed against laminin 332 found that 10 patients had an associated malignancy.

This finding gives further credence to the need to characterize individual patients' antigen-binding profiles. Testing for specific antigen binding is only available in research laboratories at present, but indirect immunofluorescence on basement membrane split skin is a standard technique in immunopathology laboratories, and can suggest the presence of antibodies to laminin 332 on the basis of the uncommon dermal binding pattern.

BP has been reported in association with a wide variety of other disorders, including psoriasis, diabetes mellitus, lupus erythematosus, pernicious anemia, thyroiditis, polymyositis, and rheumatoid arthritis. It seems unlikely that any of these associations is important in pathogenesis, but the reasons for the associations remain unclear. In a case–control study in 1984 Chuang and associates found 20% of BP patients had diabetes, compared to 2.5% of controls. This association remained significant even after correcting for age differences. The association with rheumatoid arthritis seems to be significant, and it has been hypothesized that the two disorders may share similar pathogenetic mechanisms.

Lichen planus pemphigoides has been described on many occasions. It is characterized by the typical outbreak of lichen planus followed by a bullous eruption with the histological and immunopathological findings of BP. It is unclear whether these patients have coexistent lichen planus and BP, or whether this is a distinct entity in which the inflammatory process of lichen planus stimulates an immune response to BP antigens.

Differential Diagnosis

The initial diagnostic approach to blistering disorders is reviewed under the differential diagnosis of pemphigus. If biopsy suggests that the blister is subepidermal, direct immunofluorescence microscopy of perilesional tissue is indicated. BP characteristically demonstrates linear deposition of IgG along the basement membrane. Some cases of pemphigoid have also been described as having IgG and IgA along the basement membrane, making the separation from linear IgA bullous dermatosis somewhat arbitrary.

Dermatitis herpetiformis is differentiated by its clinical appearance (see later discussion), as well as by the characteristic deposition of granular IgA in perilesional tissue. Linear IgA bullous dermatosis shows characteristic deposition of IgA along the basement membrane as the predominant and usually the only immunoglobulin. Linear IgA disease is sensitive to sulfone therapy.

Erythema multiforme may also show a subepidermal blister. Characteristic involvement of the palms and soles with target lesions (minor type) or involvement of mucous membranes and skin (major type) in an acute fashion is characteristic of erythema multiforme. Biopsy of erythema multiforme reveals individually necrotic keratinocytes, and direct immunofluorescence fails to reveal anti-BMZ antibody. Occasionally, patients with erythema multiforme may have immunoglobulins in superficial dermal blood vessels.

Bullous lupus erythematosus usually occurs in patients who fulfill the American Rheumatism Association (ARA) criteria for systemic lupus erythematosus (SLE). In addition, the disorder shows granular deposition of immunoglobulin along the BMZ. Such deposition may be sufficiently intense to give a band-like pattern that can be confused with BP. However, patients with bullous lupus erythematosus histopathologically demonstrate a neutrophilic infiltrate similar to that of dermatitis herpetiformis.

Bullous forms of lichen planus exist that are distinguished by an intense mononuclear infiltrate adjacent to the BMZ, absence of anti-BMZ antibodies, and characteristic epidermal changes of lichen planus, which allow differentiation.

Epidermolysis bullosa of the junctional and dystrophic types may show a blister at the dermoepidermal junction. Such cases are characterized by onset of blistering early in childhood, absence of the inflammatory infiltrate, and negative direct immunofluorescence. The scarring, progressive nature of these disorders is easily distinguishable clinically.

Porphyria cutanea tarda also shows pauci-inflammatory subepidermal blistering, which occurs in sun-exposed areas. Histologically, the dermal papillae irregularly extend into the bulla cavity. Direct immunofluorescence microscopy may be positive, further confusing this differentiation. The diagnosis of porphyria cutanea tarda is ultimately made on the basis of elevated 24-hour uroporphyrins. Pseudoporphyria related to the use of nonsteroidal anti-inflammatory drugs (NSAIDs) may give a clinical, pathologic and immunopathologic pattern identical to that of porphyria cutanea tarda, but the 24-hour uroporphyrin level is normal. Epidermolysis bullosa acquisita is discussed in detail later.

The mucous membrane lesions of cicatricial pemphigoid must be differentiated from those of oral lichen planus, erythema multiforme, aphthous stomatitis, Behçet's syndrome, and pemphigus. The differentiation from oral lichen planus and erythema multiforme can usually be made histopathologically. Aphthous stomatitis lesions tend to be small and punched out. Behçet's syndrome need only be considered if other components of the syndrome, including genital ulceration, pustular dermatosis, and iritis, are present. None of these disorders demonstrates anti-BMZ antibodies.

Patient Evaluation

Close examination of all mucosal and cutaneous surfaces is necessary. Esophageal involvement may produce stricture, and patients with esophageal complaints should be considered for endoscopy and possible biopsy. In the presence of symptoms and/or signs found by the general physical examination that suggest the possibility of internal malignancy, those findings should be evaluated. However, no detailed evaluation to rule out the possibility of malignancy is otherwise necessary. Potentially infected lesions should be cultured. Evaluation of the patient's general status, including CBC, chemistry profile, and urinalysis, is advisable because many patients will have associated complicating clinical problems attendant upon their age. Chest X-ray and tuberculosis skin testing should be undertaken prior to starting corticosteroid and/or immunosuppressive therapy.

Initial study attempts to correlate the titers of BP antibody with disease activity were unsuccessful. However, it had been observed that the disappearance of antibody from the serum usually heralded the onset of spontaneous remission. Recently an association between disease activity and antibody titers has been seen when antibody levels to the BPAG2 antigen are followed specifically by highly sensitive ELISA assays.

Treatment

The majority of patients with BP have a complete clinical remission following effective therapy. The mainstay of therapy for BP is parenteral corticosteroids. Oral prednisone, 40 to 60 mg daily, is generally adequate for initial treatment, and may be the only treatment necessary. With this agent, individual blisters generally resolve within 2 to 3 weeks and new blister formation ceases. A major complication of treatment is related to corticosteroid side effects, including increased susceptibility to infection, potential gastrointestinal bleeding, onset of diabetes mellitus, and the possible development of psychiatric symptoms. These problems may well be severe, in view of the elderly age group afflicted. Consequently, close attention to complications is necessary. Oral therapy with bisphosphonates is indicated to prevent steroid-induced osteoporosis if steroids are to be used for more than a few days. Some reports suggest a beneficial effect of the combination of tetracycline and niacinamide as initial therapy in mild cases.

Azathioprine, 1 to 3 mg/kg/day, is an especially effective agent when used to spare corticosteroid dosage in patients with BP. The onset of effect is slow; thus, after 4 to 6 weeks of treatment with azathioprine, corticosteroid doses can be gradually tapered. Cyclophosphamide and mycophenolate mofetil are effective and may be used in the manner described for pemphigus.

As with pemphigus, IVIg appears to be effective, especially in recalcitrant disease. Doses similar to those used in pemphigus vulgaris have been effective in some patients, but definitive studies on its efficacy in pemphigoid are lacking.

Mucous membrane pemphigoid, if localized, may be treated with topical corticosteroid preparations, but usually requires systemic corticosteroid therapy. Dapsone may be helpful in controlling the oral lesions, but is often ineffective in preventing progressive ocular disease. Therapy with dapsone should be given in doses similar to those described for dermatitis herpetiformis (see later section on dermatitis herpetiformis). Eye involvement in cicatricial pemphigoid is particularly serious and warrants aggressive therapy. If initial response to oral corticosteroid therapy is not forthcoming, aggressive treatment with cyclophosphamide is indicated. However, ophthalmic involvement may be resistant to all therapies.

Localized BP of the extremities as well as some mucosal disease may be successfully treated with intradermal injections of small amounts of triamcinolone acetonide (2.5 mg/mL) used in combination with potent topical corticosteroids.

EPIDERMOLYSIS BULLOSA ACQUISITA

Epidermolysis bullosa acquisita (EBA) is a rare acquired bullous disease that generally occurs in adults and is distinguished by the involvement of extensor surfaces with blisters that heal slowly, leaving atrophic scars. Blisters appear mechanically induced and may lead to secondary milia formation (Fig. 16-7). Immunoglobulin and complement are deposited in a dense, linear pattern along the BMZ, as seen on direct immunofluorescence microscopy, and circulating IgG anti-BMZ antibody is present in about 50% of patients. Serologic studies demonstrate that this anti-BMZ antibody reacts with a 290-kDa antigen that is type VII collagen, the same antigen as for bullous SLE.

Pathogenesis

Histopathologically, EBA is characterized by a subepidermal blister with or without a neutrophilic inflammatory infiltrate. There is dense deposition of IgG and frequently complement components along the basement membrane. The majority of cases have a circulating IgG antibody that reacts on indirect immunofluorescence with the dermal side of salt-split skin (skin that has been separated in the lower lamina lucida by incubation with 1M sodium chloride). This is in contrast to BP sera, which react with the epidermal side or both epidermal and dermal sides of such preparations. Blister formation has been reported to occur either below the lamina lucida or below the lamina densa. On immunoelectron microscopy the immune deposits of EBA are localized to the anchoring fibrils of the sublamina densa region. Lapiere and colleagues have identified the BMZ protein that is antigenic in the sublamina densa region as the noncollagenous (NC-1) domain of type VII collagen. Specifically, antibodies to the fibronectin-like repeats within collagen VII seem to be preferentially formed and probably interfere with collagen VII–laminin 332 interaction. Passive transfer experiments of IgG anticollagen VII autoantibody have produced an EBA-like clinical picture in mice.

Preparations of EBA patients' anti-BMZ antibodies show both complement-activating and noncomplement-activating subclasses. However, the presence of complement-fixing antibodies does not correlate with the inflammatory or noninflammatory clinical subtypes. Additionally, when the complement-fixing ability of EBA patients' serum is measured, it is absent to weak; therefore, it is unlikely that complement plays a major role in blister formation. Nevertheless, an organ culture system utilizing EBA antibody, tissue injury, and BMZ separation can be produced. Eventually, antibody deposition and the inflammatory process may produce sufficient damage to the anchoring fibrils such that minor trauma will produce a loss of dermoepidermal adhesion in the absence of the inflammatory process.

Classification

EBA is a sharply defined entity on the basis of its immunopathologic findings. However, there is a spectrum of clinical and histopathologic manifestations of EBA. Blisters may arise on an inflammatory or a noninflammatory base. Milia may or may not be present. The inflammatory variant is frequently associated with nail dystrophy.

EBA has been reported to be associated with a variety of disorders, including rheumatoid arthritis, multiple myeloma, chronic thyroiditis, diabetes mellitus, lymphoma, amyloidosis, inflammatory bowel disease, and cryoglobulinemia. Many of these may be chance occurrences. The strongest associations appear to be with diabetes mellitus and Crohn's disease. The mechanism for these associations is unclear.

The distinction between EBA and bullous lupus erythematosus is complex. Cases with the clinical criteria for SLE and immunopathologic findings of EBA may well represent a subset of lupus patients in whom the immune dysregulation of lupus results in the production of antibodies to type VII collagen.

Differential Diagnosis

The differential diagnosis of subepidermal blistering disease is described under BP. However, EBA may be impossible to separate from BP on the basis of clinical findings alone. If circulating antibody is present,

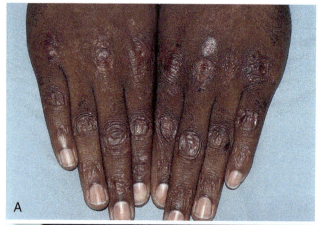

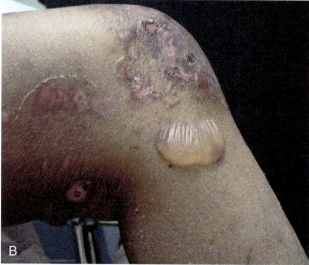

FIGURE 16-7 ■ **A,** Epidermolysis bullosa acquisita. Scars and milia are present in this patient who had multiple traumatically induced blisters on the dorsal hands. **B,** Epidermolysis bullosa acquisita in a patient with systemic lupus erythematosus.

indirect immunofluorescence utilizing BMZ split skin as described above should be utilized. In the absence of circulating antibody, immunoelectron microscopy is the only reliable way to separate BP from EBA. In this situation EBA will demonstrate deposition of IgG in the sublamina densa area of the anchoring fibrils, whereas BP IgG deposition will be in the lamina lucida.

The classic clinical and histopathologic presentation of EBA closely resembles that of porphyria cutanea tarda, but EBA patients have normal uroporphyrins. Differentiation of EBA from other forms of epidermolysis bullosa includes the adult onset, as well as a negative family history of EBA. The inflammatory variant may also closely mimic drug-induced bullous erythema multiforme, which, however, lacks the characteristic findings of EBA on direct immunofluorescence.

Patient Evaluation

The evaluation of patients with EBA is essentially the same as that for patients with BP. However, because EBA can cause scarring on mucosal surfaces, a multidisciplinary approach involving gastroenterology, otolaryngology, ophthalmology, dentistry, and speech therapy may be required to deal with these complications. Correlation of antibody titer with disease activity has not been well evaluated.

Treatment

The treatment of EBA is similar to that for BP. However, EBA tends to be progressive and unrelenting, and is much more resistant to treatment with systemic corticosteroids than is BP. In a review by Engineer, small series and case reports were summarized showing promising results with cyclosporine, colchicine, and IVIg.

DERMATITIS HERPETIFORMIS

Dermatitis herpetiformis (DH), or Duhring's disease, is characterized by involvement of extensor surfaces with grouped, pruritic, erythematous papulovesicles (Fig. 16-8). Biopsy demonstrates a blister at the basement membrane with accumulation of neutrophils in the dermal papillary tips. Perilesional skin demonstrates the pathognomonic deposition of granular IgA in dermal papillary tips. More than 90% of patients with DH have the HLA-DQ2 genotype, compared to 20% of controls. This offers a unique background on which gluten sensitivity and the subsequent IgA immune response develop. Virtually all DH patients have gluten-sensitive enteropathy on small bowel biopsy, but gastrointestinal symptoms occur in only about 25% of cases. The skin disease as well as the associated gluten-sensitive enteropathy improves with dietary restriction of gluten.

Pathogenesis

The skin disease as well as the intestinal lesions respond to a strict gluten-free diet, although it may take 3 to 6 months for clinical improvement. IgA also clears from the skin

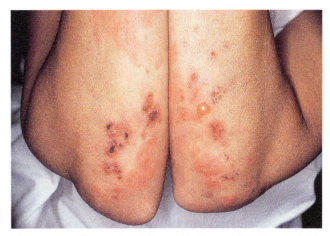

FIGURE 16-8 ■ Grouped vesicles and bullae on the elbows of this patient with dermatitis herpetiformis. (Reprinted with permission from Callen JP, Greer KE, Paller A, Swinyer L, editors. Color atlas of dermatology: a morphological approach. 2nd ed. Philadelphia: WB Saunders; 2000.)

with prolonged gluten restriction. This indicates a central role for gluten ingestion and IgA in the pathogenesis.

The HLA-DQ2 antigen is found in 90% of celiac disease and DH patients and only 20% of controls. It is believed that this genetic background is essential to presentation of the gluten antigen to the mucosal immune system. The intestinal lesion is then produced by an intestinal inflammatory infiltrate of mononuclear cells. However, it is unknown how gluten triggers IgA binding to skin, and how IgA triggers neutrophil infiltration and the inflammatory cascade. An antigen to which the IgA antibodies bind in the skin has been identified as epidermal transglutaminase (TG3).

The proposed pathogenesis of DH and celiac disease is an immune response to gliadin antigen, a digestion product of gluten, which is present in rye, barley, and wheat. Glutamine residues within gliadin are absorbed into the lamina propria of the small intestine and deamidated by tissue transglutaminase (TG2). Deamidated gliadin then binds to the groove on dendritic antigen-presenting cells and the antigen is presented to T-helper cells. Plasma cells then produce IgA antibodies to multiple antigens, including gliadin, tissue transglutaminase, and epidermal transglutaminase. Natural killer lymphocytes cause villous atrophy. Circulating IgA antibodies to TG2 and TG3 result from this process and are an index of the severity of the intestinal inflammatory response. These antibodies decrease with adherence to gluten restriction.

The cutaneous lesions are probably produced by the IgA present in dermal papillae in combination with the epidermal transglutaminase (TG3) antigen. The intestinal inflammatory process is important for the activation of neutrophils, which infiltrate into the dermal papillae where the IgA immune complexes reside. Degranulation of neutrophils releases neutrophilic enzymes, which induce degradation of the lamina lucida and a basement membrane blister.

Clinical Features

Thyroid disorders have been reported in many cases of DH. These disorders include hyperthyroidism, hypothyroidism, thyroid nodules, and asymptomatic goiter. Thyroid peroxidase antibodies are seen in 40% of patients with DH. The abnormal findings are especially prominent in females, and some thyroid abnormality may occur in as many as 40% of female DH patients.

Lymphoma is known to occur with increased prevalence in patients with gluten-sensitive enteropathy. There are many case reports of abdominal lymphoma in patients with DH, but the only controlled study of this phenomenon was performed by Leonard and suggested a slight increase in the incidence of lymphoma (4%) in patients with DH. It was suggested that this incidence may be reduced by a gluten-free diet, although at present there are insufficient data to support this conclusion. An extremely large study would be necessary to evaluate the statistical validity of the association between DH and lymphoma. Consequently, it is best to assume that the incidence is approximately that of celiac disease, and appropriate evaluation should be performed if signs of lymphoma develop.

Differential Diagnosis

The differential diagnoses are those of subepidermal blistering disease, reviewed under the heading of bullous pemphigoid. The main clinical differentiation is with linear IgA disease. Direct immunofluorescence is essential to distinguish between linear IgA disease and DH. Also helpful in differentiating the two is the fact that DH is closely associated with HLA-B8-DR3, whereas linear IgA disease has no HLA associations and does not respond to a gluten-free diet.

Patient Evaluation

Immunofluorescence is essential in diagnosis. Noninflamed perilesional skin harbors the greatest amount of IgA and is therefore the preferred biopsy site for direct immunofluorescence when DH is suspected. IgA anti-tissue transglutaminase antibodies are found in the serum of DH patients as well as those with celiac disease, and are an indication of gluten sensitivity. However, serum antibody tests should not be used for diagnosis in the absence of direct immunofluorescence.

Close clinical examination for thyroid nodules and thyromegaly is indicated as a baseline and at return visits. Detailed history of bowel symptoms, including bloating after eating, recurrent abdominal pain, diarrhea, and steatorrhea, is indicated. Patients who do not have obvious signs of gluten-sensitive enteropathy may frequently note improvement in these minimal symptoms when a gluten-free diet is instituted.

A CBC, chemistry profile, and urinalysis are necessary as baseline studies in all patients with DH. This approach not only screens for the malabsorption problems discussed previously, but also represents a baseline for subsequent abnormalities that may be induced by dapsone therapy. Serum thyroxine and thyrotropin hormone levels are evaluated as a baseline in view of the high incidence of thyroid abnormalities. Glucose-6-phosphate dehydrogenase levels should be checked as a baseline in patients who are black or of southern Mediterranean origin, as catastrophic hemolysis may result from the administration of dapsone in deficient patients. Evaluation for associated malabsorption is reviewed in Chapter 25.

Treatment

Dapsone is the drug of choice in the therapy of DH. Treatment with dapsone will adequately suppress (but not cure) the disease. Dapsone treatment requires continued monitoring and may be associated with significant side effects. Dapsone is available in 25- and 100-mg tablets. Initial treatment with 25 mg of dapsone by mouth daily usually improves symptoms within 24 to 48 hours in adults. Correspondingly smaller doses should be used in children. When taken daily, dapsone levels reach a steady state within 7 days. Maintenance therapy is then adjusted on a weekly basis to maintain adequate suppression of symptoms; the average maintenance dose is 100 mg daily (range 1 to 3 mg/kg/day). Occasional new lesions (two or three per week) are to be expected and are not an indication for altering daily dosage. Minor fluctuations in disease severity do occur and are probably related to oral gluten intake. Application of potent topical corticosteroid gel may be helpful in relieving symptoms of individual lesions. Hemolysis is the most common side effect of treatment. Dapsone is a strong oxidizer and produces a dose-related oxidant stress on normal aging red blood cells. Initial reduction of hemoglobin by 2 to 3 g is common, but subsequent partial compensation by reticulocytosis is the rule. Methemoglobinemia is seldom a severe problem, but it may be tolerated poorly in patients with cardiopulmonary decompensation. Other dose-related side effects are rare with doses <200 mg daily. These include toxic hepatitis, cholestatic jaundice, psychosis, and both motor and sensory neuropathy. Hypoalbuminemia may occur after chronic use. Carcinogenicity of dapsone has been reported in mice and rats, but has not been documented in humans. Rarely, infectious mononucleosis syndrome with fever and lymphadenopathy occurs.

Treatment with a gluten-free diet is successful in more than 90% of cases if the diet is adhered to for a minimum of 3 to 12 months. In such cases, initial suppression of symptoms with dapsone is usually necessary. When gluten restriction allows a decrease in dapsone requirement, the patient can gradually taper the dosage. Complete control of skin disease on a gluten-free diet obviates the need for hematologic follow-up. It also serves to treat the cause rather than the symptoms of the disease. Disadvantages of a gluten-free diet include the inconvenience of the diet, which some patients may find unappetizing. It must be stressed that the patient should actively participate in the decision to start a gluten-free diet, as individual patients vary in their willingness to take medications or adhere to diets over a prolonged period.

After initial baseline information is collected, a CBC should be checked weekly for 1 month, monthly for 6 months, and semiannually thereafter. Chemistry profile should be checked at 6 months and then annually to monitor for possible hepatotoxicity, changes in renal function, and hypoalbuminemia. IgA tissue transglutaminase antibodies can be monitored as an index of adherence to gluten restriction and improvement of the small intestinal inflammatory process.

LINEAR IgA BULLOUS DERMATOSIS

Linear IgA bullous dermatosis (LABD) is a chronic bullous disorder characterized by erosions and tense blisters, often on an erythematous base (Fig. 16-9). As many as 80% of patients with LABD have oral involvement. It is also known as linear IgA disease, IgA pemphigoid, and linear DH. The distinction between LABD, BP, and DH was made in 1979 by Chorzelski et al. based on direct immunofluorescence findings, which demonstrated linear depositions of IgA along the BMZ in LABD.

Classification

Chronic bullous disease of childhood (CBDC) and LABD share the same histology and immunofluorescence findings. Although they have different clinical presentations, they are considered by most experts to be the same disease.

CBDC occurs in children, with a peak incidence at 4.5 years, and tends to remit by age 13. The characteristic distribution is the lower abdomen and perineum, although the extremities can be involved. Blisters occur in the so-called "cluster of jewels" configuration, because new lesions appear at the periphery of old ones. Mucosal involvement is reported in 64% of cases.

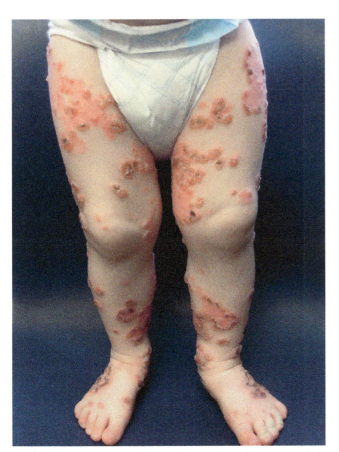

FIGURE 16-9 ■ Grouped bullae representative of linear IgA bullous dermatosis in this child.

LABD shows a slight female preponderance, with peak incidence at 60 to 65 years. Its clinical picture often resembles DH, with pruritic papules and vesicles on the extremities; however, larger vesicles and bullae similar to those of BP may occur. These may be linear or "sausage shaped." In about 60% of patients LABD may remit over several years.

LABD is unique in that it may be induced by drugs, and may remit after withdrawal of the offending drug. Vancomycin is the most common association, but others include amiodarone, ampicillin, captopril, childhood vaccinations, diclofenac, interferon-γ, interleukin-2, iodine, lithium, penicillin G, phenytoin, piroxicam, rifampin, somatostatin, and trimethoprim–sulfamethoxazole. The pathogenesis of this reaction is not understood.

Pathogenesis

In 1990 Zone et al. identified a 97-kDa protein antigen recognized in adult and childhood sera from LABD patients. This protein is identical to the extracellular portion of collagen XVII (BPAG2, BP180). This protein represents a proteolytic fragment of the shed ectodomain of BPAG2. The mechanism by which IgA basement membrane antibodies cause blistering is yet to be elucidated.

Some patients show linear IgA and linear IgG along the basement membrane, and this is thought to represent an immunologic overlap of LABD and BP. These patients should be treated according to the predominant antibody pattern.

Numerous case reports link LABD to Hodgkin's disease and other B-cell lymphomas. Transitional cell cancer of the bladder and esophageal cancer have also been reported in association with LABD. Because IgA is among the antibodies deposited at the basement membrane in SLE, it is not clear whether the association between LABD and SLE is a true one. There is a real association between ulcerative colitis and LABD: in fact, one study showed ulcerative colitis present in five of 70 patients with LABD. Other disease associations include multiple sclerosis, dermatomyositis, Crohn's disease, hydatidiform mole, and rheumatoid arthritis.

Multiple drugs have been reported to induce LABD. The reaction usually occurs within days to weeks of ingestion. The most common medication is vancomycin, although penicillins, cephalosporins, ACE inhibitors, and NSAIDs have been reported. Several other medications have been described to produce LABD on rare occasions. A detailed medication history is indicated for all patients with LABD. Most cases resolve in 2 to 6 weeks after discontinuation of the offending drug.

Differential Diagnosis

The differential diagnosis of LABD is similar to that of the other immunobullous diseases discussed in this chapter. An important differentiation is between LABD and DH, and the key to this distinction is the direct immunofluorescence findings in LABD of linear IgA along the basement membrane. Based on histology alone, without clinical history and examination, LABD can be difficult to distinguish from the bullous eruption of SLE. Bullous lupus tends to affect patients already carrying the diagnosis of lupus, or who have other stigmata associated with the disease.

Patient Evaluation

Direct immunofluorescence is the cornerstone to making the diagnosis of LABD. Perilesional skin will show linear deposition of IgA (usually IgA_1 subclass, but occasionally IgA_2) along the basement membrane. Indirect immunofluorescence is positive in about 60% to 70% of cases. BMZ split skin is a somewhat more sensitive substrate for indirect immunofluorescence. Not surprisingly, most of the antibodies in LABD bind to the epidermal side of BMZ split skin, similar to the situation seen in BP, with which LABD shares a major pathogenic antigen, BPAG2.

Treatment

As with other IgA and neutrophil-mediated diseases, the mainstay of treatment for LABD is dapsone. Dosage and management are similar to those used in DH, and the reader is referred to the discussion of this drug in that section of the chapter. As with DH, patients intolerant of dapsone may be controlled with sulfapyridine. There is evidence for the use of colchicine, combination tetracycline and nicotinamide, as well as IVIg in recalcitrant cases. Prednisone and immunosuppressive therapy as described for pemphigus and BP is successful in resistant cases. LABD is rarely associated with gluten sensitivity, and a gluten-free diet is not indicated unless celiac disease can be documented.

SUGGESTED READINGS

Alonso-Llamazares J, Gibson LE, Rogers 3rd RS. Clinical, pathologic, and immunopathologic features of dermatitis herpetiformis: review of the Mayo Clinic experience. Int J Dermatol 2007;46:910.

Culton DA, Diaz LA. Treatment of subepidermal immunobullous diseases. Clin Dermatol 2012;30:95.

Czernik A, Camilleri M, Pittelkow MR, Grando SA. Paraneoplastic autoimmune multiorgan syndrome: 20 years after. Int J Dermatol 2011;50:905.

Daniel BS, Borradori L, Hall 3rd RP, Murrell DF. Evidence-based management of bullous pemphigoid. Dermatol Clin 2011;29:613.

Getsios S, Waschke J, Borradori L, et al. From cell signaling to novel therapeutic concepts: international pemphigus meeting on advances in pemphigus research and therapy. J Invest Dermatol 2010;130:1764.

Gürcan HM, Ahmed AR. Current concepts in the treatment of epidermolysis bullosa acquisita. Expert Opin Pharmacother 2011;12:1259.

Hall RP, Mickle CP. Dapsone. In: Wolverton SE, editor. Comprehensive dermatologic drug therapy. 2nd ed. Philadelphia: Elsevier Inc; 2007. p. 239.

Kasperkiewicz M, Shimanovich I, Ludwig RJ, et al. Rituximab for treatment-refractory pemphigus and pemphigoid: a case series of 17 patients. J Am Acad Dermatol 2011;65:552.

Murrell DF, Marinovic B, Caux F, et al. Definitions and outcome measures for mucous membrane pemphigoid: recommendations of an international panel of experts. J Am Acad Dermatol January 2015;72(1):168–74.

Ruocco V, Ruocco E, Lo Schiavo A, et al. Pemphigus: etiology, pathogenesis, and inducing or triggering factors: facts and controversies. Clin Dermatol 2013;31:374.

Saha M, Cutler T, Bhogal B, et al. Refractory epidermolysis bullosa acquisita: successful treatment with rituximab. Clin Exp Dermatol 2009;34:e979.

Woodley DT, Chang C, Saadat P, et al. Evidence that anti-type VII collagen antibodies are pathogenic and responsible for the clinical, histological, and immunological features of epidermolysis bullosa acquisita. J Invest Dermatol 2005;124:958.

CHAPTER 17

Skin Signs of Internal Malignancy

Edward W. Cowen • Jeffrey P. Callen

> **KEY POINTS**
>
> - Curth's postulates provide a group of criteria that are helpful to determine whether a skin condition is likely to be related to an internal malignancy.
> - Individual paraneoplastic skin conditions tend to be associated more frequently with certain types of cancer (e.g., Bazex syndrome and upper aerodigestive cancer).
> - The pathogenesis of many paraneoplastic skin conditions remains unclear. Tumor-secreting hormones, paracrine factors, and the immune response may contribute to variable cutaneous findings.
> - Cancer-related genodermatoses, such as hereditary leiomyomatosis and its association with renal cell cancer, may present with skin findings before the internal malignancy. Therefore, early diagnosis can prompt screening to detect occult malignancy.
> - A family history of cancer and a personal or family history of cancer of the same type, particularly of earlier onset of malignancy than expected, should prompt consideration of an inherited cancer syndrome.

The skin often reflects internal processes, and patients' awareness of this leads them to consider malignancy as a potential cause for many cutaneous abnormalities. Indeed, there are many skin conditions that have been linked to internal malignancy in a specific and/or nonspecific manner. This chapter considers those cutaneous disorders that have been linked to internal malignancy, the precise manner in which the cutaneous disease and the neoplasm are related, and the evaluation necessary for the patient with a cutaneous sign of internal malignancy.

Curth previously suggested criteria by which to gauge the potential relationship of two disorders, in this case a cutaneous finding and neoplasia (Table 17-1). The disorders may occur concurrently or follow a parallel course; there may be a specific tumor site or cell type associated with the cutaneous disease; there may be a statistical association between the two processes; or there may be a genetic association between the two disorders. In this chapter, we examine these factors to determine whether a "true" association exists for three categories of skin disease: (1) proliferative and inflammatory dermatoses; (2) hormone-secreting tumors; and (3) inherited syndromes.

PROLIFERATIVE AND INFLAMMATORY DERMATOSES

Acanthosis Nigricans

The characteristic clinical feature of acanthosis nigricans (AN) is hyperpigmented, velvety thickening of the skin on intertriginous surfaces. The eruption usually affects the axillary vault (Fig. 17-1), neck, inguinal crease, nipples, and umbilicus, but may also involve areas of trauma, such as the elbows, knees, and knuckles. Frequently, the oral mucosa has a papillomatous thickening. In rare instances, the eruption can become generalized (Fig. 17-2). Verrucous or papillary lesions may accompany the typical lesions of AN. Patients may develop multiple seborrheic keratoses simultaneously.

AN can occur in many clinical scenarios, including obesity and insulin resistance, and as a manifestation of a number of heritable diseases (e.g., Crouzon syndrome, congenital lipodystrophy). Once other associations have been excluded, the possibility of an underlying neoplasm must be considered, particularly with widespread AN skin involvement. In general, patients with "malignant AN" are older adults with a history of associated weight loss.

AN most often occurs simultaneously with the underlying malignancy; however, it may precede or follow a malignancy diagnosis. Approximately 90% of the tumors associated with AN arise within the abdominal cavity,

TABLE 17-1 Criteria Used to Associate Dermatoses and Neoplasia

Concurrent onset
Parallel course
Uniform neoplasm (site or cell type)
Statistical association
Genetic association

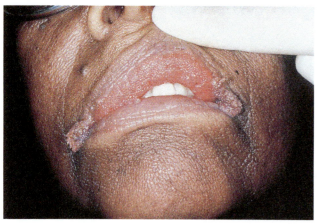

FIGURE 17-1 ■ Mucosal surfaces may be involved in acanthosis nigricans, as demonstrated by this woman with gastric adenocarcinoma. (Courtesy of Dr Mark Holzberg, Atlanta, GA.)

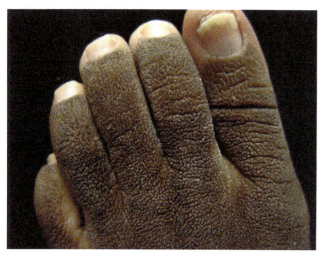

FIGURE 17-2 ■ Acanthosis nigricans, generalized in a patient who also had erythema gyratum repens.

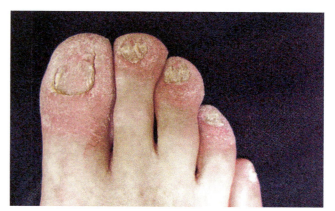

FIGURE 17-3 ■ Acrokeratosis paraneoplastica. This patient developed an acral violaceous erythema almost simultaneously with a squamous cell carcinoma of his tonsillar pillar.

particularly the gastrointestinal and genitourinary tracts. Gastric adenocarcinoma is the most commonly described cancer associated with malignant AN. However, malignancies outside the abdomen and nonadenocarcinomas have been reported. The course of malignant AN parallels the course of the tumor, which tends to be aggressive in nature. Malignant AN is a prototypic dermatological condition associated with malignancy, fulfilling all of Curth's "postulates" except for having a genetic association.

Bazex Syndrome

Acrokeratosis paraneoplastica, or Bazex syndrome, is by definition always associated with an underlying malignancy. Acrokeratosis paraneoplastica develops progressively through three stages. The initial cutaneous signs consist of erythematous to violaceous, poorly defined macules with a fine adherent scale that occur over the acral areas of the body, including the fingers, toes, ears, and nose. A paronychial reaction is also common. In the second stage, skin lesions begin to generalize and keratoderma develops. In the third stage, the eruption generalizes but still maintains its violaceous nature and predilection for acral involvement (Fig. 17-3). The three stages of the cutaneous disease parallel the growth and spread of the underlying tumor. Bazex syndrome is more common in men, and the underlying tumors are most often squamous cell carcinomas of the upper aerodigestive tract; however, a variety of other solid malignancies and lymphomas have also been associated. Therefore, a comprehensive head, neck, and pelvic examination with laboratory, radiographic, and endoscopic evaluation is needed. As with acanthosis nigricans, the course of cutaneous involvement in Bazex syndrome typically parallels the course of the tumor, thereby fulfilling the criteria to consider it a marker of internal malignancy.

Bullous Dermatoses

Several bullous dermatoses have been reported to be associated with malignancy. Although the association between bullous pemphigoid and cancer may be related primarily to the increased incidence of both conditions in elderly patients, certain other autoimmune bullous dermatoses with dermal epidermal junction pathology appear to be associated with an increased risk of malignancy, in particular those with negative immunofluorescence results, those with prominent mucosal lesions, and those with linear IgA disease. Egan and colleagues reported solid organ malignancies in 10 of 35 patients with antiepiligrin cicatricial pemphigoid (AECP). In eight cases the cancer was discovered within 14 months of the diagnosis of AECP. AECP is an uncommon, severe, and often scarring mucosal variant of pemphigoid associated with an IgG antibody directed against laminin 5. In contrast, two reviews of mucous membrane pemphigoid associated with antibodies to the $\beta 4\alpha 6$ integrin subunits did not identify an increased risk of cancer. Furthermore, although a wide variety of neoplasms have been associated with bullous pemphigoid, there does not appear to be a specific course relating the pemphigoid to the malignancy. Thus, at present the data do not support a relationship between bullous pemphigoid and malignancy, with the possible exception of certain pemphigoid subsets, particularly AECP.

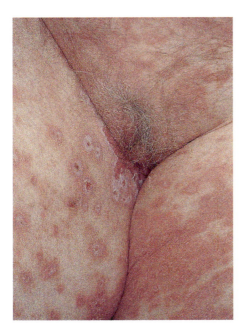

FIGURE 17-4 ■ Paraneoplastic pemphigus. Multiple erythematous papules and vesicles in the groin of this patient. (Reprinted with permission from Callen JP, Greer KE, Paller A, Swinyer L. Color atlas of dermatology: a morphological approach. 2nd ed. Philadelphia: WB Saunders; 2000.)

Epidermolysis bullosa acquisita (EBA) has very rarely been associated with malignancy, most commonly of hematologic origin. However, several such reports describe patients with features of both EBA and cicatricial pemphigoid.

The pemphigus group of disorders is most commonly associated with thymoma and lymphoproliferative malignancies. Patients with thymomas also often develop myasthenia gravis. The pemphigus course does not coincide with that of the neoplasm. However, careful review of chest X-ray findings may be prudent to ensure a possible thymoma is not missed. In the early 1990s, Anhalt and coworkers reported an entity that they termed "paraneoplastic pemphigus" (PNP). Patients with PNP develop severe mucosal erosions and ulcerations, polymorphic cutaneous lesions that may resemble erythema multiforme, and antibodies targeting a number of proteins, particularly desmoplakin, envoplakin, and periplakin (Fig. 17-4). However, several cases of lichenoid paraneoplastic pemphigus in patients treated with rituximab have been reported in which autoantibody detection was delayed or antibodies were not identified. The term paraneoplastic autoimmune multiorgan syndrome (PAMS) has been proposed in order to reflect the multiorgan system involvement now appreciated with PNP. Patients often also develop disease involving their bronchi and may die of respiratory failure (see Chapter 16 for further discussion of PNP/PAMS). The prognosis is poor, with very few survivors.

Dermatitis herpetiformis (DH) is associated with a risk of non-Hodgkin's lymphoma (NHL), particularly enteropathy-associated T-cell lymphoma and B-cell NHL. In a recent meta-analysis, one in 2000 persons with gluten-sensitive enteropathy develops NHL each year. In DH patients who develop intestinal lymphoma, the removal of the tumor does not appear to affect the course of the cutaneous disease.

Porphyria cutanea tarda (PCT) has been associated with hepatic tumors, in particular with primary hepatoma. This association is most likely a coincidental phenomenon, as hepatitis C virus infection is a risk factor for both PCT and hepatic carcinoma. The exact frequency of hepatic tumors in patients with PCT is not known; however, there are reports of concurrent onset and a parallel disease course. Careful evaluation of the liver, including hepatitis C antibody testing, is advised in all patients with PCT.

Dermatomyositis and Other Collagen–Vascular Disorders

As discussed in Chapter 2, dermatomyositis (DM) is clearly associated with malignancy, which affects approximately one-quarter of patients with adult-onset DM; however, only rarely do patients with DM have a concurrent onset and a parallel course of their tumors. The malignancy work-up of an adult with a new diagnosis of DM is reviewed in detail in Chapter 2, but goes beyond traditional age-appropriate evaluation. Women should be carefully evaluated for malignancy of the breast and gynecologic system. Ethnicity should also be considered: nasopharyngeal carcinoma was the most common malignancy in a study of DM in Taiwan. All patients should have a chest X-ray and probably a CT scan of the chest, abdomen, and pelvis, as well as a stool hematest. Malignancy risk appears to decrease with time from DM diagnosis, but repeat examinations should be performed annually for at least the first 3 years of the disease course, as malignancies such as ovarian cancer may not be easily detected by physical examination and imaging. At all times, unexplained symptoms or signs should be thoroughly evaluated.

Malignancies appear to be a coincidental occurrence in patients with lupus erythematosus. Several reports of lymphoreticular malignancies in patients with systemic lupus erythematosus likely reflect a complication of immunosuppressive therapy. Myeloma and paraproteinemias have been reported in patients with chronic cutaneous lupus erythematosus, but the frequency and significance of these findings are not clear.

An increased risk of malignancy in patients with scleroderma has been confirmed in two recent meta-analyses. Increased risk of lung cancer, NHL, and other hematopoietic cancers was found. One study suggested that men are at higher risk of developing cancer than women, possibly due to the greater number of men who use tobacco. Although breast cancer is frequently reported in women with scleroderma, the risk of breast cancer in scleroderma was found to be equivalent to that of the general population.

The coexistence of cutaneous small-vessel vasculitis and malignant neoplasms has been noted and reported as paraneoplastic vasculitis. Cutaneous small-vessel vasculitis is a common finding, as are cutaneous and systemic polyarteritis nodosa. Most of the tumors reported with vasculitis are of the lymphoreticular system (particularly hairy cell leukemia), but sporadic cases associated with solid tumors have also been described. Occasionally, the cutaneous disease is the initial finding in these patients, and a parallel course may also occur. A patient presenting with cutaneous vasculitis probably does not require a specific evaluation for malignancy.

Eruptive Angiomas, Telangiectases, and Seborrheic Keratoses

Reports linking the sudden appearance of angiomas or telangiectases with internal malignancies have been published in the dermatological literature. Angiomatous lesions are common in the adult population and are seen as small, cherry-colored papules. It is not clear whether a rapid onset of lesions should prompt a malignancy evaluation. The situation in regard to telangiectases is similarly unclear.

The sudden appearance or growth of multiple seborrheic keratoses is known as the sign of Leser–Trélat (see Fig. 17-1). Numerous reports have linked this condition to various malignancies. Many patients also have AN, and the sign of Leser–Trélat is similarly associated with intraabdominal adenocarcinoma, albeit to a lesser extent than with malignant AN. Population studies have not demonstrated a link between multiple seborrheic keratoses and internal malignancy. However, a patient has been described who had demonstrable epidermal growth factor receptors on the seborrheic keratosis, with evidence that a melanoma produced this factor. In this patient, when the melanoma was excised, the keratoses regressed. Although all the criteria for an association with malignancy are not fulfilled, it seems reasonable to carefully evaluate patients with a sudden onset or growth of multiple seborrheic keratoses, including evaluation for other epidermal features associated with internal malignancy, such as AN and tripe palms. The work-up should include a history and physical examination, and imaging studies of the gastrointestinal and genitourinary systems.

Erythroderma

Erythroderma (exfoliative dermatitis) is a cutaneous reaction characterized by general erythema, edema, and scaling (see Chapter 14). The reaction may be accompanied by fever, lymphadenopathy, organomegaly, and/or leukocytosis. Malignancy may be present in approximately 10% to 15% of patients. In most instances, the malignancy is in the lymphoreticular system, but several reports of solid tumors have also been published. The course of the cutaneous disease often follows that of the tumor, and the discovery of the malignant process has often been linked to the diagnosis of the cutaneous disorder. Therefore, the possibility of an underlying neoplasm must be considered in all patients with erythroderma of unknown etiology.

Figurate Erythemas

There are multiple figurate erythemas, but the only one that appears to be truly related to malignancy is erythema gyratum repens. In this eruption, erythematous lesions form gyrate or serpiginous bands that rapidly

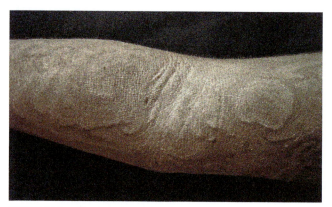

FIGURE 17-5 ■ Erythema gyratum repens. Multiple bands of erythema in a dark-skinned individual.

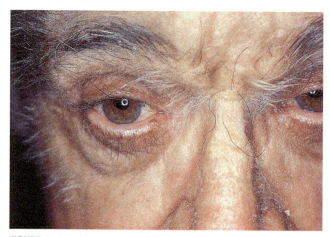

FIGURE 17-6 ■ Hypertrichosis lanuginosa. This man developed fine lanugo hairs at the same time as he was discovered to have a squamous cell carcinoma of the lung.

spread across the cutaneous surface (Fig. 17-5), producing a "wood-grain" appearance. Nearly all patients with erythema gyratum repens have an associated malignancy, which is often discovered concurrently. The course also frequently parallels that of the neoplasm. Although any malignancy may be associated, lung cancer is the most common, followed by breast, genitourinary (GU), and gastrointestinal (GI) tumors. The presence of erythema gyratum repens mandates an extensive internal evaluation for malignancy.

Hypertrichosis Lanuginosa (Malignant Down)

Hypertrichosis is the excessive growth of hair without signs of virilization (Fig. 17-6). The sudden development of fine downy hair has been linked to the presence of an underlying neoplasm in all patients thus far reported. The malignancies are of varied sites and cell types, and are often discovered at the time of the diagnosis of hypertrichosis lanuginosa. Glossitis has also accompanied the malignancy-associated down, but it is believed to be a manifestation of vitamin deficiency rather than a related finding. Patients with this type of hair growth who do not have another clear explanation for their condition, such as a medication (e.g., cyclosporine, minoxidil), porphyria cutanea tarda, or endocrinopathy, should be evaluated for the possibility of an internal malignancy.

Acquired Ichthyosis

Acquired ichthyosis resembles ichthyosis vulgaris, and is characterized by rhomboidal scales with margins that are lifted off the surface of the skin. Acquired ichthyosis is most frequently associated with lymphoreticular disorders, particularly Hodgkin's lymphoma. It is also associated with other paraneoplastic conditions, such as AN and the sign of Leser–Trélat. However, several other nonmalignant conditions have been associated with acquired ichthyosis, including hypothyroidism and sarcoidosis. When acquired ichthyosis is related to a malignancy, the cancer diagnosis precedes the diagnosis of acquired ichthyosis in most cases.

Keratoacanthoma

Keratoacanthoma is a rapidly growing epidermal neoplasm that may be locally invasive but otherwise exhibits a benign course. In association with sebaceous neoplasms, keratoacanthomas are one of the cardinal features of Muir–Torre syndrome, a variant of hereditary nonpolyposis colorectal cancer (HNPCC) Lynch syndrome II. Additional sporadic cases describing an association between multiple keratoacanthomas and internal malignancy have been described. However, because patients with keratoacanthoma tend to be elderly, this association may be an age-related phenomenon.

Migratory Thrombophlebitis (Trousseau Syndrome)

Although superficial thrombophlebitis is a relatively common medical condition, migratory thrombophlebitis (Trousseau's syndrome) is associated with a risk of an underlying occult malignancy, most frequently of the pancreas, stomach, or lung. The veins of the chest, abdomen, and lower extremities are involved either sequentially or simultaneously. The hypercoagulable state associated with cancer is probably multifactorial in origin, and may be induced by inflammatory cytokines, acute-phase reactants, circulating tissue factor, and cancer microparticles. Patients with migratory thrombophlebitis without a known underlying cause should have a thorough evaluation, including a CT scan of the chest and abdomen.

Multicentric Reticulohistiocytosis

Multicentric reticulohistiocytosis (MRH) is a rare disorder characterized by polyarthritis and nodular cutaneous lesions. Oropharyngeal lesions, ocular involvement, pulmonary effusions and fibrosis, pericardial effusions and myocardial disease, and hepatic, gastrointestinal tract and urogenital involvement may also occur. The cutaneous lesions are skin-colored to red or violaceous nodules on the scalp, ears, face,

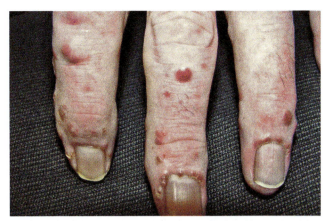

FIGURE 17-7 ■ Multicentric reticulohistiocytosis. This man did not have a malignancy, but the lesions would be identical. Note the classic "coral bead" appearance of the lesions at the nailfolds.

extremities, trunk, and mucous membranes. There is a known predilection for lesions to affect the hands, and the presence of multiple lesions at the nailfolds may give a characteristic "coral-bead" appearance, which is considered pathognomonic for MRH (Fig. 17-7). The arthritis involves the joints of the hands and is destructive, eventually resulting in severe deformities of the fingers. Multicentric reticulohistiocytosis has been associated with autoimmune disease (Sjögren's, systemic lupus erythematosus, scleroderma), endocrine disease (diabetes mellitus, thyroid disease), and cancer. Roughly one-quarter of patients have an underlying internal malignancy, and a variety of solid organ (GU, GI, pulmonary, sarcoma) and lymphoreticular malignancies have been described. The exact relationship—specifically the manner in which the disorder is associated with cancer—is not clear.

Cutaneous T-Cell Lymphoma (Mycosis Fungoides)

Cutaneous T-cell lymphoma (CTCL) is often a chronic disease characterized by poikiloderma or erythematous patches, plaques, or tumors (see Chapter 20). The disease is characterized histopathologically by epidermotropic malignant T cells. Second primary malignancies have been reported to occur in patients with CTCL more frequently than would be predicted. Data from the Surveillance, Epidemiology, and End Results program identified a significantly elevated risk for Hodgkin's disease and non-Hodgkin's lymphoma in patients with CTCL. New signs or symptoms in patients with CTCL must be carefully and thoroughly evaluated.

Necrobiotic Xanthogranuloma

The term necrobiotic xanthogranuloma with paraproteinemia was coined by Winkelmann to describe destructive cutaneous lesions associated with the histopathologic finding of an inflammatory granuloma with xanthomatosis and panniculitis, along with an associated paraproteinemia. Clinically, the lesions are yellow to red papules, nodules, or plaques that enlarge and

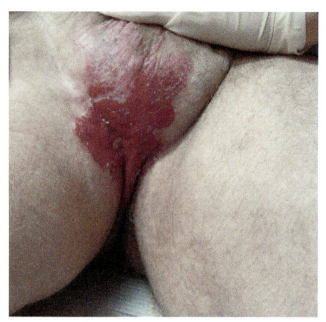

FIGURE 17-8 ■ Extramammary Paget's disease. Chronic, scaly erythematous plaque in the groin. This patient did not have an underlying neoplasm.

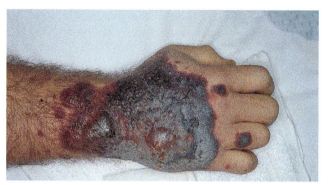

FIGURE 17-9 ■ Sweet's syndrome (acute febrile neutrophilic dermatosis) in a patient with acute myelogenous leukemia. At the time that this picture was taken he was severely thrombocytopenic, hence the massive hemorrhage.

may become ulcerative. They have a predilection for periorbital skin. By definition, these lesions are associated with paraproteinemia, most commonly an IgG kappa monoclonal gammopathy, and infrequently with myeloma.

Paget's Disease of the Breast and Extramammary Paget's Disease

Paget's disease of the breast is characterized by an erythematous, eczematous plaque surrounding the nipple and areola. This condition occurs in conjunction with a ductal adenocarcinoma of the breast, which has frequently metastasized to the axillary lymph nodes. Paget's disease is believed to be caused by an upward migration of malignant cells, and hence it is not truly a paraneoplastic sign but rather a specific malignant infiltrate.

Extramammary Paget's disease is the same clinicopathologic lesion as that found in Paget's disease of the breast, but on a nonmammary surface, most often the genital, axillary, or perianal skin (Fig. 17-8). Roughly 30% to 50% of patients with this condition have an underlying neoplasm, which generally underlies the area of skin involvement, most commonly of the genitourinary or gastrointestinal tract. In patients with extramammary Paget's disease, an evaluation of the areas contiguous to the disease should be undertaken.

Pityriasis Rotunda

Pityriasis rotunda is an unusual, round, noninflammatory lesion that occurs on the trunk and results in hyperpigmentation. Various malignancies have been reported to occur in conjunction with pityriasis rotunda. The condition has also been reported with numerous other potential etiologic agents. In a study from South Africa, 7 of 10 patients with pityriasis rotunda had hepatocellular carcinoma. The relationship of this cutaneous condition to malignancy when present is not known. To date, there have not been reports of patients whose pityriasis rotunda has followed the course of their neoplasm. Despite the lack of confirmatory data, it seems prudent to at least consider cancer in anyone with this rare cutaneous disease.

Punctate Keratoses and Arsenical Keratoses of the Palms and Soles

Punctate keratoses are discrete, skin-colored, hyperkeratotic papules that occur on the palms and soles, most commonly in African-Americans. The lesions often have a central plug or a depressed, crater-like center. They are often numerous, but remain distinct from one another. Symptoms are uncommon. Arsenical keratoses, albeit histopathologically distinct, may be clinically indistinguishable from punctate keratoses. Although the relationship between punctate keratoses and malignancy is controversial at best, chronic arsenic exposure in contaminated drinking water has been associated with bladder and lung carcinoma in addition to nonmelanoma skin cancer.

Pyoderma Gangrenosum and Other "Neutrophilic" Dermatoses

Cases of various malignancies have been reported infrequently in patients with classic pyoderma gangrenosum. Patients with atypical bullous pyoderma gangrenosum in particular may have myeloid leukemia or be in a preleukemic state. Similarly, many patients with Sweet's syndrome (acute febrile neutrophilic dermatosis) have been reported to have myeloid leukemia (Fig. 17-9). Paraneoplastic neutrophilic lesions on the face may simulate erysipelas. In patients with malignancy-associated neutrophilic dermatoses, the discovery of the leukemia often occurs simultaneously with the recognition of the cutaneous abnormality. The cutaneous lesions disappear when the leukemia is in remission, and may recur when the leukemia relapses. It seems

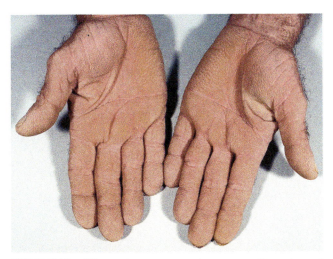

FIGURE 17-10 ■ Tripe palms: rugose changes on the palms of both hands. (Courtesy of Jon Dyer, MD, Columbia, MO.)

reasonable to evaluate all patients with atypical pyoderma gangrenosum or Sweet's syndrome with careful hematologic studies, including a bone marrow examination in selected patients.

Pachydermoperiostosis

Acquired pachydermoperiostosis manifests as thickening of the skin, hypertrophic osteoarthropathy, and clubbing of the nails. The condition may result in a coarse facial appearance resembling acromegaly. In addition, the skin of the distal extremities is frequently involved. The palms and soles may also become hyperkeratotic. Clubbing may occur without the other features of the syndrome, but has the same malignancy implications.

These disorders are most frequently associated with lung neoplasia. However, the changes are not exclusively paraneoplastic and may also occur in the setting of benign pulmonary and cardiac disease. The incidence of malignancy in patients with pachydermoperiostosis is unknown. Also, it is not clear whether tumor therapy affects the course of the skin or nail disease. Thus, clubbing with or without pachydermoperiostosis should be considered to be a sign of cardiopulmonary disease, and the possibility of lung cancer should be considered.

Tripe Palms

Tripe palms is a cutaneous paraneoplastic syndrome characterized by a thickened, moss-like, velvety texture of the palms (Fig. 17-10). The appearance of the palmar surface is similar to the intertriginous changes found in AN. Some patients with tripe palms also manifest AN, but the majority do not. Often, a malignancy is found concurrently with the recognition of the cutaneous disease. Most of the associated cancers have been found in the stomach and lungs. In the absence of AN, tripe palms is most often associated with lung cancer. It is not known whether the cutaneous disease course parallels that of the malignancy.

Vitiligo

Vitiligo or a vitiligo-like leukoderma has been reported in conjunction with malignant melanoma. Furthermore, a report linked vitiligo in individuals over 40 years with various malignant neoplasms. This association has not been confirmed. In the authors' view, the onset of vitiligo in an adult warrants a full skin examination, including a Wood's light examination.

HORMONE-SECRETING SYNDROMES

Carcinoid Syndrome

Carcinoid syndrome is produced by tumors that secrete 5-hydroxytryptamine and other vasoactive amines. The tumors are most common in the gastrointestinal tract, but may also occur in the lungs or ovaries. Clinically, flushing, diarrhea, abdominal pain, wheezing, and occasionally shortness of breath occur. Tumors from the gastrointestinal tract do not produce symptoms until they metastasize to the liver because under normal circumstances, the liver is able to detoxify the amines responsible for the production of symptoms. Tumors in other locations are capable of producing symptoms prior to metastasis. The diagnosis of carcinoid syndrome is made by finding elevated levels of 5-hydroxyindoleacetic acid (or other metabolites or vasoactive amines) in the urine. Removal of the tumor results in cessation of symptoms.

Ectopic Adrenocorticotropic Syndrome

Certain tumors are capable of amine precursor uptake and decarboxylation and are therefore known as APUDomas. These tumors usually originate in the lungs (bronchial adenoma or oat cell carcinoma), gastrointestinal tract (carcinoid), or glandular tissues. Ectopic adrenocorticotropic hormone (ACTH)-producing tumors result in many of the typical signs and symptoms of Cushing's syndrome, with the exception of obesity. Intense hyperpigmentation is rare in Cushing's disease, but is common in patients with ectopic production of ACTH. The most common tumor that produces this syndrome is oat cell carcinoma of the lung.

Necrolytic Migratory Erythema (Glucagonoma Syndrome)

Necrolytic migratory erythema is an eruption strongly associated with glucagon-producing pancreatic neoplasms. The characteristic cutaneous eruption begins in the groin area as irregular erythematous patches studded with superficial flaccid erosions, vesicles, and bullae. The erythema and bullous lesions may coalesce into circinate and/or polycyclic psoriasiform plaques. The eruption may be confused with seborrheic dermatitis, intertrigo, or candidiasis. Erythematous, scaly patches at the corners of the mouth (angular cheilitis) and glossitis also develop. Other findings include new-onset diabetes mellitus, anemia, weight loss, and diarrhea.

The clinical and histological similarity of necrolytic migratory erythema to acrodermatitis enteropathica and vitamin B deficiencies suggests that necrolytic migratory erythema may be a skin manifestation of nutritional deficiency induced by excessive glucagon secretion by the pancreatic tumor. In fact, iatrogenic necrolytic migratory erythema has been induced by the administration of glucagon to treat persistent hypoglycemia. Although removal of the glucagonoma results in resolution of skin symptoms, more than 50% of patients have hepatic metastases at the time of diagnosis, generally resulting in a poor prognosis.

INHERITED SYNDROMES ASSOCIATED WITH INTERNAL CANCER

Birt–Hogg–Dubé Syndrome (OMIM #135150)

Birt–Hogg–Dubé (BHD) syndrome was first described in 1977 as a triad of fibrofolliculoma, trichodiscoma, and acrochordon. Subsequent to this description, BHD syndrome was linked to a risk of spontaneous pneumothorax and renal cell cancer. Mutations in the BHD gene, *FLCN*, on chromosome 17p11.2, were identified in 2002, but the function of the folliculin protein remains unclear. Characteristic fibrofolliculoma facial lesions begin in the third decade as small white to skin-colored flat papules, and may range from a few scattered lesions to near-confluent involvement of the face and neck (Fig. 17-11). Affected individuals may develop multiple renal neoplasms of variable histology simultaneously in both kidneys, including unusual oncocytic–chromophobe hybrid tumors. Initial screening should include chest CT and abdominal CT or MRI to evaluate for pulmonary and renal disease, respectively.

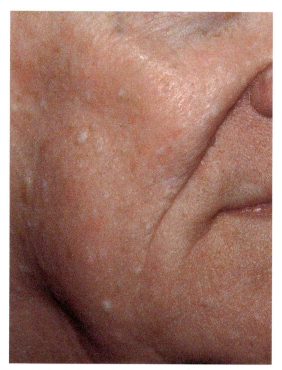

FIGURE 17-11 ■ Birt–Hogg–Dubé syndrome. Multiple white fibrofolliculomas on the face.

Cowden Disease (OMIM #158350)

Cowden disease, Bannayan–Ruvalcaba–Riley syndrome, and Lhermitte–Duclos disease share overlapping clinical features, including macrocephaly, hamartomatous gastrointestinal polyps, and lipomas, and are collectively referred to as *PTEN* hamartoma tumor syndromes. The most characteristic findings of Cowden disease are trichilemmomas located around the nose and central face, multiple keratotic papules on the face, neck, ears, and hands, and multiple papules on the oral mucosa that coalesce to form a cobblestone appearance. Systemic manifestations include polyposis of the gastrointestinal tract, tumors of the thyroid gland, ovarian cysts, and fibrocystic disease of the breast. All of these syndromes are associated with germline mutations in the *PTEN* gene (10q23.3) and an increased risk of malignancy in several organ systems. Women are at very high risk of breast cancer, often bilateral, but men with Cowden disease are at risk of breast malignancy as well. The overall prevalence of malignant tumors may be as high as 40% to 50%, specifically adenocarcinoma of the breast (20%), adenocarcinoma of the thyroid (7%), squamous cell carcinoma of the skin (4%), and cancers of the colon, prostate, uterus, cervix, bladder, or blood (<1% each). A careful evaluation for underlying malignancies is necessary in both patients with this syndrome and all family members. Some authorities have even gone so far as to suggest prophylactic mastectomy in women with this disease.

Gardner's Syndrome (OMIM #175100)

Gardner's syndrome is a variant of familial adenomatosis polyposis. Patients with Gardner's syndrome develop epidermoid cysts, fibromas, lipomas, and desmoid tumors. Multiple osteomas may develop. Bilateral congenital hypertrophy of the retinal pigment epithelium is an early ocular finding. Epidermoid cysts appear in early childhood on the face, trunk, and scalp, and may precede the identification of colonic polyposis by many years. Concern for malignant transformation of the polyps often leads to prophylactic total colectomy in childhood. Patients are also at risk of neoplasia of other organ systems, particularly central nervous system malignancy (Turcot syndrome).

Hereditary Leiomyomatosis and Renal Cell Cancer (OMIM #150800)

Hereditary leiomyomatosis and renal cell cancer is an autosomal dominant cancer syndrome characterized by cutaneous leiomyomas, uterine leiomyomas (fibroids), and renal cell cancer. Germline mutations in fumarate hydratase (FH), a Krebs cycle enzyme, predispose to this syndrome. Cutaneous leiomyomas are ovoid pink nodules that often cluster together. They are frequently

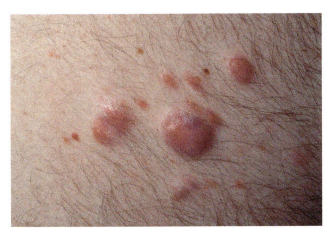

FIGURE 17-12 ■ Hereditary leiomyomatosis and renal cell cancer. Cluster of painful red nodular leiomyomas on the upper back.

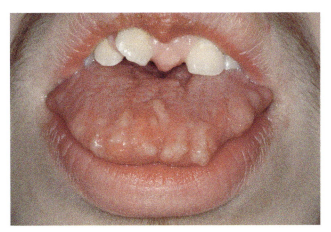

FIGURE 17-13 ■ MEN 2b. Thickened lips and multiple neuromas of the tongue in a young man with metastatic medullary thyroid carcinoma.

described as painful or sensitive to touch (Fig. 17-12). Uterine fibroids are nearly universal in women with FH mutations, leading to hysterectomy in most cases. The penetrance of renal cell cancer in affected individuals is lower than that of cutaneous and uterine leiomyomas. However, FH mutation-related renal cell cancer typically follows an aggressive clinical course, and regular screening is necessary for early detection of these tumors.

Multiple Endocrine Neoplasia (OMIM #131100 (Type 1); #171400 (2a); #162300 (2b))

The multiple endocrine neoplasias (MEN) are discrete dominantly inherited genetic disorders associated with a very high prevalence of benign and malignant endocrine neoplasms. MEN type 1 is associated with parathyroid adenoma in nearly all patients, as well as pituitary tumors and a variety of pancreatic neoplasms. Multiple facial angiofibromas are common in MEN 1. Collagenomas, café-au-lait macules, gingival papules, and lipomas are less frequent cutaneous findings. Patients with MEN 2a develop parathyroid adenoma, pheochromocytoma, and medullary thyroid carcinoma. The only cutaneous manifestation of MEN 2a is lichen amyloidosis. MEN 2b is associated with mucosal and intestinal neuromatosis, pheochromocytoma, and medullary thyroid carcinoma. Affected individuals present with a marfanoid habitus and coarse facial features, the latter due to neuronal infiltration of the eyelids, lips, and tongue (Fig. 17-13).

Muir–Torre Syndrome (OMIM #158320)

Muir–Torre syndrome is a variant of HNPCC Lynch syndrome II with multiple sebaceous tumors, including adenomas, adenocarcinomas, and epitheliomas. It is associated with deleterious mutations in DNA mismatch repair genes, including MLH1 and MSH2. The presence of two or more sebaceous tumors or a single sebaceous neoplasm in a person younger than 60 years with a personal or family history of Lynch-related cancer (GI, endometrial, ovarian, urothelial, or bilial) confers a high

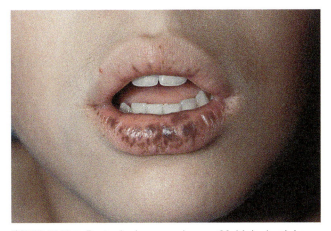

FIGURE 17-14 ■ Peutz–Jeghers syndrome. Multiple lentiginous macules on the lips.

likelihood of Muir–Torre syndrome. If suggestive features are identified, mismatch repair immunohistochemistry and microsatellite instability testing of the skin tumors may be helpful to confirm the diagnosis. Although the visceral tumors in patients with Muir–Torre syndrome appear to behave in a more benign fashion than similar sporadic tumors, 60% of patients with Muir–Torre will develop metastatic disease. In addition, 50% of patients with Muir–Torre syndrome present with an internal malignancy prior to manifesting skin lesions. Therefore, careful screening of other at-risk family members is important.

Peutz–Jeghers Syndrome (OMIM #175200)

Mucocutaneous pigmented macules (Fig. 17-14) and hamartomatous polyps of the gastrointestinal tract are characteristic of Peutz–Jeghers syndrome. Lentigines tend to cluster around the lips, on the oral mucosa, and on acral areas of the body. This disorder is inherited in an autosomal dominant pattern, but spontaneous mutations account for 50% of cases. Peutz–Jeghers syndrome is associated with germline mutations in the *LKB1* gene (19p13.3), which encodes a multifunctional

TABLE 17-2 Paraneoplastic Disorders

Disorders that Fit Curth's Criteria
Acanthosis nigricans and possibly the sign of Leser–Trélat
Acute febrile neutrophilic dermatosis (see Chapter 5)
Bazex syndrome
Carcinoid syndrome
Ectopic ACTH syndrome
Erythema gyratum repens
Glucagonoma syndrome
Hypertrichosis lanuginosa
Neutrophilic dermatoses
Paraneoplastic pemphigus

Disorders Associated Statistically with Cancer
Arsenical keratoses
Cutaneous T-cell lymphoma
Dermatomyositis
Scleroderma
Erythroderma
Extramammary Paget's disease
Generalized pruritus without a primary cutaneous eruption
Pityriasis rotunda
Porphyria cutanea tarda

Dermatoses Possibly Associated with Cancer
Acquired ichthyosis
Antiepiligrin cicatricial pemphigoid
Multicentric reticulohistiocytosis
Necrobiotic xanthogranuloma
Classic pyoderma gangrenosum
Tripe palms
Vasculitis
Vitiligo

ACTH, adrenocorticotropic hormone.

serine–threonine kinase. Affected individuals may present in adolescence with anemia, bloody stools, or intermittent abdominal pain due to intussusception from intestinal polyps. Increased aromatase activity resulting from calcifying Sertoli cell testicular tumors may induce gynecomastia as another presenting sign of the syndrome in boys. Patients are at an increased risk of both intestinal and extraintestinal malignancies, including breast, pancreatic, ovarian, testicular, and cervical cancer, mandating yearly cancer screening beginning at age 10.

Von Recklinghausen's Disease (OMIM #162200)

Von Recklinghausen's disease (neurofibromatosis) is an autosomal dominant disorder that is discussed elsewhere (see Chapter 40). Approximately 2% to 5% of the patients with this syndrome will develop a malignancy, many of which represent a malignant degeneration of the neurofibroma. However, these patients may also develop astrocytomas, glioblastomas, meningiomas, and bilateral pheochromocytomas. If the patient with neurofibromatosis develops symptoms of headache, backache, or hypertension, the potential for internal malignancy must be considered, and appropriate tests should be ordered.

CONCLUSIONS

The cutaneous disorders associated with malignancy are reviewed in Table 17-2. They are classified as: (1) those that fit Curth's postulates and thus warrant specific investigation; (2) those that are statistically related to internal malignancy but do not require extensive malignancy investigations; and (3) those with only a possible association with cancer. Further work is needed to delineate the exact relationship of these cutaneous disorders with their potentially associated internal neoplasms. Epidemiologic studies are needed to further evaluate many of the syndromes that may be malignancy related.

SUGGESTED READINGS

Abreu Velez AM, Howard MS. Diagnosis and treatment of cutaneous paraneoplastic disorders. Dermatol Ther 2010;23(6):662–75.
Anhalt GJ. Paraneoplastic pemphigus. Adv Dermatol 1997;12:77–96.
Curth HO. Skin lesions and internal carcinoma. In: Andrade R, Gumport SL, Popkin GL, Reed TD, editors. Cancer of the skin. Philadelphia: WB Saunders; 1976. p. 1308–43.
Egan CA, Lazarova Z, Darling TN, et al. Anti-epiligrin cicatricial pemphigoid and relative risk for cancer. Lancet 2001;357:1850–1.
Fernia AN, Vleugels RA, Callen JP. Cutaneous dermatomyositis: an updated review of treatment options and internal associations. Am J Clin Dermatol 2013;14:291–313.
Moore RL, Dever TS. Epidermal manifestations of internal malignancy. Dermatol Clin 2008;26:17–29.
Nguyen VT, Ndoye A, Bassler KD, et al. Classification, clinical manifestations, and immunopathological mechanisms of the epithelial variant of paraneoplastic autoimmune multiorgan syndrome: a reappraisal of paraneoplastic pemphigus. Arch Dermatol 2001;137:193–206.
Ponti G, Ponz de Leon M. Muir–Torre syndrome. Lancet Oncol 2005;6:980–7.
Ruocco E, Wolf R, Caccavale S, et al. Bullous pemphigoid: associations and management guidelines: facts and controversies. Clin Dermatol 2013;31:400–12.
Thiers BH, Sahn RE, Callen JP. Cutaneous manifestations of internal malignancy. CA Cancer J Clin 2009;59(2):73–98.
Zhang JQ, Wan YN, Peng WJ, et al. The risk of cancer development in systemic sclerosis: a meta-analysis. Cancer Epidemiol 2013;37:523–7.

CHAPTER 18

DERMATOLOGIC ADVERSE EVENTS OF CANCER THERAPY

Zhe Hou • Viswanath Reddy Belum • Mario E. Lacouture

KEY POINTS

- Dermatologic adverse events (AEs) of cancer therapies can cause patient discomfort and impair their quality of life, increase the cost of medical care, and even result in dose modifications, all of which can negatively impact clinical outcomes.
- The traditional cytotoxic chemotherapies are commonly associated with dermatologic AEs such as alopecia, hypersensitivity reactions, xerosis, skin hyperpigmentation, nail changes, and hand-foot syndrome (HFS).
- Targeted therapies encompass drugs that inhibit selective molecules and pathways critical for carcinogenesis, tumor growth, and survival. The ensuing dermatologic AEs tend to vary depending on the entity targeted (e.g., epidermal growth factor receptor [EGFR], vascular endothelial growth factor/vascular endothelial growth factor receptor, immune checkpoints, mammalian target of rapamycin), although there is overlap.
- Acneiform rash, xerosis, skin hyperpigmentation, alopecia, hair disorders (e.g. dyspigmentation, hypertrichosis, trichomegaly, textural changes), paronychia, and mucosal inflammation are characteristic dermatologic AEs of the EGFR inhibitors. Treatment with inhibitors of angiogenesis often leads to HFS, exanthems, hair disorders (alopecia, dyspigmentation, and textural changes), xerosis, mucositis, and in the case of bevacizumab/aflibercept, impairment of wound healing. The immune checkpoint inhibitors often result in pruritus and maculopapular cutaneous eruptions, although their AE profile, as with other newly developed drugs, is emerging and pending further characterization.
- Timely recognition, prompt management of dermatologic AEs related to cancer treatment, and appropriate counseling are crucial for optimal clinical outcomes, and require a multidisciplinary approach involving oncologists, dermatologists, and nurses.

INTRODUCTION

Over the last few decades, treatment of cancer has evolved to include therapies that may be broadly categorized as traditional cytotoxic chemotherapies, hormonal therapies, targeted therapies, and immunotherapies (Table 18-1). From the dermatologic perspective, cytotoxic chemotherapies have long generated much interest because of the potential to cause alopecia, their hallmark adverse event (AE). The introduction of various targeted therapies and immunotherapies in recent years, however, has led to the recognition of a broad spectrum of dermatologic AEs (Table 18-2). Besides the physical and emotional impact, impairments in patients' quality of life, and financial burden, these AEs may also disrupt cancer treatments. Therefore, their timely recognition and prompt management are crucial for optimal clinical outcomes.

In this chapter, we provide an overview of the dermatologic AEs associated with major classes of cancer therapies, as well as the management options for common entities. To indicate severity, we have utilized the Common Terminology Criteria for Adverse Events (CTCAE), which is a descriptive tool with unified standards for physicians to communicate AEs using common language. The current version, CTCAE v4.0, was issued by the National Cancer Institute in May 2009, and reflects updates on the new AEs seen with targeted therapies, and grading to guide management (Chen et al., 2012).

Cytotoxic Chemotherapeutic Agents

Alkylating Agents

The alkylating agents cause arrest of cell proliferation by forming covalent bonds within DNA bases. The main dermatologic AEs include hyperpigmentation, mucositis, alopecia, hypersensitivity reactions (HSRs), and xerosis associated with pruritus.

Nitrogen Mustards

Mechlorethamine is used intravenously to treat Hodgkin's disease (MOPP regimen—mechlorethamine (mustargen) [M], vincristine [O], procarbazine [P], and prednisone [P]), and as part of topical formulations to treat cutaneous malignancies (early-stage mycosis fungoides,

TABLE 18-1 Overview of Drugs Currently Approved in the Treatment of Various Cancers

Cytotoxic Chemotherapeutic Agents

Alkylating agents	Nitrogen mustards	Aziridines and epoxides	Alkyl sulfonates	Nitrosoureas	Hydrazines and triazine derivatives	
	Mechlorethamine	ThioTEPA	Busulfan	Carmustine	Procarbazine,	Hydroxyurea
	Cyclophosphamide	Mitomycin-C		Streptozocin	Dacarbazine	
	Ifosfamide				Temozolomide	
	Melphalan					
	Chlorambucil					

Antimetabolite agents	Folate Antagonists	Pyrimidine Analogs	Purine Analogs
	Methotrexate	5-Fluorouracil	Mercaptopurine
	Pemetrexed	Capecitabine	Thioguanine
		Cytarabine	Fludarabine
		Gemcitabine	Cladribine

Topoisomerase-interacting agents	Topoisomerase I inhibitors	Topoisomerase II inhibitors
	Irinotecan, Topotecan	Anthracyclines
		Etoposide, Tenoposide
		Mitoxantrone

Antimicrotubule agents	Taxanes	Vinca alkaloids	
	Paclitaxel	Vinblastine	Estramustine phosphate sodium
	Docetaxel	Vincristine	
	Nab-paclitaxel	Vinorelbine	
		Vindesine	
		Vinflunine	

Epigenetic modulators	Histone deacetylase inhibitors	Proteasome inhibitors	Demethylating agents
	Vorinostat	Bortezomib	5-Azacitidine
	Romidepsin	Carfilzomib	Decitabine
Retinoids	Bexarotene		
	All-trans retinoic acid		
Arsenicals	Arsenic trioxide		

Targeted Anticancer Agents

EGFR inhibitors	EGFR inhibitors	EGFR/HER2 inhibitors	EGFR/VEGFR inhibitors
	Erlotinib	Afatinib	Vandetanib
	Cetuximab	Lapatinib	
	Panitumumab		
	Gefitinib		

Angiogenesis inhibitors	VEGF inhibitors	VEGFR inhibitors
	Bevacizumab	Sorafenib
	Aflibercept	Sunitinib
		Pazopanib
		Axitinib
		Regorafenib
		Cabozantinib

BRAF inhibitors	Vemurafenib, Dabrafenib
BCR-ABL inhibitors	Imatinib, Nilotinib, Dasatinib, Ponatinib, Bosutinib
mTOR inhibitors	Everolimus, Temsirolimus
MEK inhibitors	Trametinib
SMO inhibitors	Vismodegib
JAK inhibitors	Ruxolitinib
PI3K inhibitors	Idelalisib
BTK inhibitors	Ibrutinib
ALK inhibitors	Crizotinib
Immune checkpoint inhibitors	Ipilimumab, Nivolumab, Pembrolizumab

Other monoclonal antibodies	HER-2	CD20	CD30	CD-52
	Trastuzumab	Rituximab	Brentuximab	Alemtuzumab
	Ado-trastuzumab emtansine	Ofatumumab		
	Pertuzumab	Obinutuzumab		

TABLE 18-1 Overview of Drugs Currently Approved in the Treatment of Various Cancers—cont'd

Other Anticancer Agents

Endocrine agents	SERMs	ERDs	Aromatase inhibitors	LHRH agonists	Androgens	Antiandrogens		Somatostatin analogs
	Tamoxifen	Fulvestrant	Exemestane	Leuprolide	Fluoxymesterone	Flutamide	Megestrol acetate	Octreotide acetate
	Toremifene		Anastrozole			Bicalutamide		
	Raloxifene		Letrozole					

Miscellaneous

						Thalidomides		
	L-Asparaginase		Bleomycin			Thalidomide		
						Lenalidomide		
						Pomalidomide		

EGFR, epidermal growth factor receptor; HER, human epidermal growth factor receptor; VEGF, vascular endothelial growth factor; VEGFR, VEGF receptor; BRAF, B-rapidly accelerated fibrosarcoma; BCR-abl, breakpoint cluster region-abelson; mTOR, mechanistic target of rapamycin; MEK, MAPK/ERK (extracellular signal-regulated kinase) Kinase; SMO, smoothened; JAK, janus kinase; Pi3K, phosphoinositide 3-kinase; BTK, Bruton's tyrosine kinase; ALK, anaplastic lymphoma kinase; CD, cluster of differentiation; SERMs, selective estrogen receptor modulators; ERDs, estrogen receptor downregulators; LHRH, luteinizing hormone-releasing hormone.

Langerhans cell histiocytosis, and cutaneous B-cell lymphoma). The dermatologic AEs include infusion-related reactions (phlebitis and chemical cellulitis), pruritus, alopecia, and angioedema. Other less frequent AEs include urticaria, erythema multiforme (EM)-like eruption, and hyperpigmentation (without preceding inflammation). With the topical formulation, irritant or allergic contact dermatitis is the most common acute complication. An increased risk of nonmelanoma skin cancers (NMSCs) with both systemic and topical use of mechlorethamine has also been reported.

Management of the cutaneous eruption includes topical corticosteroids (mild/moderate cases); oral corticosteroids and dose reductions may improve tolerability in a majority of patients with severe reactions. Topical retinoids, hydroquinones, and corticosteroids are effective in treating skin hyperpigmentation.

Cyclophosphamide is widely used in the treatment of various cancers, autoimmune diseases, and also during bone marrow transplantation (preparative stage). The most common dermatologic AE is alopecia (40% to 60%), which develops 3 to 6 weeks after the start of therapy. Other frequent AEs include injection site complications (erythema, swelling, and pain), mucositis, and reversible hyperpigmentation (diffuse or localized to palms and soles, or nails). Facial flushing, toxic erythemas, pruritus, hand-foot syndrome (HFS), and urticarial and anaphylactoid reactions have also been reported.

Ifosfamide, a structural isomer of cyclophosphamide, is indicated in the treatment of various solid tumors, lymphomas, sarcomas, and some pediatric tumors. Since the drug is infused, extravasation reactions can occur, and lead to local cellulitis. Patients may also commonly experience alopecia and hyperpigmentation. Of note, ifosfamide, in combination with other agents such as gemcitabine and etoposide, can result in severe oral mucositis and an extensive sunburn-like erythema with accentuation in the intertriginous and genito-anal areas.

Melphalan is used for the treatment of multiple myeloma (MM), as well as high dose myeloablative treatment prior to stem cell transplantation (SCT). It has been associated with radiation recall, urticarial and anaphylactoid reactions, and nail hyperpigmentation. When used in isolated limb perfusion to treat localized tumors (e.g., melanoma and sarcoma), it may lead to erythema, edema, blistering, temporary loss of nails, and hair growth arrest on the perfused extremity. Localized scleroderma has been reported as a rare complication.

Chlorambucil is used for the treatment of B-cell chronic lymphocytic leukemia (CLL) and lymphomas. Reported dermatologic AEs include HSRs presenting as urticaria and angioedema, erythematous eruptions, and toxic epidermal necrolysis (TEN).

Aziridines and Epoxides

ThioTEPA is used in the treatment of adenocarcinoma of the breast, ovary, and in post-transurethral resection of bladder tumor for papillary bladder cancer, myeloablation prior to SCT, and treatment of cavitary malignant effusions. Allergic reactions and immediate hypersensitivity reactions, alopecia, mucositis, and pruritus are common, while acute-onset, intense erythema of the palmoplantar surfaces, and hyperpigmentation of occluded skin have also been reported. As compared to adults, pediatric patients experience a higher rate of skin erythema progressing to desquamation and hyperpigmentation.

Mitomycin C is an antitumor antibiotic derived from the soil fungus, *Streptomyces caespitosus*. It is available for systemic use in the treatment of upper gastrointestinal, anal, and breast cancers, and topically for the treatment of ocular surface neoplasias. Intravesical instillation has also been used to treat noninvasive bladder tumors. Extravasation-related tissue injury, mucositis, immediate hypersensitivity reactions, and allergic contact dermatitis have been reported.

Alkyl Sulfonates

Busulfan is a component of many of the myeloablative regimens administered prior to autologous or allogeneic bone marrow transplantation, and is used to treat the chronic phase of chronic myeloid leukemia (CML). It has been associated with immediate hypersensitivity reactions, injection site reactions, toxic erythemas, pruritus, EM, and vasculitis. Hyperpigmentation ("dusky") is the most characteristic dermatologic AE of busulfan, which presents as diffuse-bronze discoloration, most prominent on the neck, upper portion of the trunk, nipples, abdomen, and palmar creases.

TABLE 18-2 Common and Clinically Significant Dermatologic Adverse Events from Targeted Anticancer Agents

Primary Molecular Target	EGFR	Multikinase	VEGF	VEGFR/PDGFR	BRAF	mTOR/PI3K	CD20	HER-2	CTLA-4	PD-1
Anticancer agents	Cetuximab, Panitumumab, Erlotinib, Afatinib, Lapatinib	Imatinib (I), Nilotinib (N), Dasatinib (D)	Bevacizumab (B), Aflibercept (A)	Sorafenib (So), Sunitinib (Su), Pazopanib (P), Axitinib (Ax), Regorafenib (R), Cabozantinib (C)	Vemurafenib, Dabrafenib	Everolimus (E), Temsirolimus (T), Idelalisib (I)	Rituximab, Ibritumomab tiuxetan	Trastuzumab (Tr), Trastuzumab emtansine (T-DM1)	Ipilimumab	Nivolumab (Nv), Pembrolizumab (P)

Dermatologic adverse event

Skin

Cutaneous eruptions

	EGFR	Multikinase	VEGF	VEGFR/PDGFR	BRAF	mTOR/PI3K	CD20	HER-2	CTLA-4	PD-1
Maculopapular	+++	+++	+++ (B)	++	++	+++ (E, T) ++ (I)		+ (Tr)	+++	+++
Papulopustular ("acneiform")	+++*				++	+++ (E, T)				+ (Nv)
Keratosis pilaris-like	+	+								
Xerosis	++	++		++	++	++ (E, T)				
Fissures (fingertips, toes)	++									
Skin infections (Bacterial, viral, fungal)	+						+			
Pruritus	++	++	++ (B)	++	+	+++ (E, T)			+++	+++
Hand-foot skin reaction			+	+++	+					
Photosensitivity	+++	+	+ (A)		+++					+ (Nv)

Pigmentary changes

	EGFR	Multikinase	VEGF	VEGFR/PDGFR	BRAF	mTOR/PI3K	CD20	HER-2	CTLA-4	PD-1
Hyperpigmentation		+ (I)		+ (Su)						
Hypopigmentation		++ (I)								
Depigmentation (vitiligo)			+++						++	+
Impaired wound healing	+		+++							
Skin neoplasms (KA/cuSCC)†				+ (So, R)	+++					
Psoriasis exacerbation or psoriasiform eruptions		++ (I)								
Lichenoid eruptions				+ (So)						
Eruptive nevi				++ (Su)						
Facial edema	+++	+++								

Primary Molecular Target	EGFR	Multikinase	VEGF	VEGFR/PDGFR	BRAF	mTOR/PI3K	CD20	HER-2	CTLA-4	PD-1
Appendages										
Hair										
Alopecia	++	+	+	++ (So, Su); + (P)	++			++ (Tr)	+	
Hypertrichosis, trichomegaly	+++									
Curling	++			++	++					
Hyperpigmentation										+ (P)
Hypopigmentation		+		+ (Su); ++ (P)						+ (P)
Nail										
Paronychia	++					++ (E, T)				
Nail abnormalities	++			++						
MUCOSAE										
Mucositis, stomatitis	++	++	+	+		+++ (E, T)				
Bleeding, hemorrhages			+ (B)							
Cutaneous and mucosal telangiectasia	+									
Geographic tongue			+ (B)							
Mucocutaneous reactions‡							+	+++ (T-DM1)		

*Incidence: + <10%, ++ 10% to 30%, +++ >30%.

†KA/cuSCC: keratoacanthoma/cutaneous squamous cell carcinoma.

‡Mucocutaneous reactions include paraneoplastic pemphigus, lichenoid or vesiculobullous eruptions, Stevens–Johnson syndrome, and toxic epidermal necrolysis.

EGFR, epidermal growth factor receptor; BCR-abl, breakpoint cluster region-abelson; VEGF, vascular endothelial growth factor; VEGFR, VEGF receptor; PDGFR, platelet derived growth factor receptor; CD, cluster of differentiation; BRAF, B-rapidly accelerated fibrosarcoma; mTOR, mechanistic target of rapamycin; HER, human epidermal growth factor receptor; CTLA-4, cytotoxic T-lymphocyte antigen-4; PD-1, programmed cell death.

Nitrosoureas

Carmustine (bischlorethylnitrosourea) is used systemically in the treatment of lymphoma, brain tumors, and myeloma, and locally for cutaneous T-cell lymphoma (CTCL) and melanoma. Most of the AEs are related to topical administration, and include erythema, burning, irritant or allergic contact dermatitis, and/or hyperpigmentation. The erythema may be accentuated in the intertriginous areas, and in severe cases, it is followed by telangiectasias, which may be transient or permanent. Secondary skin cancers are rare with topical carmustine.

Streptozocin is used to treat surgically incurable insulinomas and malignant carcinoid tumors. The commonly reported AEs include extravasation reactions leading to local inflammation, allergic dermatitis, and alopecia.

Hydrazines and Triazine Derivatives

Procarbazine is used as part of the MOPP regimen for Hodgkin's disease, and also for brain tumors and bronchogenic carcinomas. The common dermatologic AEs include alopecia, immediate hypersensitivity reactions, and alcohol-triggered flushing, which is accompanied by headache and diaphoresis.

Dacarbazine is used in the treatment of melanoma, soft tissue sarcomas, neuroblastoma, rhabdomyosarcoma, and medullary thyroid carcinoma. Intravenous infusion may lead to chemical cellulitis and phlebitis. Alopecia and HSRs are common, although pruritic maculo-urticarial erythemas (on sun-exposed areas), and radiation recall dermatitis can occur. Reactions leading to hepatic and hematologic dysfunction can be fatal.

Temozolomide is an oral medication indicated for the treatment of brain tumors and melanoma. Erythematous eruptions, pruritus, immediate hypersensitivity reactions, alopecia, xerosis, erythema multiforme-like eruptions and Stevens–Johnson syndrome (SJS) have been reported.

Hydroxyurea

Hydroxyurea is administered orally in the treatment of myeloproliferative disorders. Dermatologic AEs are common and dose dependent, presenting as xerosis, localized or generalized hyperpigmentation, and painful cutaneous ulcerations (over microtrauma sites). With long-term use, characteristic dermatomyositis-like skin changes (self-limiting Gottron-like papules and streaky erythema, without muscular symptoms), and an increased risk of NMSCs in sun-exposed areas, have been observed. In addition, cutaneous atrophy, cutaneous vasculitis, fixed drug eruption (FDE), and mucositis have also been reported.

Antimetabolite Agents

Antimetabolites are cytostatic agents that block cell division by inhibiting the biosynthesis of nucleotides.

Folate Antagonists

Methotrexate is a common component of regimens that target both solid and hematologic malignancies. It has been associated with a number of dermatologic AEs (especially when used as daily chemotherapy rather than as low dose weekly therapy) including tender palmoplantar erythema and edema with fissures and blisters. These inflamed lesions may also be accompanied by bullous changes. Cutaneous ulcerations within preexisting plaques of psoriasis have been reported commonly with the use of methotrexate, although normal skin may also be affected. Ultraviolet (UV) recall phenomenon is common and presents with erythema on areas of skin that previously developed UV-induced solar erythema. Oral mucositis is a common complication, which significantly impairs the quality of life. Patients may benefit from therapy with systemic corticosteroids, high dose folic acid supplementation, dose modification, and alternative intravenous or intramuscular administration.

Pemetrexed is indicated in the treatment of mesothelioma and non-small cell lung cancer (NSCLC), in combination with cisplatin. Dermatologic AEs include drug eruptions, acute generalized exanthematous pustulosis (AGEP), and SJS/TEN. Radiation recall dermatitis is frequent, and varies from mild blanchable erythema to severe soft tissue necrosis within fields of previous irradiation. Anecdotal reports of topical corticosteroid have suggested benefits; however, there is no effective treatment yet. Edema of the eyelids and limbs, which may be striking and resemble fibrosis, has also been frequently reported.

Pyrimidine Analogs

5-Fluorouracil (5-FU) inhibits thymidylate synthase, and results in the depletion of deoxythymidine triphosphate. It is approved for use in gastroenterologic malignancies. Most patients experience dermatologic reactions, which may lead to discontinuation of therapy in 5% of patients (due to intolerability). Xerosis, alopecia, UV recall reaction, hyperpigmentation, melanonychia and immediate hypersensitivity reactions, and inflammation of actinic keratosis are the most common dermatologic AEs. It can also cause lupus-like lesions with systemic or topical use.

Capecitabine is a prodrug of 5-FU, and is used for the treatment of metastatic breast, pancreatic, and colon cancer. HFS is the most commonly cited dermatologic AE (Fig. 18-1, *A* and 18-1, *B*), which may represent a surrogate marker of antitumor efficacy. It may also result in dose reductions, although it can be prevented by celecoxib use. Treatment includes high potency topical corticosteroids and salicylic acid. In addition, hyperpigmentation, mucositis/stomatitis, alopecia, onychodystrophy, and cutaneous lupus have also been reported.

Cytarabine is indicated for acute and chronic leukemias and lymphomas. The most common dermatologic AEs include morbilliform eruptions and HFS. In addition, neutrophilic eccrine hidradenitis (NEH, presenting with asymptomatic erythematous plaques), SJS/TEN, mucositis/stomatitis, alopecia, dystrophy, and transient acantholytic dermatosis/Grover's-like eruptions have all been reported.

Gemcitabine is used in the treatment of breast, ovarian, pancreatic cancers, and NSCLC. Morbilliform erythemas, leg edema (Fig. 18-2), pruritus, alopecia, and photo recall are frequently noted. A specific pseudocellulitis or erysipeloid eruption (confined to edematous skin), radiation recall, HFS, localized skin sclerosis, linear immunoglobulin A (IgA) bullous dermatosis, mucositis, pseudolymphoma, and anal pruritus may occur. In rare instances, patients may experience distal necrosis and SJS/TEN.

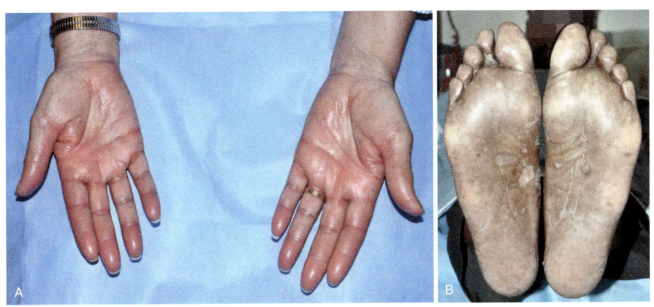

FIGURE 18-1 ■ **A,** Grade 2 hand-foot syndrome affecting the palms and soles (not shown) in a 62-year-old woman being treated with capecitabine for metastatic breast cancer. The patient also reported pain, burning, tingling sensations, and tightness of skin. **B,** Grade 2 hand-foot syndrome affecting the palms (not shown) and soles in a 74-year-old man, during treatment with capecitabine for metastatic pancreatic cancer. Note the peeling of skin and hyperkeratotic areas.

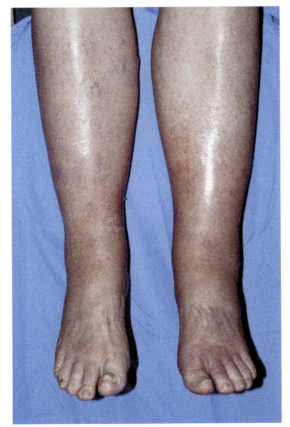

FIGURE 18-2 ■ Grade 2 leg edema in a 73-year-old woman, 1 month into treatment with gemcitabine and Abraxane® for unresectable pancreatic cancer. Note the erythema, edema, and peeling of skin ("pseudocellulitis").

Purine Analogs

Mercaptopurine is used in the treatment of acute lymphocytic leukemia (ALL). HFS, alopecia, eruptive nevi, hypersensitivity, and occasional mucositis have been reported. The risk of developing secondary skin cancers (either melanoma or nonmelanoma) may be increased.

Thioguanine is used in the treatment of certain leukemias. The dermatologic AEs include skin eruptions, alopecia, and photosensitivity (UVA) eruptions. There is an increased risk of developing NMSCs, which may be a reflection of skin damage exacerbated by photosensitivity.

Fludarabine is used in the treatment of B-cell CLL, and in some conditioning regimens for acute myeloid leukemia. Mucositis, exacerbation of psoriasis, transfusion-associated graft-versus-host disease (GVHD), and worsening of skin cancers have been reported in low incidences.

Cladribine is indicated for hairy cell leukemia. Erythema, pruritus, morbilliform erythemas (with or without eosinophilia), and injection site reactions have been reported. Rarely, skin necrosis (at the site of infusion) and TEN may develop.

Topoisomerase Inhibitors

These drugs interfere with the action of the topoisomerase enzymes (topoisomerase I and II) and cause DNA strand breaks, leading to checkpoint arrest and apoptosis. They are important components in chemotherapy regimens for the treatment of various cancers.

Topoisomerase I Inhibitors

Irinotecan is a component of first-line therapy (in combination with 5-FU and leucovorin) for metastatic colorectal cancer (mCRC). It is associated with alopecia (~60%), hyperhidrosis (16%), rash (13%), and HFS (5%).

Topotecan is indicated for the treatment of metastatic ovarian, small cell lung, and cervical cancers in their advanced stages. The most common dermatologic AEs include alopecia (~49%) and rash (16%), with pruritus and severe dermatitis being rare. Mucositis is common with both irinotecan and topotecan (88% and 32%, respectively).

Topoisomerase II Inhibitors

Anthracyclines, including doxorubicin, liposomal doxorubicin, epirubicin, and idarubicin, are widely used in the treatment of hematologic malignancies (e.g., leukemias, Hodgkin's disease, MM, and other solid tumors, e.g., thyroid, breast, lung, stomach, ovarian, and bladder cancers, and soft tissue sarcomas). The most common dermatologic AEs include alopecia, morbilliform eruptions, perifollicular erythema and scaling, HFS, nail changes, and photo/radiation recall dermatitis.

Etoposide and **teniposide** are common components of chemotherapy for hematologic malignancies and many solid tumors. Alopecia, flushing, burning erythema on the face, upper back and chest, and mucositis are common. Rare dermatologic AEs include erythema multiforme-like eruptions SJS/TEN, hyperpigmentation, and radiation recall dermatitis.

Mitoxantrone is indicated for advanced hormone-refractory prostate cancer and acute non-lymphocytic leukemia in adults. The most common dermatologic AEs include alopecia, mucositis, and nail bed changes. Immediate hypersensitivity reactions, including urticaria and angioedema, have been reported.

Antimicrotubule Agents

Taxanes

Paclitaxel and **docetaxel** are derived from the bark of the pacific yew tree (*Taxus brevifolia*), and needles of the European yew tree (*Taxus baccata*), respectively. They disrupt normal microtubule functions by rigidifying guanosine diphosphate-bound tubulin units. They have been used for head and neck squamous cell carcinoma, advanced breast, NSCLC, gastric adenocarcinoma, and prostate and ovarian cancers.

HSRs are a major AE, characterized by respiratory distress, hypotension, angioedema, urticaria, and morbilliform erythemas. Symptoms may manifest during the first few minutes of infusion, and present in a dose-dependent pattern. Interestingly, the solvents used in taxane formulations (e.g., Cremophor EL® and Tween 80®) are thought to contribute to immediate hypersensitivity reactions. In contrast, a new formulation of paclitaxel, the nanoparticle albumin-bound (nab) paclitaxel, is solvent free and not associated with these reactions. Premedication consisting of dexamethasone, cimetidine, and diphenhydramine can reduce the incidence of immediate hypersensitivity reactions by 20%, but cannot abrogate them completely. Therefore, close monitoring during the first 5 minutes of infusion is recommended. A 12-step slow infusion method may be adopted to minimize the incidence of these reactions.

Alopecia is a common dermatologic AE of paclitaxel and docetaxel use. Scalp cooling to a level ≤25 °C, prior to and during infusion, has been shown to be effective in preventing hair loss. Nail changes, mostly presenting as subungual hemorrhages, hyperkeratosis, paronychia, onycholysis, hyperpigmentation (Fig. 18-3), and cessation of nail growth are common. The incidence of grade 3 nail changes is high, however, it is dependent on cumulative dose and number of treatment cycles. A distinct form of taxane-related HFS has been reported, which presents with periarticular thenar erythema and onycholysis (PATEO syndrome), including violaceous plaques or blisters, over the dorsum of hands, Achilles tendon, and

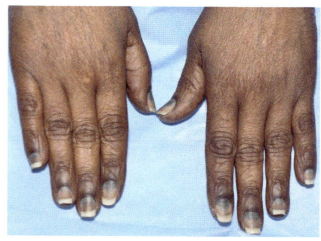

FIGURE 18-3 ■ Hyperpigmentation of the nails in a 61-year-old woman receiving paclitaxel for breast cancer.

malleoli. Frozen gloves have been shown to be effective in preventing taxane-induced HFS and onycholysis.

Maculopapular erythemas, bullous FDEs, erythema multiforme-like lesions, and AGEP have also been reported. Rarely, scleroderma-like lesions in the extremities, photosensitivity, subacute cutaneous lupus erythematosus in photodistributed areas, and radiation recall dermatitis may be encountered.

Vinca Alkaloids

The naturally occurring alkaloids **vinblastine** and **vincristine**, as well as their semisynthetic analogs **vinorelbine**, **vindesine**, and **vinflunine**, target tubulin and microtubules, eventually leading to mitotic arrest. They have been used in treating Hodgkin's and non-Hodgkin's lymphomas, ALL, MM, metastatic breast cancer, NSCLC, Kaposi's sarcoma, Wilms' tumor, neuroblastoma, rhabdomyosarcoma, Ewing's sarcoma of childhood, testicular cancer, and gestational trophoblastic carcinoma. Alopecia is a frequently reported dermatologic AE of vindesine and vinorelbine, especially when used as monotherapy. Erythematous macules over intravenous injection sites, and local injection reactions have been reported. Cutaneous eruptions, although rarely reported, present as widespread erythematous papular eruptions, rapidly resolving upon treatment discontinuation. These drugs may cause skin necrosis and ulcerations upon extravasation; local hyaluronidase infusion or a subcutaneous injection is usually effective.

Estramustine Phosphate Sodium

This drug inhibits microtubule motility and leads to cell cycle arrest. It is mainly indicated in the treatment of androgen-independent prostate cancers. The main major AEs include edema, thrombosis, and breast tenderness, although alopecia, fatigue, bruising, pruritus, and xerosis may be infrequently encountered.

Histone Deacetylase Inhibitors, Proteasome Inhibitors, Demethylating Agents

Histone Deacetylase Inhibitors

Vorinostat and **romidepsin** inhibit histone deacetylation, an important step in DNA replication, and eventually lead to cell cycle arrest and apoptosis. Vorinostat is indicated for treatment-resistant or recurrent CTCL. Alopecia and leukonychia are two common dermatologic AEs of vorinostat; they regress after discontinuation of treatment.

Romidepsin is approved for refractory CTCL, and is associated with rare dermatologic AEs such as oral candidiasis, mild drug eruptions, hypersensitivity, anticoagulant-induced skin necrosis, vasculitis, serum sickness, angioedema, SJS, and TEN.

Proteasome Inhibitors

Bortezomib inhibits the proteosomal degradation of NF-κB, activates cell signaling to induce apoptosis, and inhibits various pro-proliferative cytokines. It is indicated in the treatment of MM and mantle cell lymphoma. Erythematous papules, nodules, and plaques, with a varied distribution have been reported with bortezomib; ulcerations and morbilliform exanthems may also occur. Low dose prednisone, with or without antihistamines, has been utilized to treat the erythematous eruptions. Bortezomib is also associated with non-necrotizing small vessel cutaneous vasculitis and Sweet's syndrome. While the former may respond to topical corticosteroids, the latter may be so severe that it may necessitate intravenous methylprednisolone.

Demethylating Agents

5-Azacitidine (5-AzaC) and **decitabine** inhibit DNA methylation, thereby leading to cell proliferation abnormalities and triggering of apoptosis. They are indicated in the treatment of myelodysplastic syndrome and acute/chronic leukemia. 5-AzaC is associated with injection site reactions, presenting as erythematous plaques, and Sweet's syndrome (Trickett et al., 2012). Decitabine-associated dermatologic AEs are rare, with only one case of NEH having been reported in the literature.

Retinoids

Bexarotene and **all-trans retinoic acid (ATRA)** are retinoids used in the treatment of various cancers. For e.g., bexarotene is indicated in CTCL, in both the oral and topical formulations. ATRA is used to treat acute promyelocytic leukemia (APL) characterized by the presence of t(15;17) translocation. Retinoids are commonly associated with dermatitis (xerosis, pruritus, and cheilitis) and skin irritation. ATRA can induce neutrophilic eruptions such as Sweet's syndrome, or more specifically scrotal ulcers, which are often neutrophilic on biopsy. On the other hand, topical bexarotene has been associated with pain, vesiculobullous lesions, irritant reactions, and "sticky skin."

Arsenicals

Arsenic trioxide (ATO) is used in the treatment of nonresponsive or relapsed APL (refractory to ATRA), MM, myelodysplastic syndrome, and some solid tumors. It can induce a mild to moderate nonspecific dermatitis, and has been reported to increase the susceptibility to (localized) herpes zoster infection possibly via immunosuppression.

Targeted Anticancer Therapies

Molecularly targeted agents are relatively new additions to the (oncologic) therapeutic armamentarium. These

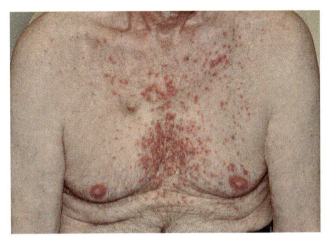

FIGURE 18-4 ■ Grade 2 epidermal growth factor receptor inhibitor-induced acneiform rash in a 68-year-old man, 1 week after initiation of treatment with panitumumab and irinotecan for colorectal cancer. The patient's face, scalp, and back (not shown) were also involved, and the rash was painful.

therapies are designed to inhibit specific oncoproteins/enzymes essential in various signaling cascades and cell proliferation. Although remarkably successful in treating cancers, their use has also been associated with a number of dermatologic AEs among others (Table 18-2; Balagula et al., 2010).

Epidermal Growth Factor Receptor (EGFR) Inhibitors

The approved EGFR inhibitors (EGFRIs) may be grouped into: (1) monoclonal antibodies (mAbs, e.g., **cetuximab**, **panitumumab**) that bind to the extracellular domain of EGFR and result in receptor internalization and subsequent degradation; and (2) small molecule inhibitors (e.g., **erlotinib**, **afatinib**) that target the intracellular tyrosine kinase domain by competing with the binding of adenosine triphosphate. Dual inhibitors against EGFR and ErbB2 (Her2/neu) have also been developed (e.g., **lapatinib**). These drugs primarily target tumor cells expressing EGFR; however, cells in the skin where EGFR signaling regulates keratinocyte proliferation, differentiation, migration, and survival are also targeted. Consequently, a number of dermatologic AEs may be encountered during treatment (Lacouture, 2006); the most common examples and their management are discussed below.

Acneiform eruption is the most clinically significant AE that manifests within the first 2 to 4 weeks of starting an EGFRI (e.g., cetuximab, panitumumab, erlotinib, and afatinib). The eruption may be preceded by dysesthesias, erythema, and edema, and is characterized by erythematous papules and/or pustules affecting the sebum-rich areas (scalp, face, upper trunk) (Fig. 18-4), with sparing of the palms and soles. Aseptic purulent material and debris may also accumulate over the lesions. In contrast to acne vulgaris, comedones and cysts are not seen, and the lesions may extend beyond the areas typically affected by acne. The rash may spontaneously improve during the course of treatment, but persistent erythema, hyperpigmentation, and telangiectasias may be noted (without permanent sequelae) in most patients. The associated symptoms, such as pain, pruritus, burning, and irritation, may all significantly impact patients' quality of life.

Lesional biopsy may reveal thinning of the stratum corneum with loss of the normal basket-weave-like configuration, superficial perifolliculitis (with an inflammatory infiltrate surrounding ectatic and hyperkeratotic follicular infundibula), or a neutrophilic suppurative folliculitis. The pilosebaceous glands may portray changes notable for decreased size, poorly differentiated sebocytes and keratinocytes, and an inflammatory cell infiltrate. However, these changes may also be seen in normal-appearing skin.

The pathogenesis is largely secondary to the direct inhibition of EGFR leading to dysregulated keratinocyte differentiation and proliferation, as well as a cell-mediated inflammatory response. Absence of a smoking history, younger age, male gender, and fair skin tone portend a greater risk for eruptions of higher severity. Prophylactic therapy is recommended and consists of oral doxycycline 100 mg twice daily or minocycline 100 mg once daily, along with topical hydrocortisone cream 1%, sunscreen, and a moisturizer. As an alternative, treatment may be initiated at the onset of eruption and is based on the severity. A combination of topical and/or oral corticosteroids and antibiotics is usually employed. Severe eruptions (grade 3 or higher) often result in dose modifications or even cessation of treatment.

Clinicians should remain vigilant of the possibility of secondary bacterial, viral, or fungal superinfections (observed in 38% of patients), and promptly initiate appropriate antimicrobial therapy. Telangiectases overlying the areas affected by the rash are late sequelae. Discontinuation of EGFRIs typically leads to resolution, but treatment with a pulsed-dye laser may improve cosmesis.

Xerosis usually manifests later than acneiform rash, typically after 4 to 6 weeks of treatment with an EGFRI, but affects up to 100% of patients when treated for more than 6 months. In severe cases, the skin may become erythematous, inflamed, and ichthyotic; painful fissuring of the skin that most commonly affects the distal tufts of fingers and toes, periungual skin, dorsal surface of the interphalangeal joints, and heels may be noted. The pruritus may be localized (accompany the acneiform eruption) or generalized.

Hyperpigmentation is a late development during the course of treatment with EGFRIs (after 1 to 2 months), and is mostly postinflammatory in nature, although cases of de novo hyperpigmentation have been reported. An African-American ethnicity and UV exposure are predisposing factors. While gradual improvement over weeks to months is the usual course, the use of hydroquinone, azelaic acid, or laser treatments may hasten resolution.

Hair changes affect many patients receiving EGFRI treatment. These include alopecia, dyspigmentation, hypertrichosis, trichomegaly (Fig. 18-5), and textural changes. The alopecia typically develops after several months of treatment with an EGFRI. Significant inflammation and pustular lesions on the scalp may result in patchy hair loss, predominantly affecting the crown. Paradoxical darkening, thickening, or curling of hair on the face and extremities may be noted. Trichomegaly and curling of eyelashes are common and may result in significant corneal inflammation (presenting as

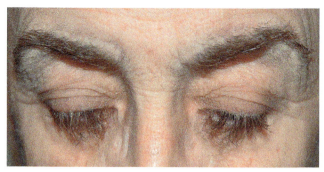

FIGURE 18-5 ■ Trichomegaly in a 69-year-old woman, 2.5 months after treatment with erlotinib for metastatic epidermal growth factor receptor inhibitor-mutant lung adenocarcinoma. Patient was advised trimming of eyelashes as necessary.

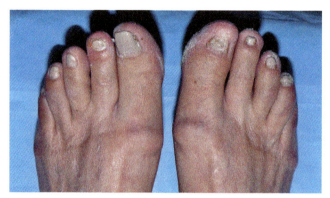

FIGURE 18-6 ■ Grade 2 paronychia in an 82-year-old woman being treated with afatinib for lung cancer.

xerophthalmia, meibomitis, and squamous blepharitis), especially when the eyelash growth is directed toward the eye (trichiasis). Manual epilation (waxing, threading, plucking), topical eflornithine, and laser epilation may be used in the management of hypertrichosis.

Paronychia usually develops after several months of therapy, and is a typically characterized by inflammation (erythema, swelling) of the lateral nail fold(s) (Fig. 18-6). Pyogenic granuloma-like lesions with friable granulation tissue are prone to bleeding (with minimal trauma) and secondary bacterial superinfections. Treatment with a combination of moisturizing creams, topical antibiotics or antiseptics, vinegar soaks, and silver nitrate may be indicated based on the severity. Electrodesiccation, cryosurgery, and nail plate avulsion are reserved for severe cases. Brittle nails may be managed with biotin and nail-plate strengtheners.

Inflammation of the oral (mucositis/stomatitis, aphthous ulcers), nasal (nasal vestibulitis), and genital mucosae can occur during treatment. A corticosteroid (dexamethasone)-containing mouthwash provides symptomatic improvement. For aphthous ulcerations, 0.1% triamcinolone acetonide in an emollient dental paste (Orabase) may be beneficial. Treatment of nasal vestibulitis is warranted, and promptly responds to intranasal mupirocin ointment.

Prophylactic treatment with a combination regimen consisting of a skin moisturizer, sunscreen, topical corticosteroid, and doxycycline in patients receiving an EGFRI such as panitumumab leads to a more than 50% decrease in dermatologic AEs as compared to controls (Lacouture et al., 2010). The preemptive regimens are recommended to patients at the time of initiation of treatment with an EGFRI.

Treatment with EGFRIs in conjunction with other cytotoxic chemotherapeutic agents and/or radiation therapy may result in an increased incidence and severity of dermatologic AEs, such as morbilliform erythema, radiation dermatitis, and mucositis. It is noteworthy that high potency topical corticosteroids have been shown to reduce the incidence and severity of radiation dermatitis in randomized trials.

Multikinase Inhibitors

Imatinib, **nilotinib**, and **dasatinib** are small molecules designed to target the Bcl-Abl fusion protein, c-kit, and platelet-derived growth factor receptor (PDGFR), expressed by gastrointestinal stromal tumors, besides CML and a few hypereosinophilic syndromes.

Imatinib generally causes facial edema (63% to 84%), maculopapular eruptions (up to 50%), and pigmentary disturbances, all of which are usually mild in severity. The clinical spectrum of AEs also includes erythroderma, SJS, AGEP, exacerbations of psoriasis or psoriasiform eruptions, lichenoid eruptions, and drug reaction with eosinophilia and systemic symptoms (DRESS) syndrome. Patients may experience reversible vitiligo-like depigmentation of the skin and hair, hyperpigmentation (Fig. 18-7), or even repigmentation of previously depigmented areas. Certain AEs such as urticaria, neutrophilic dermatoses, vascular purpura, pseudolymphoma, and photosensitivity appear to be dose dependent.

Nilotinib is reported to cause cutaneous eruptions (17% to 35%), pruritus (13% to 24%), alopecia (10%), and xerosis (13% to 17%), the majority of which are low-grade and dose dependent. Less frequent AEs include edema, pigmentary disturbances, and Sweet's syndrome. On the other hand, maculopapular eruptions (13% to 27%) and mucositis/stomatitis (16%) are common with dasatinib. Less frequent AEs include hyperhidrosis, xerosis, alopecia, photosensitivity, pigmentary disorders, and panniculitis.

Treatment is symptomatic with antihistamines, topical emollients, keratolytics, and/or topical corticosteroids being usually effective. For more severe eruptions, dose reduction accompanied by a short-acting systemic corticosteroid may be considered.

Angiogenesis Inhibitors

The vascular endothelial growth factor (VEGF)/VEGF receptor (VEGFR) pathway is an important regulator of angiogenesis. Both VEGF (**bevacizumab**, **aflibercept**) and VEGFR/PDGFR (**sorafenib**, **sunitinib**, **pazopanib**, **axitinib**, **regorafenib**, **cabozantinib**) inhibitors have been developed for the treatment of various advanced cancers including renal cell carcinoma, hepatocellular carcinoma, and colon cancer.

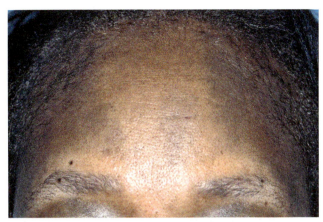

FIGURE 18-7 ■ Grade 1 skin (facial) hyperpigmentation in a 62-year-old woman, during treatment with imatinib for a gastrointestinal stromal tumor.

Hand-foot skin reaction (HFSR) is one of the major dermatologic AEs of targeted antiangiogenic drugs, which appears to be a "class-effect" (Wozel et al., 2010). Other targeted agents infrequently causing HFSR include the BRAF inhibitor, vemurafenib. HFSR is a distinct entity from HFS. The latter is associated with cytotoxic chemotherapies such as capecitabine, 5-FU, gemcitabine, cytarabine, and taxane-related agents. HFS is also synonymously referred to as palmar plantar erythrodysesthesia, acral erythema, and toxic erythema of chemotherapy. The onset is 14 to 21 days after initiation of cytotoxic chemotherapy, and in addition to affecting palms, soles, dorsal hands, and feet, it can also involve the intertrigenous regions.

On the other hand, the onset of HFSR is usually during the first 5 weeks of treatment with the development of a dysesthetic prodrome; eventually there is rapid formation of painful hyperkeratotic plaques, associated with erythema, desquamation, and even bullous lesions, often with a peripheral rim of erythema. Preventive measures include frequent podiatric care, moisturizers (ammonium lactate), keratolytic creams (topical 10% to 50% urea or 3% to 6% salicylic acid), topical anesthetics (e.g., lidocaine), and orthopedic soles or shoes, all of which have shown benefit. Patients should be counseled to use comfortable and flexible shoes with the aim of minimizing friction. Grade 1 HFS/HFSR should receive topical high potency corticosteroid twice daily and urea 10% three times a day without any dose modification of the anticancer treatment. Grade 2 reactions necessitate topical high potency corticosteroid cream twice daily (with or without topical moisturizer/keratolytics under occlusion), and pain control with nonsteroidal anti-inflammatory drugs/gamma-aminobutyric acid agonists/narcotics. Intolerable grade 2 or grade 3 reactions mandate interruption in anticancer treatment until the clinical severity reverts to grades 0/1; the treatment is same as in grade 2 reactions.

If blistering and erosions develop, secondary bacterial infection should be excluded, and antimicrobial treatment should be promptly initiated.

The hair changes include alopecia, dyspigmentation, and textural changes. Alopecia may develop gradually over several weeks or months, and is usually reversible, even with continued VEGF/PDGFR inhibitor treatment. The hair may become dryer and curlier.

Several other dermatologic AEs have also been reported and include reversible, painless, subungual splinter hemorrhages (presenting as painless longitudinal black bands on the nail), erythematous rashes, xerosis, mucositis/stomatitis, and genital eruptions with erythematous, desquamative psoriasiform or lichenoid lesions. In addition, sorafenib and regorafenib may cause eruptive nevi, early facial erythema, and squamous cell proliferations (e.g., keratoacanthomas and squamous cell carcinoma). Sunitinib may be associated with pigmentary disorders and facial edema.

Bevacizumab is a chimeric mouse-human mAb that binds to circulating VEGF, thus preventing its binding to the VEGFR. It is approved in the treatment of mCRC, nonsquamous NSCLC, metastatic breast cancer, and glioblastoma. Although it interferes with the VEGF/VEGFR pathway, the resultant dermatologic AE profile is dissimilar to that of small molecule VEGFR inhibitors (e.g., sorafenib, sunitinib). Bevacizumab mainly causes pruritus and nonspecific cutaneous eruptions, but notably it interferes with wound healing and can induce spontaneous ulcerations, particularly in damaged sites such as striae. Therefore, it is recommended that invasive surgeries and/or procedures be scheduled at least 5 weeks after discontinuing the drug. In a small case series, the occurrence of geographic tongue has been reported (Gavrilovic et al., 2012).

BRAF Inhibitors

Vemurafenib and **dabrafenib** are selective inhibitors targeting activating mutations of the *BRAF* oncogene. Vemurafenib has been approved for the treatment of unresectable or metastatic melanoma harboring the $^{V600E}BRAF$ mutation. **Sorafenib** also nonselectively targets BRAF. BRAF inhibition can result in xerosis, pruritus, keratosis pilaris-like eruptions, photosensitivity, HFSR or palmoplantar thickening, and hair changes (e.g., curling) (Fig. 18-8; Belum et al., 2013). Less commonly, milia, acantholytic dyskeratosis, panniculitis-like lesions, and toxic erythema-like reactions may occur.

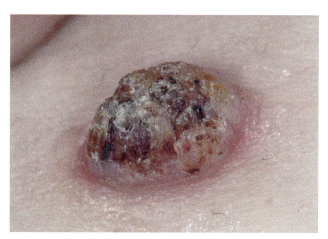

FIGURE 18-8 ■ A cutaneous squamous cell carcinoma (invasive, well differentiated with keratoacanthomatous features) on the leg of a 61-year-old woman, presenting after 3 weeks of treatment with vemurafenib for metastatic lung cancer.

Mammalian Target of Rapamycin Inhibitors

Everolimus and **temsirolimus** inhibit the serine/threonine protein kinase, mechanistic target of rapamycin (mTOR), thus blocking signaling in the PI3K/AKT/mTOR pathway, which is deregulated in renal cell carcinoma. The incidence of all-grade dermatologic eruptions has been estimated to be 27.3%, with the most common presentation being an eruption comprising erythematous papules and pustules (Balagula et al., 2012; Ramirez-Fort et al., 2014; Shameem et al., 2015). Management is symptomatic, with topical and systemic analgesics/corticosteroids forming the crux. Stomatitis is another well-recognized and common dermatologic AE that is amenable to treatment with topical corticosteroids. In addition, paronychia and/or pyogenic granulomas localized to the lateral nail folds of the fingers/toes may be noted. While topical antibiotics and antiseptics usually suffice, cryotherapy, silver nitrate chemical cauterization, or even partial nail avulsion may be needed for refractory cases.

Idelalisib, a PI3K inhibitor that blocks upstream signaling in the PI3K/mTOR pathway, has recently been approved for the treatment of relapsed CLL (in combination with rituximab), relapsed follicular B-cell non-Hodgkin's lymphoma, and relapsed small lymphocytic lymphoma. A maculopapular rash associated with pruritus was noted in 13% patients treated for relapsed indolent lymphoma (Gopal et al., 2014).

Other Monoclonal Antibodies

Trastuzumab

Trastuzumab is a humanized anti-HER2 receptor mAb, approved in the treatment of HER2-positive breast cancer. Alopecia and morbilliform erythemas appear to be the most frequently reported dermatologic AEs, although papulopustular acneiform eruptions, radiation recall dermatitis, and carotenoderma (yellow-orange skin discoloration due to carotenemia) have been described in sporadic case reports.

Trastuzumab emtansine (T-DM1) is an antibody-drug conjugate that is composed of trastuzumab conjugated to the cytotoxic agent, mertansine (DM1), via a stable linker. It delivers DM1 specifically to HER2-overexpressing cancer cells, where an antimicrotubule effect is generated. T-DM1 was initially studied in the treatment of breast cancer, and subsequently in many other types of cancers. It has been shown to cause infusion and hypersensitivity reactions, HFS, and cutaneous/mucosal telangiectasias (Krop et al., 2015). Along with underlying thrombocytopenia, it may predispose patients to mucosal hemorrhage (e.g., epistaxis and gastrointestinal) (Sibaud et al., 2014).

Rituximab

Rituximab and **ibritumomab tiuxetan** (radioisotope-linked antihuman CD20 mAb) both target the B-lymphocyte antigen CD20. They are used in the treatment of CD20-positive non-Hodgkin's lymphoma, follicular lymphoma, diffuse large B-cell lymphoma, and CLL. Rare cases of severe mucocutaneous reactions have been reported; these include paraneoplastic pemphigus, lichenoid or vesiculobullous dermatitis, serum-sickness-like reaction, SJS, and even TEN. In addition, the immunosuppressive effects of B-cell inhibition may predispose patients to transfusion-associated GVHD and skin infections.

Immune Checkpoint Inhibitors
Ipilimumab (anti-CTLA-4 mAb) and, at the time of this writing, **nivolumab** and **pembrolizumab** (both anti-PD1 inhibitors) were among the latest additions to the anticancer therapeutic armamentarium. These drugs inhibit immune "checkpoints", thereby stimulating the immune system in a nonspecific fashion to bypass the immunosuppressive environment maintained by tumor cells. While currently approved in the treatment of unresectable metastatic melanoma and NSCLC, their efficacy is being explored in clinical trials various solid tumors. The dermatologic AEs reported with ipilimumab include pruritus and a maculopapular erythema (22% to 46.5%) (Lacouture et al., 2014). The eruption usually presents 1 to 2 weeks after the initiation of treatment, and usually regresses within a few weeks to several months. Other ipilimumab-related dermatologic AEs include erythematous scaly papules/plaques (on the trunk and extensor surfaces), alopecia, vitiligo-like lesions, and TEN.

The dermatologic AEs reported to date with nivolumab and pembrolizumab include cutaneous eruptions, pigmentary changes, and pruritus. With nivolumab, vitiligo, acneiform lesions, and photosensitivity have been reported as well (Topalian et al., 2014). Pembrolizumab has been shown to cause vitiligo, eczema, erythema, and hair color changes (Hamid et al., 2013). The dermatologic AE profile of these agents, however, continues to emerge and awaits further characterization.

Other Anticancer Agents

Besides cytotoxic agents and targeted therapies, a variety of other drugs, such as endocrine-based therapies, L-asparaginase, bleomycin, and thalidomide, represent important members of the oncologic armamentarium. Their dermatologic AE profiles vary greatly and are discussed below.

Endocrine Agents

Endocrine and endocrine-based therapies are used for the treatment of advanced (metastatic) cancer, especially in the adjuvant and neoadjuvant settings. Hot flashes, hyperhidrosis, pruritus, allergic reactions, injection site reactions, and alopecia may be encountered, albeit relatively infrequently.

Selective Estrogen Receptor Modulators (SERMs)
Tamoxifen and other SERMs (**toremifene, raloxifene**) are used in the treatment of estrogen-receptor-positive (ER-positive) cancers. Mild flushing, as a result of estrogen deprivation, is common with tamoxifen (incidence, 38.6% to 40.9%), but less frequent with other SERMs. The incidence of all-grade and grade 2 alopecia with tamoxifen is estimated to be 9.3% and 6.4%, respectively.

Estrogen Receptor Downregulators
Estrogen receptor downregulators (e.g., **fulvestrant**) antagonize the ER and result in its degradation. They are used in the treatment of ER-positive metastatic breast cancer in postmenopausal women. Hot flashes can occur in up to 21% of treated patients, while all-grade alopecia (incidence of about 7.9%), injection site reactions, and vaginitis occur less frequently.

Aromatase Inhibitors
The highly selective aromatase inhibitors **exemestane, anastrozole**, and **letrozole** exert their action by preventing the synthesis of estrogen, and are thus indicated in the treatment of ER-positive breast cancers. They commonly cause hot flashes, morbilliform eruptions, alopecia, and pruritus. The alopecia encountered could be all-grade (anastrozole, 2.5%; letrozole, 2.5%; exemestane, 2.2%), or grade 2 (letrozole, 0.2%; exemestane, 1.3%) in severity. The incidence is higher (all-grade, 14.7%) in patients who receive anastrozole after treatment with tamoxifen. In addition, exemestane is associated with cutaneous eruptions (both acneiform and a nonspecific "allergic" type) and hypertrichosis. The morphology of dermatoses reported in clinical trials with anastrozole and letrozole, however, is not known. Nail changes and a few cases of erythema nodosum have been reported with letrozole.

Luteinizing Hormone-Releasing Hormone (LHRH) Agonists
Leuprolide acts as a LHRH agonist and ultimately results in androgen and estrogen deprivation, which is beneficial for the treatment of advanced prostate cancer and breast cancer (off-label use). Hot flashes, hyperhidrosis, injection site reactions, and alopecia (all-grade, 9.5%; grade 2, 1.0%) have been described, besides rare instances of "skin rash with blisters" and psoriasiform exanthems.

Androgens
Fluoxymesterone is a synthetic anabolic steroid used in the palliative treatment of female breast cancer. The AEs mimic the ones noted with other natural/synthetic androgens (testosterone), and include acne, furunculosis, male-pattern alopecia, and hirsutism.

Antiandrogens
Flutamide and **bicalutamide** are potent, nonsteroidal antiandrogens indicated in the treatment of metastatic prostate cancer. While both drugs have been associated with hot flashes, in the case of flutamide, the metabolite (2-hydroxyflutamide) appears responsible for the (UVA) photosensitizing properties; the spectrum appears to include photosensitivity, phototoxicity, lupus, and pseudoporphyria.

Megestrol Acetate
Megestrol acetate is a progestin used in the palliative treatment of breast and endometrial cancers. It is associated with hot flashes, dermatoses, alopecia (all-grade, 2.6%; grade 2, 0.5%), and hirsutism, but the incidence is low.

Somatostatin Analogs
In oncology, **octreotide acetate** is primarily used in the treatment of carcinoid tumors, vasoactive intestinal peptide (VIP) secreting VIPomas, GVHD, and treatment-related diarrhea. Reversible alopecia (all-grade, 6.7%),

probably as a result of direct action of the drug on hair follicles, is the most frequently reported dermatologic AE.

Miscellaneous

L-Asparaginase
L-Asparaginase hydrolyzes L-asparagine to L-aspartic acid and ammonia to inhibit protein synthesis. It is used in treating pediatric ALL and some mast cell tumors, and is available as an injection. While pain and edema at the injection site are common, a hypersensitivity reaction associated with *Escherichia coli*- or *polyethylene glycol*-asparaginase is the main dermatologic manifestation, which may manifest with pruritus and urticaria (often in the context of dyspnea and hypotension) at a rate of 3% to 45%. On rare occasions, TEN may develop. The hypersensitivity reactions may lead to discontinuation of therapy. The newly developed asparaginase produced from an alternate bacteria source, *Erwinia chrysanthemi*, has low cross-reactivity rate to the *E. coli*-asparaginase. Switching to *E. chrysanthemi*-asparaginase in patients who cannot tolerate *E. coli*-asparaginase has a hypersensitivity rate of 6% to 33%, with limited high grade reactions (3.6%) (Burke, 2014).

Bleomycin
Bleomycin is an antibiotic isolated from the bacterium *Streptomyces verticillus*, which is used in the treatment of various solid tumors and leukemias. It induces DNA strand breaks. However, the exact mechanism of action has not been fully delineated. Hyperpigmentation, Raynaud's phenomenon, gangrene, fibrosis, NEH, alopecia, edema, nail changes, and a characteristic "flagellate" erythema (erythemato-violaceous linear streaks on the trunk and/or shoulders) have been reported. Less frequently encountered AEs include angioedema, AGEP, and SJS.

Thalidomides
The antiangiogenic and immunomodulatory and anti-inflammatory effects of the thalidomide class of drugs (prototype, **thalidomide**; analogs, **lenalidomide, pomalidomide**) have prompted evaluation of the latter in the treatment of cancer. Currently, thalidomide is approved strictly for the treatment of MM, in combination with dexamethasone. These otherwise highly teratogenic drugs are associated with exfoliative rash, erythroderma, allergic vasculitis, thrombocytopenic purpura, TEN, and exacerbation of psoriasis. Lenalidomide is approved for myelodysplastic syndromes besides MM, and its use is commonly associated with a cutaneous eruption (morbilliform, urticarial, dermatitis, acneiform). Other AEs include facial edema, erythema, xerosis, pruritus, folliculitis, skin hyperpigmentation, hyperhidrosis, and alopecia. Various other dermatologic AEs can occur, albeit at very low rates. A newer analog, pomalidomide, appears to induce similar AEs that, however, are pending characterization.

CONCLUSIONS

Cancer treatment-related dermatologic AEs bear the potential to cause discomfort, impair patients' quality of life, increase the cost of medical care, and even result in dose modifications—all of which can negatively impact clinical outcomes. Therefore, it is imperative that clinicians be cognizant of these AEs for their timely recognition, and to initiate appropriate treatment and/or preventive strategies. Dermatologic AEs represent a problem long overlooked and underestimated, and one that requires a multidisciplinary approach involving oncologists, dermatologists, and nurses, besides effective pharmacovigilance systems.

SUGGESTED READINGS

Balagula Y, Lacouture ME, Cotliar JA. Dermatologic toxicities of targeted anticancer therapies. J Support Oncol 2010;8(4):149–61.

Balagula Y, Rosen A, Tan BH, Busam KJ, Pulitzer MP, Motzer RJ, et al. Clinical and histopathologic characteristics of rash in cancer patients treated with mammalian target of rapamycin inhibitors. Cancer 2012;118(20):5078–83.

Belum VR, Fischer A, Choi JN, Lacouture ME. Dermatological adverse events from BRAF inhibitors: a growing problem. Curr Oncol Rep 2013;15(3):249–59.

Burke MJ. How to manage asparaginase hypersensitivity in acute lymphoblastic leukemia. Future Oncol 2014;10(16):2615–27.

Chen AP, Setser A, Anadkat MJ, Cotliar J, Olsen EA, Garden BC, et al. Grading dermatologic adverse events of cancer treatments: the common terminology criteria for adverse events version 4.0. J Am Acad Dermatol 2012;67(5):1025–39.

Gavrilovic IT, Balagula Y, Rosen AC, Ramaswamy V, Dickler MN, Dunkel IJ, et al. Characteristics of oral mucosal events related to bevacizumab treatment. Oncologist 2012;17(2):274–8.

Gopal AK, Kahl BS, de Vos S, Wagner-Johnston ND, Schuster SJ, Jurczak WJ, et al. PI3Kδ inhibition by idelalisib in patients with relapsed indolent lymphoma. N Engl J Med 2014;370(11):1008–18.

Hamid O, Robert C, Daud A, Hodi FS, Hwu WJ, Kefford R, et al. Safety and tumor responses with lambrolizumab (anti-PD-1) in melanoma. N Engl J Med 2013;369(2):134–44.

Krop IE, Lin NU, Blackwell K, Guardino E, Huober J, Lu M, et al. Trastuzumab emtansine (T-DM1) versus lapatinib plus capecitabine in patients with HER2-positive metastatic breast cancer and central nervous system metastases: a retrospective, exploratory analysis in EMILIA. Ann Oncol 2015;26(1):113–9.

Lacouture ME, Mitchell EP, Piperdi B, Pillai MV, Shearer H, Iannotti N, et al. Skin toxicity evaluation protocol with panitumumab (STEPP), a phase II, open-label, randomized trial evaluating the impact of a pre-Emptive Skin treatment regimen on skin toxicities and quality of life in patients with metastatic colorectal cancer. J Clin Oncol 2010;28(8):1351–7.

Lacouture ME, Wolchok JD, Yosipovitch G, Kähler KC, Busam KJ, Hauschild A. Ipilimumab in patients with cancer and the management of dermatologic adverse events. J Am Acad Dermatol 2014;71(1):161–9.

Lacouture ME. Mechanisms of cutaneous toxicities to EGFR inhibitors. Nat Rev Cancer 2006;6(10):803–12.

Ramirez-Fort MK, Case EC, Rosen AC, Cerci FB, Wu S, Lacouture ME. Rash to the mTOR inhibitor everolimus: systematic review and meta-analysis. Am J Clin Oncol 2014;37(3):266–71.

Shameem R, Lacouture M, Wu S. Incidence and risk of rash to mTOR inhibitors in cancer patients - a meta-analysis of randomized controlled trials. Acta Oncol 2015;54(1):124–32.

Sibaud V, Vigarios E, Combemale P, Lamant L, Lacouture ME, Lacaze JL, et al. T-DM1-related telangiectasias: a potential role in secondary bleeding events. Ann Oncol 2015;26(2):436–37.

Topalian SL, Sznol M, McDermott DF, Kluger HM, Carvajal RD, Sharfman WH, et al. Survival, durable tumor remission, and long-term safety in patients with advanced melanoma receiving nivolumab. J Clin Oncol 2014;32(10):1020–30.

Trickett HB1, Cumpston A, Craig M. Azacitidine-associated Sweet's syndrome. Am J Health Syst Pharm 2012 May 15;69(10):869–71. doi: 10.2146/ajhp110523

Wozel G, Sticherling M, Schön MP. Cutaneous side effects of inhibition of VEGF signal transduction. J Dtsch Dermatol Ges 2010;8(4):243–9.

CHAPTER 19

METASTATIC DISEASE

Courtney R. Schadt • Jeffrey P. Callen

> **KEY POINTS**
> - Cutaneous metastases are not uncommon, and are usually a late finding with poor prognosis.
> - Cutaneous metastases can be the first sign of an internal malignancy or of extranodal disease in a known malignancy.
> - Breast cancer is the most common cause of cutaneous metastases in women, whereas melanoma and lung cancer are the most common causes in men.
> - Cutaneous metastases most often present with solitary or multiple skin-colored or erythematous to violaceous dermal nodules.
> - Cutaneous metastases can have a wide variety of clinical presentations, particularly in breast cancer.

Metastatic disease to the skin is not uncommon. Skin metastases may be the first sign of an internal malignancy and may offer the most accessible site for diagnosis. In addition, in patients with a known underlying cancer, skin metastasis may be the presenting symptom of extranodal disease, thus impacting therapeutic decisions.

EPIDEMIOLOGY

Studies regarding cutaneous metastases vary greatly in methodology (case reports, series, meta-analyses) and in the patient populations investigated (autopsies, cancer registries). Furthermore, some studies exclude particular cancers, such as melanoma or hematopoietic malignancies, while others exclude tumors with local extension or direct invasion, including only local or distant metastases. The incidence of cutaneous metastases in the literature ranges from 0.2% to 10%. In a retrospective study of 7316 patients with carcinoma (excluding melanoma, leukemia, lymphoma, and sarcoma), 5% of patients developed cutaneous metastases. In the follow-up study of 4020 patients that included melanoma, 10% of patients had cutaneous metastases. The average age of patients with locally invasive and/or cutaneous metastases in one study was 62 years.

Skin metastases were the presenting sign of an internal malignancy in 0.8% of patients, and were the presenting sign of extranodal metastatic disease in patients with a known underlying malignancy in 7.6% of patients (6.4% if melanoma was excluded).

The most frequent neoplasm associated with cutaneous metastases varies by study and inclusion of particular cancers. In most studies, breast cancer has the highest incidence of skin metastases. However, some studies include direct extension, while others include only local or distant metastases. In one series, metastasis occurred in 6.3% of patients with breast cancer and was the presenting sign in 3.5% of patients. In another study, skin involvement occurred in 23.9% of patients with breast cancer and was the presenting sign in 8% of patients. In patients who developed cutaneous infiltration or metastases after the diagnosis of breast cancer, it was a late finding, occurring an average of 101 months after diagnosis. In another study of 1287 patients with internal malignancy, hematologic cancers were the most frequent source of cutaneous metastases, while in another that included melanoma (but excluded hematologic malignancies), melanoma was the most frequent. Cancers of the upper respiratory tract metastasized to the skin at a high incidence as well. Lung, colon, and rectal cancers uncommonly metastasize to the skin, but given the high prevalence of these cancers, they are a common cause of metastases. Cutaneous metastases are often the presenting sign in lung cancer, and it is proposed that this type of malignancy spreads more quickly to the skin than many other cancers. Based on gender, breast, colon, and ovarian cancer are the most common causes of cutaneous metastases in women, whereas lung and colon cancer are the most common causes in men. However, if melanoma is included, it has been reported to be the most frequent source of cutaneous metastases in men, and second in women (preceded by breast cancer). The primary malignancies for cutaneous metastases based on percentage and gender are shown in Table 19-1. Prostate cancer has a very low incidence of cutaneous metastases even with its high prevalence. Neuroblastoma and leukemia are the most frequent cause of cutaneous metastases in children. In neonates, leukemia, multisystem Langerhans cell histiocytosis, and neuroblastoma, in order of rank, were the most frequent cause of cutaneous metastases.

PATHOGENESIS

Cutaneous metastases may result from hematogenous and lymphatic spread, direct tissue invasion, or iatrogenic implantation. Metastatic cells may be produced from a minor specialized subpopulation of cells, be clonal, and be genetically less stable than the nonmetastatic tumor cells. These cells must develop a blood supply through angiogenesis and cross a basement membrane to reach

TABLE 19-1 Cutaneous Involvement by Carcinoma (Including Melanoma)* (Lookingbill et al., 1993)

Distribution in Men (n = 127)		Distribution in Women (n = 300)	
Primary Site	Rounded (%)	Primary Site	Rounded (%)
Melanoma	32	Breast	71
Lung (13/19 adenocarcinoma, 2/19 oat cell carcinoma)	12	Melanoma	12
Colon/rectum	11	Ovary, unknown primary, oral cavity, lung†	5-2
Oral cavity	9	Colon/rectum, endometrium, bladder, uterine cervix, stomach, bile duct, pancreas, endocrine†	<2
Unknown primary	9	—	—
Larynx	6	—	—
Kidney, upper digestive tract, breast, nasal sinuses, bladder, esophagus†	5-2	—	—
Endocrine, stomach, pancreas, liver†	<2	—	—

*Carcinoma accounts for the overwhelming majority of cutaneous metastastes (see text).
†Listed in descending order of frequency.

the extracellular space. Through cell motility, they invade lymphatics or vasculature while evading apoptosis, attach to and invade target tissues through matrix degradation, and proliferate. Chemokine expression by tumor cells has been implicated in organ-specific metastases. Melanomas can express the chemokine CCL27, which is site-specific for skin and could explain the high incidence of cutaneous metastases in this cancer. Other factors may be related to locations for metastases as well. In one study, the face and scalp were involved preferentially in distant metastases, possibly secondary to the high vascularization of these sites.

CLINICAL MANIFESTATIONS

Site

Internal malignancies can directly invade surrounding tissues or metastasize locally or to distant sites. Direct invasion is most commonly seen with breast, followed by oral cavity cancer. Most skin metastases are local, within the anatomic vicinity of the primary malignancy, and not infrequently involve scars of surgical excisions. The chest is the most common site, followed by the abdomen. The high incidence of breast and lung cutaneous metastases account for the chest involvement, and bowel, ovary, and bladder cancers often involve the abdomen. The marked predominance of cutaneous metastases from breast cancer may also be related to the proximity of breast tumors to the skin. Although distant metastases are less common, they are seen with melanoma, lung and breast cancers, and may occur with most types of malignancy. The scalp is a frequent site, occurring in 6.9% of patients with distant metastases, regardless of histologic subtype. Renal cell carcinoma in particular is disproportionately associated with scalp metastases. Sister Mary Joseph's nodule is a well-described metastasis to the umbilicus, most commonly of gastric origin, but is a rare phenomenon. The extremities are unusual locations for cutaneous metastases, but are most frequently seen with melanoma.

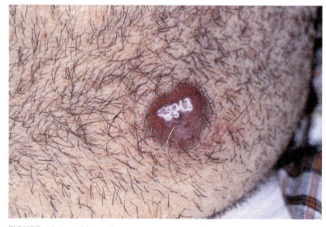

FIGURE 19-1 ■ Vascular appearance of metastatic renal cell carcinoma to the face.

Appearance

Cutaneous metastases most commonly have a nonspecific appearance, and are frequently described as asymptomatic, skin colored to erythematous or violaceous, dermal nodules. These are usually multiple but can also be solitary. In one study, solitary nodules were most commonly seen with metastatic lung cancer, followed by unknown primary malignancy. Metastatic renal cell carcinoma in particular has been described as presenting with violaceous or "vascular" nodules (see Fig. 19-1). Metastatic melanoma is often described as pigmented nodules, but is presented in this way only in 36% of cases in one study. Metastatic cutaneous breast cancer can have a wide variety of clinical appearances (see Figs. 19-2 and 19-3). Ulcerated nodules were described in 10% of patients with metastatic breast cancer and in a small number of those with metastatic melanoma. In 10% of breast cancer

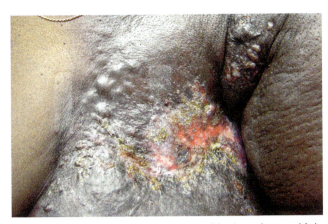

FIGURE 19-2 ■ Metastatic breast cancer with ulceration, multiple nodules, and peau d'orange appearance.

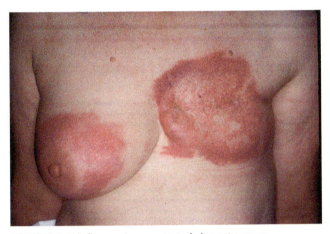

FIGURE 19-3 ■ Inflammatory metastatic breast cancer.

cutaneous metastases, inflammatory plaques resembling cellulitis occurred, often referred to as carcinoma erysipeloides. This clinical presentation is somewhat unique to breast cancer and has only rarely been reported with other primary malignancies. Metastatic breast cancer has also been described as having the following appearances: bullous, zosteriform, peau d'orange-like, erythematous patch with prominent telangiectases, lymphangioma circumscriptum-like pseudovesicular lesions, chalazion-like lesions or resembling firm swelling of the eyelid, and cicatricial plaques. Alopecia neoplastica is a cicatricial metastasis to the scalp seen most often with breast cancer. Carcinoma en cuirasse has also been reported with breast cancer and describes fibrotic metastases that resemble encasement in armor.

Other clinical appearances of cutaneous metastases include ulcers, described in three patients in one series with oral cavity carcinoma with direct extension to the skin, inflammatory abscesses misdiagnosed as hidradenitis suppurativa, cutaneous horns or keratoacanthomas, pyogenic granuloma-like lesions, pedunculated nodules, facial lymphedema, infiltration of surgical scars, morpheaform lesions, and cyst-like nodules. In neonates, cutaneous metastases usually present as multiple bluish nodules, resembling a "blueberry muffin baby."

DIFFERENTIAL DIAGNOSIS

Given the nonspecific clinical presentation of cutaneous metastases, the differential diagnosis is broad. Any patient with a history of internal malignancy presenting with a new nodule or cluster of nodules, nonhealing ulcer, or eruption should have a biopsy performed. For skin-colored or erythematous papules or nodules, benign growths, such as fibromas, lipomas, or cysts, may be considered, whereas vascular lesions should be considered for lesions more erythematous to violaceous in color. When inflammatory or indurated plaques are present, they may resemble cellulitis, other infections, or panniculitides. In a neonate with bluish nodules, infections, including the TORCH (toxoplasmosis, other agents, rubella, cytomegalovirus, herpes simplex) infectious agents, hemolytic disease of the newborn, and twin–twin transfusion syndrome must also be considered, along with the numerous neoplastic causes.

HISTOPATHOLOGIC FINDINGS

Cutaneous metastases typically resemble the primary malignancy but are often less differentiated, and definitive identification may be difficult. The histology of these tumors can broadly be classified into adenocarcinomas, squamous cell carcinomas, undifferentiated carcinomas, and a miscellaneous category that includes malignancies of the liver, endometrium, kidney, and bladder, along with small cell carcinomas. In general, the histology of most tumors demonstrates a "bottom heavy" appearance, with tumor growth confined to the deep dermis and sparing the epidermis. In some cases, however, there is ulceration, pagetoid spread, or abutment of the epidermis.

Immunohistochemistry has become increasingly valuable in determining the primary site of cutaneous metastases. For example, cytokeratin 7 and 20 immunostaining can be helpful in distinguishing colorectal and pulmonary adenocarcinomas. Most colonic cancers are CK7–/CK20+, while most adenocarcinomas of pulmonary origin are CK7+/CK20–, as are breast cancers. Most prostate cancers are CK7–/CK20–. Gross cystic disease fluid protein-15 is often positive in apocrine-derived tumors, such as ductal and lobular breast carcinoma. Antithyroid transcription factor antibody can be positive in lung adenocarcinoma and small-cell lung cancer, in addition to papillary thyroid cancer. Positivity of p63 and CK5/6 can distinguish primary cutaneous adnexal neoplasms from metastatic carcinomas. Her-2 protein expression may help differentiate metastatic breast cancer from primary cutaneous appendageal neoplasms, and androgen receptor positivity can distinguish metastatic breast cancer from primary eccrine tumors. In renal cell carcinoma, CD10 positivity is helpful in distinguishing tumor metastases from primary cutaneous adnexal tumors with eccrine and apocrine differentiation, but not from those with sebaceous differentiation.

Some morphologic clues can also be helpful in determining the primary site. Nodular metastatic breast cancer shows characteristic aggregates of neoplastic cells arranged in glandular structures surrounded by fibrosis or distributed linearly between collagen bundles in an "Indian file" pattern. In inflammatory metastases, the superficial lymphatics are dilated and plugged with metastatic cells, and there is some surrounding inflammatory infiltrate. Signet ring cells are frequently seen with adenocarcinomas of the stomach or gastrointestinal tract, but have also been described in bladder carcinoma and melanoma. Lobules of clear-staining cells with glycogen and highly vascular stroma can be seen with renal cell carcinoma, but clear cells can also originate from other sites, including the liver, lung, and ovary. Metastatic ovarian, thyroid, stomach, and certain lung cancers can also have a papillary pattern.

EVALUATION AND PROGNOSIS

In patients with an unknown primary tumor, a work-up including a complete history and physical examination, review of systems, hematologic and biochemical profiles, chest radiography, computed tomography of the chest, abdomen and pelvis, and mammography in women may yield helpful information. Cutaneous metastases are typically a late finding and portend a poor prognosis. Skin metastases from colorectal carcinomas have a better prognosis compared to other carcinomas. Prognosis varies based on cancer type, but in one study, the average survival time of patients with skin metastasis was 7.5 months.

THERAPY

When cutaneous metastases herald the onset of extranodal disease in a patient with a known internal malignancy, more aggressive intervention for treatable forms of cancer can be utilized. Solitary nodules can be excised or radiated depending on the underlying cancer. Chemotherapy for internal disease may also treat cutaneous metastases and may be more likely to induce a treatment response in certain cancer types.

SUGGESTED READINGS

Alcaraz I, Cerroni L, Rutten A, et al. Cutaneous metastases form internal, malignancies: a clinicopathologic and immunohistochemical review. Am J Dermatopathol 2012;34:347–93.

Isaacs H. Cutaneous metastases in neonates: a review. Pediatr Dermatol 2011;28:85–93.

Krathen RA, Orenga IF, Rosen T. Cutaneous metastasis: a meta-analysis of data. South Med J 2003;96:164–7.

Lookingbill DP, Spangler N, Sexton FM. Skin involvement as the presenting sign of internal carcinoma. J A Acad Dermatol 1990;22:19–26.

Lookingbill DP, Spangler N, Helm KF. Cutaneous metastases in patients with metastatic carcinoma: a retrospective study of 4020 patients. J Am Acad Dermatol 1993;29:228–36.

Marcoval J, Moreno A, Peyri J. Cutaneous infiltration by cancer. J Am Acad Dermatol 2007;57:577–80.

Saeed S, Keehn CA, Morgan MB. Cutaneous metastasis: a clinical, pathological, and, immunohistochemical appraisal. J Cutan Pathol 2004;31:419–30.

Ulker GUL, Kilic A, Muzeyyen G, et al. Spectrum of cutaneous metastases in 128 cases of internal malignancies: a study from Turkey. Acta Derm Venereol 2007;87:160–2.

CHAPTER 20

Cutaneous Lymphomas and Cutaneous Signs of Systemic Lymphomas

Lorenzo Cerroni

KEY POINTS

- Cutaneous lymphomas represent a heterogeneous group of malignant lymphomas arising primarily in the skin.
- Most cutaneous lymphomas are listed as separate entities in the World Health Organization classification of hematologic malignancies.
- Differentiation of primary cutaneous lymphomas from extracutaneous lymphomas with secondary skin manifestations is paramount, as management of patients is different.
- In some cases, only accurate staging investigations allow differentiation of primary cutaneous lymphomas from their nodal counterparts, as clinical, histological, and phenotypic features may be similar.
- In extranodal lymphomas, besides specific skin manifestations the skin may be the site of several nonspecific symptoms and/or disorders (e.g., generalized pruritus, Sweet's syndrome, pyoderma gangrenosum, etc.).

Malignant lymphomas may affect the skin both primarily (i.e., without extracutaneous disease at presentation) and secondarily (i.e., as specific manifestations of a primary extracutaneous—usually nodal—lymphoma). Differentiation of primary from secondary cutaneous lymphomas is paramount, as staging investigations, treatment modalities, and prognosis are different. In fact, the World Health Organization (WHO) classification of hematologic neoplasia recognizes several types of primary cutaneous lymphomas, the most frequent being mycosis fungoides (MF) (Table 20-1). In addition to specific skin manifestations of hematologic malignancies, many non-neoplastic cutaneous conditions may be variably associated with systemic lymphomas, the most important of them being briefly discussed at the end of this chapter and summarized in Table 20-2.

PRIMARY CUTANEOUS LYMPHOMAS

Primary cutaneous lymphomas represent a heterogeneous group of lymphoproliferative disorders affecting the skin.

By definition a primary cutaneous lymphoma does not show extracutaneous involvement at presentation (Sézary syndrome [SS] represents an exception, as involvement of the blood is a prerequisite for the diagnosis). Table 20-1 summarizes the entities included in the WHO classification. Precise diagnosis and distinction from similar entities involving the skin secondarily is crucial in order to manage patients properly.

Primary Cutaneous T-Cell Lymphomas

Mycosis Fungoides

MF represents by far the most common type of primary cutaneous T-cell lymphoma (CTCL) and of cutaneous lymphoma in general, accounting for almost half of all cases. It is defined as a tumor composed of small/medium-sized, epidermotropic T-helper lymphocytes.

TABLE 20-1 Cutaneous Lymphomas Included in the World Health Organization (WHO) Classification

Mycosis Fungoides

Sézary syndrome
Adult T-cell leukemia/lymphoma*
Primary cutaneous CD30+ lymphoproliferative disorders
 Lymphomatoid papulosis
 Primary cutaneous anaplastic large cell lymphoma
Subcutaneous panniculitis-like T-cell lymphoma
Extranodal NK/T-cell lymphoma, nasal type*
Primary cutaneous CD8+ aggressive epidermotropic cytotoxic T-cell lymphoma
Primary cutaneous gamma/delta T-cell lymphoma
Primary cutaneous CD4+ small/medium T-cell lymphoma
Extranodal marginal zone lymphoma of mucosa-associated lymphoid tissue (MALT lymphoma)†
Primary cutaneous follicle center lymphoma
Primary cutaneous diffuse large B-cell lymphoma, leg type
Intravascular large B-cell lymphoma*
Blastic plasmacytoid dendritic cell neoplasm*

*These entities are not always primary cutaneous, but may arise in the skin in the absence of systemic manifestations (i.e., negative staging at presentation).
†This category includes cases commonly classified as cutaneous marginal zone lymphoma, which in the WHO classification has been lumped together with other extranodal variants of the disease.

TABLE 20-2 Mucocutaneous Signs and Symptoms Frequently Associated with Systemic Lymphomas and Leukemias*

Associated with Tumor-Induced or Treatment-Related Bone Marrow Suppression and Resulting Cytopenia
Pallor
Purpura, especially petechial
Gingival hemorrhage; epistaxis; prolonged bleeding after minor injuries
Oral ulcerations in neutropenic patients

Associated with either Tumor-Specific or Treatment-Related Immune Dysregulation
Opportunistic infections; unusual presentations of common infections (e.g., vegetating lesions, prolongued duration of self-limited disease, severe manifestations of otherwise banal infections)

Associated with Autoantibodies Produced by the Hematologic Neoplasm
Paraneoplastic pemphigus[†]

Associated with Deposition of Amyloid Protein
Cutaneous amyloidosis
Crystal storing histiocytosis

Associated with Paraproteinemia but without Deposition of M-protein
Scleromyxedema
Scleredema
Normolipemic plane xanthoma
Necrobiotic xanthogranuloma
POEMS syndrome
AESOP syndrome
Schnitzler's syndrome

Other Conditions (Exact Mechanism and Pathogenesis of Skin Lesions Not Known)
Generalized idiopathic pruritus[‡]
Sweet's syndrome (acute febrile neutrophilic dermatosis)[§]
Bullous pyoderma gangrenosum
Acquired ichthyosis
Cutaneous and/or systemic sarcoidosis[ǁ]

*Many of these conditions may be observed in different settings other than hematologic neoplasms; some are mostly, but not invariably, associated with an underlying lymphoproliferative disorder.
[†]Associated mostly with B-cell lymphomas and leukemias.
[‡]May be observed in Hodgkin's lymphoma (HL), as well as less frequently in other types of non-Hodgkin's lymphoma (NHL); it may represent the first clinical manifestation of the disease.
[§]As paraneoplastic disorder observed mostly in patients with myelogeneous leukemia and related conditions; skin lesions may harbor neoplastic cells of the underlying condition.
[ǁ]Sarcoidosis may antedate the diagnosis of NHL ("sarcoidosis-lymphoma syndrome") or arise during the course of the disease.

The disease is characterized by a chronic course with prolonged survival. The incidence is around 6–7 cases/10^6, with regional variations and with a regular increase in recent decades. Although adults, especially elderly, are usually affected, MF represents the most common cutaneous lymphoma in children and adolescents as well.

Clinically, lesions of MF can be divided morphologically into patches, plaques, and tumors. Morphology is commonly used to classify the disease in three clinical stages according to the presence of corresponding lesions (patch, plaque, and tumor stage), with a good correlation with prognosis (this is a good "rule of thumb" to discuss with patients and guides discussion of available treatment options, but of course a more precise staging system should be applied—see below). So-called plaque and tumor stages probably should be considered together as a more aggressive phase of the disease, compared to the chronic course of patch-stage disease. Pruritus is often a prominent symptom in all stages of the disease, and may be very difficult to treat. The diagnosis of MF is based mainly on clinicopathologic correlation. Immunohistochemical and molecular analyses offer adjunctive information that should be integrated with the clinicopathologic assessment.

The precise characterization of the early phases of MF is still a matter of debate, and terms such as "parapsoriasis en plaques" or large plaque parapsoriasis are used differently to denote either a non-neoplastic condition that may progress to MF, or an early manifestation of the disease. In this stage the disease presents with variably large erythematous patches commonly located in sun-protected areas. Loss of elastic fibers and atrophy of the epidermis may confer on the lesions a wrinkled appearance. Notwithstanding the discussion on the nosology of "parapsoriasis en plaques," patients with early MF should not undergo extensive staging investigations (only clinical examination with assessment of percentage of body involvement and of superficial lymph nodes), and should be managed in a nonaggressive way.

Plaques of MF are characterized by infiltrated, variably scaling, reddish-brown, indurated lesions. Typical patches are usually observed contiguous to plaques or at other sites of the body. Tumors in MF may be observed in the absence of other lesions, or in combination with patches and plaques. They may be solitary or, more often, localized or generalized. Tumors, as the sole manifestation of MF, except as relapsed disease are highly unusual,

TABLE 20-3 Staging of Mycosis Fungoides (MF) and Sézary Syndrome (SS) according to the International Society of Cutaneous Lymphoma (ISCL) and the European Organization for Research and Treatment of Cancer (EORTC) Cutaneous Lymphoma Task Force

Skin
T1 Limited patches*, papules, and/or plaques[†] covering <10% of the skin surface. May further stratify into T1a (patch only) versus T1b (plaque ± patch)
T2 Patches, papules, or plaques covering >10% of the skin surface. May further stratify into T2a (patch only) versus T2b (plaque ± patch)
T3 One or more tumors[‡] (≥1 cm diameter)
T4 Confluence of erythema covering ≥80% body surface area

Lymph Nodes
N0 No clinically abnormal peripheral lymph nodes[§]; biopsy not required
N1 Clinically abnormal peripheral lymph nodes; histopathology Dutch grade 1 or NCI LN0-2
   N1a Clone negative[#]
   N1b Clone positive[#]
N2 Clinically abnormal peripheral lymph nodes; histopathology Dutch grade 2 or NCI LN3
   N2a Clone negative[#]
   N2b Clone positive[#]
N3 Clinically abnormal peripheral lymph nodes; histopathology Dutch grades 3–4 or NCI LN4; clone positive or negative
Nx Clinically abnormal peripheral lymph nodes; no histologic confirmation

Visceral
M0 No visceral organ involvement
M1 Visceral involvement (must have pathology confirmation[∥] and organ involved should be specified)

Blood
B0 Absence of significant blood involvement: ≤5% of peripheral blood lymphocytes are atypical (Sézary) cells[¶]
   B0a Clone negative[#]
   B0b Clone positive[#]
B1 Low blood tumor burden: >5% of peripheral blood lymphocytes are atypical (Sézary) cells but does not meet the criteria of B2
   B1a Clone negative[#]
   B1b Clone positive[#]
B2 High blood tumor burden: ≥1000/μL Sézary cells[¶] with positive clone[#]

Stage
IA T1N0M0B0,1 IB T2N0M0B0,1
II T1,2N1,2M0B0,1 IIB T3N0–2M0B0,1
III T4N0–2M0B0,1 IIIA T4N0–2M0B0 IIIB T4N0–2M0B1
IVA1 T1–4N0–2M0B2 IVA2 T1–4N3M0B0–2 IVB T1–4N0–3M1B0–2

*For skin, patch indicates any size skin lesion without significant elevation or induration. Presence/absence of hypo- or hyperpigmentation, scale, crusting, and/or poikiloderma should be noted.
[†]For skin, plaque indicates any size skin lesion that is elevated or indurated. Presence or absence of scale, crusting, and/or poikiloderma should be noted. Histologic features such as folliculotropism or large cell transformation (>25% large cells), CD30+ or CD30–, and clinical features such as ulceration are important to document.
[‡]For skin, tumor indicates at least one 1-cm diameter solid or nodular lesion with evidence of depth and/or vertical growth. Note total number of lesions, total volume of lesions, largest size lesion, and region of body involved. Also note if histologic evidence of large cell transformation has occurred. Phenotyping for CD30 is encouraged.
[§]For node, abnormal peripheral lymph node(s) indicates any palpable peripheral node that on physical examination is firm, irregular, clustered, fixed, or 1.5cm or larger in diameter. Node groups examined on physical examination include cervical, supraclavicular, epitrochlear, axillary, and inguinal. Central nodes, which are not generally amenable to pathologic assessment, are not currently considered in the nodal classification unless used to establish N3 histopathologically.
[∥]For viscera, spleen and liver may be diagnosed by imaging criteria.
[¶]For blood, Sézary cells are defined as lymphocytes with hyperconvoluted cerebriform nuclei. If Sézary cells cannot be used to determine tumor burden for B2, then one of the following modified International Society of Cutaneous Lymphoma criteria along with a positive clonal rearrangement of the T-cell receptor may be used instead: (1) expanded CD4+ or CD3+ cells with CD4:CD8 ratio of 10 or more, (2) expanded CD4+ cells with abnormal immunophenotype including loss of CD7 or CD26.
[#]A T-cell clone is defined by polymerase chain reaction or Southern blot analysis of the T-cell receptor gene.
Adapted from Olsen et al. Blood 2007;110:1713–1722.

and a tumor d'emblee diagnosis would require exclusion of cutaneous anaplastic large cell lymphoma, or a nodule of lymphomatoid papulosis, or pleiomorphic small/medium CD4+ lymphoma, NK/T cell lymphoma, etc. Ulceration is common. Erythroderma can develop in the course of the disease, rendering distinction from SS difficult. Patients with infiltrated plaques, tumors, or erythroderma should be screened for extracutaneous involvement (laboratory investigations, sonography of lymph nodes, computed tomography and/or positron emission tomography scan of chest, abdomen and pelvis, bone marrow biopsy, examination of the peripheral blood).

Staging for MF is performed according to a system proposed by a joint working group of the International Society of Cutaneous Lymphoma (ISCL) and the European Organization for Research and Treatment of Cancer (EORTC) Cutaneous Lymphoma Task Force (Table 20-3).

Many clinical and/or histopathologic variants of MF have been described. Three of them are mentioned in the WHO classification, namely, pilotropic MF, localized pagetoid reticulosis, and granulomatous slack skin. While localized pagetoid reticulosis and granulomatous slack skin show a chronic course and good prognosis (patients with localized pagetoid reticulosis may undergo long-standing complete remission), pilotropic MF seems to be characterized by a more aggressive course than the "conventional" variants of the disease. A thorough discussion of these variants is beyond the scope of this chapter. Granulomatous slack skin may be viewed as a subset of MF, but there is ample evidence that it may be more appropriately viewed as a syndrome that may result from a variety of hematologic diseases—up to 50% are associated with Hodgkin's, and other reports include non-Hodgkin's, MF, acute myelogenous leukemia, and Langerhans histiocytosis. Granulomatous slack skin shares many features with MF but it is not clear that it should always be considered to represent MF.

Prognosis and selection of proper treatment for MF depends on the stage of the disease (as well as on previous treatments). Most patients will never require aggressive therapy and can be managed with skin-directed options (e.g., psoralen and ultraviolet A, retinoids, etc.). Systemic chemotherapy is usually effective only for short periods, and recurrences are the rule. Large numbers of systemic, partly experimental therapies have been tested in the last decades (indirectly showing that no treatment option is giving a true chance for cure). In recent years several independent studies showed that patients with advanced stage disease may be treated successfully with allogeneic stem cell transplantation.

Sézary Syndrome

SS is characterized clinically by pruritic erythroderma, generalized lymphadenopathy, and the presence of circulating malignant T lymphocytes. It is considered as a disease distinct from MF, and prognosis is much worse (5-year survival of about 20% to 30%). Diagnostic criteria include the presence of the same monoclonal population of T lymphocytes within the peripheral blood and the skin, of at least 1000 circulating Sézary cells/mm^3, of an expanded CD4+ population in the peripheral blood resulting in a markedly increased CD4:CD8 ratio, of an increased population of CD4+/CD7– cells or CD4+/CD26– in the peripheral blood, and of the loss of T-cell antigens such as CD2, CD3, and CD5. Although SS is considered a leukemic variant of CTCL, the bone marrow is usually not affected in early phases.

Patients present with a variably rapid onset of erythroderma and lymph node enlargement. The erythroderma is characterized by intense pruritus and scaling, and the pruritus may be intractable. Complete staging investigations should be performed upon a confirmed diagnosis of SS (Table 20-3). Since many non-neoplastic disorders may present with erythroderma (e.g., psoriasis, drug eruptions, etc.), accurate diagnostic investigations are crucial in order to manage patients properly. It is also crucial to remember that in a distinct proportion of patients (up to 50%) a precise diagnosis is not possible ("idiopathic" erythroderma, "red man syndrome"). Some of these patients eventually progress to clear-cut SS. At the present state of knowledge,

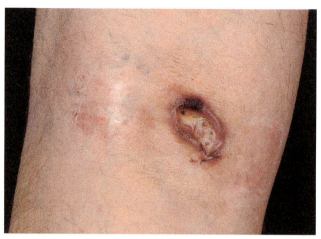

FIGURE 20-1 ■ Cutaneous anaplastic large-cell lymphoma presenting with a solitary ulcerated tumor on the leg.

however, patients with "idiopathic" erythroderma should not be treated aggressively (symptomatic treatment of associated symptoms such as pruritus, regular controls to monitor the disease). Extracorporeal photopheresis has been successfully used to treat both overt SS and idiopathic erythroderma, but the efficacy tends to be limited in time, and patients with advanced disease usually show progression in spite of treatment. As in advanced MF, allogeneic stem cell transplantation may represent a successful option for patients with SS as well.

Primary Cutaneous CD30+ Lymphoproliferative Disorders (pcCD30+LD)

pcCD30+LD include lymphomatoid papulosis (LyP) and cutaneous anaplastic large cell lymphoma (cALCL). These diseases are considered as two ends of a spectrum without clear-cut boundaries. In many cases precise classification can be achieved only upon careful clinicopathologic correlation. Both LyP and cALCL arise predominantly in adults, but LyP is the second most frequent type of cutaneous lymphoma in children after MF. pcCD30+LD are characterized by a very good prognosis, and should be clearly separated from nodal ALCL with cutaneous involvement, as treatment and prognosis are completely different.

cALCL usually presents with solitary, commonly ulcerated tumors (Fig. 20-1). Partial regression may be observed. LyP, on the other hand, is a disease characterized by recurrent crops ("waxing and waning") of papules and small nodules that may ulcerate leaving a scar (Fig. 20-2). The typical duration of each single lesion is 4 to 8 weeks, and the patients present usually with polymorphous lesions due to the appearance of new lesions while old ones are resolving. This peculiar clinical aspect represents the most important single diagnostic criterion, as histopathologic features of LyP and cALCL may overlap. In typical cases differentiation is not a problem; so-called "borderline" cases, however, may be impossible to classify precisely in one or the other category of pcCD30+LD. In particular, regional LyP (that is, LyP confined to a single area of the body) and cALCL with satellite lesions (i.e., cALCL with tumors surrounded by small "satellites") may be indistinguishable from one another both clinically and

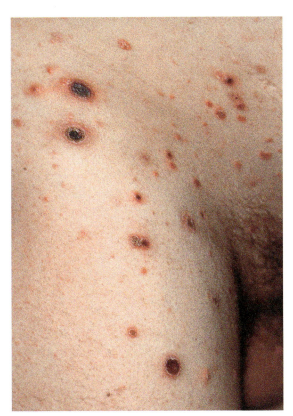

FIGURE 20-2 ■ Lymphomatoid papulosis. Multiple, partly ulcerated papules and plaques.

histopathologically. There are no phenotypic or molecular tools that allow a precise classification in these cases, and a diagnosis of pcCD30+LD is appropriate if a distinction cannot be made. Histopathologically, many cases of LyP and cALCL can be separated easily from one another, but in some instances a precise distinction may be impossible. Thus, accurate clinicopathologic correlation should be considered the standard for precise classification of pcCD30+LD.

Staging investigations are not necessary in patients with a confirmed diagnosis of LyP, but should be carried out for those with cALCL or borderline cases. Examination of the regional lymph nodes is paramount, as well as biopsy of suspicious lymph nodes.

It is particularly important to clearly separate cALCL from nodal ALCL with secondary skin involvement. In this context, anaplastic lymphoma kinase (ALK) is negative in the vast majority of cases of cALCL. It is crucial to underline that secondary skin involvement may be observed both in ALK+ and ALK– nodal ALCL, thus a negative staining for ALK is not a surrogate for staging investigations in patients with cALCL. While secondary skin manifestations of nodal ALCL are usually characterized by a bad prognosis and require aggressive treatment, cALCL is an indolent disease that should be managed by surgical excision and/or local radiotherapy.

Other Cutaneous T-cell Lymphomas

Besides the entities discussed above, many other T-cell lymphomas may arise primary in the skin (see Table 20-1).

A detailed discussion of these entities is beyond the scope of this chapter. In general, it is important to remember that clinicopathologic features similar to those of advanced MF can be observed in aggressive cytotoxic natural killer (NK)/T-cell lymphomas. However, the long "patch" stage that precedes the onset of plaques and tumors in MF is absent in cutaneous aggressive cytotoxic NK/T-cell lymphomas, and patients present with tumor stage at first diagnosis (so-called tumors "d'emblee"). Thus, accurate history is paramount for precise classification. Complete staging investigations are mandatory in cutaneous aggressive cytotoxic NK/T-cell lymphomas, with particular attention to the upper respiratory tract in cases of extranodal NK/T-cell lymphoma, nasal-type.

In some areas of the globe (particularly Japan and the Caribbean) a lymphoma caused by the human T lymphotropic virus 1 (HTLV-1, causing adult T-cell lymphoma/leukemia) may be clinically and histopathologically indistinguishable from MF, thus in endemic areas HTLV-1 testing is crucial for patients with MF-like presentation.

Subcutaneous panniculitis-like T-cell lymphoma (SPLTCL) is a low-grade T-cell lymphoma of cytotoxic T lymphocytes with a CD3+/CD4–/CD8+/TIA-1+/alfa/beta+/gamma/delta phenotype. Lesions resemble those of a panniculitis clinically (particularly lupus erythematosus panniculitis), and histopathologic diagnosis, too, may be very difficult or even impossible in biopsies of older lesions. In the past, aggressive cases with a gamma/delta phenotype were included in the group of SPTCL, but such cases are now classified as cutaneous gamma/delta T-cell lymphoma in the WHO classification. Staging investigations should be performed only in cases with a proven diagnosis of SPLTCL. Systemic corticosteroids can control the disease for long periods of time, and chemotherapy should be used only for patients with extracutaneous spread.

An entity termed primary cutaneous small/medium CD4+ T-cell lymphoma is still a provisional category in the WHO classification, as convincing data on the malignant potential of this entity are yet lacking. It seems likely that publications by different authors reported under this term either reactive processes ("pseudolymphoma"), or clonal expansions of T helper lymphocytes of undetermined significance, or aggressive cases of peripheral T-cell lymphoma, not otherwise specified, all of them sharing a histopathologic presentation characterized by a proliferation of small/medium-sized T helper lymphocytes. As a rule of thumb, patients presenting with solitary lesions located on the head and neck area have an excellent prognosis, and staging investigations or aggressive treatment should be avoided in these cases. On the other hand, patients with multiple lesions on different body areas should be managed very carefully, as these cases may represent an aggressive T-cell lymphoma.

Primary Cutaneous B-Cell Lymphomas

Most cutaneous B-cell lymphomas (CBCLs) represent diseases of low-grade malignant potential and should be managed in a nonaggressive manner. Precise classification and differentiation of aggressive versus nonaggressive entities is possible on clinicopathologic grounds in the vast majority of cases (Fig. 20-3). Some specific regional features in the incidence and etiology of CBCLs are worth mentioning, particularly the association of low-grade types with infection by *Borrelia* in endemic European countries (but not in the United States, reflecting the presence of different strains of *Borrelia*). This association has been detected particularly in the lymphoplasmacytic variant of cutaneous marginal zone lymphoma (cMZL), and has provided the rational base for antibiotic treatment in this subset of patients. This situation can be compared to the finding of *Helicobacter pylori* in a subset of patients with gastric mucosa-associated lymphoid tissue (MALT) lymphoma, and to the successful management of many such cases by antibiotic eradication of *H. pylori*. On the other hand, even in endemic European countries CBCLs associated with *Borrelia* strains represent a minority of cases, thus antibiotic treatment should be considered only in cases with proven association with *Borrelia*.

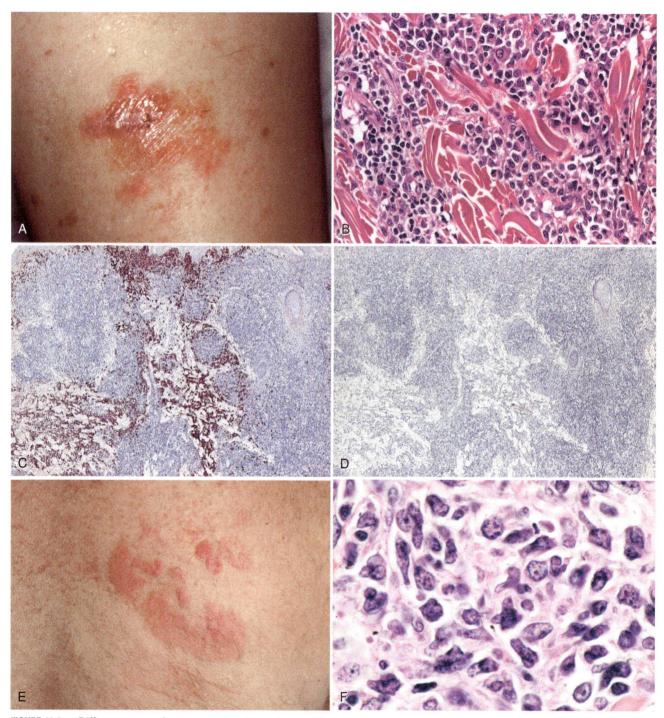

FIGURE 20-3 ■ Different types of cutaneous B-cell lymphomas. **A,** Cutaneous marginal zone lymphoma presenting clinically with a solitary plaque; **B,** histology is characterized by a population of marginal zone cells, plasmacytoid cells, and plasma cells; **C,** positive staining for immunoglobulin light-chain lambda; **D,** negativity for kappa; **E,** cutaneous follicle center lymphoma, diffuse-type presenting clinically with clustered lesions on the back (Crosti's lymphoma); **F,** predominance of large centrocytes;

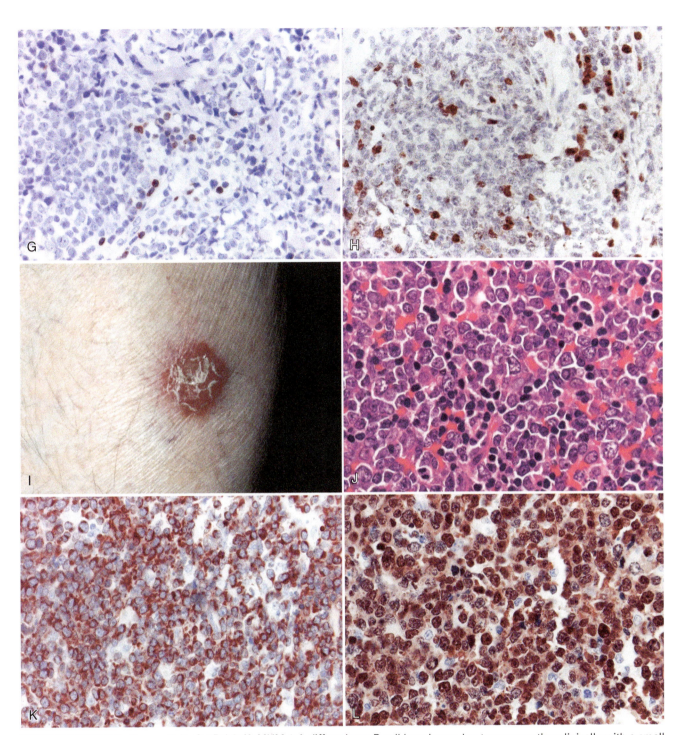

FIGURE 20-3, CONT'D ■ **G**, negativity for Bcl-2; **H**, MUM-1; **I**, diffuse large B-cell lymphoma, leg-type presenting clinically with a small tumor on the leg; **J**, predominance of large round cells; **K**, positivity for Bcl-2; and **L**, MUM-1.

Cutaneous Follicle Center Lymphoma (cFCL)

cFCL is a low-grade CBCL characterized by the proliferation of B follicular lymphocytes within the skin. It typically affects adults of both genders with papules, plaques, and tumors located on the head and neck area or on the trunk, particularly the back (the term Crosti's lymphoma has been used for a peculiar presentation on the back with plaques and tumors surrounded by erythematous macules and papules expanding centrifugally around the central tumors). Histologic examination may reveal a follicular, diffuse, or mixed (follicular and diffuse) pattern of growth. The pattern of growth does not have any prognostic significance. In this context, histopathologic differentiation of cFLC from cutaneous diffuse large B-cell lymphoma, leg-type (cDLBCL-LT) is paramount. Histopathologically, both cFCL, diffuse type, and cDLBCL-LT are characterized by a predominant population of large B lymphocytes. Morphologically, the diffuse type of cFCL shows predominance of large cleaved lymphocytes, in contrast to cDLBCL-LT, where large round cells (particularly immunoblasts) are the majority. Immunohistology reveals negativity for Bcl-2, MUM-1, IgM, and forkhead box protein 1 (FOX-P1) in cFCL, as opposed to positivity for these four markers in the vast majority of cases of cDLBCL-LT. The main problem is that in the lymph nodes the diffuse type of FCL is recognized and managed as a high-grade lymphoma, whereas in the skin it represents a morphologic variant of a low-grade CBCL. Thus, patients with the diffuse type of cFCL have been often treated with unnecessarily aggressive options. Once again, cFCL should be managed in a conservative way regardless of the histopathologic pattern, and systemic chemotherapy is required only in rare patients (those with extracutaneous dissemination). In this context, staging investigations are paramount to plan the proper treatment for any given patient, in order to rule out that the skin lesions represent a secondary manifestation of a nodal lymphoma.

Cutaneous Marginal Zone Lymphoma (cMZL)

Cutaneous cases of MZL have been lumped together with mucosal cases in the WHO classification, and are included in the group of extranodal MZL of the MALT. This group of lymphomas is characterized by several common features, particularly the association with chronic inflammation due to autoimmune disorders or infections. On the other hand, it is yet unclear whether lumping all of these entities in a single group is appropriate in terms of management of the individual patients.

cMZL occurs typically in young adults with a male predominance, but children may be affected as well (it represents one of the most frequent types of childhood cutaneous lymphoma after MF). Patients present with red to reddish brown papules, plaques, and nodules localized particularly to the upper extremities or the trunk. In the absence of extracutaneous symptoms, the need for complete staging investigations in patients with cMZL is questionable. The prognosis is excellent, and patients should be managed in a nonaggressive way (surgical excision suffices in most cases). As already mentioned, antibiotic treatment aimed at eradication of *Borrelia* infection should be carried out in patients proven to have *Borrelia*.

Cutaneous Diffuse Large B-cell Lymphoma, Leg-type (cDLBCL-LT)

This type of cutaneous lymphoma is morphologically, phenotypically, and genetically comparable to diffuse large B-cell lymphomas arising at extracutaneous sites, and is characterized by an aggressive course with a disease-specific 5-year survival of <50%. The disease predominantly affects the leg(s) of elderly patients (over 70 years of age), especially females. Complete staging investigations are mandatory, and anthracycline-containing systemic chemotherapy combined with rituximab represents the treatment of choice. Age may be a limiting factor for aggressive treatment options, and radiotherapy represents a second option. As already mentioned, differentiation of cDLBCL-LT from cFCL with diffuse pattern of growth is paramount, as treatment and prognosis are completely different. Differential diagnostic criteria have been outlined in the paragraph on cFCL earlier in this chapter. For practical purposes, a diagnosis of "primary cutaneous diffuse large B-cell lymphoma" arising on the back should be reevaluated by a center with special expertise in cutaneous lymphomas. At the same time, it must be clearly understood that the skin may be the site of secondary involvement by extracutaneous diffuse large B-cell lymphomas, thus complete staging investigations are mandatory in order to plan properly the management of each patient.

Blastic Plasmacytoid Dendritic Cell Neoplasm

Blastic plasmacytoid dendritic cell neoplasm (BPDCN) is an aggressive hematologic disorder deriving from interferon-producing plasmacytoid dendritic cells type I ("plasmacytoid monocytes"). Many patients present at onset with disease limited to the skin (i.e., staging investigations may be negative), but they should be treated similarly to those with systemic involvement. A similar situation may be observed in patients with acute myelogenous leukemia and is referred to as "aleukemic leukemia cutis." In fact, BPDCN and myelogenous leukemia are strictly related.

The disease occurs mostly in adults of both genders, but it may be observed in children and adolescents as well. Cutaneous lesions are often hemorrhagic ("bruise-like") and usually generalized, although solitary tumors may be seen. The diagnosis relies on peculiar morphologic and phenotypic features of the lesions with positivity of neoplastic cells for CD4, CD56, CD123, TCL-1, and CD303 (BDCA-2) among other markers.

Complete staging investigations are mandatory in every patient, irrespective of the clinical presentation. The disease responds well to chemotherapy but relapses are the rule (often just a few weeks after treatment), followed by rapidly progressive, intractable disease. Promising results have been reported with allogeneic stem cell transplantation.

SPECIFIC MANIFESTATIONS AND NONSPECIFIC SIGNS OF SYSTEMIC LYMPHOMAS

One of the major problems in the management of patients with cutaneous lymphomas is the proper identification of the lymphoma type and the accurate distinction between primary and secondary cutaneous cases. It should be emphasized that clinical, histopathologic, and phenotypic features may show overlaps among different entities as well as between cases arising primarily in the skin and those involving it secondarily. In particular, any lymphoma arising in the lymph nodes or within other organs as well as any leukemia may present with specific cutaneous manifestations, and skin involvement represents a frequent event for some of these entities. In some instances diagnostic criteria used in the skin and in other organs are different. As already mentioned, a paradigmatic example is represented by the diffuse type of FCL, which is classified as a large B-cell lymphoma in the lymph nodes but as an FCL in the skin, with important consequences in terms of therapy and prognosis. Another typical example is represented by ALCL. Prognosis in nodal cases depends heavily on ALK expression, with ALK+ cases showing a disease-specific 5-year survival approaching 80%, and ALK– ones characterized by a 5-year survival of approximately 50%. By contrast, cALCL is characterized by an excellent prognosis (5-year survival >90%) in spite of ALK-negativity in the vast majority of cases. In short, cutaneous lymphomas should be evaluated keeping in mind that distinction of primary from secondary cases is paramount for proper management of most patients. Accurate history, clinical examination of the entire skin, and histopathologic, phenotypic, and molecular analyses are required for a precise diagnosis (see also the paragraphs on primary cutaneous lymphomas earlier in this chapter).

In general, specific skin manifestations of extracutaneous lymphomas retain the histopathologic and phenotypic features of the original tumor. Dedifferentiation or blastic progression, however, may be observed in some cases (e.g., in cutaneous Richter's syndrome, representing in many cases large cell transformation of B-cell chronic lymphocytic leukemia [B-CLL]). In these instances, the cutaneous manifestations show different morphology and phenotype compared to the original extracutaneous tumor.

Clinical features of extracutaneous lymphomas presenting with specific skin manifestations are mostly nondescript papules and nodules, often ulcerated, and usually do not present features pathognomonic of a specific disease. In some cases lesions may be located in the skin areas drained by affected lymph nodes, but in most instances they are disseminated or localized at sites unrelated anatomically to the original tumor.

Most cases of secondary specific skin manifestations of extracutaneous lymphomas represent a marker of progression of the disease with poor prognosis (stage IV). One exception is represented by cutaneous lesions of B-CLL, which may be observed at sites of skin tumors or of other inflammatory conditions, representing recruitment of neoplastic cells in the course of immunologic responses. For example, infection by *Borrelia burgdorferi* in patients with B-CLL can be characterized by the onset of specific cutaneous manifestations at sites typical for *Borrelia*-associated lymphocytoma cutis (i.e., nipple, earlobe, genital area). Although the infiltrate shows histopathologic, phenotypic, and molecular features of the leukemic disease, these specific manifestations are not associated with a poor prognosis, and patients should be managed conservatively.

A discussion of clinicopathologic features of specific skin manifestations of each extracutaneous lymphoma is beyond the scope of this chapter, thus only a few remarks on some entities will be provided in what follows.

Cutaneous B-cell Chronic Lymphocytic Leukemia (B-CLL)

The skin is a frequent site of specific manifestations in patients with B-CLL. As already mentioned, in many instances cutaneous lesions should not be considered as a sign of progression and/or of poor prognosis, as they represent migration of neoplastic leukemic cells to sites of skin inflammation. Large cell transformation (Richter's syndrome, representing either the same neoplastic clone with morphologic transformation or an unrelated second large B-cell lymphoma) can be observed in the skin, and can represent the first sign of progression of the disease. In contrast to most skin manifestations of B-CLL, cutaneous Richter's syndrome (as Richter's syndrome arising at extracutaneous sites) is invariably associated with very poor prognosis.

Patients with specific skin manifestations of B-CLL should be managed according to the hematologic features. As already mentioned, specific infiltrates located at sites of cutaneous inflammation do not require aggressive treatment.

Cutaneous Myelogenous Leukemia (cML)

Specific skin lesions can be observed in all subtypes of ML, including both acute and chronic forms of the disease, as well as myelodysplastic syndromes (MDS). In some patients cutaneous lesions arise before the leukemia is known, and represent the first manifestation of the disease. In a small subset of these patients staging investigations are negative in spite of extensive search ("aleukemic leukemia cutis"). These cases should be managed in the same way as those with positive staging, as the prognosis is similar. Prognosis of specific skin involvement by chronic or acute ML is poor. In contrast to B-CLL, cutaneous manifestations of ML represent a sign of progression of the disease. Treatment should always be given according to hematologic guidelines for the specific type of ML.

The exact prognostic value of specific skin lesions in patients with MDS is yet unclear. Although it is supposed that they represent a sign of progression of the disease to a more aggressive phase, eventually evolving into overt leukemia, in many cases skin lesions are not associated with signs of progression in the peripheral blood and/or bone marrow. The best management for these patients is yet unclear, and a conservative approach may be indicated if clear-cut signs of leukemia are lacking.

Cutaneous Angioimmunoblastic T-cell Lymphoma (cAITL)

cAITL is a nodal lymphoma deriving from T-follicular helper lymphocytes. Specific skin manifestations can be observed and may be very difficult to diagnose, as the lymphoma is characterized by a prominent background of B lymphocytes and other inflammatory cells. In some cases, the accompanying population of B lymphocytes can progress to a second lymphoma, clonally unrelated but tightly connected with the original AITL. These AITL-related B-cell lymphomas are often associated with infection by Epstein–Barr virus (which, on the other hand, is never found in the neoplastic cells of the AITL). The skin may be infiltrated by specific cells of the AITL or of the second B-cell lymphoma; in exceptional cases the second lymphoma can be observed in the skin only, arising in the context of the specific skin manifestations of AITL, thus representing onset of the B-cell lymphoma in the skin. Management of patients with cAITL should be performed in a hematologic setting, as the disease always represents a secondary manifestation of a primary extracutaneous lymphoma.

Cutaneous Hodgkin's Lymphoma (HL)

Specific skin manifestations of HL are exceedingly rare, whereas nonspecific dermatological signs are more common. As a rule, a diagnosis of cutaneous HL should be made only in patients with known extracutaneous disease (that means, primary cutaneous cases are extremely rare, if they exist at all). As management of patients with HL has improved considerably over the last decades, the incidence of specific skin manifestations has decreased dramatically, and nowadays they are observed only exceedingly rarely. Skin involvement is found usually in the drainage area of affected lymph nodes and more rarely in a generalized fashion. Histologic examination of cutaneous infiltrates shows morphologic and phenotypic features similar to those observed in the lymph nodes. Treatment should be given according to guidelines for the nodal disease.

Nonspecific Signs of Systemic Lymphomas

Patients with systemic lymphomas may present different skin diseases unrelated to direct colonization by neoplastic cells (that is, "nonspecific" cutaneous manifestations of systemic lymphomas). The most common conditions are listed in Table 20-2. These skin disorders may precede, arise concomitant with, or follow the systemic lymphoma. Some of them are very common skin conditions observed often in nonparaneoplastic settings, and thus do not represent helpful diagnostic clues. Other conditions, on the other hand, are frequently related to nodal HL or other non-Hodgkin's lymphomas (NHLs), and may represent useful clues for diagnosis and/or monitoring of disease activity.

Pruritus is a very common cutaneous symptom and can be associated with myriads of cutaneous and systemic disorders. Chronic pruritus without evidence of skin lesions ("pruritus sine materia") may be a cutaneous sign of HL or NHL, and can antedate the diagnosis of the nodal disease by several months or years. Although idiopathic pruritus may be observed also in several other conditions unrelated to hematologic malignancies, screening for an underlying lymphoma belongs to the standard management of these patients.

Sweet's syndrome (acute febrile neutrophilic dermatosis) is characterized by the sudden onset of tender or painful cutaneous erythematous, edematous papules, or plaques accompanied by fever, malaise, and neutrophilic leukocytosis. Systemic symptoms are not invariably present, and several clinicopathologic variants have been described. Sweet's syndrome may be associated with malignancies, particularly ML or MDS (10% to 15% of cases). In some cases neoplastic cells may be observed within the inflammatory infiltrate, particularly in some variants of the disease (e.g., "histiocytoid" Sweet's syndrome). Sweet's syndrome may also be associated with the use of colony-stimulating factors and with several other neoplastic and non-neoplastic disorders. In absence of other signs and/or symptoms, extensive screening investigations in search of an underlying hematologic disorder are not necessary (with the possible exception of histiocytoid Sweet's syndrome).

Pyoderma gangrenosum (PG) is characterized by the rapid development of pustules evolving into large, undermined ulcerative lesions, often following minor trauma or after surgical procedures (so-called "pathergy"). In some cases, PG may be associated with hematologic malignancies (particularly ML and variants). In these patients lesions may have a bullous appearance and may show overlapping features with bullous Sweet's syndrome. As for Sweet's syndrome, for patients with PG extensive screening investigations in search of an underlying hematologic disorder are not necessary if other signs and/or symptoms are not present (bullous PG, though, is more frequently associated with hematologic malignancies than other variants of the disease, and these patients should be screened more carefully).

Paraneoplastic pemphigus is an autoimmune blistering disorder mainly associated with NHLs (particularly B-cell NHLs and leukemias, but also other types, as well as thymoma and Castleman's disease). It is characterized by polymorphous skin lesions with features of both erythema multiforme and pemphigus vulgaris. Paraneoplastic pemphigus may precede the diagnosis of the underlying hematologic condition. Antibodies directed against multiple skin antigens can be detected, including members of the plakin family as well as the desmogleins. Besides skin lesions, severe involvement of the oral mucosa can often be observed in these patients, as well as the presence of ocular involvement and of severe pulmonary manifestations.

Patients with paraneoplastic pemphigus should always be screened for a hematologic malignancy. The therapy is very difficult and the disease is resistant to most treatment options. Management of the underlying NHL is paramount, and the anti-CD20 antibody (rituximab) has been used in cases of B-NHL-associated paraneoplastic pemphigus in order to target specifically the antibody-producing tumor cells (although with variable efficacy).

Acquired ichthyosis is a skin condition similar to ichthyosis vulgaris both clinically and histopathologically, but appearing during adult life and usually associated with an underlying malignancy, particularly an NHL. A similar clinicopathologic presentation may be observed also as a drug eruption (clofazimine, pravastatin, allopurinol, and cimetidine among others), or in association with other conditions such as malnutrition, hypothyroidism, and infections among others. As acquired ichthyosis can be observed in several settings, in the absence of other signs and/or symptoms patients should not undergo extensive screening investigations for an underlying hematologic disorder.

The onset of **sarcoidal granulomas** may be observed in patients with NHL. The term "sarcoidosis-lymphoma syndrome" has been used for patients with systemic sarcoidosis who subsequently developed NHL, but sarcoidal granulomas may develop also after the diagnosis of the NHL, and the skin may represent one of the sites of involvement. Cutaneous sarcoidal granulomas may represent a sign of activity of the underlying lymphoma, and in some cases may be used to monitor the disease.

Patients with **paraproteinemia** due to hematologic conditions (e.g., Waldenström's macroglobulinemia, monoclonal gammopathy of undetermined significance [MGUS], etc.) may present with peculiar skin conditions, some of which are rarely, if ever, observed in other settings (e.g., necrobiotic xanthogranuloma and scleromyxedema among others). **Schnitzler's syndrome** (chronic urticarial lesions, intermittent fever, malaise, bone pain, arthralgia, and monoclonal IgM gammopathy) is another disorder with peculiar skin manifestations ("neutrophilic urticaria") associated with paraproteinemia, possibly representing an autoinflammatory condition related to the paraproteinemia. **POEMS syndrome** (polyneuropathy, organomegaly, endocrinopathy, monoclonal gammopathy [M protein], and skin changes) and **AESOP syndrome** (adenopathy and extensive skin patch overlying a plasmacytoma), too, are almost always related to paraproteinemia. **Type I cryoglobulinemia** is due to a monoclonal protein (IgG, IgM, IgA, or rarely a light chain) that precipitates when cooled. It is usually seen in association with MGUS, Waldenström's macroglobulinemia, multiple myeloma, or rarely other immunoglobulin-producing B-NHLs. Cutaneous lesions are usually characterized by purpuric lesions and/or hemorrhagic crusts and ulcerations in areas of small infarctions due to clotted vessels. Due to the lower temperature, purpuric lesions on the earlobe are a typical manifestation of the disease (Fig. 20-4).

Crystal storing histiocytosis (CSH) is characterized by crystalloid intracytoplasmic inclusions within histiocytes and macrophages, representing intracellular deposits of immunoglobulins with peculiar geometric shapes. CSH is mostly related to multiple myeloma, but may be observed occasionally also in association with other systemic hematologic conditions such as lymphoplasmacytic lymphoma, MALT lymphoma, and MGUS, and rarely without an underlying lymphoproliferative disorder.

Many other nonspecific cutaneous manifestations may be observed in patients with hematologic malignancies, either related to substances produced by the malignant tumor (e.g., amyloidosis, etc.), or to bone marrow suppression due to the neoplasm (e.g., pallor, purpura, etc.), or to the decreased immune competence related to both the hematologic malignancy and the treatment (e.g., opportunistic infections such as aspergillosis, disseminated candidiasis, etc.), or to the side effects of treatment (e.g., exanthematic drug eruptions, palmar erythema, etc.). These conditions are summarized in different chapters in this book.

SUGGESTED READINGS

Balaraman B, Conley JA, Sheinbein DM. Evaluation of cutaneous angioimmunoblastic T-cell lymphoma. J Am Acad Dermatol 2011;65:855–62.

Beltraminelli H, Leinweber B, Kerl H, Cerroni L. Primary cutaneous CD4+ small-/medium-sized pleomorphic T-cell lymphoma: a cutaneous nodular proliferation of pleomorphic T lymphocytes of undetermined significance? A study of 136 cases. Am J Dermatopathol 2009;31:317–22.

Botros N, Cerroni L, Shawwa A, Green PJ, Greer W, Pasternak S, et al. Cutaneous manifestations of angioimmunblastic T-cell lymphoma: clinical and pathological characteristics. Am J Dermatopathol 2015;37:274–83.

Cerroni L. Skin lymphoma – the illustrated guide. 4th ed. Oxford: Wiley-Blackwell; 2014.

Cerroni L, Arzberger E, Pütz B, Höfler G, Metze D, Sander CA, et al. Primary cutaneous follicle center cell lymphoma with follicular growth pattern. Blood 2000;95:3922–8.

Cerroni L, Höfler G, Bäck B, Wolf P, Maier G, Kerl H. Specific cutaneous infiltrates of B-cell chronic lymphocytic leukemia (B-CLL) at sites typical for *Borrelia burgdorferi* infection. J Cut Pathol 2002;29:142–7.

Cerroni L, Zenahlik P, Höfler G, Kaddu S, Smolle J, Kerl H. Specific cutaneous infiltrates of B-cell chronic lymphocytic leukemia. A clinicopathologic and prognostic study of 42 patients. Am J Surg Pathol 1996;20:1000–10.

Cerroni L, Zöchling N, Pütz B, Kerl H. Infection by *Borrelia burgdorferi* and cutaneous B-cell lymphoma. J Cut Pathol 1997;24:457–61.

Ferreri AJ, Govi S, Ponzoni M. Marginal zone lymphomas and infectious agents. Semin Cancer Biol 2013;23:431–40.

Fried I, Artl M, Cota C, Müller HG, Bartolo E, Boi S, et al. Clinicopathologic and molecular features in cutaneous extranodal natural killer/T-cell lymphoma, nasal type, with aggressive and indolent course. J Am Acad Dermatol 2014;70:716–23.

Gulia A, Saggini A, Wiesner T, Fink-Puches R, Argenyi Z, Ferrara G, et al. Clinicopathologic features of early lesions of primary cutaneous follicle center lymphoma, diffuse type: implications for early diagnosis and treatment. J Am Acad Dermatol 2011;65:991–1000.

Kempf W, Pfaltz K, Vermeer MH, Cozzio A, Ortiz-Romero PL, Bagot M, et al. EORTC, ISCL, and USCLC consensus recommendations

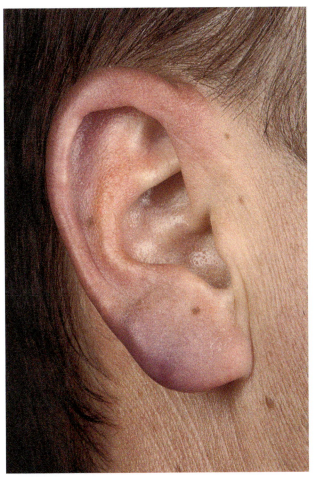

FIGURE 20-4 ■ Purpuric lesions on the ears due to lower temperature at this site are a typical sign of cryoglobulinemia and may be the first symptom of an underlying systemic B-cell lymphoma.

for the treatment of primary cutaneous CD30-positive lymphoproliferative disorders: lymphomatoid papulosis and primary cutaneous anaplastic large-cell lymphoma. Blood 2011;118(15):4024–35.

Kodama K, Massone C, Chott A, Metze D, Kerl H, Cerroni L. Primary cutaneous large B-cell lymphomas: clinicopathologic features, classification, and prognostic factors in a large series of patients. Blood 2005;106:2491–7.

Olsen E, Vonderheid E, Pimpinelli N, Willemze R, Kim Y, Knobler R, et al. Revisions to the staging and classification of mycosis fungoides and Sezary syndrome: a proposal of the International Society for Cutaneous Lymphomas (ISCL) and the cutaneous lymphoma task force of the European Organization of Research and Treatment of Cancer (EORTC). Blood 2007;110:1713–22.

Requena L, Kutzner H, Palmedo G, Pascual M, Fernández-Herrera J, Fraga J, et al. Histiocytoid Sweet syndrome: a dermal infiltration of immature neutrophilic granulocytes. Arch Dermatol 2005;141:834–42.

Sapienza MR, Fuligni F, Agostinelli C, Tripodo C, Righi S, Laginestra MA, et al. Molecular profiling of blastic plasmacytoid dendritic cell neoplasm reveals a unique pattern and suggests selective sensitivity to NF-kB pathway inhibition. Leukemia 2014;28:1606–16.

Senff NJ, Noordijk EM, Kim YH, Bagot M, Berti E, Cerroni L, et al. European Organization for Research and Treatment of Cancer and International Society for Cutaneous Lymphoma consensus recommendations for the management of cutaneous B-cell lymphomas. Blood 2008;112:1600–9.

Swerdlow SH, Campo E, Harris NL, et al., editors. WHO classification of tumors of haematopoietic and lymphoid tissues. Lyon: IARC Press; 2008.

Vitte F, Fabiani B, Benet C, Dalac S, Balme B, Delattre C, et al. specific skin lesions in chronic myelomonocytic leukemia a spectrum of myelomonocytic and dendritic cell proliferations. A study of 42 cases. Am J Surg Pathol 2012;36:1302–16.

Willemze R, Jaffe ES, Burg G, Cerroni L, Berti E, Swerdlow SH, et al. WHO-EORTC classification for cutaneous lymphomas. Blood 2005;105:3768–85.

Willemze R, Jansen PM, Cerroni L, Berti E, Santucci M, Assaf C, et al. Subcutaneous panniculitis-like T-cell lymphoma: definition, classification, and prognostic factors: an EORTC Cutaneous Lymphoma Group Study of 83 cases. Blood 2008;111:838–45.

CHAPTER 21

Dysproteinemias, Plasma Cell Disorders, and Amyloidosis

Warren W. Piette

KEY POINTS

- The presence of a monoclonal gammopathy may be an incidental finding, but there are many cutaneous disorders that are due to or are strongly associated with the presence of a monoclonal gammopathy.
- A usual way to organize thinking around the syndromes divides them into diseases directly related to the monoclonal protein, diseases frequently associated with a monoclonal protein without a clear causative role, and disorders of amyloid deposition, the most common systemic form being due to light-chain synthesis into amyloid protein.
- The diagnosis and treatment of these disorders will be addressed within this framework.

A wide variety of diseases associated with monoclonal immunoglobulin or light-chain production may cause cutaneous lesions, and these will be addressed by category: those directly related to monoclonal protein (e.g., cryoglobulin), those frequently associated with gammopathy (e.g., scleromyexedema), and those resulting from abnormal metabolism of monoclonal proteins (e.g., light-chain-related amyloidosis).

Commonly, monoclonal immunoglobulin production is simply a monoclonal gammopathy of undetermined significance (MGUS). MGUS is defined as a serum monoclonal protein <30 g/L; <10% plasma cells in the bone marrow; and the absence of end-organ damage (hypercalcemia, renal insufficiency, anemia, and/or bone lesions [CRAB]). Although this disorder is uncommon in young individuals, its incidence increases with age, reaching 3% in those 50 years of age or older, and 5% in those over 70 years. The risk of progression to multiple myeloma or a related disorder is 1% per year. Three risk factors are useful in predicting the likelihood of progression (as measured at 20 years' follow-up): (1) an increase in serum-free light chains; (2) an MGUS of nonimmunoglobulin G (IgG) origin; or (3) a serum M protein of 15 g/L or more. The risk of multiple myeloma at 20 years was 58% with all three risk factors, 37% with two risk factors, 21% with one risk factor, and 5% when no risk factors were present. Smoldering myeloma is a term used to describe an asymptomatic phase of myeloma characterized by a serum IgG or IgA monoclonal protein >30 g/L and/or >10% plasma cells in the bone marrow, but no evidence of myeloma-related end-organ damage. In this group, the cumulative probability of progression to active multiple myeloma or amyloidosis was 51% at 5 years, 66% at 10 years, and 73% at 15 years, with a median time to progression of 4.8 years.

DISORDERS DIRECTLY RELATED TO MONOCLONAL PROTEINS

Pathogenesis

Monoclonal proteins may cause disease directly by acting as cryoglobulins, by raising serum viscosity, or by acting as cold agglutinins. Cryoglobulins are immunoglobulins with temperature-dependent conformational change leading to water insolubility and precipitation on exposure to cold. They may be unstable in other settings, such as in the hyperosmotic environment found in the kidneys, or in microvascular areas with a slow blood flow. The most critical factor that determines the behavior of the cryoglobulin in vivo is the temperature at which it begins to precipitate. If that temperature approaches those found in the cutaneous microvasculature on cold exposure, cold-induced disease is usually significant. If it precipitates only at a temperature well below room temperature, symptoms, if any, will not be cold-related. Cryoglobulins are divided into three categories, depending on their composition. Type I cryoglobulins consist of a single monoclonal protein; type II are composed of a monoclonal immunoglobulin with anti-IgG (rheumatoid factor) activity that binds to polyclonal serum IgG; and type III cryoglobulins consist of polyclonal immunoglobulins, usually with anti-IgG activity, that bind to polyclonal serum IgG (a polyclonal rheumatoid factor). Types I and II cryoglobulinemia are often (but not always) associated with a lymphoproliferative disorder or plasma cell dyscrasia. Patients with type II cryoglobulinemia may have IgM, IgG, or IgA as their monoclonal rheumatoid factor. Only IgM rheumatoid factor testing is routinely available. Since the monoclonal protein is bound to a polyclonal IgG antigen, serum protein electrophoresis may not show a discrete M-spike, and if the specimen is allowed to cool before sampling, all studies will be negative.

The hyperviscosity syndrome results from a significant increase in whole blood viscosity. Such an increase may be related to an increase in the cellular elements in the blood, as in polycythemia vera, but most often results from a change in serum viscosity due to large amounts of monoclonal protein in the blood.

Cold agglutinin disease is a cold antibody-induced autoimmune hemolytic anemia. The antibody, usually IgM, binds to the red cell in the cold and initiates complement activation; it then elutes at body temperature while the complement activation proceeds to red cell lysis. The cold agglutinin also promotes temperature-dependent agglutination of red cells, leading to sludging or occlusion of the blood flow in the microvasculature exposed to cold temperatures.

Clinical Manifestations

Cryoglobulinemia

Roughly 5% to 10% of myeloma proteins and macroglobulins are cryoprecipitable. Type I cryoglobulins are usually IgM and therefore primarily intravascular; however, they can also be composed of IgG. To be symptomatic they should precipitate at temperatures easily attained in the cutaneous microvasculature. Such disease may present as Raynaud's phenomenon, livedo reticularis, digital infarcts, peripheral gangrene, or purpura; the latter may be palpable (Fig. 21-1A and B), exhibit central necrosis, or have a livedoid or retiform component (Fig. 21-1C).

Cold sensitivity is more variable with types II and III cryoglobulins because these are usually bound to normal IgG. The classification of essential mixed cryoglobulinemia is now known to include primarily patients with hepatitis C viral infection. Mixed cryoglobulins may be detected as cryoproteins or as rheumatoid factor in the laboratory; in the patient, they are more likely to cause disease as an immune complex than as a cryogelling protein. For this reason, mixed cryoglobulinemias tend to present with features of leukocytoclastic (necrotizing) vasculitis that affect both small- and medium-sized vessels in the skin and elsewhere. Palpable purpura, digital infarcts, arthralgias and arthritis, and glomerulonephritis are the usual clinical features. Some patients with an underlying lymphoproliferative disease may develop angioedema with urticaria as a result of C1 esterase inhibitor depletion; the monoclonal protein in such patients may also behave as a cryoglobulin in the test tube. Finally, some cases of cold-induced urticaria are caused by a circulating cryoglobulin without evidence of any associated disease.

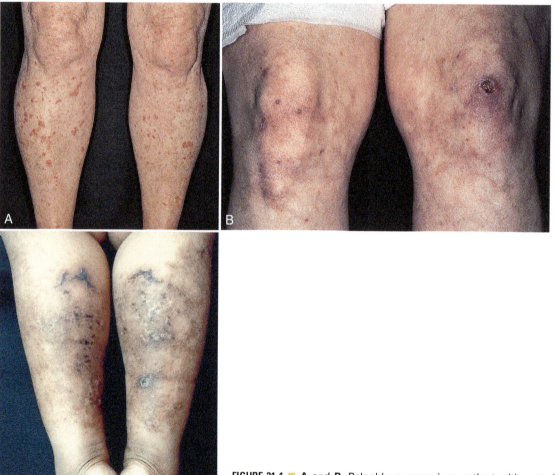

FIGURE 21-1 ■ **A** and **B**, Palpable purpura in a patient with cryoglobulinemia. **C**, Retiform necrotic lesions in a patient with type I cryoglobulinemia.

Hyperviscosity Syndrome

Hyperviscosity syndrome may present as macular hemorrhage, mucous membrane bleeding, retinopathy, neurologic disturbances, hypervolemia, or cardiac failure, and, if caused by a cryoglobulin, Raynaud's phenomenon. Symptoms require a four- to fivefold increase in blood viscosity, usually associated with >3 g/dL IgM (or >15 g/dL IgG, >4 to 5 g/dL polymerized IgG3, >10 to 11 g/dL IgA, >6 to 7 g/dL polymerized IgA) and can also be seen with chylomicronemia syndrome, and with cellular causes of hyperviscosity in polycythemia vera, sickle cell disease, leukemia, and spherocytosis. Hyperviscosity alone may not fully explain the increased bleeding tendency in these patients. Additional factors in some patients are antibody activity against clotting factors, platelet dysfunction as a result of surface coating by immunoglobulin, and other poorly understood clotting defects.

Cold Agglutinin Disease

Cold agglutinin disease is characterized clinically by episodes of hemolytic anemia, hemoglobinuria, and cold-mediated vaso-occlusive phenomena. Patients may develop acrocyanosis, Raynaud's-like phenomenon, or generalized livedo reticularis, but cutaneous ulcerations or necrosis are unusual. Jaundice or pallor may follow a severe episode of hemolysis. Cold agglutinin disease occurs in two forms: primary (idiopathic) and secondary. Patients with primary cold agglutinin disease may develop features diagnostic of Waldenström's macroglobulinemia, whereas secondary forms follow certain infections. Cold agglutinins can also be categorized by their red cell antigen affinity. The antibodies are usually directed against the I/i antigen system, and, rarely, against Pr group antigens. Anti-I antibodies occur primarily in association with idiopathic disease, *Mycoplasma* pneumonia, and some lymphomas; anti-i-specific antibodies are associated with infectious mononucleosis and some lymphomas. The cold agglutinins are monoclonal in primary and lymphoma-associated disease and polyclonal in postinfectious disease. The rare cases of IgA cold agglutinin disease are also characterized by red cell agglutination in the microvasculature, but hemolytic anemia does not develop because the cell-bound IgA does not fix complement.

Waldenström's Macroglobulinemia

This is a disease characterized by a serum monoclonal IgM spike and by malignant lymphoplasmacytoid proliferation, primarily in the bone marrow, liver, spleen, and lymph nodes. In some patients the IgM paraprotein may behave as a monoclonal (type I) cryoglobulin or a cold agglutinin. Urticarial vasculitis associated with an IgM monoclonal protein, bone pain with hyperostosis, and intermittent fever is known as Schnitzler syndrome.

Cryofibrinogenemia

Cryofibrinogen is a plasma complex of fibrin, fibrinogen, and fibronectin that can precipitate on cooling and clot when combined with thrombin. Cryofibrinogenemia occurs as a primary disorder, or as an associated disorder in patients with neoplasia, acute infections, collagen vascular disorders, or thromboembolic disease. Patients with cryofibrinogenemia may present with recurrent painful cutaneous ulcerations of the lower leg and foot. Purpura, often nonpalpable, may accompany the ulcers, which are usually small. The ulcerations heal with ivory stellate scars, resembling the cutaneous features of livedoid vasculopathy (Fig. 21-2).

Differential Diagnosis

In cases of mixed cryoglobulinemia presenting as leukocytoclastic vasculitis, the differential diagnosis primarily includes other necrotizing vasculitides. Hyperviscosity syndrome is usually caused by a clonal lymphoproliferative disorder, but it can result from other hematologic disorders, such as polycythemia vera. Raynaud's phenomenon may be idiopathic (Raynaud's disease), or may be secondary to an autoimmune connective tissue disease, including scleroderma, lupus erythematosus, rheumatoid arthritis, or Sjögren's syndrome. Other diseases may resemble Raynaud's phenomenon; in addition to those mentioned in this section, conditions such as ergotism, Buerger's disease, chilblains (pernio), and acrocyanosis should be considered. In patients presenting with lesions of dermal vessel occlusion, disorders that must also be considered are many (see Chapter 15).

Histopathologic Findings

Early cutaneous lesions of monoclonal cryoglobulinemia demonstrate intravascular amorphous eosinophilic material composed principally of precipitated cryoglobulin. There is often red blood cell extravasation into the dermis. Inflammation is usually minimal, and appears to be a response to, rather than a cause of, necrosis, which results from vessel occlusion. Biopsy of a late lesion of occlusion with necrosis may show changes of secondary leukocytoclastic vasculitis. By contrast, early cutaneous lesions of mixed cryoglobulinemia show histopathologic changes of leukocytoclastic (necrotizing) vasculitis. Immunoreactant deposition in vessel walls can be seen on direct immunofluorescence microscopy.

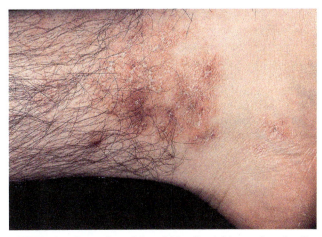

FIGURE 21-2 ■ Purpuric nodules within a livedoid vasculopathy-like eruption in a patient with hepatitis-C-related cryoglobulinemia.

Cutaneous lesions that are the result of cryofibrinogenemia, cold agglutinin disease, or paroxysmal nocturnal hemoglobinuria should show histologic evidence of multiple dermal vessel thrombosis, usually in the absence of significant inflammatory infiltrate.

Evaluation

Although the detection and analysis of a serum or urine monoclonal immunoglobulin or Bence Jones protein (i.e., light chain) was classically accomplished via serum or urine protein electrophoresis, immunofixation techniques have proved to be significantly more sensitive. The serum-free light-chain assay has emerged as the most sensitive method for the detection of plasma cell dyscrasias characterized by overproduction of light chains. When a patient is suspected of having a cryoprotein-related disease, blood can be drawn for both serum and plasma sampling and kept at body temperature until the cellular elements have been removed. Following at least overnight refrigeration, each sample is then examined for evidence of a cryoprecipitate. A cryoglobulin should appear in both the serum and the plasma sample, whereas cryofibrinogen will appear in only the plasma fraction. Immunofixation of the precipitated cryoglobulin can then define its composition. Patients found to have type I or II cryoglobulins should be examined for an underlying plasma cell dyscrasia or lymphoproliferative disorder. Patients with type II or III cryoglobulins should be evaluated for hepatitis C viral infection; non-hepatitis-related disease may be secondary to an underlying connective tissue or autoimmune disease, or to other chronic infections or inflammatory diseases.

Vessel occlusion caused by cold agglutinins is rare, despite their low-level presence in many different acute and chronic diseases. If hyperviscosity syndrome is suspected, serum viscosity measurements are usually easily obtained from clinical laboratories, but whole-blood viscosity measurements remain a specialized research procedure.

Treatment

The treatment of cryoglobulinemia depends on the clinical features. If clinically relevant cold sensitivity is present, adequate clothing and avoidance of cold exposure are essential and may be all that is required. For those with more severe disease, treatment of the underlying plasma cell dyscrasia or lymphoproliferative disorder is indicated. In patients with type II or III cryoglobulinemia, in whom necrotizing vasculitis is the usual presenting finding, cutaneous lesions may respond to oral dapsone or colchicine therapy. Aggressive therapy with systemic corticosteroids in combination with immunosuppressive or cytotoxic agents may be required in severe systemic disease. In hepatitis-C-related cryoglobulinemia, interferon regimens of antiviral therapy may reduce the vasculitis but can occasionally induce flaring. Published data are rare with regard to the effect of new specific antihepatitis C agents; vasculitis remission is reported. Patients with specific underlying etiologic disorders may respond to effective treatment of that disorder. Plasmapheresis may provide temporary but rapid relief of symptoms in patients with high levels of circulating cryoglobulins, and it may be synergistic when combined with chemotherapy in appropriate cases. Intravenous γ-globulin therapy is occasionally successful in cryoglobulinemia and refractory vasculitis.

Cold agglutinin disease is best treated by keeping the patient (particularly the extremities) warm. Cytotoxic agents may be useful in some patients, but plasmapheresis is contraindicated because it may induce severe hemolytic anemia. Postinfectious cases of cold agglutinin disease are usually self-limiting.

For patients in whom simple measures do not address the clinical manifestations of cryofibrinogenemia, the use of an oral anabolic steroid such as stanozolol (4 to 8 mg/day) or danazol may prove beneficial, with rapid pain relief and ulcer healing observed in a number of patients. Stanozolol and danazol are androgenic steroids with fibrinolytic properties. Stanozolol has been removed from the market in the United States, but apparently can be obtained through compounding pharmacies. Other therapies for livedoid vasculopathy associated with cryofibrinogenemia include heparin, warfarin, streptokinase, plasmapheresis, immunosuppressive agents, and tissue plasminogen activator.

DISORDERS ASSOCIATED WITH MONOCLONAL PROTEIN PRODUCTION

Pathogenesis

This group of disorders is united by the frequent finding of an associated monoclonal gammopathy. Some diseases are almost always associated with a monoclonal gammopathy (e.g., POEMS syndrome, scleromyxedema), whereas others are frequently associated with a monoclonal gammopathy (e.g., normolipemic plane xanthoma). Many diseases have a greater than chance association with the presence of a serum or urine monoclonal protein, but this is not required for typical disease expression (e.g., scleredema).

Clinical Manifestations

POEMS Syndrome

This was recognized as a distinct entity in Japan in 1968 and is also known as the Crow–Fukase or Takatsuki syndrome. POEMS is an acronym for polyneuropathy, organomegaly, endocrinopathy, M-protein, and skin changes. In a large series men were affected twice as frequently as women, and patients were young to middle-aged adults with a mean age of 46 years (compared to mean age of myeloma presentation of 62 years). All patients had peripheral polyneuropathy (usually sensorimotor), 97% had elevated cerebrospinal fluid protein, and 62% had papilledema. Organomegaly was manifested as hepatomegaly in 82% of the patients, lymphadenopathy in 65%, and splenomegaly in 39%. The most common endocrine abnormalities were impotence (78%) and gynecomastia (68%) in men, and amenorrhea (68%) in women. Additional endocrine findings in this and other series include glucose intolerance (28% to 48%), hyperthyroidism (10% to 24%), and hyperprolactinemia, adrenal insufficiency, or hypercalcemia (rare).

Most patients (75%) have had a serum or rarely a urine monoclonal spike. Of these spikes, approximately 55% were IgG1 and 40% were IgA1. Although in some of these patients the disease may ultimately progress to multiple myeloma, this does not always occur. Slightly more than half of patients with POEMS syndrome had bone lesions, and 85% of patients with bone lesions had osteosclerotic lesions, with or without osteolytic lesions; this is in contrast to a large series of patients with myeloma in whom osteosclerotic lesions comprised only 0.5% to 3.0% of bone lesions. Also, unlike the findings in osteolytic multiple myeloma, anemia, hypercalcemia, and renal insufficiency are uncommon, and extensive bone marrow infiltration by plasma cells is rare.

Cutaneous changes are common in this disorder, and reported changes include diffuse hyperpigmentation (93% to 98%); peripheral edema (92%); and sometimes anasarca, hypertrichosis (78% to 81%), a poorly characterized skin thickening (77% to 85%), and digital clubbing (56%). Cutaneous angiomas occur in 24% to 44% of patients and include cherry, verrucous, subcutaneous, or "glomeruloid" angiomas (Fig. 21-3). The histopathological finding of a glomeruloid angioma is highly indicative of this syndrome. That circulating levels of vascular endothelial growth factor (VEGF) are markedly increased in these patients may provide some explanation for the vascular changes in POEMS. This increase in VEGF may come from aggregating platelets overly rich in VEGF, which could provide very high local microcirculatory concentrations of VEGF. In patients with POEMS in association with multicentric Castleman's disease, viral interleukin (IL)-6 produced by human herpesvirus-8 could also lead to increased circulating levels of VEGF. Sclerodermoid changes, facial atrophy, flushing, Terry's nails, acrocyanosis, Raynaud's phenomenon, and sicca syndrome have also been described. Biopsy findings of the skin are often nonspecific, but include hyperpigmentation, dermal thickening caused by edema and an increase in collagen and proteoglycan, microvascular proliferation, and occasional large fibroblasts in the dermis.

Variable findings include ascites, pleural effusions, fever, polycythemia, leukocytosis, thrombocytosis, and an elevated erythrocyte sedimentation rate. POEMS syndrome may predispose to arterial and venous thromboses and stroke. Associations with Castleman's disease have been reported, as have presentations such as flushing, hypotension, and bronchial spasm, mimicking carcinoid. The AESOP (adenopathy and extensive skin patch overlying a plasmacytoma) syndrome describes a distinctive presentation of a slowly extending violaceous skin patch overlying a solitary plasmacytoma of bone, associated with enlarged regional lymph nodes. Of the four reported patients, all had neuropathy and two developed POEMS syndrome.

Primary Cutaneous Marginal Zone Lymphoma of Mucosa-Associated Lymphoid Tissue Type (PCMZL-MALT): Formerly Cutaneous Plasmacytoma

In the WHO-EORTC and current WHO classifications, cutaneous plasmacytomas and cutaneous immunocytomas are considered to be variants of PCMZL. These are rare and may be solitary or multiple. Most of these cutaneous lesions are smooth, nontender, cutaneous, or subcutaneous nodules, skin-colored to violaceous, and 1 to 5 cm in diameter, and they may be crusted or ulcerated. They are usually located on the trunk, extremities, or face. All immunoglobulin classes have been associated with PCMZL, but most are IgG- or IgA-producing cells. True cutaneous plasmacytomas indicate a large tumor cell burden in patients with multiple myeloma, and therefore usually occur late in the course of the disease, either as an extension from underlying bone or as distinct cutaneous metastases. Although IgD myeloma is rare, patients with this disease have a higher incidence of extramedullary lesions, including cutaneous plasmacytomas (up to 18%). The IgD subset of myeloma usually develops in young men and has an aggressive course.

A lesion of PCMZL may be an isolated finding, even with long-term follow-up. Because the number of plasma cells in such a lesion is small and the amount of immunoglobulin synthesized is directly related to cell numbers, such patients are unlikely to have a serum monoclonal antibody spike. Conversely, the presence of a monoclonal spike suggests extracutaneous disease.

Cutaneous and Systemic Plasmacytosis

Plasma cell-rich lesions have been described in cutaneous and systemic plasmacytosis as well as plasma cell orificial mucositis. Cutaneous and systemic plasmacytosis is a rare disorder reported almost exclusively in patients of Japanese descent, and is characterized by widespread reddish-brown macules (due to polyclonal plasma cell infiltration), polyclonal hypergammaglobulinemia, peripheral adenopathy (~60%), and sometimes infiltration of the lung, liver, spleen, or kidneys. Although rare, these disorders present with so extensive an infiltration of

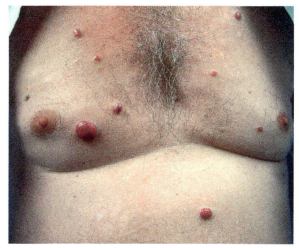

FIGURE 21-3 ■ Multiple angiomas in this patient with POEMS syndrome.

plasma cells that, on biopsy, they may mimic cutaneous plasmacytomas.

Necrobiotic Xanthogranuloma with Paraproteinemia

This is a distinctive entity, typically presenting with yellowish periorbital plaques or nodules that tend to ulcerate and heal with scar formation. Lesions may also develop on the trunk or proximal limbs, especially in flexural areas (Fig. 21-4). The lesions often extend deeply into the dermis and subcutis and, on biopsy, show both Touton and foreign body giant cells, broad areas of altered collagen, and necrobiosis on a background of extensive granulomatous inflammation. Most patients have a monoclonal gammopathy (IgG, often κ), many have leukopenia, bone marrow plasmacytosis is common, but multiple myeloma or other lymphoproliferative disorders are rare. In one series, hepatomegaly or splenomegaly was reported in 20 of 48 patients.

Other Xanthomatous Diseases

Other xanthomatous disorders may occasionally indicate an underlying plasma cell disorder. Xanthoma disseminatum is a disorder that usually develops in patients 25 years old or younger and is associated with an increased incidence of monoclonal gammopathy or multiple myeloma in adults (see Table 17-2). Generalized plane xanthomatosis has also been associated with multiple myeloma. Lesions in this disorder are yellow to yellow-brown flat plaques, and, when generalized, they typically involve the head, eyelids, neck, and upper trunk. Rarely, patients with multiple myeloma have an antilipoprotein antibody as their monoclonal protein, and this may result in an abnormal lipid profile and, occasionally, in the development of xanthomas.

Benign Hypergammaglobulinemic Purpura of Waldenström

This is characterized by flat, petechial or small purpuric lesions on the lower extremities in association with polyclonal hypergammaglobulinemia. New lesions may develop in cycles and may be preceded by a burning sensation. Most patients have an IgG anti-IgG rheumatoid factor that is not demonstrated by current standard rheumatoid factor testing. Some of these IgG rheumatoid factors have been shown by specialized tests to be monoclonal, and this may relate to the small but increased incidence of multiple myeloma or lymphoproliferative disorders in some patients after several years of disease. Both primary and secondary forms of this disease have been described. At least half the patients with primary disease in one series who were followed for 5 years developed evidence of an associated disease, occasionally malignant but usually autoimmune. Such autoimmune diseases include keratoconjunctivitis sicca, Sjögren's syndrome, lupus erythematosus (particularly anti-Ro [SS-A]-positive disease), undifferentiated connective tissue disease, or sarcoidosis.

Scleromyxedema

This is a type of generalized lichen myxedematosus (also known as papular mucinosis) that presents with coalescent erythematous to yellow papules and plaques (Figs 21-5 and 21-6). Usually located on the face, neck, and forearms, these plaques may mimic the facial features of

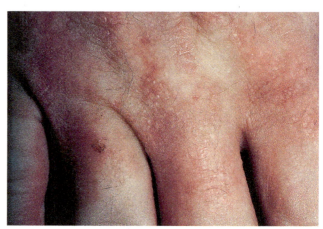

FIGURE 21-5 ■ Multiple small papules in a linear array in a patient with papular mucinosis and paraproteinemia.

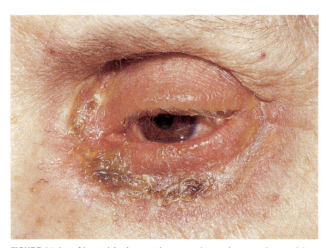

FIGURE 21-4 ■ Necrobiotic xanthogranuloma in a patient with a paraproteinemia.

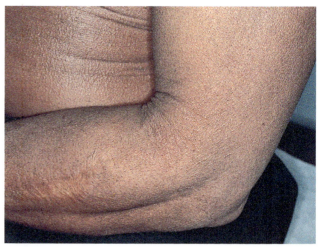

FIGURE 21-6 ■ Multiple papules that have formed linear bands in a patient with lichen myxedematosus.

acromegaly or generalized myxedema. These patients may suffer from intense pruritus. They may also have esophageal dysmotility, myopathic changes, arthritis, neuropathy, central nervous system disease, or cardiac disease.

Patients with scleromyxedema frequently have an associated monoclonal gammopathy and may have a characteristic finding on serum protein electrophoresis of a "slow γ-region" migrating protein (extreme migration toward the negative electrode). Evidence suggests that this unusual migration pattern is not caused by a response to a common antigen, with different idiotype characteristics from patient to patient. Some studies found that sera from these patients produced a mucin-stimulatory effect on fibroblasts in vitro, and one study suggested that the abnormal protein was not the stimulatory factor. Despite the frequent (albeit not obligatory) presence of monoclonal protein in this disease, associated lymphoproliferative malignancies are rare.

Other Disorders

Other cutaneous diseases may have a rare, but apparently real, association with monoclonal gammopathies due to plasma cell dyscrasias or lymphoproliferative diseases. Such diseases include scleredema adultorum, erythema elevatum diutinum, subcorneal pustular dermatosis, pyoderma gangrenosum, some forms of acquired angioedema (patients can develop a monoclonal protein with anti-C1 esterase activity, for example), and, more rarely, dermatomyositis, dermatitis herpetiformis, cutaneous T-cell lymphoma, and Kaposi's sarcoma. Although IgG paraprotein-associated disorders are usually the most common, some of these disorders (erythema elevatum diutinum, subcorneal pustular dermatosis, and pyoderma gangrenosum) appear to have a strong IgA association, which is as yet unexplained. Dermatitis herpetiformis is frequently associated with polyclonal IgA gammopathy, but the increased incidence of malignancies in this disease is due to enteropathy-associated T-cell lymphoma, not myeloma. Spicule-like hyperkeratosis (follicular > nonfollicular) has been reported as a rare but distinctive cutaneous finding in patients with myeloma (Fig. 21-7), as has crystal-storing histiocytosis; the latter is also associated with lymphoproliferative disorders. Although skin involvement is rare in crystal-storing histiocytosis, the histologic findings are distinctive: macrophages with thin crystalloid structures in the cytoplasm, consisting of phagocytosed crystals of immunoglobulins. Additional rarely reported associations include possible increased sensitivity to developing halogenoderma, pityriasis rotunda, and linear IgA bullous dermatosis.

Treatment

The therapy of these disorders is aimed largely at controlling the underlying disease process when present. Multiple myeloma usually responds to thalidomide, lenalidomide, or bortezomib (a proteasome inhibitor), either alone or in combination with weekly systemic corticosteroids. Autologous hematopoietic stem cell transplantation is considered the standard of care for patients under the age of 60 years after they have responded to medical therapy. Treatment of POEMS syndrome in younger healthy individuals is currently by stem cell transplantation. In older or infirm patients melphalan and corticosteroids can be helpful.

Primary cutaneous marginal zone lymphoma (formerly cutaneous plasmacytoma) is treated with radiation, intralesional corticosteroids, and/or chemotherapy. Patients with Schnitzler syndrome have been reported to respond to anakinra therapy. Therapy of xanthoma disseminatum is often ineffective, but cutaneous lesions may respond if systemic cytotoxic therapy is otherwise indicated. Individual lesions may respond to cryotherapy. The therapy of hypergammaglobulinemic purpura in the absence of a lymphoproliferative disorder is largely symptomatic. Necrobiotic xanthogranuloma may respond to therapy with alkylating agents such as melphalan, but the benefits must outweigh the risks, including the long-term risk of leukemogenesis. Scleromyxedema is usually treated with corticosteroids or intravenous immunoglobulin therapy, but frequently relapses. Autologous hematopoietic stem cell transplantation has been reported as successful in a number of patients with scleromyxedema, but the durability of the response is uncertain.

AMYLOIDOSIS

Amyloidosis is a general term used to describe a group of conditions characterized by the extracellular deposition of an abnormal protein that has a specific set of staining properties and a fibrillar ultrastructure.

Pathogenesis

The amyloidoses are now understood to be a subset of misfolded protein disorders. Loss of function misfolding disorders are due to elimination of a needed protein because of clearing of the protein (e.g., cystic fibrosis). Gain-of-toxic function results from the inability to successfully clear misfolded proteins as in the amyloidoses. In amyloidosis, the misfolded proteins form toxic oligomers en route to fibril formation, and these oligomers seem to trigger much of the organ dysfunction by triggering oxidative stress and inflammatory pathways. The body has a number of specialized molecules—chaperones, disaggregases, heat shock

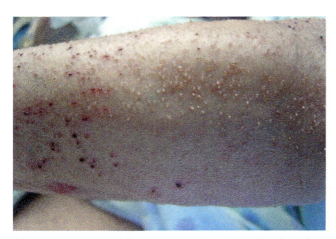

FIGURE 21-7 ■ Multiple follicular keratotic lesions in this patient with myeloma.

proteins—which are vital to the normal transport of molecules from the endoplasmic reticulum through the cell membrane, and during transit to final destination. These pathways are overwhelmed in amyloidosis syndromes. Although most proteins in humans and other species are synthesized in an α-helical structure, amyloid proteins are among the few that are ultimately assembled in a much less biodegradable β-pleated sheet structure.

There are 27 known precursor proteins for amyloid, and at least eight known proteins that can serve as precursors for amyloid fibril deposition in the skin: (1) light chain monoclonal protein; (2) serum protein A; (3) β_2-microglobulin; (4) plasma transthyretin (prealbumin); (5) gelsolin; (6) cystatin C; (7) keratin or keratin-related proteins; and (8) injected insulin. The pattern of amyloid deposition correlates with the precursor protein type, which in turn depends on the underlying syndrome.

Clinical Manifestations (Table 21-1)

Light-Chain-Related Systemic Amyloidoses

The age-adjusted incidence of light-chain-related amyloidosis is between 5.1 and 12.8 per million person-years, accounting for 1300 to 3200 new cases annually in the United States. This is roughly one-fifth the incidence of multiple myeloma, and about the same incidence as Hodgkin's disease or Ph1-positive chronic granulocytic leukemia. Men account for 60% to 65% of cases, and only 1% of patients are under the age of 20 years. Fatigue and weight loss are the most common presenting symptoms. Light-headedness is also common, and may be secondary to nephrotic syndrome with volume contraction, to cardiac amyloidosis with low stroke volume, or to autonomic neuropathy with orthostatic hypotension.

The light-chain-derived systemic amyloidoses (amyloid light-chain fibril, or AL) occur in the setting of primary systemic amyloidosis and an associated plasma cell dyscrasia. True myeloma-associated amyloidosis is uncommon. Even when patients with AL amyloidosis have >10% plasma cells in the bone marrow, lytic bone lesions, myeloma cast nephropathy, and anemia secondary to marrow replacement are rare. It is assumed that all AL fibril-type systemic amyloidoses are caused by a monoclonal protein. Blood or urine immunofixation studies for monoclonal immunoglobulin or light-chain protein are positive in nearly 90% of cases, and both should be obtained if AL amyloidosis is suspected. Even in those instances in which no monoclonal abnormality can be detected, the problem is thought to be one of test sensitivity. More recently, the serum-free light-chain assay, which is nearly 100% sensitive, has improved diagnostic accuracy; in contrast to immunofixation, it is a quantitative assay. Subcutaneous fat aspiration is positive in 70% to 80% of patients with AL amyloidosis.

The reported incidence of cutaneous lesions in AL-derived systemic amyloidosis ranges from 10% to 40%. The most common lesions include purpura, papules, plaques, and nodules, but bullous eruptions (sometimes mimicking porphyria cutanea tarda or epidermolysis bullosa acquisita), scleroderma-like cutaneous infiltration, pigmentary changes, nail dystrophies, acral localized acquired cutis laxa, and alopecia have been reported. Purpura is most common (Figs 21-8 and 21-9) and is usually attributed to amyloid infiltration of the dermal blood vessels and supporting tissue, resulting in problems with

TABLE 21-1 Characteristics of Systemic Amyloidoses

Feature	Light-Chain-Related AL	Secondary/Reactive AA	Dialysis-Associated A β-Microglobulin	ATTR
Underlying disease	Almost always? associated with monoclonal protein	Usually associated with chronic infection or inflammatory disease	Usually occurs after long-term dialysis	Senile due to wild-type transthyretin. Familial due to mutations in transthyretin
Major clinical presentation	Cardiac, renal, gastrointestinal, carpal tunnel	Renal	Chronic arthralgias, destructive arthropathy, carpal tunnel syndrome	Senile ATTR: cardiomyopathy most common. Mutant ATTR: familial polyneuropathy or cardiomyopathy syndromes most common
Renal	Expected	Expected	Already on dialysis	
Hepatic	Usually	Usually	Uncommon	
Spleen	Often	Often	Uncommon	
Cardiac	Frequently impaired	Deposits common, but impairment very rare	Uncommon	
Periarticular	Occurs, carpal tunnel common	Rare	Expected, carpal tunnel common	
Neurologic	Common, often autonomic	Rare		
Macroglossia	12%-15%	No	One case reported	
Cutaneous findings	Clinical lesions 10%-40%, subclinical deposits frequent	Clinical lesions rare, subclinical deposits frequent	Clinical skin lesions rare, subclinical deposits occasional	Syndrome-dependent: clinical lesions occur in several, subclinical deposits expected in some syndromes

AL, Amyloid light chain; *AA*, amyloid A; *ATTR*, transthyretin (TTR) amyloidosis.

hemostasis following mild trauma. Rare causes of hemorrhage in AL amyloidosis include depletion of factor X by adsorption to splenic amyloid deposits, and acquired von Willebrand syndrome, apparently secondary to the plasma cell dyscrasia. Deposition of AL amyloid is most prominent on the upper body. Stroking or pinching the skin may induce purpura in lesions in these areas, and spontaneous periorbital hemorrhage is commonly seen following Valsalva-like maneuvers (coughing or vomiting) or a dependently positioned head. Papules and plaques are most often yellow to skin colored, nonpruritic, and frequently hemorrhagic. A waxy or translucent character in such papules is strongly suggestive of AL-type amyloid deposition. Papular deposition of amyloid is most common on the central face, eyelids, lips, tongue, buccal mucosa, postauricular areas, neck, and intertriginous zones. There are reports of acquired cutis laxa, often presenting as bulbous soft distal enlargement of the fingertips, as well as pseudoxanthma elasticum changes, with altered elastin histology or function, Rarely, tissue infiltration by amyloid may present as proptosis, ophthalmoplegia, periarticular soft tissue enlargement, or skeletal muscle pseudohypertrophy. Infiltration of lacrimal or parotid glands may cause keratoconjunctivitis sicca or may mimic Sjögren's syndrome. Deposits of AL amyloid can involve almost any internal structure, but the most characteristic associated features include peripheral neuropathy, carpal tunnel syndrome, orthostatic hypotension as a result of autonomic neuropathy, macroglossia, congestive heart failure (secondary to a restrictive cardiomyopathy), and nephrotic syndrome.

Reactive or Secondary Amyloidosis

Acquired systemic amyloidosis of the amyloid A (AA) protein fibril type is usually seen in association with a chronic inflammatory process, such as rheumatoid arthritis, leprosy, tuberculosis, syphilis, chronic osteomyelitis, or chronic inflammatory bowel disease. It may also be associated with certain long-standing cutaneous disorders that may be the source of chronic inflammation, such as decubitus ulcers, stasis ulcers, thermal burns, neglected basal cell carcinomas, hidradenitis suppurativa, dystrophic epidermolysis bullosa, psoriasis and psoriatic arthritis, and reactive arthritis (previously referred to as Reiter's disease). In the United States, secondary amyloidosis is rare because chronic inflammation secondary to infection is rare. Amyloid fibrils in this setting are derived from chronically elevated serum protein A, an apolipoprotein. This protein increases with inflammation, during pregnancy, and with advancing age. Any organ may be involved, but significant hepatic, splenic, and renal infiltration is most typical. Also, unlike systemic AL fibril disease, cardiac infiltration in AA fibril disease almost never results in cardiac dysfunction.

Deposition of amyloid in the skin is common in AA amyloidosis and may be detected by subcutaneous fat aspiration or, less often, by blind skin biopsy. However, clinically apparent skin lesions are rare. Macular purpura is one of the few reported manifestations. The rarity of skin lesions in this syndrome distinguishes it from AL amyloidosis. The presence of cutaneous lesions in a patient with systemic amyloidosis strongly suggests AL rather than AA amyloidosis.

Hemodialysis-Related Amyloidosis

Hemodialysis-related amyloidosis is dependent on β_2-microglobulin. This single polypeptide chain (length 100 amino acids) is normally present on all cell membranes, except erythrocytes and trophoblastic cells, and is the constant β-chain portion of the class I histocompatibility antigen molecule. The β_2-microglobulin molecule is constantly shed from cell membranes, and like many proteins it is freely filtered through the glomerulus and reabsorbed in the proximal tubule, where it is catabolized. In renal failure this major catabolic pathway is lost, and serum levels rise. Most β_2-microglobulin-associated amyloidosis occurs in patients dialyzed for 8 or more years. The amyloid is deposited primarily in perineural and periarticular structures, joints, bones, skin, and subcutaneous tissue. Patients typically present with shoulder periarthritis, carpal tunnel syndrome, and flexor tenosynovitis of the hands. The incidence of carpal tunnel syndrome in this group ranges from 2% to 31%. Other major clinical manifestations of this deposition are chronic arthralgias and destructive arthropathy. Less frequent sites of involvement

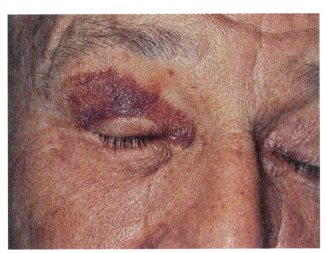

FIGURE 21-8 ■ "Pinch purpura" in a patient with multiple myeloma. This represents amyloidosis of the skin.

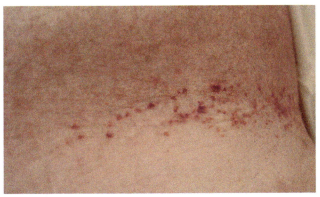

FIGURE 21-9 ■ Widespread purpura due to amyloidosis occurring as a late manifestation of myeloma.

include the rectal mucosa, liver, spleen, kidneys, prostate, and blood vessels. Macroglossia is rare. In one series, 16 of 16 skin biopsy specimens were negative for amyloid, but subcutaneous abdominal fat aspiration was positive in nine of 25 (36%) of these patients. Subcutaneous amyloid masses (amyloidomas) have been reported. The incidence of this complication of chronic dialysis appears to be declining due to changes in dialysis membrane function.

Senile and Mutant Transthyretin (TTR) Amyloidoses (ATTR)

TTR, long known as prealbumin, is a large tetrameric molecule which transports both retinol and thyroid T4 hormone. Amyloid protein can be derived both from the wild-type molecule (senile systemic amyloidosis) and from more than 100 known mutations (familial ATTR, mostly as familial amyloid polyneuropathy, familial amyloid cardiomyopathy [FAC], and central nervous system-selective amyloidoses). In developed countries, light-chain amyloidosis is the most common form, and ATTR in wild and familial forms are next; amyloidosis due to serum protein A elevation secondary to chronic infectious or inflammatory states is very uncommon. Wild-type or senile systemic amyloidosis (SSA) usually presents as late-onset sporadic cardiomyopathy, which may affect as many as 15% of men >80 years of age, and may present by age 60 years in some. Familial syndromes of amyloidosis due to mutation of TTR typically present much earlier, at 20 to 30 years of age for some of the polyneuropathy forms.

Familial Syndromes of Systemic Amyloidosis

Most familial syndromes of amyloidosis are now known to result from mutations in transthyretin and comprise roughly 10% of systemic amyloidosis in developed countries. Inheritable autoinflammatory syndromes may result in AA-type amyloidosis. Familial Mediterranean fever, inherited in an autosomal recessive fashion, results in an AA fibril type of systemic amyloidosis that is secondary to the frequent inflammatory episodes characteristic of this disease. Patients with the Muckle–Wells syndrome, a familial disorder characterized by repeated febrile episodes, a painful urticarial eruption, and progressive deafness, develop an amyloid nephropathy due to AA fibril deposition. The remaining familial amyloidosis syndromes that may cause skin lesions are rare. Gelsolin (an actin-modulating protein) is now known to be the fibril source in hereditary gelsolin amyloidosis (AGel amyloidosis). Cutis laxa is a principal clinical manifestation of this disease, along with skin fragility and intracutaneous bleeding. In Iceland there is a hereditary cerebral hemorrhagic disease secondary to the deposition of amyloid fibrils derived from cystatin C, a proteinase inhibitor. In 12 of 12 patients with this disorder who were tested, prominent subclinical cutaneous deposition of cystatin C-derived amyloid was demonstrated by light microscopy of punch biopsy specimens.

Skin-Limited Amyloidoses

A variety of primary cutaneous amyloidoses have been described, including lichen amyloidosis; macular amyloidosis; biphasic amyloidosis; and amyloidoses of the anosacral, bullous, poikiloderma-like, and dyschromic types. These syndromes are seen uncommonly in the United States, lichen amyloidosis being seen the most frequently. Patients with lichen amyloidosis develop pruritic, hyperkeratotic, skin-colored or hyperpigmented papules, particularly on the anterior lower extremities, although other areas may be involved. Those with macular amyloidosis have pruritic, oval, grayish-brown macules that may coalesce to rippled or reticular hyperpigmented patches on the lower extremities or back. Patients with both macular and papular lesions are sometimes classified as having biphasic amyloidosis, but macular, biphasic, and lichen amyloidoses probably represent a continuum of the same process. These cutaneous amyloidoses are thought to have a keratin protein as the amyloid fibril precursor and are considered an amyloid keratin (AK) protein type of amyloidosis. The biopsy specimens in these disorders show distinctive changes that aid in distinguishing them from systemic amyloidosis. Variants, such as poikilodermatous or vitiliginous amyloidoses, have been reported; these may develop early in life and may be associated with short stature or light sensitivity (e.g., amyloidosis cutis dyschromica). Familial syndromes of lichen amyloidosis have also been reported. Familial primary localized cutaneous amyloidosis is an autosomal dominant disorder associated with chronic pruritus and AK amyloid deposition in the dermis. This syndrome is associated with missense mutations in the oncostatin M-specific receptor β gene. Several reports now exist of a familial syndrome of multiple endocrine neoplasia type 2a associated with lichen amyloidosis.

Localized amyloid AK deposition may occur around or within a number of cutaneous growths, including actinic keratoses, basal cell carcinomas, Bowen's disease (a form of in situ squamous cell carcinoma), and seborrheic keratoses. Patients undergoing psoralen–ultraviolet A light treatment also may have subclinical cutaneous amyloid deposition, presumably of the AK type.

Although nodular (tumefactive) cutaneous amyloidosis is also considered to be a form of primary cutaneous amyloidosis, it is not the result of AK disease. Amyloid deposition in nodular cutaneous amyloidosis is thought to derive from a light chain precursor produced at the site by surrounding clonally restricted plasma cells. This type of amyloidosis presents as nodules on the face, extremities, trunk, or genitalia. These nodules are usually skin colored and frequently have overlying epidermal atrophy or features resembling anetoderma. The mean age at diagnosis is 55 years, with a range of 20 to 87 years, and there is no gender predilection. Patients with nodular cutaneous amyloidosis require regular follow-up because some may develop systemic amyloidosis. Initial reports suggested a 50% progression rate to systemic amyloidosis, but more recent data suggest that the rate is less than 10%. Local light chain production and conversion to AL amyloid should not result in a detectable serum or urine monoclonal protein; its presence should suggest the need for further work-up and close follow-up.

A second form of skin-limited nodular amyloidosis may develop at sites of repetitive subcutaneous insulin injection, with insulin serving as the precursor protein for amyloid. In addition to recognizing its cause, recognition of this syndrome is also important because it may lead to poor glucose control despite increasing doses of insulin, and risk of hypoglycemia if the higher dose is now administered to a normal skin site. Given 20 earlier and 52 recently reported cases, this should always be considered in the differential diagnosis of nodules in diabetic patients in typical areas of insulin administration.

Differential Diagnosis

The differential diagnosis for systemic amyloidoses depends on the syndrome, but AL amyloidosis should always be considered in the differential diagnosis of cephalad-distributed waxy papules or unexplained hemorrhage induced by mild trauma. Patients with the AA or familial syndromes of amyloid frequently have no specific cutaneous amyloid lesions. Lichen and macular amyloidosis may be confused with localized pigmentary disorders, lichen simplex chronicus, notalgia paresthetica, and prurigo nodularis.

Histopathologic Findings

Skin Biopsy

A biopsy of clinical lesions in AL-derived systemic amyloidosis should provide diagnostic evidence of amyloid deposition. Amyloid deposits are usually located in the superficial dermis and dermal vessels. Epidermal atrophy (or at least the loss of rete ridges) is an associated finding. Congo red staining with green birefringence under polarized light is the most specific stain for amyloid, although other stains, such as methyl violet, crystal violet, or thioflavine T, may be more sensitive.

Despite the rarity of clinical lesions in AA fibril-type (secondary) systemic amyloidosis, a biopsy of apparently normal skin may yield evidence of amyloid deposition. The pattern of amyloid deposition differs from that seen with the AL type. The deposits are usually deep in the dermis and subcutaneous fat, and are occasionally in a perivascular or periappendageal distribution. Amyloid deposition in hemodialysis-related amyloidosis and in several familial amyloid syndromes (dependent on transthyretin, gelsolin, or cystatin C) has been similar to that described for AA fibril-type amyloidosis. As discussed previously, subcutaneous fat pad aspiration is frequently positive in AL, AA, and perhaps other systemic amyloidoses, but this test requires experience to interpret and to avoid overstaining the tissue with Congo red.

Lichen amyloidosis and macular amyloidosis have a biopsy appearance unlike that of AL or AA amyloidosis. Amyloid is deposited in the papillary tips, with rete ridge elongation and sparing of dermal blood vessels. The changes in macular amyloidosis are sometimes minimal. Cutaneous tumor-associated amyloidosis is a pathologic curiosity; its recognition as an entity is important primarily to prevent its misinterpretation as evidence of a more serious amyloid disorder. The cutaneous deposits in nodular cutaneous amyloidosis are localized to the nodules. Extensive dermal and subcutaneous deposits within the lesions are typical, as is blood vessel wall infiltration. Plasma cells are usually prominent; giant cells and focal calcification may be seen.

Subcutaneous Fat Aspiration

Subcutaneous abdominal fat aspiration may be helpful in confirming a diagnosis of systemic amyloidosis in patients with AL, AA, senile ATTR, or some familial amyloid syndromes. However, in the absence of laser microdissection with mass spectrometry of any amyloid present on the slide, it is not specific. AL, AA, and familial ATTR may each involve the kidneys; AL, senile (wild-type ATTR), and familial ATTR frequently result in cardiac dysfunction, AL and senile ATTR both involve carpal tunnel, and AL and familial ATTR syndromes may cause neuropathy. Wild-type ATTR can induce a sporadic late-onset cardiomyopathy that may affect up to 15% of men >80 years of age, and is not rare beginning with men >60 years of age. The familial syndromes of ATTR that result from any of at least 100 mutations in transthyretin can result in cardiomyopathy in patients as young as 20 years of age. Even the presence of a gammopathy may be misleading. In one series, 20 of 81 patients with ATTR had a monoclonal protein, making a misdiagnosis of AL-type amyloid a possibility. The combination of ATTR and MGUS is increased in black patients because of an increase in the Val122I transthyretin mutation, which leads to cardiomyopathy and an incidence of MGUS by age 80 years nearly twice that of white individuals. Incidence of amyloid on subcutaneous fat aspirate is 80% to 90% in AL, perhaps 50% in AA, 67% in FAC-type ATTR, and 14% in SSA (wild-type) ATTR. Biopsy of the abdominal fat pad to a depth and width of 1.5 cm may increase the finding of amyloid deposition to roughly 75% in some types of ATTR.

Evaluation

The evaluation of a patient with biopsy-proven cutaneous amyloid deposition must be directed by the setting. The presence or absence of clinical lesions, the site sampled (lesional or nonlesional skin, subcutaneous fat), the presence of associated systemic findings, and the specific histologic features seen on the biopsy specimen are all important in determining the most appropriate evaluation for an individual patient. For example, the presence of waxy hemorrhagic facial papules with histologic features of epidermal atrophy, significant dermal amyloid deposition, and amyloid infiltration of vessel walls is nearly diagnostic of AL-type systemic amyloidosis. In such a case, a thorough search for an associated plasma cell dyscrasia is mandatory. By contrast, the presence of skin-colored pruritic papules on the lower extremity that, when sampled, show features of papillary tip amyloid deposition, sparing of vessels, and rete ridge elongation would be sufficient for the diagnosis of lichen amyloidosis and would obviate the need to search for a systemic cause. Currently, the gold standard to establish the type of amyloid involvement involves the use of laser microdissection of a tissue section, followed by mass spectrometry of the dissected material.

Treatment

The prognosis and treatment of systemic AL amyloidosis is now focused on three indicators. One point is assigned for each of the following: serum N-terminal pro-brain natriuretic peptide (NT-proBNP) ≥1800 pg/mL, serum troponin T ≥0.025 ng/mL, and the difference between involved and uninvolved serum-free light chains >180 mg/L. Median survival in months by total point score of 0 to 3 is as follows: 94.1, 40.3, 14, and 5.8. Stem cell transplantation (SCT) offers up to 25% 10-year survival, and up to 52% 10-year survival for complete responders, but only 20% of patients qualify. Patients not qualifying for SCT may benefit from melphalan-dexamethasone, cyclophosphamide-thalidomide/lenalidomide-dexamethasone or bortezomib-based regimens.

Familial ATTR syndromes have been treated with liver transplantation to replace the mutant TTR protein with wild type, but this has appreciable risk and limited availability. Tafamidis is a kinetic transthyretin stabilizer that works to prevent dissociation of the tetramer; it is available in Europe but not approved by Food and Drug Administration. Diflunisal, a salicylate, is thought by some to help in mitigating familial ATTR, but has not reached phase III trial status.

The therapy of AA (reactive) systemic amyloidosis is directed toward treating or eliminating the underlying disorder leading to chronic inflammation. Colchicine can prevent or greatly diminish attacks and AA amyloid deposition in patients with familial Mediterranean fever and some other autoinflammatory syndromes. The treatment of lichen and macular amyloidosis is often unsatisfactory. Nonetheless, attempts should be made to control the pruritus, and occasional good results have been reported with the use of topical or intralesional corticosteroid therapy, corticosteroid-impregnated tape, topical pramoxine, topical retinoic acid, topical dimethyl sulfoxide, and systemic retinoid. Treatment of nodular cutaneous amyloidosis includes monitoring for development of a serum gammopathy, along with usually local measures such as excision, corticosteroid injection, or lesional radiotherapy to interrupt the local light chain production.

SUGGESTED READINGS

Appiah YE, Onumah N, Wu H, Elenitsas R, Jammes W. Multiple myeloma-associated amyloidosis and acral localized acquired cutis laxa. J Am Acad Dermatol 2008;58(Suppl. 2):S32–3.

Argula RG, Strange C, Budisavljevic MN. Multiorgan system dysfunction in the chylomicronemia syndrome. J Intensive Care Med 2014;29(3):175–8.

Arita K, South AP, Hans-Filho G, Sakuma TH, Lai-Cheong J, Clements S, et al. Oncostatin M receptor-beta mutations underlie familial primary localized cutaneous amyloidosis. Am J Hum Genet 2008;82(1):73–80.

Blancas-Mejia LM, Ramirez-Alvarado M. Systemic amyloidoses. Annu Rev Biochem 2013;82:745–74.

Burnside NJ, Alberta L, Robinson-Bostom L, Bostom A. Type III hyperlipoproteinemia with xanthomas and multiple myeloma. J Am Acad Dermatol 2005;53(5 Suppl. 1):S281–4.

Colaco SM, Miller T, Ruben BS, et al. IgM-λ paraproteinemia with associated cutaneous lymphoplasmacytic infiltrate in a patient who meets diagnostic criteria for POEMS syndrome. J Am Acad Dermatol 2008;58(4):671–5.

D'Souza A, Theis JD, Vrana JA, Dogan A. Pharmaceutical amyloidosis associated with subcutaneous insulin and enfuvirtide administration. Amyloid 2014;21(2):71–5.

Dispenzieri A. POEMS syndrome. Blood Rev 2007;21(6):285–99.

Fine NM, Arruda-Olson AM, Dispenzieri A, Zeldenrust SR, Gertz MA, Kyle RA, et al. Yield of noncardiac biopsy for the diagnosis of transthyreting cardiac amyloidosis. Am J Cardiol 2014;113(10):1723–7.

Garcia T, Dafer R, Hocker S, et al. Recurrent strokes in two patients with POEMS syndrome and Castleman's disease. J Stroke Cerebrovasc Dis 2007;16(6):278–84.

Gertz MA. Immunoglobulin light chain amyloidosis: 2014 update on diagnosis, prognosis, and treatment. Am J Hematol 2014;89(12):1132–40.

Johnson SM, Connelly S, Fearns C, Powers ET, Kelly JW. The transthyretin amyloidoses: from delineating the molecular mechanism of aggregation linked to pathology to a regulatory-agency-approved drug. J Mol Biol 2012;421(2–3):185–203.

Kalajian AH, Waldman M, Knable AI. Nodular primary localized cutaneous amyloidosis after trauma: a case report and discussion of the rate of progression to systemic amyloidosis. J Am Acad Dermatol 2007;57(Suppl. 2):S26–9.

Kempf W, Kazakov DV, Mitteldorf C. Cutaneous lymphomas: an update. Part 2: B-cell lymphomas and related conditions. Am J Dermatopathol 2014;36(3):197–210.

Kiuru-Enari S, Keski-Oja J, Haltia M. Cutis laxa in hereditary gelsolin amyloidosis. Br J Dermatol 2005;152(2):250–7.

Kos CA, Ward JE, Malek K, Sanchorawaia V, Wright DG, O'Hara C, et al. Association of acquired von Willebrand syndrome with AL amyloidosis. Am J Hematol 2007;82(5):363–7.

Landgren O, Graubard BI, Katzmann JA, Kyle RA, Ahmadizadeh I, Clark R, et al. Racial disparities in the prevalence of monoclonal gammopathies: a population-based study of 12,482 persons from the National Health and Nutritional Examination Survey. Leukemia 2014;28(7):1537–42.

Lee MR, Choi HJ, Lee EB, Baek HJ. POEMS syndrome complicated by extensive arterial thromboses. Clin Rheumatol 2007;26(11):1989–92.

Leonard AL, Meehan SA, Ramsey D, et al. Cutaneous and systemic plasmacytosis. J Am Acad Dermatol 2007;56(Suppl. 2):S38–40.

Lipsker D, Rondeau M, Massard G, Grosshans E. The AESOP (adenopathy and extensive skin patch overlying a plasmacytoma) syndrome: report of 4 cases of a new syndrome revealing POEMS (polyneuropathy, organomegaly, endocrinopathy, monoclonal protein, and skin changes) syndrome at a curable stage. Medicine 2003;82(1):51–9.

Pock L, Stuchlik D, Hercogova J. Crystal storing histiocytosis of the skin associated with multiple myeloma. Int J Dermatol 2006;45(12):1408–11.

Retamozo S, Brito-Zeron P, Bosch X, Stone JH, Ramos-Casals M. Cryoglobulinemic disease. Oncology 2013;27(11):1098–105. 1110–6.

Rongioletti F, Patterson JW, Rebora A. The histological and pathogenetic spectrum of cutaneous disease in monoclonal gammopathies. J Cutan Pathol 2008;35(8):705–21.

Rongioletti F, Merlo G, Cinotti E, Fausti V, Cozzani E, Cribier B, et al. Scleromyxedema: a multicenter study of characteristics, comorbidities, course, and therapy in 30 patients. J Am Acad Dermatol 2013;69(1):66–72.

Rubinow A, Cohen AS. Skin involvement in generalized amyloidosis. Ann Intern Med 1978;88(6):781–5.

CHAPTER 22

CUTANEOUS MANIFESTATIONS OF THE HISTIOCYTOSES

Warren T. Goodman • Joshua R. Bradish • Terry L. Barrett

KEY POINTS

- Langerhans cell histiocytosis (LCH) is a clonal neoplastic disorder.
- LCH represents a spectrum of disease from asymptomatic skin-limited self-resolving lesions to systemic multisystem disease with high mortality.
- The majority of LCH cases harbor the BRAF V600E mutation, suggesting a potential role for BRAF inhibitors as treatment.
- LCH cells express S100, CD1a, CD207 (Langerin), and Fascin.
- The LCH-III trial confirmed a combination of vinblastine and prednisone as effective therapy for multisystem LCH both with and without risk of organ involvement.
- The cells in the non-LCH disorders express CD68 and CD163 and are always negative for Langerin (CD207).
- Juvenile xanthogranuloma is by far the most common of the non-LCH disorders.
- Leukemia, lymphoma, or a paraproteinemia are observed, sometimes frequently, in association with many of the non-LCH disorders.

INTRODUCTION

This chapter focuses on disorders commonly referred to as the "histiocytoses." These conditions can be unpredictable and present in a wide variety of ways, from harmless self-resolving skin lesions to systemic disease with a high mortality rate. According to the Writing Group of the Histiocyte Society in 1987, the histiocytoses can be broadly classified into three groups: Langerhans cell histiocytosis (LCH, class I), non-Langerhans cell histiocytosis (non-LCH, class II), and malignant histiocytosis (class III).

Histiocytes of cutaneous importance are derived from bone marrow CD34+ progenitor cells. These cells can mature into Langerhans cells (which reside in the epidermis) or alternatively into monocytes, macrophages, or dendritic cells (which reside in the dermis or deeper soft tissues). Lesional tissue of LCH is composed of LCH cells (which have a similar immunophenotype to Langerhans cells) while the non-LCH disorders are comprised of monocytes, macrophages, and/or dendritic cells.

The malignant histocytic disorders are very rare and most are aggressive. These will be discussed briefly at the conclusion of this chapter.

CLASS I: LANGERHANS CELL HISTIOCYTOSIS

Pathogenesis

The pathogenesis of LCH was uncertain until recently and there was much debate as to whether to classify LCH as a reactive or neoplastic condition. Studies have not shown evidence of an infectious etiology, and demonstrated elevated levels of multiple cytokines and interleukins in LCH are believed to be produced by the LCH inflammatory cell infiltrate rather than being responsible for causing the disease.

The recent major discovery of recurrent BRAF 600E mutations provides strong evidence to regard LCH as a neoplastic condition. Rare cases of familial LCH have been documented as well, and several older studies have demonstrated consistent clonality in LCH tissue. Given these later findings, LCH appears to represent a clonal neoplastic disorder.

Clinical Manifestations

Langerhans cell histiocytosis (LCH) is a rare disorder. Although it most commonly presents in children from ages 1 to 3 years it can occur at any age and is more common in males. The disease ranges from mild asymptomatic involvement of a single organ to severe, multiorgan system involvement with a high mortality. Given the wide range of disease expression, it is not surprising that the etiology of the disease was uncertain until later in the twentieth century, with four previously described syndromes found to represent overlapping clinical variants of LCH. These variants include Letterer–Siwe disease, Hand–Schuller–Christian disease, eosinophilic granuloma, and Hashimoto–Pritzker (congenital self-healing reticulohistiocytosis). While it is well recognized that LCH is one disease with a broad clinical spectrum, it is still helpful to note the older variants for perspective.

The acute form of LCH with diffuse and multisystem involvement was previously referred to as Letterer–Siwe disease. While it usually presents in infants less than 2 years of age, it can occur at any age. It presents as erythematous to skin-colored crusted 1 to 2-mm vesiculopustules,

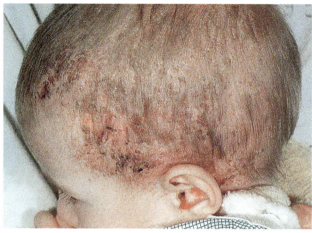

FIGURE 22-1 ■ Acute form of LCH (Letterer–Siwe disease). Erythematous, slightly scaly plaques are present on the scalp of this child.

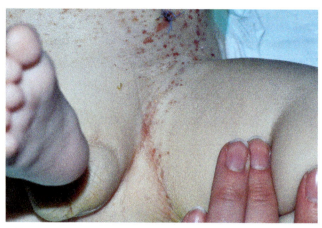

FIGURE 22-2 ■ Acute form of LCH (Letterer–Siwe disease). Petechial and minimally scaly eruption involving the bathing trunk distribution in this child. (Photo courtesy of Kristen Hook, MD.)

sometimes with secondary impetiginization, involving the scalp (Fig. 22-1), neck, intertriginous areas, and bathing trunk area (Fig. 22-2). Coalescing areas can become fissured, and petechia and purpura are also common. Soft tissue nodules can occur and rare presentations include ulcerative lesions and a papular form imitating molluscum contagiosum. Nail changes have also been described. The lungs, liver, spleen, and bone are commonly involved during the disease course. Lytic bone lesions are painful and primarily affect the cranium, vertebrae, and flat bones. So-called risk organ involvement includes the marrow (hematopoietic system), liver, lungs, and spleen. The prognosis of this form of LCH is variable. In those patients with risk organ involvement, especially in children less than 2 years of age, there is a high risk of mortality and systemic treatment is required.

Some patients present with a chronic and progressive form of disease. This form most often presents during childhood. Although LCH in adults is very uncommon, a chronic progressive course is a common mode of presentation in adults. Bone lesions are very frequent in this form (at least 80%) and approximately one-third of patients develop skin or mucous membrane lesions. LCH cells also infiltrate the posterior pituitary gland in approximately 30% of patients causing diabetes insipidus. Rarely, exophthalmos develops as a late finding. The triad of diabetes insipidus, bone lesions, and exophthalmos was previously referred to as Hand–Schuler–Christian disease. The skin lesions, favoring the scalp, upper trunk, and intertriginous areas, are initially similar to those described in the acute form, but ulcerating nodules can develop especially in the gingival and genital areas. Lesions can occur in crops, older lesions can become xanthomatous, and some may spontaneously regress leaving scars. The cranium is the most common site of bone involvement. Chronic otitis media is also common and can be a clue to the presence of cranial involvement. Although patients with this variant tend to have persistent or progressive disease, most will survive with treatment.

Eosinophilic granuloma is a localized variant of LCH with a striking predilection for the bone. It most commonly occurs in older children. The most common presentation is a single, often asymptomatic granulomatous cranial lesion, though any bone can be affected. The lung can also be involved, which may be confused with but likely overlaps with a separate variant of LCH, pulmonary Langerhans cell histiocytosis (PLCH). Development of PLCH has a strong association with cigarette smoking and usually occurs in young adult males, with a predilection for Caucasian men. In eosinophilic granuloma, skin and mucous membrane lesions are rare although mucocutaneous nodules can present in the periorofacial, genital, or perianal regions. Patients with this variant can have a prolonged course but have an overall good prognosis.

Congenital self-healing reticulocytosis (Hashimoto–Pritzker) presents in newborn infants as a solitary lesion, multiple, or diffuse 2-mm to several centimeter red-brown papules or nodules, which may, over time, ulcerate and crust. Vesicular lesions can also occur. The vast majority of cases are limited to the skin but, uncommonly, involvement of the liver, colon, marrow, and spleen have been described. The prognosis is excellent as the lesions spontaneously regress over 2 to 3 months. However, postlesional scars can be permanent sequelae.

Differential Diagnosis

The differential diagnosis is extensive and includes seborrheic dermatitis, eczema, diaper dermatitis, Darier's disease, urticaria pigmentosa, arthropod bites, scabies, leukemia, B- and T-cell lymphomas, and some of the non-Langerhans cell histiocytoses (especially indeterminate cell histiocytosis, benign cephalic histiocytosis, generalized eruptive histiocytosis, and xanthoma disseminatum). Ear involvement can easily be mistaken for chronic otitis media or otitis externa. As this is predominantly a disease of the pediatric population, it may not be suspected in adults leading to delay in diagnosis.

Histopathologic Findings

In the skin, an infiltrate of LCH cells is most often observed in the papillary dermis (Fig. 22-3), but can also present in a nodular fashion in the dermis or in a perifollicular distribution. The epidermis is also

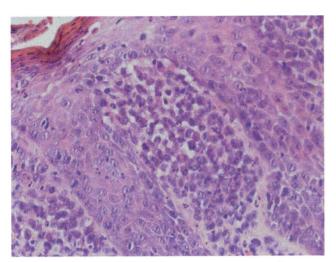

FIGURE 22-3 ■ High-power histopathology view of LCH (Letterer–Siwe disease) on an H&E (hematoxylin and eosin)-stained section. Note the aggregates of large LCH cells in the papillary dermal tips.

typically infiltrated by LCH cells, sometimes giving a pagetoid appearance. LCH cells are large, and often have a reniform-shaped nucleus with abundant eosinophilic cytoplasm. The infiltrate commonly occurs along with eosinophils (sometimes numerous) and lymphocytes, and sometimes scattered plasma cells, mast cells, and neutrophils. Giant cells can occasionally be observed. LCH cells are confirmed by their expression of CD1a, S100, and Langerin (CD207), and their typical lack of expression for CD68, CD163, and factor XIIIa.

It is important for the dermatopathologist, dermatologist and nondermatologist clinician to recognize that reactive conditions can occasionally result in collections of normal Langerhans cells developing in the skin, usually in the context of mixed lymphohistiocytic inflammation with eosinophils. Examples include nodular scabies, other arthropod bite reactions, and atopic dermatitis.

Evaluation

In patients with biopsy-confirmed disease, complete blood count, liver function tests, routine metabolic panel, chest X-ray, and bone films as clinically indicated should be obtained. Additional evaluation of the CNS and bone marrow may also be necessary depending on the patient signs and symptoms and the severity of the disease.

Treatment

For patients with mild single-system involvement, conservative treatment is most often appropriate, and sometimes no treatment is needed if the patient is not symptomatic. For the skin, narrow-band ultraviolet therapy, topical corticosteroids, topical nitrogen mustard, or imiquimod cream are common options. For isolated symptomatic bone lesions, curettage, intralesional corticosteroid therapy, nonsteroidal anti-inflammatory drugs, or radiation are typical choices.

The Histiocyte Society Evaluation and Treatment Guidelines note that systemic therapy is suggested in several settings. It is indicated for patients with multisystem LCH, or single-system LCH with multifocal bone lesions, with "special site" lesions (vertebral with intraspinous extension or craniofacial bone with soft tissue involvement), or with "CNS risk" lesions. A combination of vinblastine and prednisone is the typical regimen for multisystem LCH. There are various treatment options for nonresponding patients with treatment tailored to the patient's particular situation. The website for the Histiocyte Society (www.histiocytesociety.org) should be consulted for information on current trials and treatment guidelines.

CLASS II: NON-LANGERHANS CELL HISTIOCYTOSIS

Pathogenesis and Pathology

The disorders that comprise non-Langerhans cell histiocytosis (non-LCH) include a large group of conditions, many of which involve the skin. There is clinical overlap between several of these disorders, notably between benign cephalic histiocytosis, juvenile xanthogranuloma, and generalized eruptive histiocytoma. The historical exclusion of some other histiocytic disorders (i.e., granuloma annulare and sarcoidosis) from the category appears somewhat arbitrary.

Most of these conditions are rare and the pathogenesis is unknown. A few partial exceptions exist. A familial form of Rosai–Dorfman disease, caused by mutations in the SLC29A3 gene, is now generally accepted. In necrobiotic xanthogranuloma, there is such a strong association with monoclonal gammopathies that a link seems likely. Finally, there appears to be a genetic link between leukemia (acute myelomonocytic leukemia and chronic myelomonocytic leukemia) and some cases of generalized eruptive histiocytoma.

Histologically, all of the non-LCH disorders are composed of histiocytes that stain positive for CD68 or CD163, and with just rare exceptions are negative for S100 and CD1a. Specifically, indeterminate cell histiocytosis stains positive with CD1a and S100, and Rosai–Dorfman stains positive with S100. The lack of staining with CD1a and with S100 in the non-LCH disorders are important discriminators from LCH, which clinically can mimic some of the non-LCH disorders. Although there is significant histologic overlap between the non-LCH disorders, there are subtle histologic findings often unique to the various non-LCH disorders that can assist in diagnosis. The detailed specific histologic features of these disorders are beyond the scope of this chapter.

Clinical Manifestations

When learning and organizing these disorders, it is most useful to place them in categories. In this chapter (Table 22-1), we have categorized them as follows: (1) primarily skin limited, (2) frequently mixed skin and systemic findings, and (3) systemic findings with

TABLE 22-1 Class II: Non-Langerhans Cell Histiocytoses: Primarily Skin Limited

Disease and Frequency	Age/Sex	Cutaneous Lesions	Mucous Membranes	Systemic Findings	Prognosis/Treatment	Clinical Differential Diagnosis
Indeterminate cell histiocytosis: very rare	Adults, children, and infants	*Solitary nodular form* Soft red 1-cm nodule *Multiple papulonodular form* Widespread firm few mm to 1-cm dark red to brownish asymptomatic lesions	Rare corneal and conjunctival lesions	Uncommon, but death in several cases. Multiple cases associated with hematologic malignancies	Most patients are healthy with self-resolution so treatment is usually not needed. Watch for some patients with progressive course, and for possible hematologic malignancies	Urticaria pigmentosa, lymphomatoid papulosis, other papular non-LCH disorders, LCH
Benign cephalic histiocytosis: rare	6-12 months (rarely onset not until age 3 years)	Multiple 2-8-mm red to yellow-brown papules, often becoming confluent. Upper face, head initially, then upper trunk and limbs	No	Rare—diabetes insipidus reported in one patient	Self-resolving but exacerbations can occur	LCH, papular non-LCH disorders, urticaria pigmentosa
Progressive nodular histiocytosis: very rare	Children > adults	Progressive development of hundreds of lesions Most common: yellow-brown or -pink 2–10-mm papules, widespread with flexural sparing. Less common: 1-5-cm red-brown dermal nodules with overlying telangiectasia. Face may be heavily involved; ectropion and leonine facies may result	Conjunctival, oral, and laryngeal mucosa	Seldom	Usually otherwise healthy. Persistent or progressive treatment-resistant disease is common	Other papular non-LCH disorders, sarcoidosis, generalized papular granuloma annulare
Hereditary progressive mucinous histiocytosis: very rare	Begins in childhood or adolescence; mostly women	Few to numerous skin-colored to red-brown 1–5-mm papules or dome-shaped nodules. Symmetric, primarily face, hands, forearms, legs. Autosomal dominant inheritance	Spared	None	Slowly progressive cutaneous course. No specific therapy	Other papular non-LCH disorders, sarcoidosis, papular granuloma annulare
Generalized eruptive histiocytoma: very rare	Bimodal (young children <4 and adults 20–50)	Crops of multiple 3–10-mm red-brown or flesh-colored papules symmetrically arrayed on the face, trunk (Fig. 22-5), proximal limbs	Occasional	Rare	Lesions involute completely in several months leaving hyperpigmented macules. Recurrent crops of lesions are common before condition finally resolves. More dangerous forms of non-LCH have developed in patients with this disorder	LCH, urticaria pigmentosa, generalized papular granuloma annulare, other papular non-LCH disorders

Papular xanthoma: very rare	Children and adults with a biphasic onset	Can be either a single papule or multiple 2–15-mm yellow, yellow-pink papules or nodules. No confluence, no red-brown color. Trunk, proximal extremities most common followed by face, with sparing of flexural folds	Yes	No. Rare cases associated with mycosis fungoides	Spontaneous involution over 1–5 years in most cases, but can be progressive. Patients are usually normolipemic	JXG, eruptive xanthoma, Spitz nevus, fibrous histiocytoma
JXG/Giant cell reticulohistiocytoma: most common histiocytosis	Most cases arise from birth until 2 years. Occurs uncommonly in adults	Head and neck most commonly involved followed by upper torso and extremities. Large nodular form with one or two lesions is most common presentation (Fig. 22-4) Small nodular (micronodular) form with many lesions is less common. Lesions begin brown or red and quickly become yellow. Giant cell reticulohistiocytoma likely represents a variant of JXG with a solitary lesion on the head and unique histology	Tongue and oropharynx rare	Eye most common—usually the iris and unilateral. Lung second most commonly involved noncutaneous site. Other sites of involvement include liver, spleen, lung, bone, colon, ovaries, testes, kidney, pericardium, and muscle Can be associated with NF, juvenile myelomonocytic leukemia, or both. In children with both JXG and NF, the risk of myeloid leukemia is 20–32 times higher than normal	Usual course is spontaneous resolution of lesions within 3–6 years. Although rare, symptomatic systemic disease may prove fatal	Other papular non-LCH disorders, molluscum contagiosum, Spitz nevus

LCH, Langerhans cell histiocytosis; JXG, juvenile xanthogranuloma; NF, neurofibromatosis.

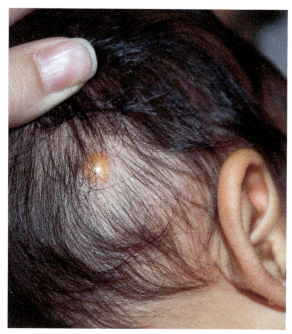

FIGURE 22-4 ■ Juvenile xanthogranuloma. Yellow dome-shaped papule on the scalp of a young child. (Photo courtesy of Kristen Hook, MD.)

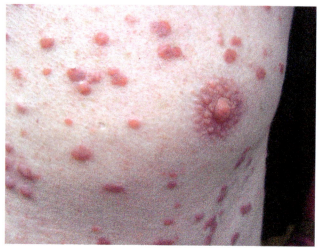

FIGURE 22-5 ■ Generalized eruptive histiocytomas. Erythematous to brown nodules on the trunk. (Photo courtesy of Jeffrey P. Callen, MD.)

infrequent or absent skin involvement. Table 22-1 provides the important features of these disorders allowing for quick comparisons.

Juvenile xanthogranuloma (JXG) is the prototypical non-LCH disorder, and is common (see Table 22-1). The other non-LCH disorders are rare. JXG presents routinely with skin lesions (Fig. 22-4), can present much less commonly with both mucous membrane lesions and systemic lesions affecting any organ, and can even lead to death in rare cases. JXG also has well-recognized associations with café-au-lait macules, neurofibromatosis type 1 and juvenile myelomonocytic leukemia. Therefore, a strong working knowledge of this disorder is a good starting place for understanding the other non-LCH conditions.

In many of the non-LCH disorders, leukemia, lymphoma, or a paraproteinemia can occasionally or frequently occur in association with the condition. These include generalized eruptive histiocytoma, indeterminate cell histiocytosis, juvenile xanthogranuloma, necrobiotic xanthogranuloma, Rosai–Dorfman, and hemophagocytic lymphohistiocytosis. Additionally, solid tumor malignancies are not uncommon in multicentric reticulohistiocytosis. The specifics are listed in Table 22-1.

Differential Diagnosis

Each of the non-LCH disorders has its own differential diagnosis, and these are briefly noted in Table 22-1. Diagnosis of these disorders requires an expert clinician with knowledge of the typical appearance and distribution of lesions.

Evaluation

Careful consideration of the appearance of the lesion(s), the distribution of the lesions, and attention to any associated systemic findings is the first step in appropriate evaluation of patients with histiocytic disorders. Although a clinical diagnosis can be strongly suspected, a skin biopsy is usually an important part of establishing a definitive diagnosis. Depending on the suspected disorder and the symptoms of the patient, various blood, serologic, bone, and urine studies may be necessary (Tables 22-2 and 22-3).

Treatment

For those disorders that are generally self-limiting, often no treatment is needed unless a lesion is causing physical impairment or is a significant cosmetic concern. For those that have associated symptomatic systemic lesions (i.e., a lesion involving the posterior pituitary causing diabetes insipidus), treatment may be required and is specific to the lesion and/or to the resulting problem (see Table 22-1). Additionally, for those patients with associated hematologic pathology (i.e., a paraproteinemia or lymphoproliferative disorder), clearly intensive hematologic subspecialty care directed at the particular problem will be required.

CLASS III: MALIGNANT HISTIOCYTOSIS

The true malignant histiocytoses are very rare. These include Langerhans cell sarcoma, histiocytic sarcoma, interdigitating dendritic cell sarcoma, and follicular dendritic cell sarcoma. With the exception of follicular dendritic cell sarcoma, which is rather indolent, these are very aggressive malignancies with a high mortality. Obviously, these patients require expert subspecialty hematologic care.

TABLE 22-2 Frequently Mixed Skin and Systemic Findings

Disease and Frequency	Age/Sex	Cutaneous Lesions	Mucous Membranes	Systemic Findings	Prognosis/Treatment	Differential Diagnosis
Necrobiotic xanthogranuloma: rare	17–60 years	100% cutaneous involvement. Yellow indurated papules, nodules, or plaques. Telangiectases, atrophy, and ulceration with subsequent scarring are common. Periorbital most common then trunk, face, extremities	Yes—conjunctiva	IgG monoclonal gammopathy in at least 80%. Hepatosplenomegaly, leukopenia, cryoglobulinemia occur, less common multiple myeloma	Skin lesions difficult to treat. Corticosteroids and chlorambucil described as most effective treatment. Presence and aggressiveness of plasma cell dyscrasia/multiple myeloma determine prognosis	Necrobiosis lipoidica, plane xanthomas, xanthelasma, other non-LCH disorders, sarcoidosis, rheumatoid nodules, granuloma annulare
Multicentric reticulohistiocytosis: rare	Usually adult Caucasian women 30–40 years	100% with cutaneous involvement. 2 mm–2-cm flesh, pink, red, brown, or yellow papules or nodules on fingers, ears, head, hands, and articular areas of extremities. Can form a "coral bead" appearance (Fig. 22-6)	Yes, ~50% with oral, pharyngeal and nasal mucosal lesions	Symmetric, chronic, destructive arthritis especially in hands, wrists, knees, which can progress to arthritis mutilans. Cartilage destruction of nose and ears can lead to disfigured face. Rare involvement of many other organs. One-third have hypercholesterolemia. Up to 28% have associated malignancy (gastric, ovarian, breast, uterine, cervical). Increased risk of autoimmune disease	Most have spontaneous remission in 5–10 years, but often left with significant disability. Medications usually given in combination (i.e., NSAIDs and glucocorticoids or methotrexate with NSAIDs, anti-TNF, glucocorticoids, bisphosphonates, or cyclophosphamide)	Rheumatoid nodules, granuloma annulare, dermatomyositis, other papular non-LCH disorders, sarcoidosis
Rosai–Dorfman: rare	Any age—but age 10–30 years most common	Skin limited disease increasingly recognized. In the systemic form, cutaneous lesions occur in only ~10% and are usually multiple. Skin is the most common extranodal site (usually face or eyelids). Lesions are red, brown, or yellow macules, papules, nodules, and plaques	Rare	In patients with systemic form, massive, painless, bilateral cervical lymphadenopathy; other nodal basins may be involved. Skin, eye, upper respiratory tract, salivary glands, CNS, and bone most common extranodal sites. Fever, anemia, neutrophilia, polyclonal hypergammaglobulinemia are common associated findings. Elevated ferritin levels can also occur	Spontaneous remission is common, but a protracted course in many patients. Patients with associated immune abnormalities, disseminated nodal disease, kidney or respiratory tract disease have unfavorable prognosis. Up to 7% mortality risk	For skin lesions: other non-LCH papular disorders, sarcoidosis, papular granuloma annulare. For nodal disease: infectious disorders, lymphoma, leukemia, metastasis, Kikuchi's disease
Xanthoma disseminatum: rare	Any age though majority before age 25	100% cutaneous involvement. Hundreds of small red-brown papules, symmetric, evolving to yellow-brown and coalescing into plaques. Face, flexural, and intertriginous areas favored	Yes, in 40–60% with upper airway and oral mucosa commonly affected. Also corneal and conjunctival lesions	Upper respiratory tract lesions can cause hoarseness and dyspnea. CNS lesions (hypothalamus and pituitary stalk) cause diabetes insipidus in 40%. Rare monoclonal gammopathies, thyroid disorders, seizures, growth retardation	Diabetes insipidus is often mild and may self resolve but is sensitive to vasopressin. Skin lesions resolve with scarring. Rare mortality in severe progressive cases with organ failure and CNS involvement	Other papular non-LCH disorders, eruptive xanthoma

LCH, Langerhans cell histiocytosis; anti-TNF, antitumor necrosis factor; NSAIDs, nonsteroidal anti-inflammatory drugs; CNS, central nervous system.

TABLE 22-3 Systemic Findings with Infrequent or Absent Skin Involvement

Disease and Frequency	Age/Sex	Cutaneous Lesions	Mucous Membranes	Systemic Findings	Prognosis and Treatment	Differential Diagnosis
HLH: rare. Primary cause (genetic): Familial HLH (most cases due to perforin abnormality), Chediak–Higashi syndrome, Griscelli syndrome type 2, and X-linked lymphoproliferative syndrome. Secondary cause (acquired): infection (i.e., EBV), malignancy-associated (T-cell lymphomas), macrophage activation syndrome (e.g., in Still's disease)	In primary: 0–2 years. In secondary: any age	20% in one series nodules or purpuric macules most frequent. May ulcerate. Generalized or localized edema may be seen	No	Caused by abnormal high levels of cytokine release by T cells leading to activation of macrophages with subsequent cytophagocytosis by macrophages. Symptoms/signs include fever, elevated ferritin, constitutional symptoms, cytopenias and coagulopathy, hypertriglyceridemia, hepatomegaly, splenomegaly, lymphadenopathy, less commonly renal failure and pulmonary infiltrates. Subcutaneous panniculitis-like T-cell lymphoma and other cutaneous T-cell lymphomas in malignancy-associated variant	If caused by infection, may reverse if immunosuppressive agents withdrawn or infection treated; if caused by malignancy, course and treatment depend on tumor response to therapy	Dependent on the cause
Erdheim-Chester disease: very rare	Adult (26–78 years)	~25% involve skin. May have erythema over long bones. Xanthoma disseminatum-like presentation: lesions either red-brown papules (Fig. 22-7) becoming more yellow, isolated but gradually coalescing into plaques, later softening or becoming atrophic. Symmetric involvement, decreasing frequency eyelids, axillae, groin, neck, trunk, face. Papular xanthoma-like presentation: less common. 2-15-mm yellow to pink-yellow papules, nodules, on back and head	Spared	Focal bone pain, especially lower extremity, is presenting symptom in 50%. Fever is common. X-ray: mixed sclerotic (common) and lytic (30%) bone lesions. Diabetes insipidus up to one-third of patients. Bilateral painless exophthalmos common, renal and retroperitoneal one-third; pulmonary 20%. Testes can also be involved	Usually progressive with high mortality. Mean survival in one study <3 years. Cases of this disease with Langerhans' cell histiocytosis reported. Recently described BRAF V600E mutations have been noted and thus BRAF inhibitors may be effective	Dependent on the presenting signs. Cutaneous lesions with diabetes insipidus can mimic xanthoma disseminatum, JXG, papular xanthoma or sarcoidosis
Sea-blue histiocytotic syndrome: rare. Name derives from histologic appearance of blue staining cytoplasmic granules in macrophages with Giemsa or May–Gruenwald treatment	Begins in adolescents or young adults; may be familial	Rare skin involvement. Macular brown hyperpigmentation of the face with waxy plaques and swelling of eyelids; nodular lesions on face, trunk, hands, or feet	Spared	Primary form: hepatosplenomegaly and bone marrow infiltration with bleeding diathesis; lung, lymph nodes > retinal or nervous system. Secondary form with marrow disorders, inherited metabolic defects such as Niemann-Pick, partial sphingomyelinase deficiency, apoE mutations, or abnormal lipid metabolism (including total parenteral nutrition); findings depend on underlying disease	Primary form relatively benign clinical course, but with progressive skin lesions. No known effective treatment. Secondary forms: course depends on underlying disease	Depends on signs and symptoms

apoE, apolipoprotein E; EBV, Epstein–Barr virus; HLH, hemophagocytic lymphohistiocytosis; JXG, juvenile xanthogranuloma.

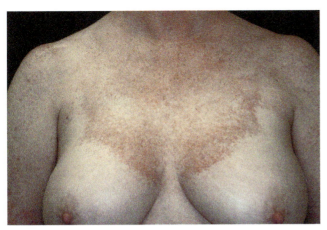

FIGURE 22-6 ■ Multicentric reticulohistiocytosis. This patient demonstrates multiple erythematous papules in a photodistribution. (Photo courtesy of Jeffrey P. Callen, MD.)

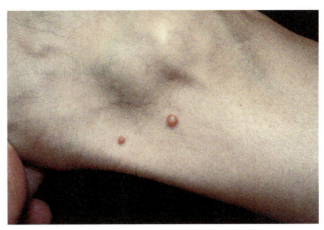

FIGURE 22-7 ■ Erdheim–Chester disease. This patient presented with multiple cutaneous nodules, but later developed bone pain and was found to have lesions on MRI (magnetic resonance imaging) of the brain. Her biopsies were found to have a BRAF V600E mutation. (Photo courtesy of Jeffrey P. Callen, MD.)

SUGGESTED READINGS

Badalian-Very G, Vergilio J, Degar BA, et al. Recurrent BRAF mutations in Langerhans cell histiocytosis. Blood 2010;116:1919–23.

Berres ML, Lim KP, Peters T, et al. BRAF-V600E expression in precursor versus differentiated dendritic cells defines clinically distinct LCH risk groups. J Exp Med 2014;211(4):669–83.

Chang MW, Frieden IJ, Good W. The risk of intraocular juvenile xanthogranuloma: survey of current practices and assessment of risk. J Am Acad Dermatol 1996;34:445–9.

Caputo R. Text atlas of histiocytic syndromes, a dermatological perspective. Mosby; 1998.

Foucar E, Rosai J, Dorfman R. Sinus histiocytosis with massive lymphadenopathy (Rosai-Dorfman disease): review of the entity. Semin Diagn Pathol 1990;7:19–73.

Gianotti R, Alessi E, Caputo R. Benign cephalic histiocytosis: a distinct entity or a part of a wide spectrum of histiocytic proliferative disorders of children? Am J Dermatopathol 1993;15:315–9.

Goodman WT, Barrett TL. Histiocytoses. In: 3rd ed. Bologna, Jorizzo, Schaffer, editors. Dermatology, vol. 2. Elsevier Limited; 2012. p. 1529–46.

Khezri F, Gibson LE, Tefferi A. Xanthoma disseminatum: effective therapy with 2-chlorodeoxyadenosine in a case series. Arch Dermatol April 2011;147(4):459–64.

Logemann N, Thomas B, Yetto T. Indeterminate cell histiocytosis successfully treated with narrowband UVB. Dermatol Online J October 16, 2013;19(10):20031.

Marie I, Pittaluga S, Dale JK, et al. Histologic features of sinus histiocytosis with massive lymphadenopathy in patients with autoimmune lymphoproliferative syndrome. Am J Surg Pathol 2005;29:903–11.

Molho-Pessach V, Ramot Y, Camille F, et al. H syndrome: the first 79 patients. J Am Acad Dermatol 2014;70:80–8.

Newman B, Weimin H, Nigro K, et al. Aggressive histiocytic disorders that can involve the skin. J Am Acad Dermatol 2007;56:302–16.

Patsatsi A, Kyriakou A, Sotiriadis D. Benign cephalic histiocytosis: case report and review of the literature. Pediatr Dermatol September 2014;31(5):547–50.

Ratzinger G, Burgdorf WH, Metze D, et al. Indeterminate cell histiocytosis: fact or fiction? J Cutan Pathol 2005;32:552–60.

Seward JL, Malone JC, Callen JP. Generalized eruptive histiocytosis. J Am Acad Dermatol 2004;50:116–20.

Vaiselbuh SR, Bryceson YT, Allen CE, et al. Meeting report: update on histiocytic disorders. Pediatr Blood Cancer 2014;61:1329–35.

Willman CL, Busque L, Griffith BB, et al. Langerhans'-cell histiocytosis (histiocytosis X) – a clonal proliferative disease. N Engl J Med 1994;331:154–60.

Wood AJ, Wagner VU, Abbott JJ, et al. Necrobiotic xanthogranuloma. A review of 17 cases with emphasis on clinical and pathologic correlation. Arch Dermatol 2009;145(No.3):279–84.

CHAPTER 23

Vascular Neoplasms and Malformations

Julie V. Schaffer • Jean L. Bolognia

KEY POINTS

- A variety of vascular lesions can serve as cutaneous signs of systemic disease.
- Telangiectasias or angiokeratomas with particular morphologies and distributions raise suspicion for an autoimmune connective tissue disease or a genetic disorder.
- Vascular anomalies are divided into two major categories: *tumors* due to endothelial cell proliferation and *malformations* that result from errors in vascular morphogenesis.
- Benign vascular tumors and vascular malformations may have associated widespread or regional extracutaneous findings.
- Kaposi's sarcoma and angiosarcoma represent two malignant vascular tumors with internal manifestations.

There are a number of vascular lesions that serve as cutaneous signs of systemic disease, from the mat telangiectasias of scleroderma and the papular telangiectasias of hereditary hemorrhagic telangiectasia (Osler–Weber–Rendu syndrome) to the angiokeratomas of Fabry disease. In addition, some vascular tumors and malformations may be associated with extracutaneous findings such as profound thrombocytopenia in Kasabach–Merritt syndrome or glaucoma and neurologic abnormalities in Sturge–Weber syndrome. Over the past several decades, increased appreciation of the differences between vascular tumors and malformations has led to improved classification and management of these lesions. This chapter concludes with a discussion of two malignant vascular tumors with potential internal manifestations: Kaposi's sarcoma and angiosarcoma.

TELANGIECTASIAS

Telangiectasias are such a common cutaneous finding that they are often overlooked or disregarded. In the head and neck region, the linear variety is most commonly due to solar damage or rosacea, whereas on the lower extremities telangiectasias are usually a sign of venous hypertension (Fig. 23-1; Table 23-1). The recurrent flushing of the face and upper trunk that occurs in patients with the carcinoid syndrome may also be accompanied by linear telangiectasias, which can result in misdiagnosis as the erythematotelangiectatic form of rosacea.

In ataxia–telangiectasia, linear telangiectasias first appear on the bulbar conjunctivae during early childhood, followed over time by similar, but often more subtle, lesions in sites such as the periocular skin, ears, and antecubital and popliteal fossae. The telangiectasias are typically preceded by the onset of cerebellar ataxia when the patient began to walk. Additional skin findings may include granulomatous dermatitis, nevoid hyper- or hypopigmentation, and progeric changes. Affected individuals usually develop recurrent pulmonary infections and are at high risk of lymphoproliferative disorders. This autosomal recessive disorder is due to mutations in the *ATM* gene, but how this relates to the formation of telangiectasias is not well understood (see Chapter 34).

A rare variant of mastocytosis (see Chapter 36) referred to as telangiectasia macularis eruptiva perstans (TMEP) is characterized by multiple clusters of telangiectasias. Although somatic activating mutations in the *KIT* gene are found in most adults with urticaria pigmentosa, to date they have not been reported in patients with TMEP. Arborizing telangiectasias are a classic feature of basal cell

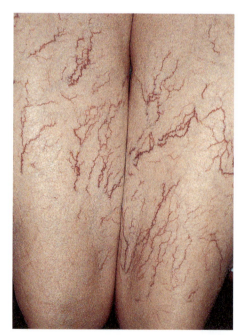

FIGURE 23-1 ■ Linear telangiectasias of the lower extremities in a patient with venous hypertension.

carcinomas, and telangiectasias are also seen within cutaneous B-cell lymphomas (Fig. 23-2).

One or two papular telangiectasias commonly occur on the face or hands of healthy individuals, especially women and children. Spider telangiectasias (also known as spider angiomas or spider nevi) represent dilations in ascending dermal arterioles and are characterized by both a punctum and radiating legs. The development of multiple spider telangiectasias can be a sign of hyperestrogenemia, such as occurs during pregnancy and in patients with hepatic cirrhosis.

The presence of multiple papular and stellate macular telangiectasias on the oral mucosa and lips (Fig. 23-3, *A*)

TABLE 23-1 Types and Causes of Telangiectasias

Primary Cutaneous Disorders
Linear
- Rosacea
- Actinically damaged skin
- Hereditary benign telangiectasia (may also have punctate lesions)
- Venous hypertension, especially of the lower extremities
- Costal fringe
- Generalized essential telangiectasia
- Cutaneous collagenous vasculopathy
- Within basal cell carcinomas or infantile hemangiomas (minimal growth or involuting lesions; see Fig. 23-16)

Papular or punctate
- Idiopathic
- Angioma serpiginosum

Spider
- Idiopathic
- Pregnancy

Stellate
- Unilateral nevoid telangiectasia

Poikiloderma
- Ionizing radiation
- Poikiloderma vasculare atrophicans

Systemic Diseases
Linear
- Carcinoid
- Ataxia–telangiectasia
- Mastocytosis (in particular telangiectasia macularis eruptiva perstans [TMEP])
- Within B-cell lymphomas of the skin

Papular
- Hereditary hemorrhagic telangiectasia (may also have stellate macules)

Spider
- Hepatic cirrhosis

Mat
- Scleroderma

Periungual
- Systemic lupus erythematosus
- Scleroderma
- Dermatomyositis
- Hereditary hemorrhagic telangiectasia
- Fabry disease

Poikiloderma
- Dermatomyositis
- Xeroderma pigmentosum
- Other genodermatoses (e.g., Kindler syndrome, Rothmund–Thomson syndrome)
- Cutaneous T-cell lymphoma
- Graft-versus-host disease

Adapted from Bolognia JL and Braverman IM. Skin manifestations of internal disease. In: Fauci AS, Braunwald E, Kasper DL et al., editors. Harrison's principles of internal medicine. 17th ed. New York: McGraw-Hill Medical; 2008. p. 324.

as well as the face, fingers (Fig. 23-3, *B*), and nailfolds (Fig. 23-3, *C*) raises the possibility of hereditary hemorrhagic telangiectasia (HHT; Osler–Weber–Rendu syndrome). These vascular lesions most often become apparent around or after puberty, and a personal or family history of epistaxis, gastrointestinal bleeding, or cerebrovascular accidents increases suspicion of this autosomal dominant condition. The vascular lesions of HHT actually represent arteriovenous malformations (AVMs), which explains their propensity to bleed. By stretching the skin, an eccentric punctum with radiating branches can be visualized.

When the clinical diagnosis of HHT is made, it is important to screen individuals with a transthoracic echocardiogram bubble study (which assesses shunting) and a brain MRI with gadolinium enhancement to exclude pulmonary and cerebral AVMs, both of which are amenable to interventional vascular procedures, e.g., embolotherapy or surgical excision. Most patients with HHT have a mutation in *ENG* or *ACVRL1*, genes that encode endoglin and activin A receptor type II-like 1, respectively. Patients with juvenile gastrointestinal polyposis in addition to HHT may

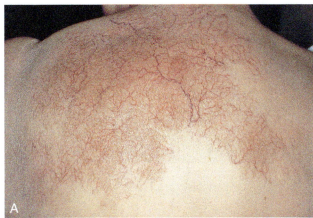

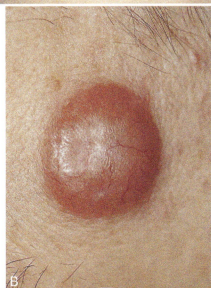

FIGURE 23-2 ■ **(A, B)** Linear telangiectasias within lesions of cutaneous B-cell lymphoma. (**A**, courtesy of Yale Residents' Slide Collection.)

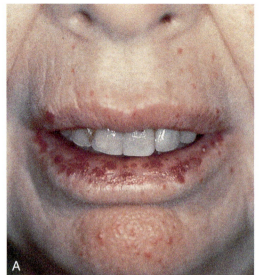
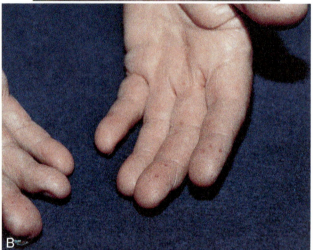
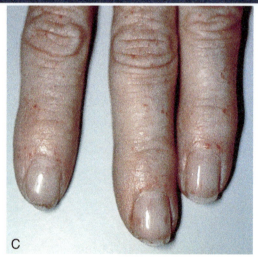

FIGURE 23-3 ■ Papular telangiectasias of the lips (**A**), fingers (**B & C**), and nailfolds (**C**) in two patients with hereditary hemorrhagic telangiectasia (HHT). (Courtesy of Yale Residents' Slide Collection.)

have mutations in the *SMAD4* gene, which encodes a protein that, like endoglin and ACVRL1, is involved in transforming growth factor-β signaling; these patients are at increased risk of early-onset colorectal carcinoma.

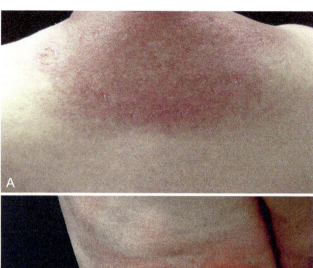
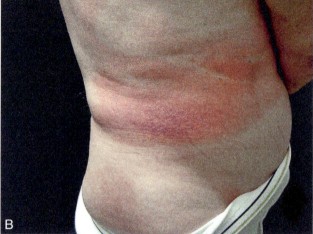

FIGURE 23-4 ■ **A,** Poikiloderma of the upper back (shawl sign) in a patient with dermatomyositis. **B,** Poikiloderma in a patient with early cutaneous T-cell lymphoma. The latter photograph was taken over 20 years ago, and this patient's disease has been controlled with the application of moderately potent corticosteroids.

Poikiloderma is defined by the presence of (1) telangiectasias; (2) wrinkling due to epidermal atrophy; and (3) reticulated areas of hypo- and hyperpigmentation. This combination of skin findings is characteristically seen years after orthovoltage irradiation. Poikiloderma can be a feature of dermatomyositis (Fig. 23-4, *A*) and cutaneous T-cell lymphoma. In the latter condition, the lesions favor the axillae and groin (Fig. 23-4, *B*).

Telangiectasias, in particular mat and periungual variants, are an important cutaneous clue to the diagnosis of autoimmune connective tissue diseases (AI-CTD). Mat telangiectasias are flat, often have a polygonal shape, and favor the face, oral mucosa, and hands (Fig. 23-5). They are a sign of scleroderma or an overlap syndrome that includes scleroderma. Of note, in the acronym for the more indolent, anticentromere antibody-positive CREST variant of scleroderma, the T stands for telangiectasias. Periungual telangiectasias are seen in systemic lupus erythematosus (SLE), dermatomyositis (DM), and scleroderma. In the latter two AI-CTD, individual telangiectasias appearing as swollen loops are admixed with avascular areas (Fig. 23-6), whereas in lupus the telangiectasias have an appearance that has been likened to that of renal glomeruli. Nailfold telangiectasias are accompanied by erythema in SLE, and both erythema and ragged cuticles in DM.

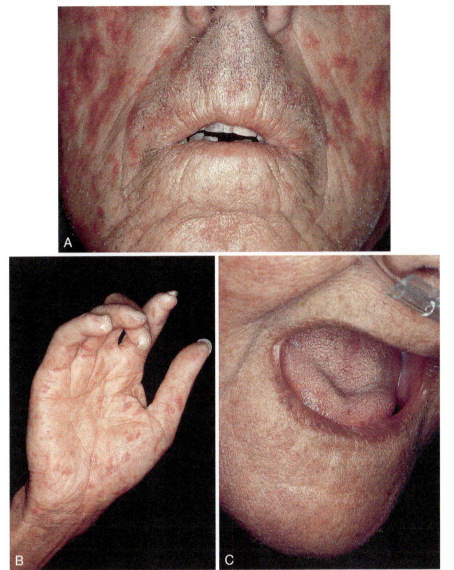

FIGURE 23-5 ■ Mat telangiectasias of the face, tongue, and hand in two patients with scleroderma. Note the perioral furrowing in **A**, and the sclerodactyly and loss of distal digits in **B**. (**A** and **C**, courtesy of Yale Residents' Slide Collection.)

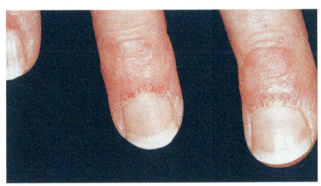

FIGURE 23-6 ■ Periungual telangiectasias in a patient with dermatomyositis; note the swollen loops alternating with avascular areas.

BENIGN VASCULAR TUMORS AND MALFORMATIONS

On the basis of biologic characteristics, vascular anomalies are divided into two major categories (Table 23-2): vascular tumors, which arise by cellular hyperplasia; and vascular malformations, which result from errors in vascular morphogenesis during intrauterine development and have normal cellular turnover. When vascular tumors are compared to vascular malformations, there are important differences in natural history, histologic features, associated findings (Table 23-3), and treatment options. However, despite the distinct processes that govern their development, occasionally vascular tumors and malformations are associated with one another, e.g., in kindreds with autosomal dominant cosegregation of infantile hemangiomas and vascular malformations. This suggests overlap in the regulation of prenatal vascular development and postnatal endothelial cell proliferation.

TABLE 23-2 **Classification of Selected Benign Vascular Tumors and Malformations**

Benign vascular neoplasms and reactive proliferations
    Infantile hemangioma (superficial and/or deep components)
    Congenital hemangiomas
        Rapidly involuting (RICH)*
        Noninvoluting (NICH)
        Partially involuting (PICH)
    Cherry angioma (senile angioma)
    Pyogenic granuloma
    Tufted angioma*
    Kaposiform hemangioendothelioma*
    Multifocal lymphangioendotheliomatosis with thrombocytopenia
    Glomeruloid hemangioma
    Spindle cell hemangioma
    Angiolymphoid hyperplasia with eosinophilia†
    Reactive angioendotheliomatosis‡
    Bacillary angiomatosis
    Infantile hemangiopericytoma (related to infantile myofibromatosis)

Vascular malformations
Low flow
    Capillary malformation (port-wine stain)
    Venous malformations
        Classic
        Glomuvenous
        Verrucous venous (verrucous "hemangioma")
    Lymphatic malformations
        Typical superficial/microcystic (lymphangioma circumscriptum)
        Targetoid hemosiderotic (hobnail "hemangioma")
        Deep/macrocystic (cystic hygroma)
        Kaposiform lymphangiomatosis (also has features of a vascular tumor)
    Combined vascular malformations (e.g., capillary–venous–lymphatic)
    Angiokeratoma circumscriptum
High flow
    Arteriovenous malformation (AVM)

*Can be associated with Kasabach–Merritt syndrome or, for RICH, a milder thrombocytopenic coagulopathy.
†Associated with peripheral eosinophilia and enlargement of regional lymph nodes.
‡Can be associated with systemic disorders such as monoclonal gammopathies (including type I cryoglobulinemia), antiphospholipid syndrome, bacterial endocarditis, and atherosclerosis (diffuse dermal angiomatosis variant).

Vascular Tumors

Infantile hemangiomas arise during the first few months of life and are the most common tumors of infancy, with an incidence of approximately 5% by 1 year of age and a female-to-male ratio of 3–4:1. Unlike other vascular tumors and malformations, infantile hemangiomas express the placental marker glucose transporter protein-1 (GLUT-1). These hemangiomas typically mark out their territory early on and subsequently expand in volume. The proliferative phase lasts until 3 to 9 months of age, with the most rapid growth in the first few months. This is followed by slow spontaneous regression during the involutional phase, which is complete by 3 to 10 years of age. Superficial hemangiomas are initially bright red in color and then become dull red to gray during involution, whereas deep hemangiomas are light blue in color and become softer and less warm as they involute. The term "cavernous hemangioma," which has been used to describe both hemangiomas with a deep component and venous malformations, has led to confusion and should be avoided. Infantile hemangiomas can be complicated by ulceration, interference with the function of vital structures such as the eyes or airway, high-output cardiac failure, and problems related to associated regional structural anomalies (Table 23-3; see Fig. 23-16). Hypothyroidism occasionally occurs in infants with large-volume proliferating hemangiomas, especially hepatic lesions, because of production of iodothyronine deiodinase within the tumors. In the past decade, use of the β-blocker propranolol has revolutionized the treatment of infantile hemangiomas that would otherwise threaten vital functions or result in disfigurement.

There are a variety of benign vascular tumors and reactive proliferations other than infantile hemangiomas (Table 23-2). Congenital hemangiomas represent relatively uncommon, GLUT-1-negative vascular neoplasms that are fully formed at birth and have a natural history of either rapid involution during the first year of life or proportionate growth and failure to involute. These lesions typically present as a pink to blue-violet nodule or plaque with central coarse telangiectasias and peripheral pallor.

Cherry angiomas are small, bright-red papules representing a benign proliferation of capillaries; commonly seen on the trunk of adults, they increase in number with age. Pyogenic granulomas are rapidly developing vascular lesions that typically appear as friable papules on the face, fingers (Fig. 23-7), or mucous membranes. Histologically resembling granulation tissue, pyogenic granulomas frequently occur at sites of minor trauma or on the gingiva during pregnancy.

Bacillary angiomatosis primarily affects patients with AIDS and most often presents as multiple red vascular papules and nodules; internal organ involvement, e.g., liver and bone, can also occur. The causative organisms, *Bartonella quintana* or *B. henselae*, can be seen with Warthin–Starry staining of tissue specimens. Kaposiform hemangioendotheliomas and tufted angiomas are two vascular tumors that can be complicated by Kasabach–Merritt syndrome, an acute, life-threatening consumptive coagulopathy with profound thrombocytopenia (Table 23-3). Spindle cell hemangiomas are unusual tumors that typically develop within existing venous malformations and may be associated with Maffucci syndrome (Fig. 23-8; Table 23-3).

Vascular Malformations

Classically, vascular malformations are present at birth and enlarge in proportion to the child's growth. However, some of these structural anomalies do not become clinically apparent for many years, and rapid expansion in size may occur as a result of hormonal fluctuations (e.g., puberty or pregnancy), trauma, thrombosis, or infection. Histologically, vascular malformations are characterized by dilated vascular channels with abnormal walls lined with quiescent endothelium. Further categorization of vascular malformations depends upon the rate of blood flow and the predominant type of vessel involved (Table 23-2). In addition, these malformations are associated with a wide

TABLE 23-3 Benign Vascular Tumors and Malformations: Syndromes and Associations

	Syndrome/Association	Features of Vascular Lesion(s)	Associated Clinical Features
Vascular tumors	Kasabach–Merritt syndrome	Kaposiform hemangioendothelioma or tufted angioma; large, rapidly growing ecchymotic mass (cutaneous or retroperitoneal)	Severe thrombocytopenia and variable consumption coagulopathy; occurs primarily in infants; possible mortality
	Multifocal lymphangioendotheliomatosis with thrombocytopenia	Multiple (often >100) red-brown papules and plaques present at birth or appearing during infancy + gastrointestinal > pulmonary involvement	Thrombocytopenia; severe gastrointestinal bleeding; occasionally hemoptysis; possible mortality
	Multifocal infantile hemangiomas with extracutaneous involvement (diffuse neonatal hemangiomatosis)	Multiple (≥5) small cutaneous hemangiomas + internal hemangiomas affecting the liver and rarely other organs (e.g., gastrointestinal tract, lungs, brain)	Hepatomegaly, high-output cardiac failure, abdominal compartment syndrome, hypothyroidism (see text)
	Airway hemangiomas	Hemangiomas in "beard" distribution	Noisy breathing, biphasic stridor, hoarseness, respiratory failure
	PHACE(S) syndrome	Large (>5cm) cervicofacial infantile hemangioma*, typically in a segmental pattern correlating with a developmental unit (e.g., embryonic facial prominences; Fig. 23-16)	Posterior fossa malformations; *H*emangiomas; cervical and cerebral *A*rterial anomalies; *C*ardiac defects (especially *C*oarctation of the aorta); *E*ye anomalies; *S*ternal or *S*upraumbilical clefting
	LUMBAR syndrome	Midline *L*umbosacral or Lower body infantile hemangioma, often large and segmental*	*L*ipoma/other skin lesions (e.g., "skin tag"): *U*rogenital anomalies, *U*lceration; *M*yelopathy (spinal dysraphism)†; *B*ony deformities; *A*norectal, *A*rterial and *R*enal anomalies
	POEMS syndrome	Cherry angiomas, glomeruloid hemangiomas	*P*olyneuropathy, *O*rganomegaly, *E*ndocrinopathy, *M*-protein (monoclonal gammopathy), *S*kin changes such as diffuse hyperpigmentation, edema, sclerodermoid changes
Vascular malformations§	Sturge–Weber syndrome (SWS)	Facial CM in V1 (±V2, V3) dermatomal distribution (uni- > bilateral) together with ipsilateral leptomeningeal ± choroidal CVM	Seizures, developmental delay, contralateral hemiparesis, characteristic "tram-track" cerebral gyral calcifications; ipsilateral glaucoma; facial soft tissue/bony hypertrophy over time; mosaic *GNAQ* mutation in affected tissues
	Bonnet–Dechaume–Blanc (Wyburn–Mason) syndrome	(Centro)facial AVM (may mimic a CM) + metameric AVM of the ipsilateral orbit and/or brain	Ipsilateral visual impairment, various contralateral neurologic manifestations
	Cobb syndrome	AVM (may mimic a CM or angiokeratomas) in a dermatomal distribution + metameric AVM in the corresponding spinal cord segment	Neurologic manifestations of spinal cord compression (e.g., paraparesis)
	Klippel–Trenaunay syndrome (KTS)	CVM/CVLM of lower extremity > upper extremity, trunk; 85% unilateral; vascular stain with a sharply demarcated, geographic pattern is a sign of lymphatic involvement	Soft tissue/bony hypertrophy (or occasionally hypotrophy‡) of affected limb(s), venous thrombosis and ulcers, lymphedema; occasionally gastrointestinal bleeding, hematuria and pulmonary embolism
	Parkes Weber syndrome (PKWS)	AVM ± CM/CLM of an extremity	Soft tissue/bony hypertrophy with progressive deformity over time, high-output cardiac failure
	Capillary malformation–arteriovenous malformation	Multifocal, small, round-to-oval pink to red-brown CM ± AVM of face, extremities, brain and/or spine	PKWS (see above); headaches, seizures, sensorimotor deficits, cerebral hemorrhage; AD inheritance of *RASA1* mutations
	Cutaneous + cerebral capillary malformations	Hyperkeratotic cutaneous CVMs + cerebral CMs; congenital red-purple plaques and red-brown macules with peripheral telangiectatic puncta	Headaches, seizures, cerebral hemorrhage; AD inheritance, usually due to *KRIT1* mutations
	Cutis marmorata telangiectatica congenita (CMTC)	Localized, segmental or generalized; broad, red-purple reticulated vascular network on extremities > trunk > face; telangiectasias, ± prominent veins, ± cutaneous atrophy	Often hypotrophy (rarely hypertrophy) of affected limb (girth > length); occasionally glaucoma, developmental delay; aplasia cutis + transverse limb defects ± cardiac malformation (Adams–Oliver syndrome)

Continued

TABLE 23-3 Benign Vascular Tumors and Malformations: Syndromes and Associations—cont'd

Syndrome/Association	Features of Vascular Lesion(s)	Associated Clinical Features
Megalencephaly–CM (macrocephaly–CM; formerly macrocephaly–CMTC)	Reticulated CM, persistent midfacial capillary stain	Macrocephaly, asymmetric overgrowth/hemihypertrophy, CNS abnormalities, developmental delay, syndactyly (especially of 2nd–3rd toes), joint laxity; mosaic *PIK3CA* mutations
CLOVES syndrome	Vascular malformations (slow- or fast-flow)	Congenital *L*ipomatous *O*vergrowth, *E*pidermal nevi, *S*keletal anomalies (e.g., scoliosis, splayed feet); mosaic *PIK3CA* mutations
PTEN hamartoma–tumor syndrome (Bannayan–Riley–Ruvalcaba syndrome > Cowden disease)	Multifocal intramuscular arteriovenous anomalies associated with ectopic fat; ± CM, LM; intracranial developmental venous anomalies	Macrocephaly, developmental delay, lipomas, genital pigmented macules, trichilemmomas, acral keratoses, oral papillomas, neuromas, sclerotic fibromas, intestinal hamartomatous polyps, breast and thyroid adenoma/carcinoma; AD inheritance of *PTEN* mutations
Proteus syndrome	CM/LM/CVM/CLM, most often of extremities	Progressive, disproportionate, asymmetric soft tissue/bony overgrowth, cerebriform connective tissue nevi of soles > palms, dermal hypoplasia, lipomas/regional absence of fat, epidermal nevi, CNS abnormalities, venous thrombosis/pulmonary embolism, lung cysts; mosaic *AKT1* mutations
Phacomatosis pigmentovascularis	CM > CMTC; ± nevus anemicus	Dermal melanocytosis and/or speckled lentiginous nevus (nevus spilus); may have extracutaneous features of SWS or KTS
Blue rubber bleb nevus syndrome (Bean syndrome)	Multiple VM of skin, gastrointestinal tract > other organs	Gastrointestinal bleeding, anemia
Multiple cutaneous and mucosal venous malformations	Multiple VM of skin, oral mucosa, and muscles	AD inheritance of *TEK* mutations
Maffucci syndrome	Multiple VM/VLM, most often of distal extremities; spindle cell hemangioma	Multiple enchondromas of long bones, especially metacarpals and phalanges of the hands; chondrosarcoma (15%–30%); skeletal deformities, short stature; somatic *IDH1*>2 mutations in enchondromas and spindle cell hemangiomas
Gorham syndrome	Multiple CVLM/LM of the skin, mediastinum, and bones	Massive osteolysis ("disappearing bones"), skeletal deformities, pathologic fractures, pulmonary complications
Fabry disease	Angiokeratoma corporis diffusum—small dark red papules symmetrically in a "bathing trunk" distribution, ± mucosal involvement	Acral paresthesias, painful crises, hypohidrosis, whorl-like corneal and lenticular opacities, progressive renal and coronary artery disease, cerebrovascular accidents; X-linked recessive lysosomal storage disease due to α-galactosidase A deficiency
Fucosidosis	Angiokeratoma corporis diffusum (as described above)	Mental retardation, spastic paresis, seizures, recurrent sinus and pulmonary infections; AR lysosomal storage disease due to α-L-fucosidase deficiency

CM, capillary malformation; VM, venous malformation; LM, lymphatic malformation; CVLM, capillary–venous–lymphatic malformation; AVM, arteriovenous malformation; AD, autosomal dominant; AR, autosomal recessive; CNS, central nervous system; *GNAQ*, guanine nucleotide binding protein (G protein); q polypeptide; *IDH*, isocitrate dehydrogenase; *PIK3CA*, phosphatidylinositol-4,5-bisphosphate 3-kinase, catalytic subunit alpha.

*PHACE(S) and LUMBAR may occur in association with a "minimal growth" hemangioma with reticulated erythema, linear telangiectasias, and often small peripheral red papules.
†Midline lumbosacral capillary malformations are also occasionally associated with spinal dysraphism, usually when present together with another skin finding.
‡Referred to as Servelle-Martorell syndrome.
§Massive osteolysis capillary stains have also been described in association with a variety of dysmorphic conditions, including Beckwith–Wiedemann, Roberts, and Rubinstein–Taybi syndromes.
‖Angiokeratoma corporis diffusum has also been reported in other lysosomal storage diseases such as galactosialidosis, GM1 gangliosidosis, and β-mannosidosis.

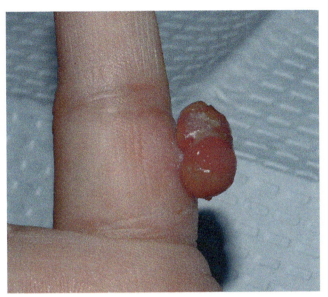

FIGURE 23-7 ■ Pedunculated pyogenic granuloma of the finger at a site of trauma. The beefy red appearance is reminiscent of granulation tissue.

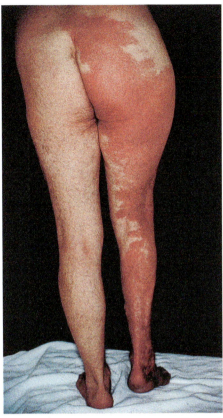

FIGURE 23-9 ■ Extensive capillary–venous malformation of the right lower extremity associated with limb-length discrepancy in a patient with Klippel–Trenaunay syndrome. (Courtesy of Yale Residents' Slide Collection.)

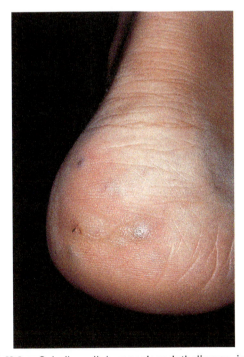

FIGURE 23-8 ■ Spindle cell hemangioendotheliomas in a patient with Maffucci syndrome. (Courtesy of Yale Residents' Slide Collection.)

variety of syndromes with localized and systemic features (Fig. 23-9; Table 23-3).

Low-flow vascular malformations may be composed of capillaries, veins, and/or lymphatic channels. Capillary malformations (port-wine stains; PWSs) appear as pink to dark red patches and can be associated with regional extracutaneous involvement, e.g., ocular and leptomeningeal in the case of facial PWSs (Table 23-3; see Chapter 34). Mosaic activating mutations in the *GNAQ* gene, which encodes a G protein α-subunit, underlie both nonsyndromic PWSs and Sturge–Weber syndrome.

PWSs are typically unilateral and/or segmental in distribution and persist throughout life, often deepening in color and becoming raised and nodular over time. In contrast, the nevus simplex (salmon patch, stork bite) is a pink-red vascular birthmark that is present in 30% to 50% of neonates and tends to fade by early childhood (glabella, eyelids, philtrum) or persist (nape) without associated complications.

Venous malformations appear as soft, compressible swellings that are blue to violaceous in color. In the blue rubber bleb nevus syndrome, multiple venous malformations are found in the skin, muscle, and gastrointestinal tract (Fig. 23-10); resultant gastrointestinal bleeding can lead to iron-deficiency anemia. In contrast, multiple glomuvenous malformations caused by heterozygous germline mutations in the *GLMN* gene typically present as blue-purple nodules and plaques that are limited to the skin and subcutis, resist full compression, and are painful upon palpation. Venous and lymphatic malformations may be associated with skeletal alterations, functional impairment of involved limbs, and a low-grade, chronic, localized consumptive coagulopathy that results in thrombosis (leading to phlebolith formation) as well as bleeding. The presence of a high-flow vascular malformation, such as an arteriovenous malformation (AVM), is suggested by clinical signs such as warmth, a bruit, a thrill, or pulsations. In the later stages, AVMs are characterized by ulceration and intractable pain; when located within an extremity,

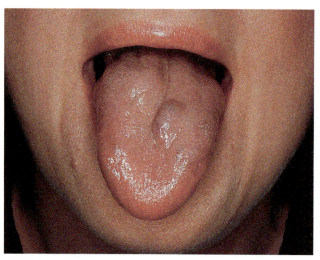

FIGURE 23-10 ■ Multiple venous malformations on the tongue in a patient with blue rubber bleb nevus syndrome and gastrointestinal bleeding.

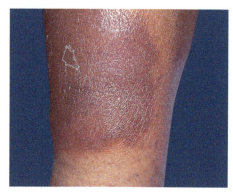

FIGURE 23-11 ■ Violaceous plaque of acroangiodermatitis ("pseudo-Kaposi's sarcoma") on the distal shin of a patient with venous hypertension and chronic lower extremity edema.

violet plaques of acroangiodermatitis ("pseudo-Kaposi's sarcoma") may develop (Fig. 23-11).

Angiokeratomas

Angiokeratomas are small (1 to 5-mm), red to dark-blue papules characterized by vascular ectasias in the superficial papillary dermis together with epidermal hyperkeratosis. When numerous, these lesions can be a sign of inborn errors of metabolism such as Fabry disease (Table 23-3). More commonly, however, angiokeratomas are a manifestation of aging, e.g., multiple dark blue to purple papules on the scrotum or vulva. Solitary angiokeratomas may be mistaken for melanoma because of their dark color, but these two entities can be readily distinguished with dermoscopy.

KAPOSI'S SARCOMA

Kaposi's sarcoma was first described in 1872 by Moritz Kaposi as "idiopathic multiple pigmented sarcoma of the skin." Over a century later, human herpesvirus 8 (HHV-8; Kaposi's sarcoma-associated herpesvirus) was determined to be the primary and necessary agent in the pathogenesis of this vascular tumor. HHV-8 is the infectious cause of all the clinical variants of Kaposi's sarcoma, which have similar histologic features but develop in distinct patient populations and clinical settings, with different sites of involvement, rates of progression, and prognoses. These variants include: (1) classic Kaposi's sarcoma, an indolent disease that primarily affects elderly men of Mediterranean, Eastern European, or Jewish heritage; (2) African-endemic Kaposi's sarcoma, a locally aggressive cutaneous disease in adults and a fulminant lymphadenopathic disease in children; (3) human immunodeficiency virus (HIV)-associated epidemic Kaposi's sarcoma, an aggressive disease most frequently affecting men who have sex with men; and (4) iatrogenic Kaposi's sarcoma occurring in the setting of immunosuppression, in particular after solid organ transplantation.

HHV-8 DNA can be detected in virtually all Kaposi's sarcoma lesions, regardless of clinical subtype. HHV-8 encodes several genes that have been shown to independently transform cells to a malignant phenotype in vitro; this herpesvirus is also clearly associated with body cavity-related B-cell lymphoma (primary effusion lymphoma) and multicentric Castleman's disease. Both the detection of HHV-8 DNA in peripheral blood and antibody seroconversion studies have shown that HHV-8 infection precedes and is predicative of the development of Kaposi's sarcoma. Antibodies to HHV-8 can be found in 80% to 95% of all patients with Kaposi's sarcoma and almost 100% of immunocompetent patients with the disease, compared to approximately 1% to 5% of the general population. The seroprevalence of HHV-8 infection parallels the incidence of Kaposi's sarcoma, and both the seroprevalence and the incidence are higher in geographic areas such as the Mediterranean regions and central Africa, as well as in subpopulations such as HIV-negative and HIV-positive men who have sex with men (approximately 20% and 40% HHV-8 seroprevalence, respectively). Approximately 40% of men who are seropositive for both HIV and HHV-8 develop Kaposi's sarcoma within 10 years. HHV-8 DNA has been detected in both the saliva and the semen of infected individuals, and epidemiologic evidence suggests a sexual mode of transmission.

Immunosuppression appears to be an important cofactor in the pathogenesis of Kaposi's sarcoma in HHV-8-infected individuals. HIV infection in particular may promote the development of Kaposi's sarcoma via mechanisms such as depletion of CD4+ T lymphocytes, stimulation of cytokine release, and production of mitogens such as the HIV tat protein. However, paradoxically, in the setting of the immune reconstitution inflammatory syndrome (IRIS) due to the institution of antiretroviral therapy (ART), new lesions can appear as well as progression of previously stable lesions.

Clinical Manifestations

Most cases of classic Kaposi's sarcoma develop after the sixth decade of life, and although the older literature reported a male:female ratio of 10–15:1, more recent population-based studies have found lower ratios of 3–4:1. Classic Kaposi's sarcoma usually begins as one or

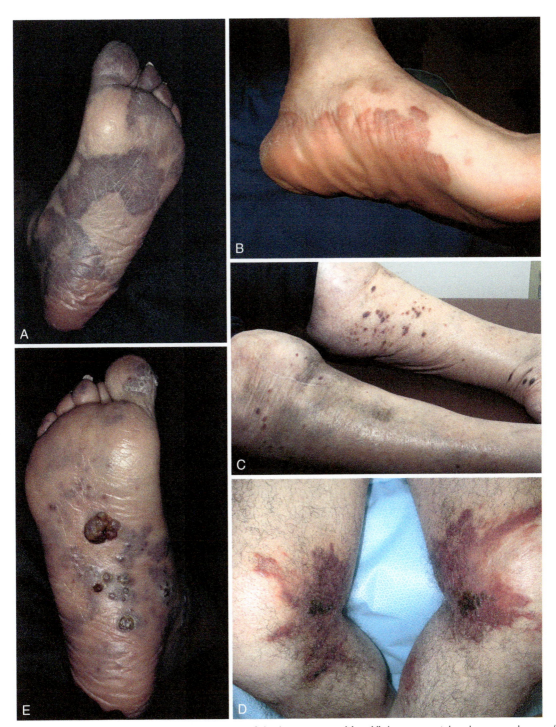

FIGURE 23-12 ■ Classic Kaposi's sarcoma with involvement of the lower extremities. Violaceous patches become plaques (**A, B**) and may develop a nodular component (**C, E**) or verrucous appearance (**D, E**). (**B**, courtesy of Frank Samarin, MD. **C**, courtesy of Kalman Watsky, MD.)

more pink to deep red-purple macules on the distal lower extremities. Lesions progress slowly, expanding and coalescing to form large plaques or developing into nodular tumors (Fig. 23-12). Older lesions may become purple-brown in color and develop keratotic surface changes. The disease spreads centrally toward the trunk and often involves both lower extremities, which may become edematous as a result of lymphatic involvement and/or cytokine release; eventually, lesions can erode, ulcerate, and cause severe pain.

Kaposi's sarcoma may involve the oral mucosa and conjunctiva, and the gastrointestinal tract is the most frequent site of visceral disease; however, these lesions are usually asymptomatic. Other potential sites of internal involvement include the lymph nodes, liver, spleen, lungs, adrenal glands, and bones. Classic Kaposi's sarcoma typically has an indolent course, with patients surviving 10 to 15 years and eventually dying of unrelated causes; however, several studies have noted an increased incidence of lymphomas in patients with classic Kaposi's sarcoma.

African-endemic Kaposi's sarcoma most commonly affects young adults in equatorial Africa (male: female ratio 13–18:1), often with an indolent course resembling that of classic Kaposi's sarcoma, but sometimes with locally aggressive disease characterized by invasion of muscle and bone. A fulminant lymphadenopathic variant occurs in African children (male: female ratio 3:1) and is generally fatal within 2 years.

Kaposi's sarcoma develops in 0.5% to 5% of solid organ transplant recipients (male: female ratio 2–4:1), most often within 2 to 3 years of transplantation, and has also been reported in patients undergoing chronic immunosuppressive therapy for autoimmune diseases and malignancies; the incidence is highest in ethnic groups at increased risk for classic Kaposi's sarcoma. Although Kaposi's sarcoma in the setting of iatrogenic immunosuppression tends to be aggressive, lesions often undergo spontaneous regression upon reduction or discontinuation of immunosuppressive therapy. Substitution of sirolimus (rapamycin) for calcineurin inhibitors can lead to resolution of cutaneous lesions of Kaposi's sarcoma in kidney and other solid organ transplant recipients without leading to rejection.

Kaposi's sarcoma had been reported to develop in approximately 20% of HIV-positive men who had sex with men and <1% to 5% of other HIV-positive patients (male: female ratio 10–20:1); however, the incidence has been decreasing over the past two decades. The clinical course of HIV-associated Kaposi's sarcoma is highly variable, ranging from stable localized lesions to rapid widespread growth. However, with the exception of flares in the setting of IRIS, the frequency and severity of HIV-associated Kaposi's sarcoma are typically proportional to the patient's degree of immune impairment. As a result, most patients have CD4+ T-lymphocyte counts <500/mm^3 and develop multicentric, progressive disease (Fig. 23-13).

In contrast to other variants of Kaposi's sarcoma, initial cutaneous lesions often develop on the face and trunk; in the latter location, lesions may be aligned with their long axes in the direction of skin folds (Fig. 23-13C). Lesions of the oral mucosa, most often involving the palate, are common and may be the first manifestation of disease. The lymph nodes are affected in approximately half of patients with HIV-associated Kaposi's sarcoma. Symptomatic gastrointestinal involvement also occurs frequently, with complications including ulceration, bleeding, perforation, and ileus. Pulmonary Kaposi's sarcoma has a poor prognosis; its clinical presentation may be similar to that of opportunistic respiratory infections, with symptoms such as dyspnea, intractable cough, and hemoptysis. Radiographic findings range from discrete parenchymal nodules to bilateral perihilar infiltrates to pleural effusions.

Histopathologic Findings

A skin biopsy can confirm the diagnosis of Kaposi's sarcoma, revealing an angioproliferative neoplasm characterized by spindle-shaped tumor cells and irregular, slit-like endothelium-lined spaces containing erythrocytes. A normal vessel or adnexal structure protruding into an ectatic vascular space (promontory sign) is a hallmark for early disease; spindle cells become more prominent as the lesions progress. An inflammatory infiltrate containing lymphocytes, plasma cells, and histiocytes is typically present. Immunohistochemical staining for the latency-associated nuclear antigen (LNA-1) of HHV-8 can help to distinguish Kaposi's sarcoma from other vascular neoplasms.

Although the precise cell of origin of Kaposi's sarcoma is still debated, the predominant expression of endothelial markers in Kaposi's sarcoma tissues suggests development from endothelial cells of vascular or lymphatic origin. In vitro, HHV-8 can infect blood as well

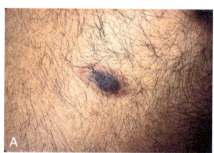
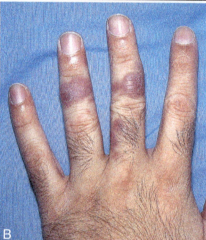
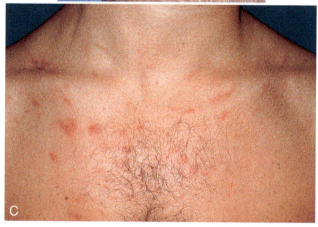

FIGURE 23-13 ■ Plaques of Kaposi's sarcoma in three men with AIDS; the lesions range in color from deep purple with a rim of hemorrhage (**A**), to violet (**B**), to pink-red (**C**). On the chest, several of the lesions are aligned with their long axes in the direction of skin folds. (**B** and **C**, courtesy of Yale Residents' Slide Collection.)

as lymphatic vascular endothelial cells, with induction of lymphangiogenic molecules in both cell types.

Evaluation and Treatment

The initial evaluation of a patient with Kaposi's sarcoma involves a thorough physical examination with careful attention to areas frequently affected by the disease (including the oral mucosa), testing of the stool for occult blood, and a chest X-ray. When gastrointestinal or pulmonary involvement is suspected, the work-up should include endoscopy or bronchoscopy. Additional studies include HIV testing, particularly in men who have sex with men and other high-risk patients, and determination of HIV-1 viral load and CD4+ T-lymphocyte count in HIV-positive patients.

Treatment options in Kaposi's sarcoma depend on the extent and rate of growth of the tumor as well as the overall medical condition of the patient. Limited cutaneous disease can be treated with local excision, topical alitretinoin gel, intralesional vinblastine, radiation therapy, laser therapy, photodynamic therapy, or cryotherapy. In patients with widespread disease in whom systemic therapy is warranted, liposomal anthracyclines (daunorubicin or doxorubicin) and taxanes (e.g., paclitaxel) are the treatments of choice, with high benefit-to-risk ratios and response rates of 50% to 80%. Vinblastine, vincristine, and bleomycin, either alone or in combination, have also been shown to produce response rates of >50%. Interferon-α therapy has been widely used for HIV-associated Kaposi's sarcoma, but requires high doses that result in significant systemic toxicity. Iatrogenic Kaposi's sarcoma often regresses with reduction or modification (e.g., switch to sirolimus) of immunosuppressive therapy; however, the risk of allograft rejection may limit the first option in organ transplant recipients. Lastly, the use of ART has been associated with a dramatic reduction in the incidence of HIV-associated Kaposi's sarcoma, as well as regression of existing lesions in most patients (see above).

Therapies currently under investigation include angiogenesis inhibitors (e.g., thalidomide, bevacizumab), tyrosine kinase inhibitors, and matrix metalloproteinase inhibitors.

ANGIOSARCOMA

Angiosarcoma represents a malignancy of endothelial cells, either vascular or lymphatic in origin, which has four clinical variants. The idiopathic form develops on the scalp and upper face, usually in older adults. The lesions range from subtle erythema of the face and scalp to obvious purple plaques and tumors the color of an eggplant (Fig. 23-14). Clinically, the more subtle forms are sometimes misdiagnosed as acne rosacea or soft tissue infections, and areas of induration can mimic cutaneous lymphoma.

In the second subtype (Fig. 23-15) tumors arise within areas of chronic lymphedema, such as the lower extremities of patients with congenital lymphedema (Milroy's disease) or the upper extremities of breast cancer patients who have undergone lymph node dissections. The latter form is sometimes referred to as lymphangiosarcoma of Stewart–Treves, but more recently use of the more general term angiosarcoma has been advocated, given the difficulty of determining whether the endothelial cells are vascular or lymphatic in origin.

The third type of cutaneous angiosarcoma arises within radiation ports in patients who have been treated for internal malignancies; the most common location for radiation-associated angiosarcoma is the anterior trunk, in particular the breast. With the increasing use of breast-conserving therapy (i.e., lumpectomy followed by radiation therapy) for the treatment of breast cancer, the incidence of the latter has increased, but it is still uncommon. This form has to be distinguished from atypical vascular proliferations

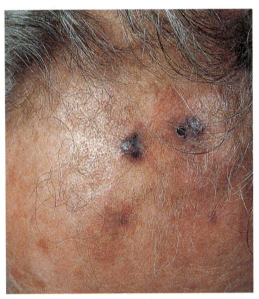

FIGURE 23-14 ■ Dark blue-purple plaques and nodules of angiosarcoma on the forehead and scalp of a 70-year-old man. The circular area is the biopsy site.

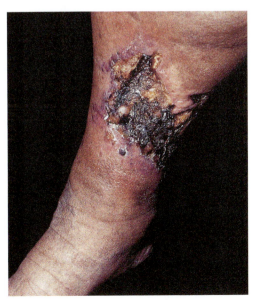

FIGURE 23-15 ■ Ulcerated plaque of angiosarcoma in a woman with chronic severe lower extremity lymphedema. (Courtesy of Yale Residents' Slide Collection.)

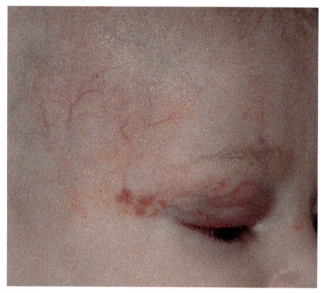

FIGURE 23-16 ■ Segmental minimal-growth infantile hemangioma associated with PHACE(S) syndrome.

following radiation therapy of the breast. The fourth type is an aggressive variant referred to as epithelioid angiosarcoma.

The diagnosis of an angiosarcoma may require the examination of several biopsy specimens. Histologically, anastomosing vascular channels lined by atypical endothelial cells are observed in the well-differentiated portions of the tumor. In the less well-differentiated areas, pleomorphic cells are seen, some of which are epithelioid in appearance. Positive staining of the tumor cells for CD31 serves as a diagnostic aid. Angiosarcoma must be differentiated from Kaposi's sarcoma as well as benign endothelial proliferations, including those within organizing thrombi (intravascular papillary endothelial hyperplasia).

Treatment of angiosarcoma is difficult because the tumor often extends beyond the clinically apparent margins. As a result, local recurrences are common following surgical excision. Although patients can develop metastases to regional lymph nodes and visceral organs, they often die of complications due to local disease. In addition to surgical excision, extended field radiation and chemotherapy, in particular taxanes (paclitaxel, docetaxel) and daunorubicin, can be used.

SUGGESTED READINGS

Antman K, Chang Y. Kaposi's sarcoma. N Engl J Med 2000;342: 1027–38.

Blockmans D, Beyens G, Verhaeghe R. Predictive value of nailfold capillaroscopy in the diagnosis of connective tissue diseases. Clin Rheumatol 1996;15:148–53.

Chang Y, Cesarman E, Pessin MS, et al. Identification of herpesvirus-like DNA sequences in AIDS-associated Kaposi's sarcoma. Science 1994;266:1865–9.

DiLorenzo G, Konstantinopoulos PA, Pantanowitz L, et al. Management of AIDS-related Kaposi's sarcoma. Lancet Oncol 2007;8: 167–76.

Garzon MC, Huang JT, Enjolras O, et al. Vascular malformations. Part I. J Am Acad Dermatol 2007;56:353–70.

Garzon MC, Huang JT, Enjolras O, et al. Vascular malformations. Part II: associated syndromes. J Am Acad Dermatol 2007;56:541–64.

Haggstrom AN, Drolet BA, Baselga E, et al. Prospective study of infantile hemangiomas: clinical characteristics predicting complications and treatment. Pediatrics 2006;118:882–7.

Iacobas I, Burrows PE, Frieden IJ, et al. LUMBAR: association between cutaneous infantile hemangiomas of the lower body and regional congenital anomalies. J Pediatr 2010;157:795–801.

Isovich J, Boffetta P, Franceschi S, et al. Classic Kaposi sarcoma. Cancer 2000;88:500–17.

Leidner RS, Aboulafia DM. Recrudescent Kaposi's sarcoma after initiation of HAART: a manifestation of immune reconstitution syndrome. AIDS Patient Care STDS 2005;19:635–44.

Léauté-Labrèze C, Hoeger P, Mazereeuw-Hautier J, et al. A randomized, controlled trial of oral propranolol in infantile hemangioma. N Engl J Med 2015;372:735–46.

Metry D, Heyer G, Hess C, et al. Consensus Statement on Diagnostic Criteria for PHACE Syndrome. Pediatrics 2009;124:1447–56.

Naka N, Ohsawa M, Tomita Y, et al. Prognostic factors in angiosarcoma: a multivariate analysis of 55 cases. J Surg Oncol 1996;61:170–6.

Shirley MD, Tang H, Gallione CJ, et al. Sturge-Weber syndrome and port-wine stains caused by somatic mutation in GNAQ. N Engl J Med 2013;368:1971–9.

Stallone G, Schena A, Infante B, et al. Sirolimus for Kaposi's sarcoma in renal-transplant recipients. N Engl J Med 2005;352:1317–23.

Wassef M, Blei F, Adams D, et al. Vascular anomalies classification: recommendations from the International Society for the Study of Vascular Anomalies. Pediatrics 2015;136:e203–14.

CHAPTER 24

DIABETES AND THE SKIN

Christine S. Ahn • Gil Yosipovitch • William W. Huang

> **KEY POINTS**
> - Diabetes mellitus (DM) is a highly prevalent, chronic, multisystem disease that affects the skin at some point of the disease in up to 70% of affected individuals.
> - Although the etiology is often unknown, the pathogenesis of many cutaneous findings is thought to be due to microangiopathy, glycosaminoglycan deposition with collagen alterations, and immune complex deposition.
> - There are numerous cutaneous manifestations of DM, which range in severity from asymptomatic, benign conditions such as acanthosis nigricans, to debilitating diseases such as diabetic foot.
> - Cutaneous manifestations such as necrobiosis lipoidica can precede the diagnosis of DM.
> - Most cutaneous conditions linked with DM will improve with optimal glycemic control.

Diabetes mellitus (DM) is characterized by abnormal carbohydrate metabolism. The prevalence of diabetes worldwide is approximately 350 million, with increased prevalence in industrialized nations. Diabetes is a complex, multiorgan disease that can impact nearly every organ system. Cutaneous manifestations of diabetes, which can be associated with significant morbidity, are reported in up to 70% of patients with DM at some point during the course of their disease. This chapter describes dermatologic manifestations of diabetes, which is divided into (1) cutaneous manifestations of DM, (2) other cutaneous findings in DM, (3) dermatologic diseases associated with DM, and (4) cutaneous complications of diabetes therapy.

CUTANEOUS MANIFESTATIONS OF DIABETES

Acanthosis Nigricans

Description

Acanthosis nigricans (AN) is a common dermatologic finding seen in insulin-resistant states such as diabetes. It is characterized by velvety to verrucous thickening and light brown to black hyperpigmentation of the skin, found predominantly in intertriginous and flexural surfaces of the body (Fig. 24-1). Flexural areas are most commonly affected areas such as the neck, axillae, and submammary regions. Involvement of the palmar hands is referred to as tripe palms. Histologically, epidermal papillomatosis, hyperkeratosis, and mild acanthosis are characteristic. The hyperpigmentation observed clinically relates to the thickness of the keratin-containing superficial epithelium, not to changes in melanocytes or melanin content. AN is considered a cutaneous marker of insulin resistance, thus clinical diagnosis of AN warrants screening for diabetes and potentially other endocrinopathies.

Epidemiology

Although observed in all ethnicities, there is a higher prevalence among Native Americans, Hispanics, Southeast Asians, and African-Americans. In addition to diabetes, AN can be observed as a paraneoplastic phenomenon, in obesity and metabolic syndrome, polycystic ovarian syndrome, Cushing syndrome, and other endocrine abnormalities involving insulin resistance.

Pathogenesis

The precise mechanism is not fully elucidated, but hyperinsulinemia may activate insulin growth factor (IGF-1) receptors on keratinocytes, leading to epidermal growth and subsequent hyperpigmentation.

Treatment

Lifestyle modifications such as weight reduction, dietary restrictions, and physical activity are most effective in the control and reversal of AN. Treatment of insulin resistance and optimizing glycemic and insulin balance will further improve this condition. Dermatologic therapies do not have a direct benefit, but topical keratolytics such as salicylic acid, ammonium lactate, or retinoid acid can help alleviate symptoms and reduce thickening of the skin.

Acquired Perforating Dermatoses

Description

Acquired perforating dermatoses (APD) are a group of chronic skin disorders characterized by pruritic, perifollicular, hyperkeratotic, dome-shaped papules or nodules with a central keratin plug. Perforating lesions can occur anywhere, but most commonly occur on the legs and trunk, and less often on the head. The eruption often demonstrates koebnerization and can be exacerbated by excoriation. Histologically these disorders are characterized by the presence of devitalization of connective tissue components of the dermis such as collagen,

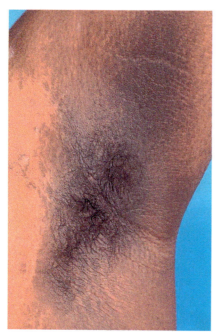

FIGURE 24-1 ■ Acanthosis nigricans in a patient with insulin resistance.

keratin, and elastic fibers, and transepidermal extrusion of the material.

Epidemiology

APD are observed nearly exclusively in patients with chronic renal failure and diabetes, although there are rare associations with malignancy and hypothyroidism. Although APD are rare in the general population, they are observed more often in African-Americans, and their incidence in diabetic patients undergoing renal dialysis is 5% to 10%. The disorder typically occurs in the context of advanced and long-standing diabetes, ranging from 10 to 30 years after diagnosis, and usually several months after initiation of renal dialysis, although lesions can occur before initiation of dialysis. In a review of patients with APD, 50% of patients had diabetes, and 91% of diabetic patients had chronic renal failure due to diabetic nephropathy.

Pathogenesis

The pathogenesis is not fully understood, though proposed theories include epidermal or dermal alterations as a result of metabolic derangements, deposition of a substance not removed through dialysis, and microtrauma as a result of chronic scratching and rubbing or as a manifestation of microangiopathy. Recent molecular studies have suggested that minor trauma or scratching in patients with DM leads to keratinocyte exposure to dermal interstitial advanced glycation end product-modified collagens, which interact and migrate upward together from the basal to the horny layers of the skin, leading to transepidermal elimination.

Treatment

Lesions are chronic and relatively unresponsive to therapy, but may resolve slowly over months if scratching and trauma are avoided. Thus, treatment is directed at symptomatic relief of pruritus. Topical and systemic retinoids, topical and intradermal corticosteroids, cryotherapy, psoralen plus UVA light (PUVA), UV light therapy, allopurinol, and doxycycline are treatment options with varying reports of efficacy. Although dialysis does not improve the disease, renal transplantation has resulted in clearance of the dermatosis.

Diabetic Bullae

Description

Diabetic bullae, or bullosa diabeticorum, present in diabetic patients as painless, noninflammatory, sterile blisters that arise on otherwise normal skin. They begin as tense bullae, but can become flaccid as they enlarge. The distal lower extremities are most commonly affected. Less often, fingers, hands, forearms, or trunk are involved. Histologic analysis of lesions reveals blisters that occur at different levels of cleavage. The most common patterns of cleavage are intraepidermal or subepidermal and nonacantholytic. These lesions can resolve spontaneously and without scarring. Less commonly, cleavage below the dermoepidermal junction is observed with destruction of anchoring fibrils, which can lead to clinical scarring and atrophy. Immunopathologic studies (immunofluorescence) are negative in patients with all forms of diabetic bullae.

Epidemiology

Diabetic bullae are a rare phenomenon, only seen in patients with DM. The overall reported prevalence of diabetic bullae is estimated to be 0.5% among diabetic patients. It is observed more often in long-standing type-1 insulin-dependent diabetes mellitus (IDDM), and the average age of onset ranges from 50 to 70 years. Bullae often occur in patients with severe DM, diabetic neuropathy, or retinopathy. Spontaneous acral bullae may be the first sign of DM.

Pathogenesis

The pathogenesis is unknown, although numerous proposed mechanisms include highly varying blood glucose levels, microangiopathy, an autoimmune phenomenon, and vascular insufficiency.

Treatment

Diabetic bullae are a self-limiting condition and lesions usually resolve within 2 to 6 weeks. There is no preventive treatment for this eruption and treatment is targeted at skin protection and prevention of secondary infection. Sterile drainage and topical antibiotics may be required for larger lesions.

Diabetic Dermopathy

Description

Diabetic dermopathy, also known as shin spots and pigmented pretibial patches, are red to brown papules or

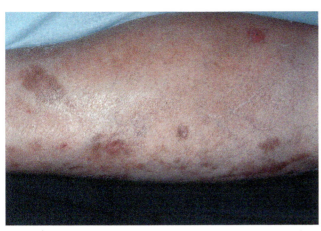

FIGURE 24-2 ■ Diabetic dermopathy.

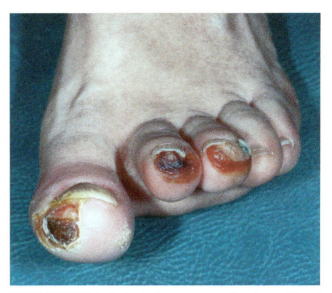

FIGURE 24-3 ■ Diabetic foot changes secondary to peripheral neuropathy.

plaques that typically range in size from 0.5 to 1.5 cm. They occur most commonly on the pretibial legs, but occasionally affect the thighs and forearms (Fig. 24-2). They are usually asymptomatic, and evolve into well-circumscribed macules that can be atrophic with a fine scale. Lesions at varied stages are seen contemporaneously. Biopsy specimens show thickening of blood vessels, perivascular lymphocytic infiltrates, and scattered hemosiderin skin deposits associated with hemorrhage, which are relatively nonspecific findings. Patients with diabetic dermopathy often have other vasculopathy-associated complications of diabetes, such as retinopathy, neuropathy, or nephropathy, thus the presence of diabetic dermopathy is a potential indication to clinicians to pursue further evaluation even in known diabetics.

Epidemiology

Shin spots are the most common cutaneous markers of DM, seen in up to 50% of diabetics, and observed twice as often in men than in women. In one report, up to 70% of men with DM older than 60 years had diabetic dermopathy. In addition, it is more prevalent in patients with longstanding disease and a history of poor glycemic control, although diabetic dermopathy can be seen preceding the onset of diabetes.

Pathogenesis

Although the exact mechanism of pathogenesis is unknown, microangiopathy with associated capillary changes is thought to cause diabetic dermopathy.

Treatment

Diabetic dermopathy is self-limited, and lesions heal spontaneously over time, leaving behind scars that are atrophic and often hyperpigmented. There is no known effective therapy aside from prevention of secondary infection, and no correlation has been established between glycemic control and the development of diabetic dermopathy.

Diabetic Foot

Description

Diabetic foot is a condition that involves neuropathic foot deformity in diabetic patients, and is characterized by the presence of peripheral neuropathy, Charcot arthropathy, and peripheral vascular disease. Peripheral neuropathy can lead to mal perforans, or neuropathic ulcers, which are nonpainful ulcerations. Typically, a thick callus forms over bony prominences and areas of repeated trauma, which breaks down over time to form an ulcer. The most common sites of involvement are the bony prominences of the foot and ankle. Infection and gangrene are potential serious complications (Fig. 24-3). Charcot arthropathy in diabetic patients involves progressive deterioration of weight-bearing joints, usually observed in the ankle and hindfoot. Clawing deformities of the toes are other sequelae of diabetic neuropathy, thought to be due to intrinsic muscle atrophy leading to muscle imbalance.

Epidemiology

Peripheral neuropathy and subsequent ulcers account for significant morbidity and mortality in the diabetic population. The lifetime risk of developing a diabetic ulcer is estimated to be 15% to 25% among diabetic patients. In addition, 80% of major nontraumatic amputations performed in the US are in diabetic patients, 85% of whom presented with a preceding foot ulcer. Neuropathic arthropathy, a significant risk for limb loss, is seen in up to 10% of patients with neuropathy, and affects bilateral lower extremities in approximately one-third of patients.

Pathogenesis

Diabetic foot is a result of atherosclerosis of lower extremity arteries, abnormalities in sensory, motor, and autonomic nervous systems, and altered gait. Chronic hyperglycemia, which leads to formation of advanced glycosylation end products, oxidative stress, and neuroinflammation, causes a loss of myelinated and unmyelinated fibers and blunted nerve production. Sensory and motor neuropathy can lead to foot deformities that increase the risk of ulcer formation. Autonomic neuropathy can lead to anhidrosis in the lower extremities, causing dryness, cracks, and callus formation, increasing the risk for ulceration and secondary infection.

Treatment

Neuropathic ulcers usually heal within weeks if treated with aggressive debridement and offloading with various devices, or most effectively, with a total contact cast. Adherence to principles of wound-healing strategies is an important component of treatment, and there is a wide range of wound-healing agents available, including saline dressings, impregnated gauze, hydrogels, hydrocolloids, calcium alginate, silver, vacuum-assisted closure, and hyperbaric oxygen. A surgical revascularization procedure can correct the ischemic state. The use of topical growth factors or bioengineered skin grafts may be helpful but cannot replace revascularization procedures, debridement, and ulcer offloading. Because of the prevalence of bacterial colonization of ulcers, the need for antibiotic therapy rests on clinical evaluation and judgment. Prevention of complications remains paramount through daily foot inspection, care guidelines, and prevention of pressure, friction, and callus formation by the use of appropriate footwear.

Eruptive Xanthomatosis

Description

Eruptive xanthomas present as yellow to red papules that appear over weeks to months (Fig. 24-4). The lesions can be tender or pruritic, and may be surrounded with mild erythema. Xanthomas have a predilection for the buttocks and extensor surfaces of the extremities, with koebnerization noted in areas of pressure. Histologically, there is infiltration of the dermis with lipid-laden histiocytic foam cells as well as lymphocytes and neutrophils. Unlike other forms of xanthomas, the lipids within the macrophages represent triglycerides rather than cholesterol esters.

Epidemiology

Although the prevalence of xanthomatosis is not well characterized, it is reported in less than 1% of patients with noninsulin-dependent DM. Concomitant dyslipidemia in addition to diabetes leads to a higher risk for developing eruptive xanthomatosis.

Pathogenesis

Eruptive xanthomas are pathognomonic of hypertriglyceridemia, and up to one-third of patients with diabetes have lipoprotein abnormalities caused by low insulin levels. The low-insulin state of diabetes leads to the inability of insulin to act as a stimulating factor for lipoprotein lipase, an enzyme with a role in metabolism of serum triglycerides and triglyceride-rich lipoproteins. Without the appropriate activity of lipoprotein lipase, there is impaired clearance of very-low-density lipoproteins and chylomicrons, which can lead to increased levels of lipids and may precipitate eruptive xanthomas.

Treatment

The eruption improves with optimization of glycemic control and insulin levels, and improved control of carbohydrate and lipid metabolism. Treatment may also be supplemented with statins and fibrates.

Necrobiosis Lipoidica

Description

Necrobiosis lipoidica (NL) is a necrotizing, granulomatous skin disease that is characterized by well-circumscribed,

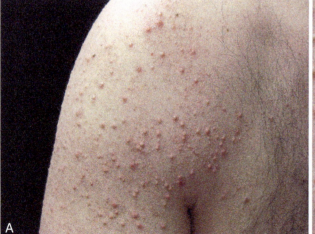
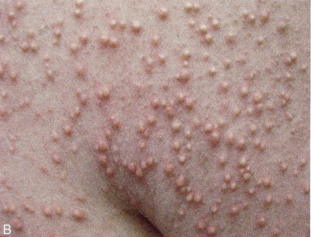

FIGURE 24-4 ■ (A) Multiple eruptive xanthomas in a patient with poorly-controlled diabetes. This patient did not know that he had diabetes mellitus when he presented for evaluation. His blood glucose was 598 mg/dL (normal = 65 to 99) and his triglyceride level was 270 mg/dL (normal = 0 to 149). (B) Characteristic yellow to red papules on the anterior shoulder and upper arm.

yellow-brown, occasionally indurated, painless plaques with pronounced epidermal atrophy and visible vasculature and frequent ulcerations within the lesions. Lesions often begin as small papules that enlarge, with an active erythematous or violaceous border. The lesions follow a chronic course, with variable progression and scarring. Unless treated, they can involve large areas of the skin surface and lead to disability and disfigurement. Most lesions occur in the pretibial region, and bilateral involvement is seen in up to 75% of patients (Figs. 24-5 and 24-6). Less commonly, NL can occur on the feet, arms, trunk, or scalp. Histologically, it is characterized by collagen degeneration surrounded by a palisading granulomatous response, thickening of blood vessel walls, and fat deposition.

Epidemiology

Less than 2% of diabetics develop NL. More than 66% of patients with NL have overt DM, and approximately 20% have glucose intolerance or a parent with diabetes. NL is observed more often in women, and usually follows the onset of diabetes by a mean of 10 years, with an average age of onset of 22 years in type 1 diabetics, and 49 years in type 2 diabetics. NL can be a presenting sign and occur concurrently with diabetes, and can even precede the diagnosis of diabetes. Thus, patients with NL and normal glucose metabolism should be evaluated and followed for the possibility of developing DM at a later date.

Pathogenesis

The specific pathogenesis of NL is unknown, although diabetic microangiopathy, collagen alterations, and immune complex deposition linked to an inflammatory process are thought to play a role. Patients with NL have higher rates of retinopathy and diabetic nephropathy, suggesting that vascular injury plays a role in NL. The role of glycemic control in the development of NL is unclear, although optimal glycemic control is recommended in the management of NL.

Treatment

Treatment of NL is challenging due to widely variable responses to therapy and the refractory nature of these lesions. Spontaneous remission is observed in less than 20% of cases over 6 to 12 years. While tight glycemic control of diabetes is recommended, it has not been specifically associated with significant improvement in NL. Topical and intralesional corticosteroids and calcineurin inhibitors are used to decrease the inflammation of early active lesions. Agents such as pentoxiphylline and low-dose aspirin may have a gradual effect on vasculopathic aspects of pathogenesis. Compression therapy is used on ulcerated plaques, with semipermeable membrane dressings. Phototherapy, particularly PUVA, has been reported as beneficial in some cases. Systemic immunomodulatory or immunosuppressive treatments have been helpful in rare reports, and recently, there have been reports of using biologic agents such as infliximab and etanercept in severe refractory cases. Local excision is usually complicated by recurrences at the borders.

Scleredema

Description

Scleredema diabeticorum is a connective tissue disorder associated with type 2 diabetes characterized by diffuse, symmetric, nonpitting induration of the skin with occasional erythema (Fig. 24-7). Rarely, an acute version of scleredema can follow streptococcal infection and an uncommon indistinguishable variant is associated with monoclonal gammopathy. Scleredema affects the neck, shoulders, and back, and rarely can involve the buttocks, abdomen, and thighs, while acral skin is almost always spared. Histopathologic examination reveals marked thickening of the reticular dermis, and thick collagen bundles and mucin infiltration in the deep dermis are hallmark findings. The clinical course is slowly progressive over years. Although the process is asymptomatic, patients may experience discomfort and decreased mobility, depending on the body region affected.

Epidemiology

Scleredema is a rare disorder, with an estimated prevalence between 2% and 15% in diabetics. It occurs more

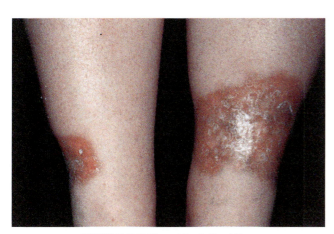

FIGURE 24-5 ■ Necrobiosis lipoidica.

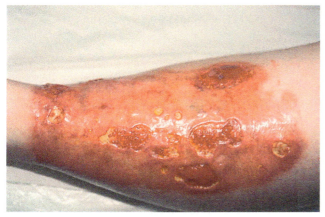

FIGURE 24-6 ■ Ulcerative necrobiosis lipoidica.

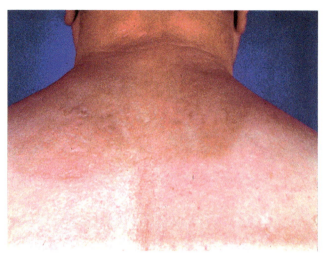

FIGURE 24-7 ■ Scleredema. Erythematous, indurated area on the upper back of this diabetic patient. (Reprinted with permission from Callen JP, Greer KE, Paller A, Swinyer L, editors. Color atlas of dermatology: a morphological approach, 2nd ed. Philadelphia: WB Saunders; 2000.)

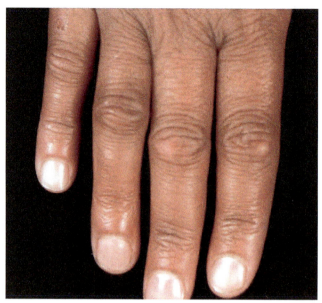

FIGURE 24-8 ■ Scleroderma-like skin changes.

in men over the age of 40 years. Patients with scleredema are more likely to have IDDM and have multiple other diabetes-related complications because of long-standing poor glycemic control.

Pathogenesis

The pathogenesis is unknown, although glycosaminoglycan deposition in the dermal connective tissue may play a role. Thickening of the reticular dermis with deposition of mucin between thickened collagen bundles is noted. This phenomenon may be similar to the more prevalent waxy induration of the skin of the extremities seen in IDDM.

Treatment

There is no effective therapy for sclerederma and the lesions are usually asymptomatic. In severely affected patients, the combination of UVA1 or PUVA and physical therapy can help improve mobility; intravenous immunoglobulin has been reported to be beneficial in severe cases. Strict glycemic control does not appear to affect the condition, although it is recommended as a preventive measure. Physical therapy benefits patients whose disease affects the shoulder girdle range of motion.

Scleroderma-like Skin Changes

Description

Distinct from scleroderma, scleroderma-like skin changes consist of thickening and induration of the skin on the dorsum of the fingers (sclerodactyly), proximal interphalangeal joints, and may involve the metacarpophalangeal joints (Fig. 24-8). It can extend to the forearms, arms, and back, and skin may have a waxy appearance. These changes are bilateral, symmetric, and painless. Extensive scleroderma-like skin changes of the torso and back occur in a subgroup of diabetic patients. Unlike scleroderma, this entity does not demonstrate dermal atrophy, telangiectasia, edema, Raynaud's phenomenon, or pain. Scleroderma-like skin change is also distinguished from scleredema diabeticorum by the greater extent of involvement, lack of mucin deposition, and the appearance in younger patients. The clinical course is progressive and leads to extensive involvement and stiffness. Patients with type 1 DM and severe scleroderma-like skin changes have a twofold increase in the occurrence of retinopathy and nephropathy compared to patients with no or mild disease. Scleroderma-like skin changes are related to disease duration but not to parameters of diabetic control.

Scleroderma-like skin findings are often seen in conjunction with diabetic hand syndrome, which consists of joint limitations (mainly an inability to fully extend the fingers), thickened skin of the hand, and the "prayer sign"—an inability to press the palms together completely, with a gap remaining between opposed palms and fingers (Fig. 24-9). Commonly, contractures begin in the fifth digit and progress radially to the other fingers. Palmar fascial thickening (Dupuytren's contractures) further complicates the diabetic hand syndrome. A strong association has been found with dry palms.

Epidemiology

Between 10% and 50% of diabetics manifest a degree of these findings. It is more common in patients with type 1 DM, and males and females appear to be equally affected.

Pathogenesis

In biochemical studies, there has been evidence to support that scleroderma-like syndrome with skin and joint involvement is due to nonenzymatic advanced glycosylation end products that can cause stiffening and alteration of turnover of collagen.

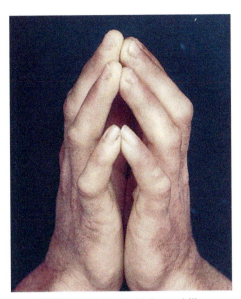

FIGURE 24-9 ■ Limited joint mobility.

Treatment

Anecdotal reports have demonstrated that tight glycemic control with an insulin pump results in reduced skin thickness. Another treatment option used in several patients with limited joint mobility is an aldose reductase inhibitor, which inhibits the accumulation of sugar alcohols. Physical therapy may be important in patients with severe disease to improve the range of motion of the joints.

OTHER CUTANEOUS FINDINGS OF DIABETES MELLITUS

Acquired Ichthyosiform Changes of the Shins

Acquired ichthyosiform changes of the shins is one of the most common skin findings seen in diabetes, with reported prevalence as high as 50% in IDDM patients. It is characterized by symmetric dryness and scaling of the anterior shins, and occurs as a result of microangiopathy, stratum corneum adhesion defects, advanced glycosylation, and accelerated skin aging. The condition improves with tight glycemic control.

Acrochordons

Acrochordons, or skin tags, are common benign skin tumors occurring on the eyelids, neck, axilla, and other flexural surfaces. In many patients, they appear in conjunction with acanthosis nigricans. Some studies have shown an increased risk of DM in patients with multiple skin tags; however, the evidence regarding a positive correlation between the total number of skin tags and the incidence of diabetes or impaired glucose tolerance is controversial.

Diabetic Cheiroarthropathy

Diabetic cheiroarthropathy is a condition of limited joint mobility that is seen in up to 40% of patients with diabetes. The most commonly affected joints are the metacarpophalangeal and interphalangeal joints, leading to joint stiffness. Limited joint mobility is caused by the thickening of periarticular connective tissue, and the disease process is positively correlated with long-standing poorly controlled diabetes. In patients with diabetic cheiroarthropathy, there is a fourfold increase in the risk of microvascular disease.

Diabetic Thick Skin

Thick skin in various clinical forms can be seen in diabetics, including waxy thickening of the dorsal hand and scleredema. The most common form is a benign condition of generalized thickening of the skin, which is usually asymptomatic. This condition often goes unrecognized, but measurement through ultrasound will reveal thicker-than-normal skin. The most common areas affected are the hands and feet.

Diabetes-Related Pruritus

Pruritus is occasionally present in diabetics and is mainly associated with diabetic neuropathy. It more commonly presents as localized pruritus in the scalp, trunk, and as part of small nerve fiber neuropathy in lower legs. It can also occur in the genitalia and perianal area, with concomitant candidiasis or intertrigo. Treatment consists of the use of oral antiepileptic agents such as gabapentin and pregabalin, and antifungal agents when there is candidiasis. Topical capsaicin may be helpful in some cases of localized neuropathic pruritus.

Finger Pebbles

Finger pebbles, also known as Huntley papules, are a variation of diabetic thick skin, and occur more in patients with type 2 DM. They appear as grouped papules on the dorsum of the hand, knuckles, and periungual areas, and over time may coalesce into confluent plaques with associated hypopigmentation. Histologically, biopsy specimens reveal marked thickening of the dermis and connective tissue. Finger pebbles are seen in up to one-third of patients with diabetic cheiroarthropathy, although both conditions can be seen independently.

Keratosis Pilaris

Keratosis pilaris is a disorder of perifollicular hyperkeratosis. It is a common benign condition that manifests as folliculocentric keratotic papules in characteristic areas of the body. Keratosis pilaris, like acquired ichthyosis, develops early in the course of diabetes (Fig. 24-10). General measures to prevent excessive skin dryness are recommended such as emollients, lactic acid, tretinoin cream, α-hydroxy acid lotions, urea-containing formulations, salicylic acid, and topical corticosteroids.

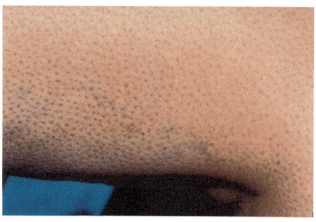

FIGURE 24-10 ■ Keratosis pilaris.

Palmar Erythema

Palmar erythema is an asymptomatic erythema seen in bilateral palms, often most prominent on the thenar and hypothenar eminences. It is a process distinct from normal physiologic mottling of the palm from inciting factors such as temperature as it is thought to be a microvascular complication of diabetes.

Periungual Telangiectases

Periungual telangiectases or nailbed erythema is a relatively common cutaneous finding in diabetic patients, seen in up to 65%. Clinically, the proximal nailfold will appear reddish in color. Slit-lamp examination will show visibly dilated capillaries around the nail bed caused by dilation of the superficial vascular plexus due to diabetic microangiopathy. It is asymptomatic, although it can be associated with cuticle changes and tenderness in the fingertips.

Pigmented Purpura

Pigmented purpura, or pigmented purpuric dermatoses, presents as asymptomatic orange to brown nonblanching patches that are often seen in the lower extremities. These skin findings, which must be distinguished clinically from stasis-associated hemosiderin deposition, are seen together with diabetic dermopathy and occur more often in elderly patients. It develops in later stages of the disease due to increasing fragility of capillary vessels associated with microangiopathy, which leads to extravasation of erythrocytes and deposition of hemosiderin in macrophages (siderophages).

Rubeosis Faciei

Rubeosis faciei is a chronic flushed appearance of the face, neck, and occasionally the extremities. It is more prominent in fair-skinned individuals, with an estimated prevalence of 8% in diabetic patients, although prevalence up to 59% has been reported in hospitalized diabetic patients. The clinical appearance is the result of microangiopathic alterations and superficial facial venous dilation, which may be due to reduced vasoconstrictor tone. Optimal glycemic control and reduced intake of vasodilators, including alcohol and caffeine, help alleviate symptoms.

Yellow Skin and Nails

Yellowish hue in the skin and nails is an asymptomatic benign finding among diabetics. The most affected areas are those of prominent sebaceous activity such as the face, areas with a thick stratum corneum such as the palms and soles, and the nails. The skin changes may be due to disproportionate accumulation of carotene in the skin caused by impairment of its hepatic conversion. Another theory attributes the yellow skin to dermal collagen glycosylation with end-stage glycosylation products. This condition improves with tight glycemic control.

Infections

Cutaneous infections occur in 20% to 50% of patients with diabetes and are more prevalent in individuals with poorly controlled type 2 diabetes than those with type 1 disease. Poor glycemic control increases the risk of infection by causing abnormal microcirculation, reduced phagocytosis, impaired leukocyte adherence, and delayed chemotaxis.

Fungal Infections

Fungal infections are the most prevalent type of cutaneous infection in diabetic patients. Candidal infections are common and often the first manifestation of DM. Candidal infections can cause angular stomatitis, paronychia, balanitis, and vulvovaginitis. Treatment requires the use of topical or oral antifungal agents, keeping the affected site dry, and, most importantly, blood glucose control.

Dermatophyte infections can present a significant threat in diabetics. Diabetic neuropathy in the distal lower extremities creates an ideal environment for dermatophyte infections, allowing benign cases of tinea pedis to become devastating. Breaks in the normal skin barrier due to tinea can lead to superficial bacterial infections such as erysipelas and cellulitis, and even sepsis or fungemia. For this reason, tinea pedis should be promptly and aggressively treated.

DM with debilitating ketosis increases the risk for life-threatening mucormycosis (Fig. 24-11). This occurs when various fungi of the Phycomycetes group produce an angiocentric necrotizing infection, particularly in the nasopharyngeal area, that may lead to cerebral involvement and death. Prompt intensive supportive care, surgical debridement, and intravenous therapy with amphotericin B are required.

Bacterial Infections

A polymicrobial etiology has been implicated in diabetic foot infections. Care must be taken to separate infection from colonization. Gram-negative infections are three times more frequent in diabetic individuals than nondiabetics. Gram-negative bacteria such as *Pseudomonas aeruginosa* may cause severe tissue damage, sepsis, and lead to amputation. As such, these organisms should not be regarded as insignificant in diabetic foot ulcers. Antibiotic resistance in *P. aeruginosa* from diabetic foot ulcers

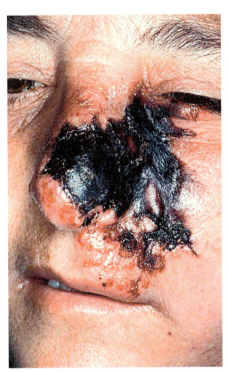

FIGURE 24-11 ■ Extensive central necrosis and associated swelling and erythema in a patient with mucormycosis.

is common, and isolates are often resistant to at least one or more antibiotics tested. β-Lactamase inhibitor antibiotics are first-line agents. Other antibiotics that can be used are clindamycin and a Gram-negative antimicrobial agent, or broad-spectrum quinolones and linezolid.

Erysipelas and cellulitis are more common in diabetic patients, as diabetics are more likely to have meticillin-resistant *Staphylococcus aureus* (MRSA) colonization and MRSA-induced bullous erysipelas. A common uncomplicated diabetic skin infection is bacterial folliculitis, which responds well to topical antibacterial treatment. Recent studies have shown a significant increase in community-acquired MRSA folliculitis.

Uncontrolled DM is a significant risk factor for necrotizing fasciitis, which is a serious skin and soft tissue infection that causes rapidly spreading necrosis of the soft tissues, often leading to systemic sepsis, multiorgan failure, and delayed cutaneous necrosis. In most patients with necrotizing fasciitis, the causative organism is not isolated or found to be polymicrobial. The mortality rate remains high despite combined treatment with antibiotics, surgical debridement, and hyperbaric oxygen.

Malignant otitis externa is an uncommon pseudomonal infection of the external ear canal. This condition occurs more frequently in elderly patients with DM, causing purulent discharge and severe external ear pain. The infection can spread to deeper tissues, causing osteomyelitis and meningitis. Despite aggressive treatment with debridement and antipseudomonal antibiotics, mortality is reported in over 50% of patients.

Erythrasma is characterized by nonpruritic, well-demarcated, red-tan scaly patches and thin plaques in intertriginous areas. Caused by *Corynebacterium minutissimum*, erythrasma is often confused with tinea cruris or candidiasis. Wood's light examination aids in diagnosis, showing characteristic coral-red fluorescence. Treatment consists of topical erythromycin, clindamycin, or clotrimazole and oral erythromycin.

DERMATOLOGIC DISEASES ASSOCIATED WITH DIABETES MELLITUS

Disseminated Granuloma Annulare

Granuloma annulare (GA) is a relatively common inflammatory disorder of unknown etiology. The most common clinical presentation is localized disease, which is not associated with diabetes. The disseminated form of GA has significant correlation with diabetes in many studies, although other studies question this association. Patients present with few to hundreds of 1- to 2-mm papules or nodules. Lesions may coalesce into annular plaques, with peripheral extension and central clearing. GA is generally asymptomatic, and does not resolve spontaneously. Although treatment is not medically necessary, patients often pursue treatment due to the physical appearance of the lesions. Disseminated GA is difficult to treat. There are reports of photochemotherapy with PUVA, isotretinoin, dapsone, antimalarial agents, and corticosteroids, with varying success.

Lichen Planus

Lichen planus is an inflammatory dermatitis with unknown etiology. It is characterized by the presence of firm, erythematous, pruritic papules that commonly affect the wrists, lower back, and ankles. Several studies have explored the relationship between the incidence of diabetes and lichen planus, and diabetes or abnormal glucose metabolism has been observed with varying rates of reported incidence in patients with lichen planus (14% to 85%). Medications used to treat diabetes have been associated with lichenoid drug eruptions.

Vitiligo

Vitiligo is an acquired disorder of depigmentation that is thought to be autoimmune-mediated. It is seen up to 10 times more frequently in diabetic patients than in the general population. It is particularly common among women with type 2 DM. In patients with IDDM, vitiligo may be associated with other autoimmune endocrine autoantibodies.

Psoriasis

Psoriasis is a chronic inflammatory skin disease with a worldwide prevalence between 1% and 3%. There is an increased risk of developing diabetes in patients with severe psoriasis, compared to the general population.

CUTANEOUS COMPLICATIONS OF DIABETIC THERAPY

Cutaneous reactions that occur with oral antidiabetic drugs include macular erythema, urticaria, and erythema multiforme. In addition, tolbutamide and chlorpropamide can produce photosensitivity. Of all the oral hypoglycemic medications, sulfonylureas most often cause allergic skin reactions. Lichenoid and rosacea-like eruptions are common with oral hypoglycemic agents, which cause a reaction in 1% to 5% of patients. The second-generation sulfonylureas cause fewer cutaneous side effects than first-generation agents.

Lipoatrophy is characterized by circumscribed, depressed areas of skin at insulin injection sites that develop 6 to 24 months after starting insulin. It occurs more often in children and women, and in areas of substantial fat deposits, such as the thighs. Several pathogenic theories are proposed, including the lipolytic components of the insulin preparation. Spontaneous improvement after rotating injection sites is rare, but has been reported. Use of purified and recombinant human insulin has resulted in reduced lipoatrophy. Substituting rapidly acting insulin may be effective.

Lipohypertrophy is described as soft dermal nodules that clinically resemble lipomas. The prevalence is 20% to 30% in type 1 and 4% in type 2 diabetics. It is more common with the use of human insulin, frequent number of injections per day, higher total daily dose of insulin, reuse of needles, and missing rotation of injection sites. It may be a response to the lipogenic action of insulin. Injection into a lipohypertrophied site can lead to a significant delay in insulin absorption, resulting in erratic glucose control and unpredictable hypoglycemia. Education of patients about correct injection techniques and the necessity for routine change of injection sites can be preventive.

Insulin allergy is relatively rare and more commonly seen with bovine insulin than with porcine insulin. Recombinant DNA-produced human insulin produces less allergy and lipodystrophy. Documented examples of insulin allergy include immediate hypersensitivity reactions, which result in urticarial, serum sickness-like reactions, often characterized by vasculitic or purpuric urticarial lesions, and delayed hypersensitivity reactions, which may present as localized nodules.

SUGGESTED READINGS

Ahmed I, Goldstein B. Diabetes mellitus. Clin Dermatol 2006;24:237–46.

Bee YM, Ng ACM, Goh SY, et al. The skin and joint manifestations of diabetes mellitus: superficial clues to deeper issues. Singapore Med J 2006;47:111.

Huntley AC. Cutaneous manifestations of diabetes mellitus. Diabetes Metab Rev 1993;9:161–76.

Murphy-Chutorian B, Han G, Cohen SR. Dermatologic manifestations of diabetes mellitus: a review. Endocrinol Metab Clin North Am 2013;42(4):869–98.

Ngo BT, Hayes KD, DiMiao DJ, et al. Manifestations of cutaneous diabetic microangiopathy. Am J Clin Dermatol 2005;6:225–37.

Tabor CA, Parlette EC. Cutaneous manifestations of diabetes. Signs of poor glycemic control or new-onset disease. Postgrad Med 2006;119:38–44.

Yosipovitch G, Hodak E, Vardi P, et al. The prevalence of cutaneous manifestations in IDDM patients and their association with diabetes risk factors and microvascular complications. Diabetes Care 1998;21:506–9.

CHAPTER 25

THYROID AND THE SKIN

Elizabeth Ghazi • Ted Rosen • Joseph L. Jorizzo • Warren R. Heymann

KEY POINTS

- When evaluating cysts and nodules of the head and neck, consider thyroglossal ductal cysts and thyroid carcinoma metastases.
- There are many syndromes associated with thyroid cancer with dermatologic manifestations (e.g., Cowden's disease, multiple mucosal neuroma syndromes, Gardner's syndrome, Carney's complex, and Werner's syndrome).
- Urticaria has been associated with papillary carcinoma and autoimmune thyroid disease although the pathogenesis remains to be elucidated.
- Pretibial myxedema, Graves' ophthalmopathy, and thyroid acropachy often exist as a triad in patients with Graves' disease.
- Hypothyroid states are characterized by myxedema and mucin deposition.
- Hair and nail changes often serve as important clues in thyroid disease (e.g., madarosis with hypothyroidism and Plummer nails in hyperthyroidism).

Thyroid hormones influence the differentiation, maturation, and growth of many different body tissues; the total energy expenditure of the organism; and the turnover of nearly all substrates, vitamins, and other hormones. Thus, it is not surprising that the thyroid gland plays an important role in both skin development and the maintenance of normal cutaneous function. In general, the biologic effects of thyroid hormones require binding to specific nuclear receptors with subsequent alteration of gene transcription and stimulation of messenger RNA synthesis. It is postulated that, in addition to nuclear receptors, subcellular receptors exist in mitochondria and plasma membranes. It has been clearly demonstrated that thyroid activity directly affects oxygen consumption, protein synthesis, mitosis, and the thickness of the epidermis. Thyroid activity is also considered essential for the formation and growth of hair, and for sebum secretion. Dermal effects are less well defined.

The impact of thyroid hormone activity on the integument, however, is more notable during deficiency or excess states than during normal physiologic processes. The prevalence of hypothyroidism is 4.6% and that of hyperthyroidism is 1.3%, therefore, the clinician will frequently observe these findings in practice. With several important exceptions (discussed later), the majority of cutaneous changes accompanying thyroid disease are neither unique nor pathognomonic. However, in patients with thyroid dysfunction, even such nonspecific cutaneous findings and associations often provide important clues that aid in the diagnosis of previously unsuspected thyroid disease. Finally, some syndromes with cutaneous or mucosal lesions are associated with an increased risk for thyroid tumors (e.g., Cowden's disease, multiple mucosal neuroma syndromes, Gardner's syndrome, Carney's complex, and Werner's syndrome).

The thyroid gland, which weighs an average of 20 to 25 g in adults, actively secretes thyroxine (T_4) and triiodothyronine (T_3) from the intraluminal thyroglobulin of its follicular cells. The follicular cells are derived primarily from median midpharyngeal tissue during embryologic development. T_3 is more active than its precursor T_4. It is worth noting that about 80% of the T_3 produced daily actually results from hepatic and renal deiodination of T_4, rather than from direct thyroid secretion. Thyroxine has a lower metabolic clearance rate and longer serum half-life than T_3 because it binds more tightly to serum-binding proteins than does T_3. The half-life of T_3 is less than a day, whereas the half-life of T_4 is about 7 days. Furthermore, although only 0.02% of the total plasma T_4 and 0.30% of the total plasma T_3 are free (i.e., not protein bound), the free forms both determine the thyroid "status" and maintain the negative feedback regulatory system involving the hypothalamic–pituitary–thyroid axis.

Calcitonin is secreted from thyroid parafollicular cells (C cells). This hormone is involved in the metabolism of calcium and phosphorus, leading to decreasing serum calcium by inhibiting osteoclast bone resorption. In comparison, parathyroid hormone increases bone resorption. The parafollicular cells are derived embryologically from the neural crest, becoming incorporated within the ultimobranchial pharyngeal pouch.

Thyroid evaluation should commence with a physical examination of the gland. Laboratory tests of direct thyroid function include total and free T_4 and T_3, free T_4 index, T_3 or T_4 resin uptake (now termed the thyroid hormone-binding ratio), and radioactive iodine uptake. An evaluation of thyroid gland function is characteristically based on thyrotropin levels (thyroid-stimulating hormone—TSH), being elevated in patients with primary causes of hypothyroidism (e.g., Hashimoto's thyroiditis) or reduced in patients with primary forms of hyperthyroidism (e.g., Graves' disease). The thyroid may undergo anatomic evaluation by a thyroid scan, ultrasonography, fine-needle aspiration, or surgical biopsy. Finally, tests for autoimmune thyroid disease include serum thyroid peroxidase (antimicrosomal), thyroid-stimulating, or antithyroglobulin antibody determination. Following thyroidectomy for carcinoma, increases in serum thyroglobulin are considered suspicious for recurrent disease. Table 25-1 shows the differences in laboratory tests for Graves' disease and Hashimoto's thyroiditis.

The cutaneous manifestations of thyroid disease may be categorized as follows: (1) specific lesions that contain thyroid tissue; (2) signs and symptoms of hyperthyroid and hypothyroid states; and (3) other skin or systemic disorders associated with thyroid disease.

TABLE 25-1 **Thyroid Function Tests**

	Graves' Disease	Hashimoto's Thyroiditis
Thyroid stimulating hormone (TSH)	Decreased	Increased
T_4, T_3, free T_4	Increased	Decreased
Thyroglobulin antibody	12–30%	50–60%
Anti-TSH receptor assay	80–100%	6%
Radioiodine uptake	Increased	Decreased

SPECIFIC LESIONS

Thyroglossal Duct Cysts

During embryonic life, the developing thyroid gland descends in the neck while possibly maintaining its connection to the tongue by a narrow tube of undifferentiated epithelium, the thyroglossal duct. Thyroglossal duct cysts can present anywhere from the tongue to the diaphragm. Movement of the cyst with tongue protrusion is only seen if the connection to the tongue is preserved. This structure may activate later in life, and the cells then differentiate into columnar, ciliated, or squamous epithelium, or even into overt glandular tissue. Thyroglossal duct cysts account for 70% of the congenital cystic abnormalities of the neck. They usually present in the first decade of life as a cystic midline mass containing mucoid material. Occasionally, part of the duct will form a sinus tract extending to the skin surface at, or just lateral to, the midline. This may present as a bullous lesion. These anomalies are classified according to their location with respect to the hyoid bone: 65% are infrahyoid; 20% are suprahyoid; and 15% are juxtahyoid. Thyroglossal duct cysts are usually mobile and nontender, unless complicated by infection. Dysphagia may occur with lesions beneath the tongue and superior vena cava syndrome may occur with lesions that are retrosternal. Malignancies develop within these structures in less than 1% of cases; 80% of such neoplasms are papillary adenocarcinomas. It is essential that clinicians be certain that these cysts are distinguished from ectopic thyroid tissue, which may be the only functioning thyroid tissue present in 75% of ectopic thyroid patients. Ectopic tissue can be detected by ultrasound or radionuclide scans. Possible treatment modalities include excision of a portion of the hyoid bone along with the cyst (the "Sistrunk" procedure decreases recurrence rate compared to simple excision) and endoscopic CO_2 laser for those lesions extending into the respiratory tract.

Cutaneous Metastases

Thyroid cancer accounts for 3.8% of new cancers and 0.3% of cancer deaths. Although the incidence of thyroid cancer has been increasing, much of this may be attributable to increased detection by ultrasound screening procedure. Papillary thyroid carcinoma accounts for the majority of thyroid malignancies in early life. It metastasizes to regional lymph nodes, but only rarely distantly (including to the skin). By contrast, follicular carcinoma usually appears in middle-aged or elderly individuals, and distant metastases are more frequent. Anaplastic tumors—the giant or spindle cell subtypes—occur almost without exception in those over 60 years of age, grow rapidly, and possess a propensity for both nodal and distant metastases. Albeit rare, all histologic types of thyroid cancer have been reported to metastasize to the skin. Such metastatic lesions tend to favor the head and neck region, may be either solitary or multiple, and are generally painless. In this respect, metastases from thyroid neoplasms do not differ significantly from those originating in other sites. Seeding of the skin has been reported after percutaneous needle biopsy. Thyroid cancer metastases have been reported from 2 to 10 years after the discovery of the primary tumor. Although such lesions usually occur in patients with a known history of malignancy, they may be the initial presentation of a cancer. In those cases where a biopsy was performed and the routine histology is equivocal, immunohistochemical stains (i.e., thyroid transcription factor and thyroglobin for most tumors, with calcitonin, synaptophysin, chromogranin, and CD56 being specific for medullary carcinoma) may allow for a precise diagnosis.

Dermatologic Syndromes Associated with Thyroid Cancer

Medullary carcinoma of the thyroid originates from parafollicular cells (C cells); these are of neural crest origin. Medullary thyroid carcinoma is familial in 20% of cases, occurring as an autosomal dominant trait as part of multiple endocrine neoplasia (MEN) syndrome type 2a or 2b, caused by mutations in the RET proto-oncogene. In this setting, thyroid cancer is associated with mucosal neuromas, pheochromocytomas, neurofibromas, diffuse lentigines, and café-au-lait macules. Cutaneous macular (or lichen) amyloidosis can occur in association with MEN 2a, making it an important clinical sign. Another autosomal dominant disorder that predisposes to thyroid carcinoma is Cowden's disease, also known as the multiple hamartoma syndrome. The syndrome shows a dominant inheritance pattern, with a variable penetrance. Various germline mutations in the *PTEN* gene have been found in more than 80% of patients. Features of this disease include facial trichilemmomas, oral papillomatosis, acral and palmar keratoses, and an increased risk of developing breast carcinoma. Thyroid involvement is common in Cowden's syndrome, with as many as 60% developing benign thyroid lesions, such as multinodular goiter, and follicular adenomas. The risk for thyroid cancer (typically follicular, but occasionally papillary) is approximately 10%. Gardner's syndrome (mutation of the *APC*

TABLE 25-2 Thyroid Cancer Syndromes

Disease	Histologic Type	Gene Mutation	Incidence	Key Associated Findings
FAP and Gardner's syndrome	PTC, including cribiform-morular classical variant	APC tumor suppressor gene	2–12%	Epidermoid cysts, pilomatricomas, desmoid tumors, CHRPE, osteomas, colorectal malignancy
Cowden's syndrome	FTC, PTC	PTEN tumor suppressor gene	>10%	Trichilemmomas, acral verrucous keratotic papules, mucosal papules, lipomas, angiomas, fibromas, malignancy
Carney's complex	FTC, PTC	PRKAR1-x	60% and 4%	Cutaneous and mucosal lentigines, blue nevi, melanocytic nevi, CALM, testicular tumors, psammomatous melanocytic schwannoma, testicular tumors, atrial myxoma
Werner's syndrome	FTC, PTC, ATC	WRN gene	18%	Short stature, premature aging, malignancy
MEN 2a	MTC	RET proto-oncogene	20%	Mucosal neuromas, pheochromocytomas, neurofibromas, lentigines, CALM, macular amyloid
McCune–Albright's syndrome	PTC, clear cell	GNAS-1	Two case reports	CALM, oral lentigines, polyostotic fibrous dysplasia, precocious puberty

FAP, Familial adenomatous polyposis; PTC, parafollicular thyroid cancer; CHRPE, congenital hypertrophy of the retinal pigment epithelium; FTC, follicular thyroid cancer; CALM, café-au-lait macules; MEN, multiple endocrine neoplasia; ATC, anaplastic thyroid cancer.
Adapted from Son EJ, Nose. Familial follicular cell-derived thyroid carcinoma. Front Endocrinol 2012;3:61.

gene), Carney complex (mutation in *PRKAR1-x*), Werner's syndrome (mutation in *WRN*), and McCune–Albright's syndrome (mutation in *GNAS1*) have also been associated with thyroid neoplasms. A recent report of clear cell thyroid carcinoma in association with Birt–Hogg–Dubé demonstrated folliculin mutation within the tumor itself. See Table 25-2 for a summary of thyroid tumor syndromes.

Hyperthyroidism may be seen in patients who develop widespread metastatic lesions from a primary thyroid malignancy, regardless of the histologic type. The occurrence of this phenomenon, albeit rare, correlates with a large tumor load. Successful therapy for the tumor and possible metastatic lesions results in a resolution of the symptoms of hyperthyroidism.

There have been rare cases of urticaria associated with papillary thyroid cancer. Resolution of urticaria associated with papillary carcinoma has been achieved with thyroidectomy.

HYPERTHYROIDISM

General

Excessive quantities of circulating thyroid hormones produce a hypermetabolic state known as hyperthyroidism or thyrotoxicosis. The prevalence of this condition is about 2.5% in women and less than 0.2% in men. Graves' disease accounts for 85% of all cases of hyperthyroidism. However, there are many other causes of this disorder, including toxic multinodular goiter, toxic follicular adenoma, subacute thyroiditis, ingestion of excess thyroid hormone (factitious thyrotoxicosis), tumors secreting hormones that stimulate the thyroid (e.g., TSH-secreting pituitary tumor, choriocarcinoma, and embryonic testicular carcinoma), and tumors that directly secrete thyroid hormone. Etiologies of hyperthyroidism are listed in Table 25-3. The most common symptoms accompanying hyperthyroidism, regardless of the exact cause, are systemic rather than cutaneous. These include nervousness, emotional disturbance, weight loss despite an increased appetite, heat intolerance, hyperhidrosis, "weakness," palpitations, and/or tremor. Patients often speak rapidly and complain bitterly about heat intolerance. Common clinical signs in thyrotoxic patients include sinus tachycardia; atrial fibrillation; increased systolic and lowered diastolic blood

TABLE 25-3 Causes of Hyperthyroidism

Autoimmune
Graves'

Inflammatory/Destructive
Postpartum thyroiditis
Painless thyroiditis
Subacute thyroiditis
Thyroid infarction
Radiation thyroiditis
Ectopic production
Struma ovarii

Hypothalamopituitary Axis Dysregulation
Thyroid-stimulating hormone (TSH)-secreting adenoma
Thyrotropic resistance to thyroid hormone
Trophoblastic tumor
Hyperemesis gravidarum
Gestational thyrotoxicosis
Autosomal dominant hyperthyroidism

Extrinsic Consumption
Exogenous thyroid consumption
Dietary iodine excess
Drug-induced thyroiditis

Intrinsic Overproduction
Thyroid carcinoma
Toxic adenoma
Toxic multinodular goiter

Reproduced with permission from Cokonis CD, Cobb CW, Heymann WR, Hivnor CM. Cutaneous manifestations of hyperthyroidism. In: Heymann WR, editor. Thyroid disorders with cutaneous manifestations. London: Springer Verlag; 2008.

TABLE 25-4	Dermatological Manifestations of Hyperthyroidism
Skin	Fine, velvety, or smooth
	Warm and moist (increased sweating), rarely dry
	Hyperpigmentation (localized or generalized)
	Vitiligo
	Urticaria or dermatographism
	Pretibial myxedema and thyroid acropachy
Hair	Fine, thin
	Alopecia (diffuse and mild; rarely severe)
	Alopecia areata
Nails	Onycholysis
	Koilonychia
	Clubbing with thyroid acropachy

pressures; fine to coarse resting or intention tremors; proximal muscle weakness; and changes in the skin, hair, and nails (Table 25-4).

The skin is described as being moist and warm, the result of vasodilation and increased cutaneous perfusion. It is further characterized as soft and velvety in texture, comparable to that of an infant. The skin is usually less oily, and hyperthyroidism in adolescence is associated with a reduced incidence of acne due to decreased sebaceous activity. Palmar erythema, episodic flushing over the face and thorax, increased capillary fragility, and persistent erythema of the elbows may also occur. Hyperhidrosis may be either generalized or localized to the palms and soles.

Diffuse hair loss is present in 20% to 40% of hyperthyroid patients, although the severity of alopecia does not correlate with the severity of thyrotoxicosis. The hair itself is typically fine, soft, straight, and unable to retain a permanent wave. Human hair follicles are direct targets of thyroid hormones. Thyrotropin-releasing hormone (TRH), TSH, T_4, and T_3 have been associated with proliferation of matrix keratinocytes. TRH, T_3, and T_4 have been shown to stimulate intrafollicular melanin synthesis.

Nail changes, present in about 5% of cases of hyperthyroidism, are often reversible following successful therapy. The nails are described as rapidly growing, soft, and friable. Although not truly pathognomonic for thyrotoxicosis, the nails often assume a "scoop shovel" configuration and/or demonstrate striking onycholysis. Such nails are referred to as Plummer nails. Any or all the fingernails and toenails may be involved.

Pigmentary changes associated with hyperthyroidism include localized hyperpigmentation (facial, in scars, or in palmar creases), generalized hyperpigmentation, which may be in an Addisonian pattern, canities, or vitiligo. Hyperpigmentation is believed to be caused by an increased release of adrenocorticotropic hormone in compensation for an accelerated rate of peripheral cortisol degradation. Vitiligo is associated with a variety of autoimmune disorders, the most frequent being autoimmune thyroid disease (including both Graves' disease and Hashimoto's thyroiditis).

Graves' Disease

Graves' disease is an autoimmune disorder that develops as a result of susceptibility genes and presumed exposure to environmental factors. Age of onset is usually between

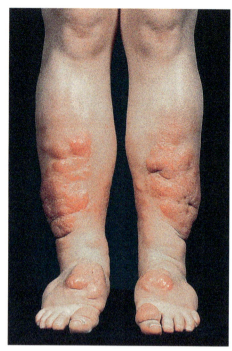

FIGURE 25-1 ■ Pretibial myxedema manifested as infiltrative plaques in a woman 10 years after thyroidectomy for Graves' disease.

20 and 50 years and the disease occurs seven to 10 times more frequently in females. To date, no unique susceptibility genes specific to pretibial myxedema or Graves' ophthalmopathy have been identified. The hyperthyroidism of Graves' disease appears to be caused by the binding of thyroid-stimulating autoantibodies to the TSH receptor. Activation of the TSH receptor by the autoantibody results in excessive production of thyroid hormones.

In addition to demonstrating the nonspecific signs and symptoms discussed previously, patients with Graves' disease often demonstrate several distinctive features, e.g., pretibial myxedema (0.5% to 10%) and thyroid acropachy (1%). Pretibial myxedema is often, albeit not invariably, associated with ophthalmopathy; 15% of those with ophthalmopathy have associated pretibial myxedema. Pretibial myxedema may also be seen with Hashimoto's thyroiditis and Graves' disease. The status of thyroid function bears no direct relation to the development of pretibial myxedema, and the condition may develop after treatment. Although the pretibial location is most typical, lesions may occur on the arm, shoulder, and thigh. For this reason, the term "thyroid dermopathy" is preferred.

Early lesions of pretibial myxedema appear as bilateral, raised, asymmetrical, firm plaques and nodules (Fig. 25-1). A peau d'orange appearance, caused by dermal infiltration by the glycosaminoglycans (GAGs) hyaluronic acid and chondroitin sulfate, may be noted. The lesions may be pink, violaceous, or flesh-colored and have a waxy translucent quality. They may enlarge and coalesce to form grotesque arrays, resembling elephantiasis. Pathogenesis is believed to be increase of GAGs stimulated by autoantibodies. Topical and intralesional corticosteroids are the mainstay of therapy. Compression therapy is valuable. Intravenous immunoglobulin, corticosteroids, octreotide, and pentoxyfylline are second-line therapies.

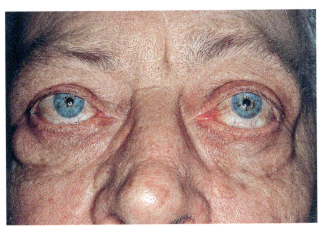

FIGURE 25-2 ■ An example of the ophthalmopathy associated with Graves' disease. (Reproduced with permission from Cokonis CD, Cobb CW, Heymann WR, Hivnor CM. Cutaneous manifestations of hyperthyroidism. In: Heymann WR, editor. Thyroid disorders with cutaneous manifestations. London: Springer Verlag; 2008.)

Plasmapheresis was reported to be of transient benefit in some patients; there has been a report of utilizing plasmapheresis with rituximab, which was successful in a patient. Surgery yields equivocal results, and is not routinely recommended. Although lesions persist, most patients will improve slowly with time, typically over many years.

Thyroid acropachy is rare, with fewer than 100 cases being reported. Ninety-five percent of patients develop acropachy after therapy for Graves' disease. This disorder consists of a triad of clubbing of the fingers and toes; periosteal proliferation of the phalanges and long bones; and swelling of the soft tissue overlying bony structures. The most common manifestation of acropachy is clubbing of the fingernails and toenails, which occurs in 19% of patients who have thyroid dermopathy. The first, second, and fifth metacarpals, the proximal phalanges of the hand, and the first metatarsal and proximal phalanges of the feet are most often affected. Bone scanning is the most sensitive objective test to detect thyroid acropachy. No therapy is indicated because the condition is usually asymptomatic. Patients who smoke should be encouraged to quit, as smoking has been associated with all extrathyroidal manifestations of Graves' disease, including thyroid acropachy.

In patients with suspected Graves' disease, examination of the neck may reveal obvious thyromegaly. Examination of the eyes will reveal mild changes (exophthalmos) to severe changes (proptosis), along with congestion of the sclera. Exophthalmos occurs in nearly all patients with Graves' disease and may be the first sign of hyperthyroidism (Fig. 25-2). The complaints accompanying this problem include "protruding" eyes, lid retraction, easy tear production or dry eyes, photophobia, and the sensation of a foreign body in the eye. This disorder is caused by infiltration of retrobulbar tissues and extraocular muscles by mononuclear cells and mucopolysaccharides (MPS), but the precise factor(s) responsible remain a unidentified. Patients should be counseled to stop smoking. Potential therapies include topical lubricants, Botox injections for lid retraction, and prednisone and decompression surgery for severe disease. Rituximab, a monoclonal CD20 antibody that targets B cells, may be a promising future therapeutic alternative as it may stop the immune stimulation of MPS deposition.

Graves' disease has been associated with other findings including unilateral palpebral edema and annular lipoatrophy of the ankles (a lobular panniculitis).

HYPOTHYROIDISM

General

Hypothyroidism results from a deficiency of thyroid hormones and, like hyperthyroidism, is much more likely to be seen in women, with a female-to-male ratio of 7:1. The disorder is particularly likely to affect women between the ages of 40 and 60 years. Almost 95% of all cases can be classified as either primary acquired or idiopathic. About 5% are the result of pituitary or hypothalamic dysfunction; the remainder are caused by the congenital absence of thyroid tissue, inherited deficiency in thyroid hormone-synthesizing enzymes, or severe iodine deficit. Rarely, hypothyroidism results from drugs (e.g., lithium and sulfonamides) or from irradiation of the neck region. The cause of the disease in the majority of patients affected by primary acquired hypothyroidism is Hashimoto's thyroiditis or iatrogenic thyroid ablation (^{131}I therapy or surgical thyroidectomy). Table 25-5 lists the causes of hypothyroidism.

The term thyroiditis actually covers a number of histologically distinct entities, including acute suppurative thyroiditis, subacute granulomatous thyroiditis, and chronic sclerosing thyroiditis of Riedel. Nonetheless, the majority of patients are classified as having Hashimoto's or chronic lymphocytic thyroiditis. This disorder is believed to have an autoimmune-mediated pathogenesis, as illustrated by the many patients who have circulating antithyroglobulin or antiperoxidase (microsomal) antibodies. There is also a strong genetic predisposition to develop this disease among those with the HLA-B8 and -DR3 haplotypes, which correspond to the atrophic/fibrotic subtype, and HLA-DR5, which corresponds to the hypertrophic subtype. Hashimoto's thyroiditis is increased in trisomy 21 and Turner's syndrome.

The clinical manifestations of hypothyroidism, regardless of the exact cause, can be attributed to both a deceleration of cellular metabolic processes and/or myxedema, the accumulation of acid mucopolysaccharides in various organs, such as the skin, vocal cords, and oropharynx. The exact pathogenesis of myxedema remains obscure, but most authorities have abandoned the hypothesis that it is the result of increased levels of TSH, which occurs in response to low thyroid hormone levels. The extracutaneous features of hypothyroidism include pleural and pericardial effusions, bradycardia and reduced cardiac output, weight gain secondary to fluid retention, hoarseness, swollen lips and tongue, rheumatoid-like polyarthritis, and a wide variety of neurologic problems (such as slowed mentation). When hypothyroidism develops in adolescence, delayed sexual maturation occurs; in adults, impotence, oligospermia, and amenorrhea are common. The symptoms often include weakness and fatigue, anorexia, cold intolerance, voice changes, muscle cramps,

TABLE 25–5 Causes of Hypothyroidism

Primary	Defects in thyroid hormone biosynthesis
	Congenital defects in hormone synthesis
	Inheritable enzyme defects
	Iodine deficiency
	Iodine excess
	Antithyroid medications (lithium, amiodarone, goitrogens, bexarotene)
	Reduced functional thyroid tissue
	Hashimoto's (chronic autoimmune thyroiditis)
	Thyroid surgery
	Radioiodine (^{131}I) therapy
	Radiation to head and neck
	Infiltrative diseases: sarcoidosis, hemochromatosis, systemic sclerosis, amyloidosis, Riedel's thyroiditis, cystinosis
	Viral infections: subacute thyroiditis
	Postpartum thyroiditis
	Thyroid dysgenesis/agenesis
Central (pituitary/hypothalamic)	Reduced pituitary/hypothalamic tissue
	Tumors: pituitary adenoma, craniopharyngioma, meningioma, glioma, metastases
	Vascular: ischemic necrosis, hemorrhage (Sheehans' syndrome), internal carotid artery aneurysm, compression of pituitary stalk
	Trauma: head injury, radiation, surgery
	Infectious: brain abscess, tuberculosis, syphilis, toxoplasmosis
	Infiltrative: sarcoidosis, hemochromatosis, histiocytosis
	Chronic lymphocytic hypophysitis
	Congenital abnormalities: pituitary hypoplasia, basal encephalocele
	Genetic mutations in thyrotropin releasing hormone (TRH) receptor, thyroid-stimulating hormone (TSH) receptor, and Pit-1

Reproduced with permission from Kopp SA et al. Cutaneous manifestations of hypothyroidism. In: Heymann WR, editor. Thyroid disorders with cutaneous manifestations. London: Springer Verlag; 2008.

and swelling of the extremities. Such symptoms may easily be overlooked or mistakenly ascribed to aging.

Alterations in the skin, hair, and nails occurring in hypothyroidism are summarized in Table 25-6. In one review, coarse skin was the most common finding, followed by hair loss and edema, respectively. Generalized myxedema is caused by the dermal deposition of acid MPS (notably hyaluronic acid and chondroitin sulfate). The entire skin appears swollen, dry, waxy, and pale. The cutaneous pallor is due both to vasoconstriction and to the increased water and MPS content in the dermis, which alters the refraction of incident light. The skin is also "boggy" but nonpitting, especially around the eyes, lips, and acral portions. The skin is cool to the touch and may be so xerotic that hypothyroidism may be considered as a cause of acquired ichthyosis. The palms and soles are hypohidrotic and may demonstrate a keratoderma. Carotenemia may also be encountered on the volar and palmar surfaces as a result of reduced hepatic conversion of β-carotene to vitamin A.

The hair in patients with hypothyroidism is dull, coarse, and brittle. The growth rate is slowed, with an increase in telogen (resting) hairs. Although diffuse alopecia may be seen in patients with hypothyroidism, the classic pattern of hair loss is the loss of the lateral third of the eyebrows (madarosis). Hypertrichosis in association with hypothyroidism has been reported in children.

The nails are affected to some degree in 90% of all patients. They are typically thin, brittle, slow-growing, and striated (either in longitudinal or transverse fashion). Onycholysis, more commonly seen in hyperthyroid states, has also been reported to accompany myxedema.

TABLE 25-6 Dermatological Manifestations of Hypothyroidism

Skin	Dry, rough, or coarse; cold and pale; puffy, boggy, or edematous (myxedema)
	Yellow discoloration as a result of carotenemia
	Ichthyosis and palmoplantar hyperkeratosis
	Easy bruising (capillary fragility)
	Eruptive bruising (capillary fragility)
	Eruptive and tuberous xanthomas (rare)
Hair	Dull, coarse, and brittle
	Slow growth (increase in telogen or resting hairs)
	Alopecia (lateral third of eyebrows, rarely diffuse)
Nails	Thin, brittle, striated
	Slow growth
	Onycholysis (rare)

Congenital Hypothyroidism

When the thyroid gland fails to secrete sufficient hormone in utero or during the early perinatal period, congenital hypothyroidism (cretinism) occurs. This phenomenon appears in one of every 3000 to 4000 live births. The overwhelming majority of cases are sporadic, although some 15% are genetic, secondary to dyshormonogenesis. This disease becomes clinically apparent by 6 weeks of age, although no single clinical feature can be said to be pathognomonic.

The earliest symptoms of hypothyroidism are nonspecific and include lethargy, poor feeding, constipation, persistent neonatal jaundice, and respiratory difficulty as a result of myxedema of the oropharynx and larynx. The characteristic puffy facies, macroglossia, umbilical hernia, and hypotonia are not evident until 3 to 4 months of age. The presence of a clavicular fat pad at birth may suggest hypothyroidism. As in adult hypothyroidism, the skin tends to be cold, dry, and pale; the hair is coarse, dry, and brittle. A reduced metabolic rate causes reflex peripheral vasoconstriction, which may result in cutis marmorata. Growth retardation and mental retardation occur if therapy is not instituted at an early stage.

Infantile hemangiomas have been associated with a "consumptive hypothyroidism" due to an increase in type 3 iodothyronine deiodinase which inactivates thyroxine and triiodothyronine. This is most common with hepatic hemangiomas and cutaneous hemangiomas associated with PHACES (Posterior fossa malformations, Hemangiomas, Arterial anomalies, Cardiac defects and coarctation of the aorta, Eye abnormalities, and Sternal abnormalities or ventral developmental defects) syndrome. High doses of thyroid hormone are often required in such patients, until the "consumptive hypothyroidism" resolves; recently propranolol has been utilized to hasten resolution of hepatic and infantile cutaneous hemangiomas of infancy.

MISCELLANEOUS CUTANEOUS DISORDERS AND THE THYROID

Thyroid diseases need to be considered as contributing to the clinical picture in patients with a host of systemic and dermatologic disorders, many of which are classified as autoimmune. Alopecia areata occurs in up to 8% of patients with thyroid disease. Thyroid disease was reported in 25% of vitiligo patients. Lichen planopilaris has been associated with thyroid disease. Bullous pemphigoid and pemphigus have been linked statistically to autoimmune thyroid disease. About one-third of all patients with dermatitis herpetiformis have either clinical thyroid disease or abnormal thyroid function test results. Most connective tissue–vascular diseases have an increased frequency of autoimmune thyroid disorders. Atopic dermatitis may be linked to Graves' disease, as may acanthosis nigricans. Sweet's syndrome (acute febrile neutrophilic dermatosis) has been reported in conjunction with several different thyroid disorders. Generalized granuloma annulare has occurred in patients with autoimmune thyroiditis. In one study of patients who developed typical melasma, the frequency of thyroid dysfunction was four times that of a control group. Both myxedema and thyrotoxicosis have been reported with pseudoxanthoma elasticum. Hyperthyroidism and psoriasis may also be statistically associated.

Finally, it should be noted that pruritus may be severe in up to 5% of patients with Graves' disease, especially those with attendant chronic idiopathic urticaria associated with thyroid autoantibodies. Indeed, 12.1% of chronic urticaria patients had increased antithyroid microsomal antibodies; meta-analysis showed patients with urticaria were more likely to have thyroid autoimmunity than controls. Pruritus may also be associated with the xerotic skin that occurs in hypothyroidism, and there are a number of reports in which the urticaria resolved only when the underlying thyroid problem was treated. It is theorized that antithyroid antibodies are not pathogenic, but serve as markers of autoimmunity.

SUGGESTED READINGS

Ai J, Leonhardt JM, Heymann WR. Autoimmune thyroid diseases: etiology, pathogenesis, and dermatologic manifestations. J Am Acad Dermatol 2003;48:641–59.
Bartalena L, Fatourechi V. Extrathyroidal manifestations of Graves' disease: a 2014 update. J Endocrinol Invest 2014;37(8):691–700.
Heymann WR, editor. Thyroid disorders with cutaneous manifestations. London: Springer Verlag; 2008.
Heymann WR. Cutaneous manifestations of thyroid disease. J Am Acad Dermatol 1992;26:885–902.
Kasumagic-Halilovic E, Probic A, Begovic B, Ovcins-Kurtovic N. Association between vitiligo, and thyroid autoimmunity. J Thyroid Res 2011;2011:938257.
Puri N. A study of the cutaneous manifestations of thyroid disease. Indian J Dermatol 2012;57(3):247–8.

CHAPTER 26

Cutaneous Manifestations of Lipid Disorders

Inbal Braunstein

> **KEY POINTS**
>
> - Cutaneous xanthomas present as yellow papules, nodules, or plaques and can signal the presence of an underlying lipid, metabolic, or hematologic abnormality.
> - Xanthelasma is the most common cutaneous xanthoma and can be seen in association with dyslipoproteinemia in about half of patients.
> - Xanthomas can also occur in normolipemic patients and herald an underlying metabolic, neurologic, or hematologic disorder.
> - Treatments are available for many of the dyslipoproteinemia syndromes. Accurate dermatologic diagnosis and referral to a specialist is critical to mitigate against the predisposition for atherosclerotic, pancreatic, and other systemic comorbidities.

Cutaneous xanthomas result from intracellular and dermal deposition of lipids and can be a harbinger of underlying systemic disorders, most commonly hyperlipoproteinemias. Multiple forms of cutaneous xanthomas exist. While not entirely specific, different morphologies can point toward particular forms of primary hyperlipoproteinemia (see Table 26-1), or secondary hyperlipoproteinemias (see Table 26-2), or other normolipemic conditions. Many of the primary hyperlipoproteinemias are now defined at a molecular level with specific apoprotein or receptor mutations. A basic understanding of lipid metabolism provides insight into the pathogenesis of hyperlipoproteinemias.

LIPID METABOLISM AND PRIMARY HYPERLIPOPROTEINEMIAS

Lipids are a heterogeneous group of fats or fat-like substances that are insoluble in water, thus most plasma lipids are complexed as a lipoprotein with a hydrophilic phospholipid and apoprotein shell. Lipoproteins are classified by their density, which is a reflection of the core lipid content. Chylomicrons and very-low-density lipoproteins (VLDLs) have high triglyceride (TG) and low cholesterol ester (CE) content, while low-density lipoproteins (LDLs), intermediate-density lipoproteins (IDLs), and high-density lipoproteins (HDLs) have increasing CE and decreasing TG content. The lipoprotein structure allows the delivery of TG and CEs to peripheral cells for metabolic functions via interaction between apoproteins and specific receptors. An example is the interaction of the B100/E apoprotein found on VLDLs, IDLs, and LDLs and lipoprotein lipase on hepatocytes and capillary endothelium.

Two major pathways of lipoprotein synthesis exist: exogenous (dietary) and endogenous (hepatic production). In the endogenous pathway, ingested TGs are taken up in the intestine and packaged with a small amount of CEs into the central core of a chylomicron. These chylomicrons then enter the systemic circulation and release free fatty acids (via hydrolysis of the TGs) to the peripheral tissues. This process is mediated via the interaction between apoprotein CII on the chylomicrons and lipoprotein lipase on capillary endothelium. After release of the free fatty acids a chylomicron remnant is taken up by the liver via the apoprotein B100/E receptor.

In the endogenous pathway the liver forms VLDLs from circulating free fatty acids and hepatic TG stores. The rate-limiting enzyme is HMG-CoA, the target of the statin class of antihypercholesterolemia agents. VLDLs enter the circulation and after removal of TG content (via interaction of apoprotein CII on VLDL and lipoprotein lipase on the endothelium), an IDL is formed. IDLs are taken up by the liver or remain in circulation and become LDLs. LDLs deliver cholesterol to peripheral tissues for use in synthesis of cell membrane bilayers, myelin nerve sheaths, and for steroidogenesis and bile acid production. LDLs are ultimately taken up by the liver via apoprotein B100/E. HDLs transfer excess CEs from peripheral tissues and transfer them to other lipoproteins (LDLs, VLDLs, or chylomicrons) for transportation back to the liver. The clinical emphasis on low levels of LDL and high levels of HDL reflects appropriate levels of production and removal of cholesterols in the circulation.

Primary Hyperlipoproteinemias

Various classification schemas have been proposed for the primary hyperlipoproteinemias. The initial numerical schemes by Frederickson and Lee in 1965 are based on the serum lipoproteins present. Numerous synonyms exist and today this classification scheme is enhanced by insights from molecular biology (see Table 26-1).

TABLE 26-1 Primary Hyperlipoproteinemias

Elevated Lipoprotein Class	Fitzpatrick Type, Synonyms, and Primary Genetic Disorders	Lipid Profile	Cutaneous Xanthoma	Systemic Manifestations
Chylomicrons	Type I, familial lipoprotein lipase deficiency/Bürger–Grütz disease, familial apoprotein CII deficiencies	Hypertriglyceridemia	Eruptive	Presents in childhood or adolescence. Pancreatitis, lipemia retinalis. No increased risk of coronary artery disease
Chylomicrons and VLDLs	Type V, familial combined hyperlipidemia	Hypertriglyceridemia	Eruptive	Presents in adulthood. Association with diabetes, alcohol intake, obesity
VLDLs	Type IV, endogenous familial hypertriglyceridemia	Hypertriglyceridemia	Eruptive	Presents in adulthood. Association with diabetes, alcohol intake, obesity
LDLs	Type IIa, familial hypercholesterolemia, LDL receptor defect, defective B100/E, PCSK9 mutations	Hypercholesterolemia	Tendinous, tuberoeruptive, tuberous, planar (xanthelasma, intertringinous, interdigital web spaces*)	Atherosclerosis. Homozygous forms presents in childhood
LDLs and VLDLs	Type IIb, familial multiple lipoprotein-type hyperlipidemia, combined hyperlipidemia	Hypercholesterolemia	Tuberous, planar	Atherosclerosis, diabetes
IDLs	Type III, remnant hyperlipidemia, familial dysbetalipoproteinemia, broad beta deficiency, ApoE deficiency	Hypertriglyceridemia Hypercholesterolemia	Tuberoeruptive, tuberous, tendinous, planar, (xanthoma striatum palmares—most characteristic)	Atherosclerosis

VLDL, very-low-density lipoprotein; LDL, low-density lipoprotein; IDL, intermediate-density lipoprotein.
*Pathognomonic for homozygous form of type IIa disease.

TABLE 26-2 Secondary Hyperlipoproteinemias

Diabetes mellitus
Cholestasis: Primary biliary cirrhosis, Alagille syndrome
Biliary atresia
Hypothyroidism
Nephrotic syndrome
Pregnancy
Alcoholism
Drugs: Estrogens, systemic retinoids, olanzapine, azacitidine, corticosteroids, antiretrovirals
Paraproteinemias: Multiple myeloma, lymphoma

Hyperchylomicronemia

Two genetically determined defects of TG removal lead to hypertriglyceridemia and hyperchylomicronemia: these are autosomal recessive lipoprotein lipase deficiency (also known as type I or Bürger–Grütz disease) and familial apoprotein CII deficiency. However, the majority of patients with high levels of chylomicrons and TGs have acquired secondary forms of hyperlipidemia. Pancreatitis and bouts of abdominal pain are common in severe type I disease, often beginning in early childhood. In addition, these children develop hepatosplenomegaly, eruptive xanthomas, and lipemia retinalis, especially when the TG levels exceed 4000 mg/dL. Premature atherosclerotic vascular disease does not occur in type I disease. Patients with an absence of lipoprotein lipase activator (apoprotein CII) first develop symptoms after adolescence. Patients with type V disease have elevations of both chylomicrons and VLDLs—so-called familial combined hyperlipidemia. The symptoms usually begin in adult life, and as is true for many patients with primary hyperlipidemia, secondary factors, such as alcohol intake, obesity, associated renal disease, or diabetes mellitus, are frequently involved in exacerbation of the disease.

Increased VLDLs

Endogenous familial hypertriglyceridemia (type IV disease) results primarily from accelerated production of VLDL in the liver. This autosomal dominant disorder is common. The symptoms first appear in adulthood, frequently being precipitated by the ingestion of large amounts of carbohydrate or alcohol. Patients with this disorder are often obese, diabetic, and hyperuricemic and have an increased risk of coronary artery disease. Eruptive xanthomas are common, and xanthoma striatum palmare can also occur. VLDLs may be elevated along with chylomicrons in type V disease. Patients with elevations of both VLDL and LDL have type IIb disease.

Increased LDLs

LDLs alone are elevated in type IIa disease (familial hypercholesterolemia), and are elevated together with VLDLs in type IIb disease. There are several different phenotypic genetic conditions of familial hypercholesterolemia, and the severity of the clinical manifestations varies considerably. Xanthomas, especially the tendinous and tuberous types, are prominent, and there is a significant increase in the incidence of coronary artery disease, often beginning in early adulthood.

Elevated IDLs

Patients with high levels of cholesterol and TGs, carried in remnant lipoproteins (IDLs), have type III or broad-β disease (familial dysbetalipoproteinemia). Type III hyperlipoproteinemia is inherited as an autosomal dominant disease, although similar remnant lipoprotein accumulation in the plasma has been seen as a secondary phenomenon in hypothyroidism and multiple myeloma. The disorder appears to be related to a defect in the removal of these remnants from the circulation. Clinically, patients with broad-β disease are usually obese, glucose-intolerant, and have cutaneous xanthomas and atherosclerotic disease.

Secondary Hyperlipoproteinemias

The majority of cases of xanthomatosis are secondary, rather than the primary familial disorders listed in Table 26-1. Secondary hyperlipidemias result from disease in various organs (e.g., liver, kidney, thyroid, or pancreas) and are caused by a disturbance in the metabolism of TGs and cholesterol (Table 26-2). Eruptive xanthomas may appear when hypertriglyceridemia develops in patients with uncontrolled diabetes mellitus, and in patients with the nephrotic syndrome. Tuberous and eruptive xanthomas can be seen in patients with hypothyroidism, but only rarely. Infants with biliary atresia and adults with biliary cirrhosis may develop any of the four types of xanthoma (Figs. 26-1 and 26-2). Diffuse plane xanthomas are associated primarily with malignancies of the reticuloendothelial system, including multiple myeloma and lymphoma. Associated dyslipoproteinemias have been reported and attributed to complexes between the lipoproteins and paraproteins.

Normolipemic Xanthomatosis

Xanthomas may occur in disorders with histiocytic proliferations and secondary uptake of fat, rather than with an error of lipid metabolism. Blood lipid levels are normal in these disorders, which include nevoxanthoendothelioma, xanthoma disseminatum, cerebrotendinous xanthomatosis, and verruciform xanthoma.

Nevoxanthoendothelioma, also known as juvenile xanthogranuloma, is a benign proliferation of lipid-laden histiocytes that occurs primarily in infancy and is usually characterized by one or a few nodules that are yellow-brown and vary from a few millimeters to several centimeters in diameter. They are especially common on the scalp, face, or extensor extremities, and although they usually disappear spontaneously over several months, they may persist for many years. Involvement of visceral organs is rare, but the lesions may occur in the iris and ciliary body of the eye, and in the lung, heart, and oropharynx.

Xanthoma disseminatum is a rare and unusual disease characterized by xanthomatous nodules in the axillae, the antecubital and popliteal fossae, the intertriginous areas, and the oropharynx and upper respiratory tract. The disorder is discussed in Chapter 17. Familial cerebrotendinous xanthomatosis is a rare condition characterized by the deposition of cholestanol and cholesterol in all tissues of the body beginning in childhood. Xanthomas in the Achilles tendon are characteristic, but the major damage results from sterol deposition in the brain and lungs.

Verruciform xanthomas are benign solitary lesions characterized by lipid-laden dermal macrophages in the dermal papillae of a verrucous papule. These can occur in the mouth, anogenital, or periorificial skin and are not associated with hyperlipidemia.

Hypolipoproteinemias

Abnormally low levels of cholesterol and TG may be observed in patients with malabsorption, parenchymal liver disease, or cachexia, but primary or familial cases of hypolipoproteinemia are extremely rare and include such diseases as Tangier disease (α-lipoprotein deficiency), hypo- or abetalipoproteinemia, and lecithin-cholesterol acyltransferase deficiency. Cutaneous lesions are not specific in these disorders, but patients with Tangier disease have characteristic yellow-orange tonsils.

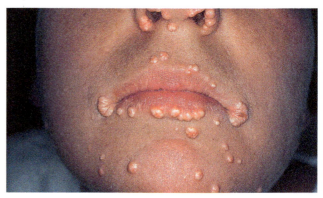

FIGURE 26-1 ■ Primary biliary cirrhosis. Multiple xanthomas are present, but in addition there is a brown color to the skin.

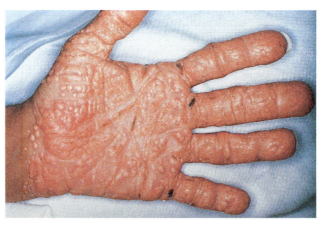

FIGURE 26-2 ■ Primary biliary cirrhosis with palmar xanthomas.

CUTANEOUS XANTHOMAS

Xanthomas are localized accumulations of intracellular or extracellular lipid found in the dermis or tendons. They are categorized as tendinous, tuberous, planar, or eruptive. Cholesterol is the major lipid, although sterols and TGs may accumulate in significant quantities in certain xanthomas. Xanthomas can occur in persons of any age, but are more common in those over 50. Males and females are equally affected. The morbidity and mortality of xanthomas are related primarily to associated atherosclerosis and pancreatitis.

Tendinous Xanthomas

Tendinous xanthomas are produced by a diffuse infiltration of lipid within tendons, ligaments, and occasionally fasciae. They appear as slowly enlarging deeply situated subcutaneous nodules, with normal overlying skin that is freely movable. Classically, they affect the extensor tendons of the hands, knees, elbows, and the Achilles tendons. They may be confused with rheumatoid nodules or gouty tophi. Trauma is thought to be a predisposing factor, although the unique distribution of the lesions in the various forms of hyperlipoproteinemia is unexplained. Tendinous xanthomas are usually associated with hypercholesterolemia and increased levels of LDL, and they may occur in association with other cutaneous xanthomas, especially xanthelasmas and tuberous xanthomas. Rarely, however, tendinous xanthomas may occur in normolipemic xanthomatosis, especially in cerebrotendinous xanthomatosis. Patients with tendinous xanthomas have an extremely high incidence of atherosclerotic vascular disease.

Tuberous Xanthomas

Tuberous xanthomas begin as small, soft, yellow, red, or flesh-colored papules, and usually develop in pressure areas such as the extensor surfaces of the body, including the elbows, knees, and buttocks. They are painless and frequently coalesce to form large globular masses (Figs. 26-3 and 26-4). Their presence usually suggests an elevation of serum cholesterol and LDL, but they may also be seen with TG elevation. They can be associated with familial dysbetalipoproteinemia (type III) and familial hypercholesterolemia (type IIa), and may be present in some of the secondary hyperlipidemias (e.g., nephrotic syndrome, hypothyroidism) and in the rare condition, sitosterolemia, associated with impaired metabolism of plant-derived lipids. As with tendinous xanthomas, patients with tuberous xanthomas also have an extremely high incidence of atherosclerotic vascular disease.

Planar Xanthomas

Planar xanthomas are by far the most commonly encountered xanthomas. These yellow, soft, macular to barely palpable lesions occur in three forms: xanthelasma, xanthoma striatum palmare, and diffuse plane xanthoma.

Xanthelasmas are soft, velvety, flat, yellow, polygonal papules that appear in the eyelid area, most commonly in the medial canthus (Fig. 26-5). At least 50% of patients with xanthelasmas will have normal plasma lipid levels. If the lipid levels are abnormal, serum cholesterol is usually elevated. This is especially true in younger patients. An associated finding in many of these patients is corneal arcus, which may also occur in the older population in the setting of normal lipid levels. Some secondary hyperlipoproteinemias, such as cholestasis, may also be associated with xanthelasmas.

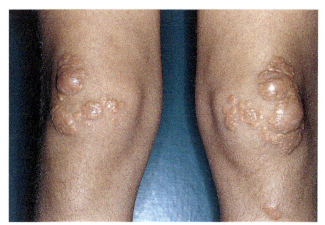

FIGURE 26-4 ■ Tuberous xanthomas of the knees.

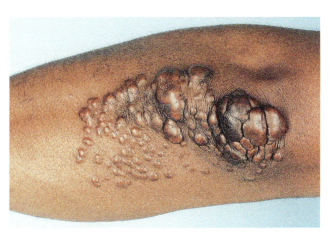

FIGURE 26-3 ■ Tuberous xanthomas of the elbows.

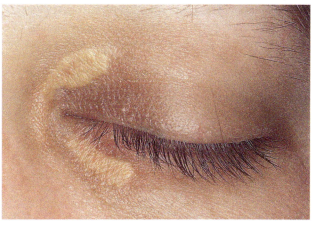

FIGURE 26-5 ■ Planar xanthomas (xanthelasmas of the eyelids).

Xanthoma striatum palmare presents as flat, yellow to orange lesions in the palmar creases (Fig. 26-2) that occur only in patients with abnormal serum lipid levels, including elevations of cholesterol and TGs. There have been a few reports in the literature of this type of xanthoma occurring in individuals with primary biliary cirrhosis.

Diffuse plane xanthomas usually cover large areas of the face, neck, thorax, and arms. Individuals may or may not have hyperlipidemia (hypertriglyceridemia in particular), but frequently have paraproteinemia, including multiple myeloma (Fig. 26-6).

Eruptive Xanthomas

Eruptive xanthomas appear suddenly, usually in crops, and unlike the other forms of xanthoma may be pruritic and/or tender. Eruptive xanthomas are characterized by their yellow color (although this may be difficult to appreciate and the diagnosis should still be considered in the appropriate setting with only eruptive red lesions), small size (1 to 4 mm in diameter), palpability, and the erythematous halo around their base. They occur most commonly over pressure points and extensor surfaces of the arms, legs, and buttocks (Fig. 26-7). Rarely, they may be diffusely scattered over the trunk or on the mucous membranes. They occur exclusively in association with elevated TG levels. A frequent circumstance is their occurrence with hypertriglyceridemia secondary to uncontrolled diabetes mellitus. Treatment of the diabetes mellitus can lead to subsequent resolution of the xanthomas.

TREATMENT

The therapy of disorders of lipid metabolism depends on the underlying lipoprotein abnormality and is directed toward returning the lipids to normal levels. Attempts should also be made to find any underlying secondary disease causing the hyperlipidemia so that it can be addressed. Dietary manipulation and lipid-lowering agents such as statins, fibrates, bile-acid-binding resins, probucol, and nicotinic acid are the mainstays of therapy for primary hyperlipidemias, but there is no effective therapy for the normo- or hypolipemic conditions unless monoclonal gammopathy is present, which can be treated with thalidomide or other agents. The lipid-lowering effects of these agents have been well studied, but few studies mention the efficacy of these drugs for resolving xanthomas. Eruptive xanthomas usually resolve within weeks of initiating systemic treatment, and tuberous xanthomas usually resolve after months, but tendinous xanthomas take years to resolve or may persist indefinitely. The main goal of therapy for hyperlipidemia is to reduce the risks of atherosclerotic cardiovascular disease, whereas in patients with severe hypertriglyceridemia the goal is to prevent pancreatitis and its complications.

Surgery or locally destructive modalities can be used for idiopathic or unresponsive xanthomas. Xanthelasmas are often treated with topical trichloroacetic acid,

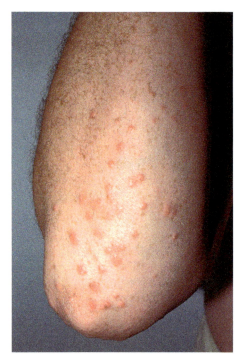

FIGURE 26-6 ■ Planar xanthoma.

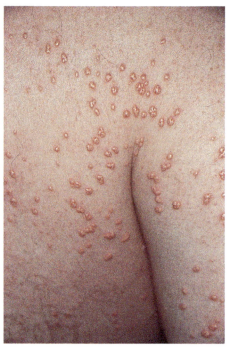

FIGURE 26-7 ■ Eruptive xanthomas: multiple yellow papules appeared over several weeks in this man with insulin-dependent diabetes mellitus.

electrodesiccation, laser therapy, and excision, but recurrences may occur. Although these therapies can be effective in clearing the xanthomas, the goal is to attempt to reverse or slow the associated atherosclerotic process (lipid-laden plaques collecting on the intima of blood vessels), the most serious complication of lipid disorders.

SUGGESTED READINGS

Abifadel M, Varret M, Rabés J-P, et al. Mutations in PCSK9 cause autosomal dominant hypercholesterolemia. Nat Genet 2003;34:154–6.

Alam M, Garzon MC, Salen G, Starc TJ. Tuberous xanthomas in sitosterolemia. Pediatr Dermatol 2001;17:447–9.

Bergman R. Xanthelasma palpebrarum and risk of arteriosclerosis: a review. Int J Dermatol 1998;37:343–5.

Borelli C, Kaudewitz P. Xanthelasma palpebrarum: treatment with the erbium:YAG laser. Lasers Surg Med 2001;29:260–4.

Burnside NJ, Alberta L, Robinson-Bostom L, Bostom A. Type III hyperlipoproteinemia with xanthomas and multiple myeloma. J Am Acad Dermatol 2005;53:S281–4.

Fujita M, Shirai K. A comparative study of the therapeutic effect of probucol and pravastatin on xanthelasma. J Dermatol 1996;23:598–602.

Garcia MA, Ramonet M, Ciocca M, et al. Alagille syndrome: cutaneous manifestations in 38 children. Pediatr Dermatol 2005;22:11–4.

Haygood LJ, Bennett JD, Brodell RT. Treatment of xanthelasma palpebrarum with bichloracetic acid. Dermatol Surg 1998;24:1027–31.

Hsu JC, Su TC, Chen MF, et al. Xanthoma striatum palmare in a patient with primary biliary cirrhosis and hypercholesterolemia. J Gastroenterol Hepatol 2005;20:1799–800.

Lee RS, Frederickson DS. The differentiation of exogenous and endogenous hyperlipemia by paper electrophoresis. J Clin Invest 1965;44:1968–77.

Marcoval J, Moreno A, Bordas X, et al. Diffuse plane xanthoma: a clinicopathologic study of 8 cases. J Am Acad Dermatol 1998;39:439–42.

Raulin C, Schoenermach MP, Werner S, Greve B. Xanthelasma palpebrarum: treatment with ultrapulsed CO_2 laser. Lasers Surg Med 1999;24:122–7.

Sato-Matsumura KC, Matsumura T, Yokoshiki H, et al. Xanthoma striatum palmare as an early sign of familial type III hyperlipoproteinemia with an apoprotein E genotype e2/e2. Clin Exp Dermatol 2003;28:321–2.

Sibley C, Stone NJ. Familial hypercholesterolemia: a challenge of diagnosis and therapy. Cleveland Clin J Med 2006;73:57–64.

Stone NJ. Secondary causes of hyperlipidemia. Med Clin North Am 1994;78:117–41.

CHAPTER 27

Adrenal, Androgen-Related, and Pituitary Disorders

Robert G. Micheletti

KEY POINTS

- Classic signs of excess cortisol (Cushing's) include moon facies, striae, atrophy, and acne.
- Cortisol deficiency (Addison's) presents with hyperpigmentation of the skin, nails, and mucous membranes.
- Excess androgens, as seen in polycystic ovary syndrome and congenital adrenal hyperplasia, cause hirsutism, acne, male-pattern alopecia, and virilization.
- Androgen insensitivity (testicular feminization) leads to ambiguous genitalia, sparse sexual hair development, and an absence of acne and male-pattern alopecia.
- Acromegaly due to excess growth hormone and insulin-like growth factor 1 causes characteristic frontal bossing and prognathia, enlarged nose, tongue, lips, and hands.
- Hypopituitarism can manifest with thin skin, scant body hair, and pale complexion.

Hormones of the steroid family (glucocorticoids, androgens and other sex steroids, and mineralocorticoids) are critical in the control of homeostasis and cell differentiation. These hormones are produced by the adrenal gland and gonads, and are regulated by pituitary secretions. They control cell growth, differentiation, and metabolism by binding to intracellular receptors that act directly at the DNA level to produce changes in gene expression.

ADRENAL DISORDERS

Excessive Glucocorticoid Activity (Cushing Syndrome)

Hypercortisolism is most commonly the result of exogenous administration of glucocorticoids, but similar findings occur in patients with endogenous hypercortisolism, e.g., excess pituitary adrenocorticotropic hormone (ACTH) production (Cushing disease), ectopic ACTH secretion, or glucocorticoid-producing adrenal tumors. These findings may be dramatic or subtle. Systemically, they include hypertension, proximal muscle weakness/myopathy, diabetes, obesity, osteopenia and osteoporosis, and psychiatric disturbances. The association of these features with characteristic cutaneous and physical changes should raise the possibility of Cushing syndrome.

Cutaneous findings in hypercortisolism include cutaneous atrophy, striae, purpura, telangiectasias, and acne. Cutaneous atrophy is caused by a reduction in both epidermal and dermal components. There is thinning of the epidermis, and collagen synthesis is reduced. There is also loss of elastic fibers and dermal mucopolysaccharides. A weakened dermis and obesity result in the development of prominent striae (Fig. 27-1). The skin is injured easily by minor trauma. Purpura, skin tears, and ulcerations result; these, in turn, heal slowly due to the inhibiting effects of cortisol on wound healing.

Subcutaneous fat deposition over the face and trunk contributes to the characteristic moon facies and body habitus—buffalo hump, supraclavicular fat pad, and central adiposity. Erythrocytosis, telangiectasias, and cutaneous atrophy also contribute to the characteristic facial appearance, which is notably round and plethoric. Steroid acne may also occur. This disorder is distinguished from typical acne vulgaris by the absence of a comedonal component as well as by the monomorphic appearance of its red papules and pustules, which are in a uniform stage of development. The usual distribution is on the upper trunk, shoulders, and arms, with relative sparing of the face. Patients with hypercortisolism are also predisposed to the development of chronic fungal infections of the skin (tinea versicolor, dermatophytosis, and candidal infections). When hypercortisolism is caused by increased ACTH production, hyperpigmentation may occur, as in adrenal insufficiency.

Cortisol levels can be increased in several disorders other than Cushing syndrome. This scenario, a kind of physiologic hypercortisolism, is known as pseudo-Cushing syndrome. Possible causes include physiologic stress, such as is seen in the setting of severe infection; significant obesity or polycystic ovary syndrome; psychological stress, such as severe major depressive disorder; and, in rare cases, chronic alcoholism. Patients with pseudo-Cushing syndrome seldom display the cutaneous findings associated with true Cushing's. Laboratory abnormalities observed in hypercortisolism include hyperglycemia and hypokalemia. After excluding exogenous glucocorticoid use, those with clinical features of Cushing syndrome should undergo initial screening using 24-hour urine free cortisol, late night salivary cortisol, or low-dose dexamethasone suppression test. The evidence-based Endocrine Society Guidelines (2008) recommend at least two of these tests be unequivocally abnormal to establish the

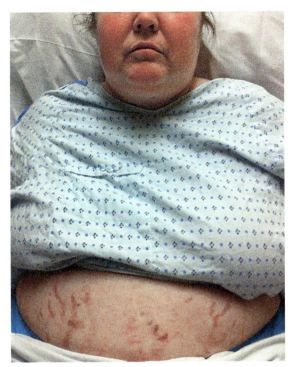

FIGURE 27-1 ■ Moon facies and abdominal striae in a patient with Cushing syndrome.

diagnosis. Because of limited sensitivity and specificity, these tests should be performed more than once, and their results should be concordant.

After the presence of hypercortisolism is confirmed, additional testing must be performed to determine the cause. Most cases of endogenous hypercortisolism are the result of excessive secretion of ACTH by a pituitary tumor. Other causes include adrenal tumors (which are ACTH-independent) and ACTH production from nonpituitary tumors, the most common of which are oat cell carcinoma of the lung, carcinoid, gastrinoma, malignant thymoma, pheochromocytoma, and medullary carcinoma of the thyroid. The treatment of hypercortisolism depends on the detection and correction of the underlying cause, such as surgical resection of a causative tumor.

Insufficient Glucocorticoid Activity (Addison Disease)

Adrenal insufficiency may result from a number of processes that cause extensive destruction or dysfunction of the adrenal cortices. Prolonged administration of synthetic glucocorticoids with subsequent discontinuation is by far the most common cause of adrenal insufficiency. Other major causes include autoimmune adrenalitis (more common in women), infections (primarily tuberculosis and deep fungal infections), and metastatic disease. Less common causes include drugs and hemorrhage. The systemic antifungal medication ketoconazole inhibits steroidogenesis but only rarely causes clinical hypocortisolism. Other medications that inhibit cortisol biosynthesis include the antiepileptic drug aminoglutethimide, the anesthetic sedative drug etomidate, and the antiparasitic drug suramin.

The clinical manifestations of Addison's are diverse. Constitutional symptoms include malaise, reduced energy, weight loss, and a feeling of ill health. Other systemic manifestations are hypotension, weakness, fatigue, gastrointestinal symptoms (anorexia, nausea, and abdominal pain), and psychiatric symptoms. Adrenal crisis (acute adrenal insufficiency) may result in life-threatening hypotension and shock.

The primary dermatologic manifestation is hyperpigmentation of the skin and mucous membranes (Fig. 27-2). The hyperpigmentation of adrenal insufficiency is the most characteristic physical finding of the disease and may precede other symptoms by months or years. Skin darkening is induced by high levels of ACTH and melanocyte-stimulating hormone, which share the prohormone pro-opiomelanocortin in common. For this reason, hyperpigmentation does not occur in those with pituitary failure but is, rather, limited to those with primary adrenal failure. Because adrenal insufficiency often has an insidious onset, the hyperpigmentation may go unnoticed by the patient. Commonly involved areas include those which are sun-exposed; those exposed to friction or pressure such as the knuckles, elbows, and knees; scars; and naturally hyperpigmented sites such as the axillae, perineum, and nipples. Darkening of the palmar creases is considered nearly specific for adrenal insufficiency in light-skinned patients. Pigmentation of the tongue, lips, and buccal mucosa is another useful sign. The hair may become darker, and pigmented longitudinal bands may develop on the nails. New nevi can appear, and old nevi darken.

Adrenal insufficiency is associated with other skin manifestations as a part of polyglandular autoimmune syndrome type I (chronic mucocutaneous candidiasis) and type II (vitiligo). A rare manifestation of adrenal insufficiency is fibrosis and calcification of the ear cartilage.

The laboratory abnormalities seen in adrenal insufficiency include hyponatremia and hyperkalemia. Screening for adrenal insufficiency includes two tests: basal plasma ACTH level and cortisol level 30 to 60 minutes following ACTH (cosyntropin) stimulation test. Primary adrenal insufficiency manifests with high basal ACTH combined with a blunted cortisol response to the ACTH stimulation test. Low cortisol and low basal ACTH levels suggest either secondary (i.e., pituitary) or tertiary (i.e., hypothalamic) adrenal insufficiency. In this instance, a corticotropin-releasing hormone stimulation test is necessary to distinguish between the two etiologies. After the diagnosis of hypocortisolemia is determined, the cause of adrenal failure must be found.

The treatment of adrenal insufficiency is long-term replacement of glucocorticoids. Prednisone and dexamethasone have replaced shorter-acting agents such as cortisone or hydrocortisone because the longer duration of action provides a smoother physiologic effect. Mineralocorticoid replacement can be achieved with fludrocortisone. In times of physiologic stress induced by illness or surgery, glucocorticoid replacement must be increased to avoid adrenal crisis.

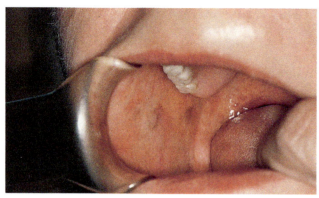

FIGURE 27-2 ■ Pigmented macules on the buccal mucosa and lips in Addison disease.

Pheochromocytoma

Pheochromocytoma is a catecholamine-producing tumor arising from chromaffin cells of the sympathetic nervous system. The majority of pheochromocytomas develop in the medulla of one or both adrenal glands. Other sites of origin include para-aortic sympathetic ganglia, the walls of the urinary bladder, the chest, and, extremely rarely, sympathetic tissue associated with intracranial branches of the vagus nerve. Some inherited disorders predispose to pheochromocytomas, including neurofibromatosis, von Hippel–Lindau syndrome, and multiple endocrine neoplasia type 2 (or Sipple syndrome). More than 90% of the tumors are benign. They occur most frequently during the fourth and fifth decades of life.

The most distinctive clinical feature of pheochromocytoma is hypertension, although it accounts for less than 0.1% of patients with diastolic hypertension. The hypertension is usually paroxysmal and occurs in association with headaches, palpitations, sweating, and a feeling of apprehension. Symptoms can be reproduced experimentally by the injection of norepinephrine (noradrenaline) and epinephrine (adrenaline). These episodes may occur at weekly intervals or as frequently as 20 times a day. They may be precipitated by emotional situations, eating, exercise, and by activities that compress the tumor, such as bending. The only significant cutaneous manifestation of pheochromocytoma is flushing, which appears to occur primarily when the tumor secretes larger amounts of epinephrine than norepinephrine. The flushing occurs paroxysmally and is most prominent on the face, chest, and upper extremities. When pheochromocytomas occur as part of a genetic syndrome, cutaneous manifestations of that syndrome may also be apparent. In some patients with hypertension, for example, recognition of café-au-lait macules of neurofibromatosis may lead to the appropriate diagnosis.

The diagnosis of pheochromocytoma can be established by assaying levels of catecholamines and their metabolites in the plasma or urine (fractionated catecholamines and metanephrines), especially during paroxysmal attacks. In patients in whom the episodes are very brief, establishing the diagnosis is much more challenging, and, occasionally, induction of attacks with intravenous glucagon or histamine is performed. Treatment involves the use of adrenergic antagonists, beginning with alpha blockers such as phentolamine and phenoxybenzamine, and surgical removal of the tumors.

ANDROGEN-RELATED DISORDERS

Excess Androgen Activity

Excess androgen activity is reflected in precocious puberty in children and degrees of virilization in women; men are asymptomatic. In women, the cutaneous signs of virilization include hirsutism, acne, and androgenic alopecia; these may have devastating psychosocial consequences. Some increase in androgen levels in women at adolescence is normal, however, and is responsible for the development of axillary and pubic hair.

Hirsutism is defined relative to cultural and environmental norms as more facial and body hair than is considered acceptable. It is a common complaint, with a prevalence estimated to be as high as one-third of menstruating and 75% of postmenopausal women. Objective measurement of hirsutism is possible using the Ferriman–Gallwey scale (Fig. 27-3), which quantifies the extent of hair growth in androgen-dependent areas. Using this scale, mild hirsutism is defined by a score of 8 to 15; >15 is considered moderate or severe. Hirsutism occurring in the absence of increased androgens is termed idiopathic hirsutism. Hirsutism must be distinguished from hypertrichosis, which is generalized excess hair growth not limited to androgen-sensitive sites. Hirsutism may or may not be associated with other signs of virilization, including worsening acne, male-pattern alopecia, and menstrual irregularity.

Acne vulgaris is a common disorder. Nevertheless, some authors recommend an evaluation of androgen levels in all women with acne; others disagree. Most women exhibit a degree of scalp hair loss over time, generally in the form of hairline recession. More extensive alopecia, with marked thinning of hair on the central scalp, may be associated with androgen excess.

Androgen excess may be caused by a wide variety of conditions of both adrenal and ovarian origin. These include adrenal tumors, Cushing syndrome, congenital (or late-onset) adrenal hyperplasia, polycystic ovaries, ovarian tumors, ovarian hyperplasia, and other nonadrenal, nonovarian neoplasms. Adrenal androgens include androstenedione, testosterone, dehydroepiandrosterone (DHEA), and DHEA sulfate (DHEAS). Androstenedione and testosterone are also produced by the ovaries.

In patients with mild hirsutism and regular menses who lack other signs to suggest androgen excess, laboratory testing may not be necessary given the high likelihood that the hirsutism is idiopathic. If hirsutism is moderate or severe or there are features of a secondary cause, then testing for androgen levels is essential. Measuring plasma-free testosterone, the bioactive portion of plasma testosterone, is more sensitive than measuring total testosterone. Testosterone is bound to albumin by sex hormone-binding globulin, low levels of which may result in an elevated plasma-free testosterone level despite a normal total testosterone. Routine testing for

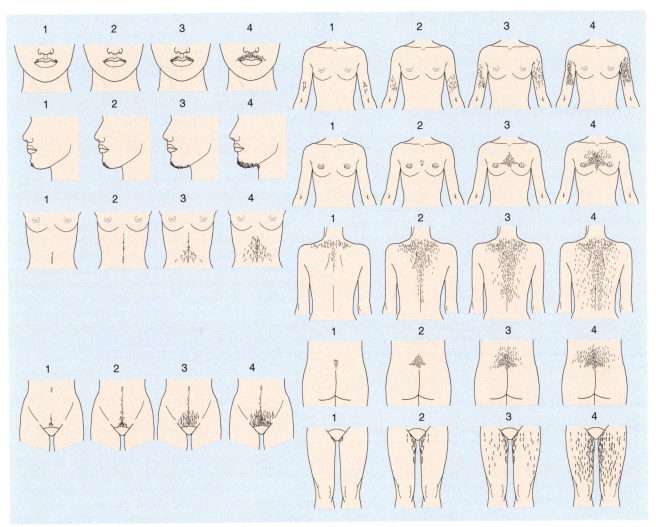

FIGURE 27-3 ■ The Ferriman–Gallwey scoring system for hirsutism. (Reproduced with permission from Hatch R, Rosenfield RL, Kim MH, Tredway D. Hirsutism: implications, etiology, and management. Am J Obstet Gynecol 1981;140:815–830.)

other androgens is of little use. If a neoplasm is suspected, ultrasonographic evaluation of the adrenal glands, ovaries, or both may be useful.

Abrupt onset of virilization, DHEAS levels >700 ng/dL, and free testosterone levels >200 ng/dL suggest an androgen-producing tumor. Patients with polycystic ovary syndrome have elevated androgen levels associated with increased luteinizing hormone (LH) and lower-than-expected follicle-stimulating hormone (FSH); this results in a high LH:FSH ratio. The laboratory investigation of congenital adrenal hyperplasia is discussed below.

The treatment of cutaneous manifestations of androgen excess is multifaceted. The most common approach includes cosmetic and physical measures. Hirsutism may be treated by bleaching; by temporary hair removal mechanisms, such as shaving, plucking, waxing, or depilatory creams; by the hair-growth-inhibitor eflornithine hydrochloride cream; by laser therapy, which is most effective in women with lightly pigmented skin and dark terminal hairs; or by electrolysis. Both laser therapy and electrolysis may result in permanent hair removal.

Systemic treatment may include estrogen–progestin oral contraceptives, antiandrogens, glucocorticoids, and other hormonal therapies. Oral contraceptives can arrest the progression of hirsutism from various causes and reduce by half the need for shaving. Contraceptives with nonandrogenic progestins are preferred. More substantial reduction of hirsutism requires the use of antiandrogens. Spironolactone is the first choice; it is started at 75 to 100 mg/day in two divided doses. Hydration must be maintained, and patients with risk factors for hyperkalemia must be closely monitored. There may be troublesome increases in menstrual bleeding. Concurrent use of spironolactone with an oral contraceptive has been shown to improve hirsutism and reduce androgen levels significantly; effective contraception is advisable anyway in women of reproductive age because of the teratogenic potential of all the antiandrogens. Other androgen antagonists include cyproterone acetate and flutamide. Flutamide is rarely used for hirsutism because of its risk for hepatotoxicity. Prednisone therapy at bedtime doses of 5 to 7.5 mg may improve hirsutism, but long-term therapy is associated with serious side effects. The 5α-reductase inhibitor finasteride may be beneficial, but its effects are considered likely to be partial compared to spironolactone. In addition to the above therapeutic options, psychosocial support is an important aspect of treatment.

Deficient Androgen Activity

The cutaneous manifestations of androgen deficiency depend on the age at onset of the deficiency, because maintenance of sexual hair is less dependent on androgen than is the development of sexual hair. If androgen deficiency occurs prior to puberty, the development of sexual hair and sebaceous and apocrine glands will be limited. Acne and androgenic alopecia do not occur. The skin shows pallor, the penis is small, the scrotum is smooth, and fine wrinkling occurs around the eyes and lips. There is poor muscle development, and delayed closure of the epiphyses results in increased height.

With the development of androgen deficiency after puberty, sexual hair remains present but grows slowly. The sebaceous glands atrophy, and acne will improve or clear. Vasomotor phenomena (hot flashes) may occur. All the cutaneous manifestations of androgen deficiency are reversible with replacement therapy.

Adrenogenital Syndromes

Adrenogenital syndromes (congenital adrenal hyperplasia [CAH]) result from genetic defects in cortisol synthesis. Defective cortisol production stimulates release of ACTH. Increased adrenal stimulation by ACTH, combined with a blocked cortisol production pathway, results in massive accumulation of adrenal androgens. This hyperandrogenism causes virilization in females, sometimes resulting in ambiguous genitalia at birth, and sexual precocity in males. Some of the genetic defects are associated with salt wasting, hypovolemia, and death due to mineralocorticoid deficiency.

Routine neonatal screening for 21-hydroxylase deficiency (which accounts for >90% of cases of CAH) is available in many countries, including the United States. Elevation of 17-hydroxyprogesterone (the substrate of 21-hydroxylase) is diagnostic of this disorder, though the test may be falsely negative. Some patients with partial activity of 21-hydroxylase (nonclassic CAH) will not be diagnosed by neonatal screening. Premature pubarche, accelerated growth, acne, and hirsutism may prompt more in-depth screening during adolescence or adulthood. Measurement of the plasma 17-hydroxyprogesterone level before and after administration of high-dose ACTH may allow detection of patients with partial 21-hydroxylase deficiency. Those with 11-beta-hydroxylase deficiency (which accounts for <10% of CAH cases) present similarly, either at birth or later in childhood or adolescence, and exhibit elevated 11-deoxycortisol levels.

The treatment of CAH is initial glucocorticoid administration to suppress completely ACTH secretion, followed by maintenance glucocorticoid doses that control the level of cortisol precursors. Surgery may be required to match the phenotypic sexual characteristics to the genotypic sex; psychosocial support is another important facet of treatment of this condition.

DISORDERS OF STEROID HORMONE RECEPTORS

Receptors for glucocorticoids, androgens, and other steroid hormones form a family of related proteins. These receptors contain a domain responsible for steroid hormone binding and a domain responsible for DNA binding and effector function. Genetic defects in both the glucocorticoid and androgen receptors have been described.

In male patients with familial glucocorticoid resistance, cutaneous findings have not been described; female patients may develop hirsutism, androgenic alopecia, and menstrual abnormalities. Both sexes have hypercortisolism and elevated ACTH levels without other features associated with Cushing syndrome. Laboratory abnormalities may also include hypertension and hypokalemic acidosis. Virilization is the result of elevated adrenal androgen levels secondary to chronic ACTH overstimulation. The treatment is dexamethasone, which normalizes the ACTH, cortisol, and androgen levels without excessive mineralocorticoid stimulation.

Androgen insensitivity syndrome is asymptomatic in female carriers. Genotypic male patients may have involvement ranging from subtle (infertility and azoospermia) to profound (a female phenotype). The latter has been termed testicular feminization syndrome. Cutaneous manifestations in these patients include sparse sexual hair development and an absence of acne and androgenic alopecia. Mild cases of androgen insensitivity can be treated with surgical repair of hypospadias, if present, and androgen supplementation. In severe cases, patients may be best treated by considering them infertile females and removing the undescended abdominal testes to prevent the development of testicular cancer.

PITUITARY DISORDERS WITH CUTANEOUS MANIFESTATIONS

Hyperpituitarism (Acromegaly)

Acromegaly most often results from hypersecretion of growth hormone by a pituitary tumor or by hyperplasia of the eosinophil cells of the anterior pituitary. The term gigantism refers to the same process occurring in prepubertal children before fusion of the epiphyses, resulting in excessively tall stature. Elevated insulin-like growth factor 1 (IGF-1), produced primarily by the liver in response to excess growth hormone, is the primary mediator of the growth-related outcomes in both conditions. Hyperpituitarism occurs more commonly in adults and leads to exaggerated growth of acral parts, especially the head, hands, and feet, although the excess growth hormone/IGF-1 affect all organs and tissues. The onset of acromegaly is usually insidious, and even before the changes in appearance are noticed, patients may complain of

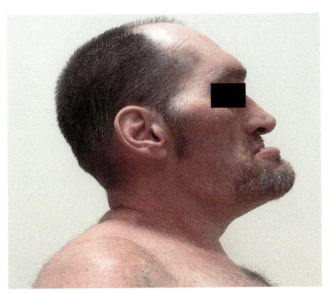

FIGURE 27-4 ■ Frontal bossing, enlarged nose and lower lip, and prognathism in a patient with acromegaly.

arthralgias, hyperhidrosis, pain, paresthesias of the slowly expanding fingers and toes, headache, visual field deficits, and loss of libido.

The clinical picture of well-developed acromegaly is easily recognized by physical examination. The skin is thickened and doughy due to an increase in connective tissue and interstitial fluid. The skin pores are unusually prominent. The skin of the face is oily as a result of increased sebum production, and there is an increase in both apocrine and eccrine sweating. Early in the course of the disease there may be an increase in coarse body and scalp hair. Additional cutaneous findings in some patients include acanthosis nigricans, hyperpigmentation, and a variety of nail changes. The face is often elongated, and there may be furrowing of the brow with accentuation of the skin folds and cutis verticis gyrata. Macroglossia is present, the jaw protrudes (prognathia), and the enlarged nose is often triangular (Fig. 27-4). One of the key diagnostic features is enlargement of the hands, and patients often note a significant increase in ring and glove sizes.

Systemic findings in acromegaly include organomegaly (e.g., liver, spleen, heart, thyroid, and kidneys); nerve entrapment, which may lead to carpal tunnel syndrome; hypertension; insulin resistance and diabetes mellitus; and galactorrhea. The course is extremely variable and may be fulminant, leading to death in a matter of a few years, or benign, lasting 50 years or longer. The diagnosis involves evaluation of IGF-1 levels; measurement of growth hormone following oral glucose challenge is less commonly used. IGF-1 is the most reliable laboratory indicator of acromegaly because of its excellent correlation with 24-hour growth hormone secretion. Once growth hormone hypersecretion has been confirmed, magnetic resonance imaging of the pituitary is recommended. Surgical removal of the pituitary tumor is first-line therapy for most patients but results in long-term cure in only about 60% of patients. Medical management as well as radiation therapy are therefore important complementary treatments. Long-acting somatostatin analogs such as octreotide are first-line medical therapy. Dopamine agonists, such as bromocriptine, and growth hormone receptor antagonists may also be beneficial.

Hypopituitarism

Hypopituitarism may manifest as an isolated deficiency of one or more anterior pituitary hormones, resulting in secondary atrophy of the gonads, thyroid, and adrenal cortex. Panhypopituitarism implies absence of all pituitary hormones, including growth hormone, thyrotropin, prolactin, corticotropin, and the two gonadotropins (FSH and LH). The most common cause of hypopituitarism in adult life is a pituitary adenoma. Other tumors, infections (syphilis or tuberculosis), sarcoidosis, basal skull fracture, infarction (such as with postpartum hemorrhage in Sheehan syndrome), and a variety of other disorders may disrupt the normal function of the gland and lead to hypopituitarism.

The endocrine manifestations of hypopituitarism vary with the type, age of development, and degree of hormone deficiency. At least 75% of the gland must be destroyed before the wide variety of signs and symptoms become clinically manifest. Cutaneous changes may be the first clue to the diagnosis. The skin and subcutaneous tissues are thin, body hair is scant, and the skin is pale or yellowish in color. Signs of hypothyroidism may be evident, and there may be symptoms of gonadotropin deficiency, especially a reduction in libido.

After the diagnosis has been established by appropriate laboratory studies, treatment includes the replacement of missing hormones.

SUGGESTED READINGS

Buzney E, Sheu J, Buzney C, Reynolds RV. Polycystic ovary syndrome: a review for dermatologists: Part II. Treatment. J Am Acad Dermatol 2014;71(5):859.e1–15.

Clark CM, Rudolph J, Gerber DA, Glick S, Shalita AR, Lowenstein EJ. Dermatologic manifestation of hyperandrogenism: a retrospective chart review. Skinmed 2014;12(2):84–8.

Därr R, Lenders JWM, Hofbauer LC, Naumann B, Bornstein SR, Eisenhofer G. Pheochromocytoma: update on disease management. Ther Adv Endo and Metab 2012;3(1):11–26.

Dekkers OM, Horváth-Puhó E, Jørgensen JO, et al. Multisystem morbidity and mortality in Cushing's syndrome: a cohort study. J Clin Endocrinol Metab 2013;98:2277.

Housman E, Reynolds RV. Polycystic ovary syndrome: a review for dermatologists: Part I. Diagnosis and manifestations. J Am Acad Dermatol 2014;71(5):847.e1–10.

Hughes IA, Davies JD, Bunch TI, Pasterski V, Mastroyannopoulou K, Macdougall J. Androgen insensitivity syndrome. Lancet 2012;380(9851):1419–28.

Jabbour SA. Cutaneous manifestations of endocrine disorders: a guide for dermatologists. Am J Clin Dermatol 2003;4(5):315–31.

Kannan S, Kennedy L. Diagnosis of acromegaly: state of the art. Expert Opin Med Diagn 2013;7(5):443–53.

Katznelson L, Laws Jr ER, Melmed S, et al. Acromegaly: an Endocrine Society clinical practice guideline. J Clin Endocrinol Metab 2014;99(11):3933–51.

Koulouri O, Conway GS. A systematic review of commonly used medical treatments for hirsutism in women. Clin Endocrinol (Oxf) 2008;68(5):800–5.

Lolis MS, Bowe WP, Shalita AR. Acne and systemic disease. Med Clin North Am 2009;93(6):1161–81.

Melmed S, Casanueva FF, Klibanski A, Bronstein MD, Chanson P, Lamberts SW, et al. A consensus on the diagnosis and treatment of acromegaly complications. Pituitary 2013;16(3):294–302.

Nieman LK, Biller BM, Findling JW, et al. The diagnosis of Cushing's syndrome: an Endocrine Society clinical practice guideline. J Clin Endocrinol Metab 2008;93:1526.

Niemann LK, Chanco Turner ML. Addison's disease. Clin Dermatol 2006;24:276–80.

Shibli-Rahhal A, Van Beek M, Schlechte JA. Cushing's syndrome. Clin Dermatol 2006;24:260–5.

Speiser PW, Azziz R, Baskin LS, Ghizzoni L, Hensle TW, Merke DP. Congenital adrenal hyperplasia due to steroid 21-hydroxylase deficiency: an Endocrine Society clinical practice guideline. J Clin Endocrinol Metab 2010;95(9):4133–60.

Witchel SF. Nonclassic congenital adrenal hyperplasia. Curr Opin Endocrinol Diabetes Obes 2012;19(3):151–8.

CHAPTER 28

PORPHYRIAS

Maureen B. Poh-Fitzpatrick

KEY POINTS

- Several porphyrias share similar photocutaneous features; sufficient testing to assure correct diagnosis must precede selection of therapies.
- Most porphyrias can be correctly diagnosed biochemically.
- Mutation analysis is the gold standard for porphyria diagnosis and family counseling.
- Clinical and biochemical remissions can be therapeutically induced in most patients with porphyria cutanea tarda.
- X-linked dominant protoporphyria, recently recognized, can be distinguished from erythropoietic protoporphyria despite many similar clinical features.
- Attacks of both variegate porphyria and hereditary coproporphyria can be rapidly diagnosed by screening for increased urinary porphobilinogen.
- Management of porphyrias with multisystem problems may be complex, requiring expert consultation.

Porphyrias are a group of inherited or acquired metabolic disorders manifested by cutaneous photosensitivity, episodic neurovisceral dysfunctions, or both (Table 28-1). Each porphyria is caused by reduced activity (or in one case, increased function) of one of eight enzymes regulating the porphyrin–heme pathway (Fig. 28-1). These enzyme anomalies produce accumulations of excess porphyrin precursors and/or porphyrins in patterns characterizing each associated porphyria.

Human heme biosynthesis occurs chiefly in hepatocytes and bone marrow erythrocyte precursors. Porphyrias are classified as "hepatic" or "erythropoietic" according to the major tissue overproducing porphyrins and/or porphyrin precursors. Reduced enzyme activity causes backup accumulation of its immediate substrate and other precursors. Irreversible spontaneous oxidation of nonphotoactive porphyrinogen precursors forms photoactive porphyrin byproducts of the pathway that can be found in urine, feces, plasma and/or erythrocytes (Table 28-2), and are disseminated throughout the body. Porphyrin molecules avidly absorb light energy of several wavelengths, maximally at 400 to 410 nm (visible violet light). Such energy can penetrate human epidermis and photoexcite porphyrins in dermal tissues. This excitation energy can then transfer to oxygen, yielding unstable, highly reactive oxidizing agents in the skin. Signs and symptoms of cutaneous photosensitivity result when lipid peroxidation and complement activation ensue, causing cell membrane disintegration and release of intravascular and cellular contents including secondary mediators of inflammation.

Four hepatic porphyrias manifest potentially fatal episodic attacks reflecting dysfunctions of central, autonomic, and peripheral nervous systems. Symptoms may include abdominal pain, limb pain and weakness, nausea, vomiting, constipation, tachycardia, hypertension, anxiety, agitation, confusion, bizarre behavior, central nerve paralysis, respiratory distress, seizures, or coma, which may be related to poorly understood effects of deranged heme synthesis on neurons. Attacks are often triggered by porphyrinogenic drugs that induce hepatic heme synthesis. Other precipitating factors include: fasting, infections, hormonal fluctuations due to menses, pregnancy or therapeutic hormones, or other stressors. Two acute attack porphyrias may also have photocutaneous features.

Many mutations in the genes encoding the protein structures of these enzymes have been identified, with various aberrations of each gene leading to clinical expression of its associated porphyria. Severity of the encoded protein defect typically determines how much, if any, residual enzyme activity remains. Degrees of phenotypic severity may be linked to variations in molecular genotype. Clinical expression of some porphyrias (Table 28-1) may also be influenced by environmental and physiologic factors.

Most porphyrias are readily diagnosed biochemically (Table 28-2). Enzyme activity assays are commercially available for only some enzymes of heme synthesis, but mutation analysis of the genes underlying any of the heritable porphyrias can be obtained. Several laboratories offering various analyses are listed at the American Porphyria Foundation website (www.porphyriafoundation.com). Only porphyrias with cutaneous manifestations will be further reviewed in this chapter.

PORPHYRIA CUTANEA TARDA

In porphyria cutanea tarda (PCT), the most common porphyria of adults, excess polycarboxylated porphyrins are produced due to reduced activity of uroporphyrinogen decarboxylase (UROD) in hepatocytes. PCT is the only porphyria with both acquired (~80%, "sporadic" or "type 1") and familial (~20%, "type 2") forms. Autosomal dominant familial PCT has a genotype of one mutated and one normal *UROD* allele. The resulting residual enzyme activity can be as low as 50% when the enzyme product of the mutant allele retains no activity

TABLE 28-1 The Porphyrias

	Cutaneous	Neurovisceral	Cutaneous and Neurovisceral
Hepatic	Porphyria cutanea tarda Hepatoerythropoietic porphyria	Acute intermittent porphyria δ-Aminolevulinic acid dehydrogenase deficiency porphyria	Hereditary coproporphyria Variegate porphyria
Erythropoietic	Erythropoietic protoporphyria X-linked dominant protoporphyria Congenital erythropoietic porphyria		

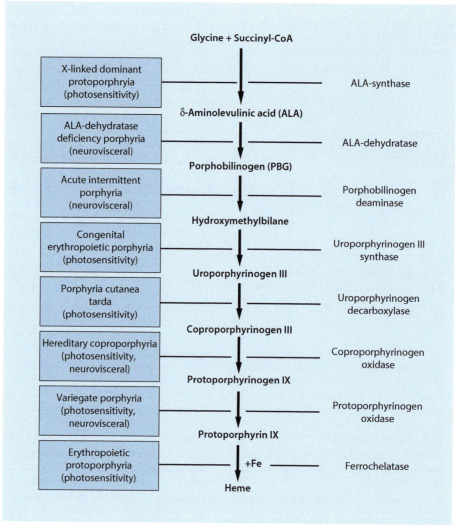

FIGURE 28-1 ■ Heme biosynthetic pathway.

whatsoever. Homozygous or compound heterozygous inheritance of two *UROD* mutations reduces residual activity to only 10% to 30% of normal, causing the more severe recessive variant "hepatoerythropoietic porphyria" (HEP). Many deleterious *UROD* mutations are known; the HEP genotype is often heteroallelic, with a different mutated allele inherited from each parent. While PCT usually presents in adulthood, HEP presents in childhood. The destructive photomutilation observed in HEP simulates that of congenital erythropoietic porphyria (CEP).

UROD sequentially decarboxylates uroporphyrinogen (eight carboxylic side groups) to coproporphyrinogen (four carboxylic side groups). Sufficiently reduced UROD activity leads to abnormally high levels of uroporphyrin and 7-carboxyl porphyrin, with lesser increases in 6- and 5-carboxyl porphyrins and coproporphyrin in urine and plasma, and abnormal fecal excretion of isocoproporphyrin, an unusual 4-carboxyl pathway by-product. In most familial PCT cases, UROD deficiency is detectable in both erythrocytes and hepatocytes; in acquired PCT, only hepatocytes have diminished UROD activity.

TABLE 28-2 Characteristic Biochemical Findings in the Porphyrias

Type of Porphyria	Urine				Feces			Erythrocytes			Plasma
	ALA	PBG	URO	COPRO	URO	COPRO	PROTO	URO	COPRO	PROTO	
Acute Porphyrias											
Acute intermittent porphyria	++ to ++++	++ to ++++	+++	++	N to +	N to +	N to +	N	N	N	N
Variegate porphyria	++ to +++	++ to +++	+++	+++	N	+++	++++	N	N	N	625–627 nm*
Hereditary coproporphyria	N to ++	N to ++	++	++++	++	++++	N to +	N	N	N	619 nm*
ALA-D deficiency porphyria	+++	N	+	++	N	+	+	N	N	++	ALA, COPRO and PROTO↑
Nonacute Porphyrias											
Porphyria cutanea tarda	N	N	++++	++	++	ISOCOPRO	+	N	N	N	URO↑
Erythropoietic protoporphyria	N	N	N	N	N	++	++ to ++++	N	N to +	+++	PROTO↑
Congenital erythropoietic porphyria	N	N	++++	++	+	+++	+	++++	+++	+++	URO and COPRO↑
Hepatoerythropoietic porphyria	N	N	+++	ISOCOPRO	N	ISOCOPRO	N	N	+	++++	URO↑
X-linked dominant protoporphyria	N	N	N	N	NA	NA	NA	NA	NA	++++†	PROTO↑

*Peak fluorometric emission.
†Approximately 40% zinc-protoporphyrin.
In patients with variegate porphyria or hereditary coproporphyria without cutaneous or systemic symptoms, urine porphyrins may not be elevated. ALA, Aminolevulinic acid; ALA-D, aminolevulinic acid dehydratase; COPRO, coproporphyrin; ISOCOPRO, isocoproporphyrin; PBG, porphobilinogen; PROTO, protoporphyrin; URO, uroporphyrin; N, normal; NA, not available; +, above normal range; ++, slightly elevated; +++, highly elevated; ++++, very highly elevated; ↑, increase.
Adapted from Frank J, Poblete-Gutiérrez P. Porphyria. In: Bolognia JL, Jorizzo JL, Schaffer JV, editors. Dermatology. 3rd ed. Elsevier; 2012.

Clinical Manifestations

Cutaneous features of PCT predominantly involve sun-exposed skin of the dorsal hands, extensor forearms, and face (Figs 28-2 to 28-5), but legs, feet, scalp, and chest (Fig. 28-6) may also be affected. Vesicles, bullae (Figs 28-2 and 28-3) and painful erosions of fragile skin (Fig. 28-4) are typical presenting complaints. Facial hypertrichosis (Fig. 28-5) frequently develops; mottled melasma-like dyspigmentation may appear in the periorbital and malar regions. Rarely, generalized melanosis simulates Addison's disease or hemochromatosis. Sclerodermoid induration of head, neck, back, and chest skin, histopathologically indistinguishable from scleroderma, may be an accompanying or sole finding (Fig. 28-7). Protracted blistering eventuates in scars, dyschromia, and milia (Figs 28-2 and 28-8), as well as alopecia with distinctive saucer-shaped scars or crater-like depressions. Indolent ulcers and dystrophic calcification may develop in chronically damaged preauricular, forehead, scalp, neck, or dorsal hand skin.

Etiologic Associations

Nongenetic factors that predispose to, precipitate, or influence clinical expression of PCT include alcohol ingestion, medicinal estrogens, excess iron intake, tobacco smoking, vitamin C depletion, and exposure to hepatotoxic polychlorinated aromatic hydrocarbons. PCT is associated with viral and sarcoidal hepatitis, hemochromatosis genes (*HFE*), lupus erythematosus, abnormal glucose metabolism, and hepatic tumors (Table 28-3).

The incidence of PCT associated with chronic hepatitis C virus infection (HCV) varies widely by geographical region. In southern Europe, 70% to 90% of PCT patients also have HCV, as do 56% in the United States, but only 20% in northern Europe, Australia, and New Zealand, where HCV is less prevalent but *HFE* mutations are more prevalent. Almost 40% of PCT patients of northern European origin harbor one or two mutated *HFE* alleles. PCT has also been associated with hepatitis B and human immunodeficiency virus (HIV) infections. Diabetes mellitus/glucose intolerance occurs more often in individuals with

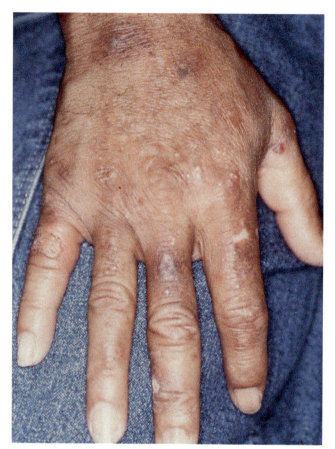

FIGURE 28-2 ■ Vesicles, bullae, crusts, milia, scars, and dyschromia of the dorsal hand in porphyria cutanea tarda (PCT).

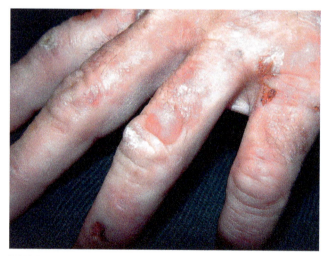

FIGURE 28-3 ■ Large bullae may occur in porphyria cutanea tarda (PCT).

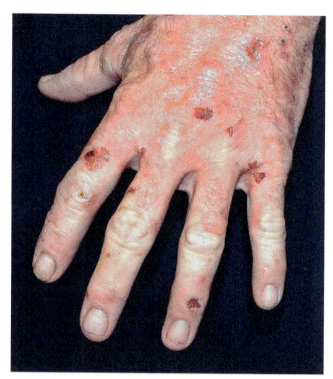

FIGURE 28-4 ■ Painful erosions result from increased skin fragility in porphyria cutanea tarda (PCT).

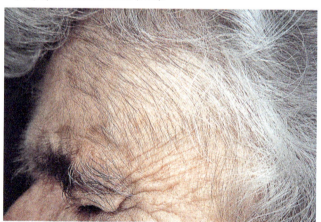

FIGURE 28-5 ■ Facial hypertrichosis in a man with porphyria cutanea tarda (PCT).

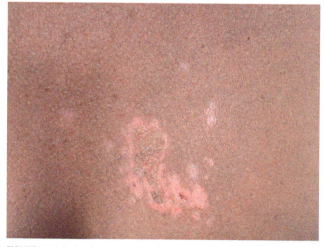

FIGURE 28-6 ■ Lesions on the chest of a woman with porphyria cutanea tarda (PCT).

PCT than in the general population. Subacute, chronic cutaneous, or systemic lupus erythematosus and PCT are comorbidities sometimes discovered when initiation of antimalarial therapy for lupus triggers latent PCT.

Mild to moderate excess hepatic iron deposition is often found in PCT, even in individuals without variant *HFE* alleles. Excess iron facilitates formation of toxic oxygen species, which enhance porphyrinogenesis by catalyzing production of oxidative inhibitors of UROD activity. Toxic

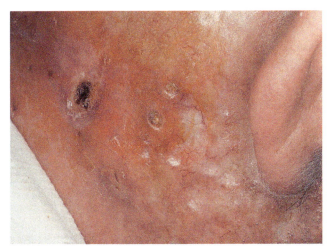

FIGURE 28-7 ■ Sclerodermoid changes with dystrophic calcification in porphyria cutanea tarda (PCT).

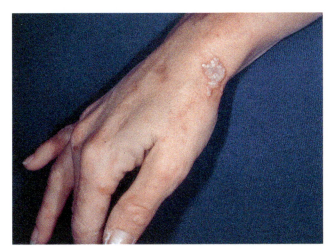

FIGURE 28-8 ■ Milia en plaque in a patient with porphyria cutanea tarda (PCT).

TABLE 28-3 Conditions and Precipitating/Aggravating Factors Associated with Porphyria Cutanea Tarda (PCT)

Alcohol Ingestion
Medications
   Estrogens
   Tamoxifen
   4-Fluoroquinolone antimalarial agents
Polychlorinated aromatic hydrocarbons
Iron overload
Hemochromatosis (homozygous or heterozygous)
Hepatitis B and C viruses
Human immunodeficiency virus
Cytomegalovirus
Tobacco smoking
Hepatic sarcoidosis
Chronic dialysis treatment for end-stage renal disease
Hepatic tumors
   Primary
   Metastatic
Abnormal glucose metabolism
Lupus erythematosus
   Chronic cutaneous
   Subacute cutaneous
   Acute cutaneous
Vitamin C depletion

effects of hepatic siderosis may aggravate liver injury and hasten development of fibrosis or cirrhosis.

PCT may lead to hepatocellular carcinoma, particularly in older men with chronic active disease, heavy alcohol intake, and cirrhosis. Screening for hepatocellular carcinoma by serum α-fetoprotein testing and hepatic ultrasonography is warranted in cases of active PCT of long duration, new-onset PCT in the elderly, unexplained recurrence after remission in the absence of other precipitating factors, or atypical urinary porphyrin profile. Some experts suggest baseline assessment at diagnosis, then annual monitoring. Surveillance for hepatocellular carcinoma at 6-month intervals is recommended in cases of HCV, cirrhosis, or other advanced hepatopathies. Liver biopsy may be indicated to assess iron burden or damage from alcohol abuse, viral infections, hemochromatosis, or suspected tumors.

Evaluation

In PCT and HEP, excess polycarboxylated porphyrins impart a red-brown color to urine, which exhibits pink fluorescence with Wood's light illumination. Quantitative urinary or plasma porphyrin fractionation demonstrates predominantly uroporphyrin and 7-carboxylic porphyrins. Fecal isocoproporphyrin is increased. In PCT, erythrocyte porphyrin levels are normal, but in HEP, increased zinc-protoporphyrin is found in erythrocytes. Reduced erythrocyte UROD activity or *UROD* mutation(s) indicate familial cases. Hematology and iron profiles including serum ferritin, a liver function panel, hepatitis and HIV serologies, and *HFE* molecular analysis are recommended at diagnosis. Antinuclear antibodies, glucose tolerance, serum α-fetoprotein, hepatic ultrasonography, and liver biopsy assessments are needed in select cases. Skin biopsy histologic changes consistent with PCT are not diagnostic; similar findings occur in other cutaneous porphyrias, pseudoporphyrias, and some primary blistering disorders.

Differential Diagnosis

Photocutaneous features of PCT and HEP are indistinguishable from those of variegate porphyria (VP), hereditary coproporphyria (HCP), or CEP. Vesiculobullous lesions of epidermolysis bullosa acquisita, amyloidosis, lupus erythematosus, or drug eruptions may resemble those of any of these porphyrias. Patients with chronic PCT may be misdiagnosed as having a host of sclerodermoid disorders. "Pseudoporphyria" refers to photoaggravated PCT-like blistering in the absence of increased porphyrin levels or other primary bullous disease; many medications have been implicated as causative (Table 28-4). Porphyria-like blistering may complicate renal failure treated with chronic dialysis (Fig. 28-9), as well as afflict individuals frequently exposed to intense artificial or natural sunlight or those receiving photodynamic therapy.

Treatment

The first step in treatment involves eliminating alcohol intake, tobacco use, medicinal estrogens (when possible), iron supplements, and environmental toxins. Sunlight exposure must be avoided until clinical remission is achieved.

A nutritious diet low in iron-rich red meats, but with adequate sources of vitamin C, should be followed. A preferred therapy for individuals with a heavy iron burden is serial phlebotomy, which rapidly reduces tissue iron, thereby normalizing heme synthesis disturbed by iron-mediated inhibition of UROD. Serum ferritin should be progressively reduced to low normal values by withdrawing up to 500 mL of whole blood at intervals ranging from twice weekly to once every 2 to 3 weeks. Intervals should be individualized to each patient's tolerance and to avoid inducing anemia (hemoglobin <10 to 11 g/dL). Diminution of photosensitivity and of porphyrin levels begins during treatment, but full clinical and biochemical remissions may not be achieved until weeks to months after low normal serum ferritin levels have been reached and phlebotomies halted. During this time, continued photoprotection and sunlight avoidance remain necessary. Improvement of hypertrichosis and dyspigmentation may be slow and incomplete. Scarring and sclerodermoid changes may be permanent. Stimulation of erythropoiesis by exogenous erythropoietin mobilizes iron in dialyzed patients with end-stage renal disease and preexisting anemia, and may allow judicious low-volume phlebotomies. The efficacy of anti-hepatitis C therapy appears enhanced if hepatic siderosis is first reduced by phlebotomy. Newer protease inhibitor therapies of hepatitis C viral infection have led to sustained remission in cases of hepatitis-C-associated PCT.

Another therapeutic option especially useful in patients with mild iron overload or when phlebotomy is inconvenient or contraindicated is hydroxychloroquine sulfate (100 to 200 mg, 2 to 3 times/week). The higher doses typically recommended for antimalarial or photoprotective indications can cause acute hepatotoxicity. An even smaller test dose may be given initially in patients perceived to be particularly at risk. Hepatic transaminases may rise transiently after institution of therapy, but tend to normalize as treatment continues. Low-dose antimalarial therapy and phlebotomy may be used concomitantly to accelerate clinical and biochemical responses. Alternative treatments (e.g., plasmapheresis, cholestyramine, vitamin E, metabolic alkalinization, iron chelators) are rarely used.

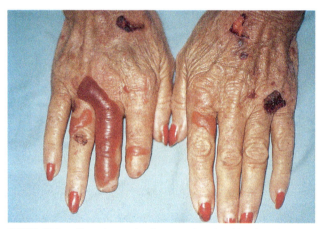

FIGURE 28-9 ■ Pseudoporphyria associated with chronic renal failure and dialysis treatment.

TABLE 28-4 Medications Associated with Pseudoporphyria

Anti-Infective Agents
 β-Lactams
 Nalidixic acid
 Tetracyclines
 Voriconazole

Diuretics
 Chlorthalidone
 Bumetanide
 Furosemide
 Hydrochlorothiazide/triamterene

Nonsteroidal Anti-Inflammatory Agents
 Diflunisal
 Ketoprofen
 Nabumetone
 Naproxen
 Oxaprozin
 Diclofenac

Retinoids
 Etretinate
 Isotretinoin

Miscellaneous
 Amiodarone
 Cyclosporine
 Imatinib
 5-Fluorouracil
 Flutamide
 Dapsone
 Pyridoxine

ERYTHROPOIETIC PROTOPORPHYRIA AND X-LINKED DOMINANT PROTOPORPHYRIA

Erythropoietic protoporphyria (EPP), the most common porphyria of children, is caused by impaired activity of ferrochelatase (FECH), the final enzyme of heme biosynthesis. Accumulation of its substrate, protoporphyrin (PP), leads to immediate cutaneous photosensitivity and to hepatobiliary disease. Overproduced primarily in bone marrow erythroid precursor cells, intracellular PP diffuses into blood plasma, thereby reaching other tissues. PP is cleared from plasma and secreted into bile by the liver, then excreted in feces. PP-rich bile facilitates gallstone formation. Hepatotoxic effects of PP can lead to fatal hepatic dysfunction. Anemia, if present, is typically mild.

The predominant EPP genotype is one mutant *FECH* allele encoding a defective enzyme protein with little or no function, paired with a relatively common polymorphic allele with low gene expression that only mildly reduces the activity of its enzyme product. Some authorities call this "pseudodominant" or "semidominant" inheritance, while others consider it autosomal recessive, in that disease expression requires anomalies in both alleles. Classical autosomal recessive inheritance of biallelic deleterious *FECH* mutations occurs in a minority of patients with EPP.

X-linked dominant protoporphyria (XLP), though clinically very similar to EPP, is now recognized as a unique disorder caused by gain-of-function mutations in the gene encoding the erythroid-specific enzyme aminolevulinic acid synthase-2 (ALAS2). Increased function of ALAS2 leads to accumulation of erythrocyte PP with a larger ratio of zinc-PP to metal-free PP than is characteristic of EPP. XLP exhibits the same childhood-onset and immediate cutaneous photosensitivity as EPP, but may have a higher risk of hepatic dysfunction.

Clinical Manifestations

Photocutaneous features of EPP and XLP are alike. Tingling, burning, and pruritus, elicited by only minutes to hours of sun exposure, are followed by photodistributed erythema and edema that slowly evolve into painful purpuric mats that fade over several days. Repeated damage can lead to indurated, weather-beaten, or cobblestoned skin, most often seen over the knuckles. Waxy induration, shallow elliptical scars, and perioral furrows are facial lesions highly suggestive of EPP or XLP. Blistering and crusting occur, but infrequently. In addition to the cutaneous findings, early onset of gallstones and progressive hepatic dysfunction may complicate the clinical course.

Diagnosis

Abnormally high PP in erythrocytes, plasma, and feces is characteristic of both disorders; in XLP, erythrocyte zinc-PP may be 15–50% of the total PP present, whereas in EPP it is typically <85%. Because PP is not water-soluble, urinary porphyrins are typically normal, however, with sufficient liver dysfunction, coproporphyrinuria appears. Blood specimens, especially plasma, must be completely protected from light during collection, transport, and processing because PP is very photolabile. Mutation analysis is available for both *FECH* and *ALAS2* genes. A hematology profile and liver function panel should be obtained at diagnosis and monitored at 6- to 12-month intervals. Since patients with EPP and XLP shun sunlight, serum vitamin D levels should be assessed. Histologic examination of chronically damaged skin reveals hyaline masses in the upper dermis and thickened upper dermal capillary walls. Ultrastructural studies show amorphous dermal deposits, replicated basal laminae surrounding dermal vessels, and degranulated mast cells.

Treatment

EPP and XLP cause lifelong cutaneous photosensitivity requiring protective clothing and lifestyle adjustments. Topical sunscreens containing zinc oxide or titanium dioxide that block long ultraviolet (UV) and visible light radiation may provide limited benefit. Glass is not an effective barrier, but plastic films that block offending wavelengths can be affixed to windows and windshields. Induction of endogenous melanin (tanning) by skin exposure to broad- or narrow-band UV-B lamps or to UV-A lamps plus psoralen may increase sunlight tolerance. Subcutaneously implantable afamelanotide, an alpha-melanocyte-stimulating hormone analog that increases skin melanin, is available in Europe. Oral β-carotene beadlets in doses of 60 to 300 mg/day reduce photosensitivity in some, but not all, patients.

Supplementation with cholecalciferol (vitamin D3) should be given if serum levels are low, and consultation for bone health assessment should be considered.

The associated anemia rarely requires specific therapy. Cholelithiasis is managed surgically, and caution is advised in using cholestatic drugs. Immunization against hepatitis viruses should be offered. Liver dysfunction is an ominous development mandating referral to a center with expertise in treating porphyric liver disorders. Progressive intractable liver insufficiency is an indication for liver transplantation, but this alone fails to cure protoporphyrias, which are due to bone marrow PP overproduction. Combined liver and bone marrow transplantations can be curative. Operating room lighting must be filtered to mitigate interoperative PP-sensitized damage to internal organs and to exposed skin during liver transplantation.

CONGENITAL ERYTHROPOIETIC PORPHYRIA

CEP is a rare autosomal recessive disorder manifested by photocutaneous lesions, hemolytic anemia, and skeletal and ocular disorders. Biallelic uroporphyrinogen III synthase (*UROS*) mutations encoding defective enzyme proteins lead to accumulation of isomer I polycarboxylated porphyrins that are useless for heme production but can photosensitize reactions in the skin, resulting in fragility, blisters, erosions, and scarring. Red-brown urine, bones, and teeth (erythrodontia), pigmented by polycarboxylic porphyrin deposition, fluoresce pink to red under a Wood's lamp.

Chronic damage to skin, eyes, bones, and nasal and auricular cartilages beginning in early childhood can progress to mutilation. Hypertrichosis, waxy indurated plaques, dyspigmentation, scarring of the face and extremities, and scarring alopecia of the scalp are often prominent. Hemolytic anemia varies from mild to severe with associated splenomegaly and osseous fragility. Ocular manifestations include conjunctivitis, blepharitis, cicatricial ectropion, and lagophthalmos, which may lead to corneal scarring and eventual blindness. Milder cases have occurred in very rare adult-onset cases.

Diagnosis

Elevated isomer I porphyrin levels in urine, plasma, feces, and erythrocytes distinguish CEP from other porphyrias (Table 28-2). Pink staining of diapers due to excreted porphyrins may signal this diagnosis in neonates. Mutation analysis for the *UROS* gene is commercially available.

Treatment

CEP is a complex multisystem disorder best managed by experts. Sun avoidance is essential; vitamin D supplementation may be needed. Oral β-carotene has little benefit. Oral α-tocopherol and ascorbic acid may reduce oxygen free radicals, thereby reducing photodamage. Oral superactivated charcoal or cholestyramine may reduce plasma porphyrins by mitigating their reabsorption; hypertransfusion or chemosuppression of marrow may slow heme production, but these therapies have many adverse effects. Splenectomy may be required. Bone marrow transplantation can be curative.

VARIEGATE PORPHYRIA AND HEREDITARY COPROPORPHYRIA

Cutaneous features of these two autosomal dominant "acute attack" porphyrias resemble those of PCT. Skin lesions afflict ~50% to 80% of patients with VP (and may be the only manifestation) and ~30% of those with HCP. Neurovisceral attacks may be triggered in either disorder by porphyrinogenic drugs, fasting, hormonal fluctuations, infections, or other stressors. Mutations in the protoporphyrinogen oxidase gene (*PPOX*) cause VP; mutations in the coproporphyrinogen oxidase (*CPOX*) gene cause HCP. Both disorders typically present after puberty in heterozygotes, but the majority of *PPOX* or *CPOX* mutation carriers never develop symptoms. Biallelic *PPOX* mutations cause childhood onset of a severe phenotype including short stature, clinodactyly, mental retardation, seizures, and photosensitivity. Biallelic *CPOX* mutations cause similar severe childhood HCP variants.

Diagnosis and Evaluation

VP is biochemically characterized by combined excess PP greater than coproporphyrin (CP) in feces and CP greater than uroporphyrin in urine (Table 28-2). Abnormally high levels of porphobilinogen and aminolevulinic acid appear in urine and plasma during attacks. Plasma fluorescence emission scanning shows a pathognomonic peak at 626 ± 1 nm. Porphyrin and porphyrin precursor levels in urine, plasma, and feces may normalize when VP is quiescent, or may remain increased at variable levels and rise during attacks. HCP is biochemically characterized by increased CP III in urine and feces as well as high urinary porphobilinogen and aminolevulinic acid during attacks. Suspected acute attacks should be rapidly assessed by urinary porphobilinogen screening tests, and medical management instituted immediately if positive.

Mutation analysis for *PPOX* and *CPOX* genes is commercially available. Since most heterozygous carriers of *PPOX* or *CPOX* mutations remain clinically silent and may also be biochemically silent, particularly in childhood, confidently identifying all family members at risk requires mutation analyses. Both VP and HCP may be complicated by hepatocellular carcinoma. Hepatic ultrasound and serum α-fetoprotein surveillance every 6 to 12 months, beginning at age 47 to 50 years, has been recommended in both patients and mutation carriers.

Treatment

Unlike PCT, VP and HCP do not improve with antimalarial therapy or phlebotomy; photoprotective measures are essential when skin lesions are active. Minimizing the risk of evoking an acute attack by avoiding porphyrinogenic drugs, carbohydrate-restricted diets, immoderate alcohol intake, and tobacco smoking is critically important for individuals with expressed disease and for silent carriers. A "Drug Safety Database" can be found at the American Porphyria Foundation website (www.porphyriafoundation.com/drug_database). When necessary, steroid hormone therapy should be initiated cautiously. Infections or other stressors should be treated promptly. An alert tag identifying an incapacitated wearer as having VP or HCP may prevent inadvertent administration of hazardous drugs. Medical management of acute attacks is complex and often involves oral or intravenous glucose and infusion of hemin; early consultation with experts is strongly recommended.

SUGGESTED READINGS

Anstey AV, Hift RJ. Liver disease in erythropoietic protoporphyria: insights and implications for management. Gut 2007;56:1009–18.
Ashwani AK, Anderson KE. Variegate porphyria. In: Pagon RA, Adam MP, Bird TD, et al., editors. GeneReviews [Internet]. Seattle (WA): University of Washington; February 14, 2013. 1993–2014. Available from: http://www.ncbi.nlm.nih.gov/books/NBK121283/.
Balwani M, Desnick R. The porphyrias: advances in diagnosis and treatment. Blood 2012;120:4496–504.
Bissell DM, Wang B, Cimino T, Lai J. Hereditary coproporphyria. In: Pagon RA, Adam MP, Bird TD, et al., editors. GeneReviews [Internet]. Seattle (WA): University of Washington; December 13, 2012. 1993–2014. Available from: http://www.ncbi.nlm.nih.gov/books/NBK114807/.
Erwin A, Balwani M, Desnick RJ. Congenital erythropoietic porphyria. In: Pagon RA, Adam MP, Bird TD, et al., editors. GeneReviews [Internet]. Seattle (WA): University of Washington; September 12, 2013. 1993–2014. Available from: http://www.ncbi.nlm.nih.gov/books/NBK154652/.
Lecha M, Puy H, Deybach JC. Erythropoietic protoporphyria. Orphanet J Rare Dis 2009;4:19. Available from: http://www.ojrd.com/content.
Poblete-Gutiérrez P, Wiederholt T, Merk HF, Frank J. The porphyrias: clinical presentation, diagnosis and treatment. Eur J Dermatol 2006;16:230–40.
Poh-Fitzpatrick MB. Porphyrin-sensitized cutaneous photosensitivity: pathogenesis and treatment. Clin Dermatol 1985;3:41–82.
Puy H, Gouya L, Deybach JC. Porphyrias. Lancet 2010;375:924–37.
Ryan Caballes F, Sendi H, Bonkovsky HL, Hepatitis C. Porphyria cutanea tarda, and liver iron: an update. Liver Int 2012;32:880–93.
Sarkany RP. The management of porphyria cutanea tarda. Clin Exp Dermatol 2001;26:225–32.
Schulenburg-Brand D, Katugampola R, Anstey AV, Badminton MN. The cutaneous porphyrias. Dermatol Clin 2014;32:369–84.
Singal AK, Parker C, Bowden, et al. Liver transplantation in the management of porphyria. Hepatology 2014;60:1082–9.

CHAPTER 29

CUTANEOUS DISEASES ASSOCIATED WITH GASTROINTESTINAL ABNORMALITIES

Mark D. Herron • John J. Zone

KEY POINTS

- Gastrointestinal hemorrhage may be associated with pseudoxanthoma elasticum or hereditary hemorrhagic telangiectasia.
- Adenomatous polyposis may be associated with epidermoid tumors, fibromas, and dermoid tumors.
- Peutz–Jeghers syndrome and Cowden's syndrome are associated with hamartomatous polyps.
- Malabsorption may be associated with dermatitis herpetiformis and celiac disease or acrodermatitis enteropathica and zinc deficiency.
- Inflammatory bowel disease is associated with neutrophilic dermatoses such as pyoderma gangrenosum, aphthosis, and Sweet's syndrome as well as erythema nodosum.
- Pancreatitis may be manifested as purpura in specific areas or as panniculitis.

There are a number of diseases of the gastrointestinal tract that feature recognizable cutaneous diseases as part of their spectrum. This discussion includes cutaneous associations of the following disorders: gastrointestinal hemorrhage, polyposis, malabsorption, inflammatory bowel disease, and pancreatic disease. The genetic basis of many of these diseases has now been elucidated (Table 29-1).

GASTROINTESTINAL HEMORRHAGE

Extensive gastrointestinal hemorrhage may occasionally be related to systemic disorders that are easily recognized by their cutaneous findings. Pseudoxanthoma elasticum and hereditary hemorrhagic telangiectasia will be discussed.

Pseudoxanthoma Elasticum

Pseudoxanthoma elasticum (PXE) is a rare inherited disorder of elastic tissue that occurs in 1:25,000–100,000 births. There is progressive calcification of tissue rich in elastin fibers, including the skin, retina, and blood vessels. There is significant heterogeneity in the age of onset as well as the severity of organ system involvement. The greatest morbidity lies in reduced vision from macular hemorrhage and scarring of the macula. Affected individuals have a normal lifespan.

Pathogenesis

PXE is inherited in an autosomal recessive manner. PXE is caused by mutation in the *ABCC6* gene, ATP-binding cassette transporter protein. The gene has been mapped to chromosome 16p13.1. At least one *ABCC6* mutation can be found in 80% of affected individuals. ABCC6 protein is largely expressed in the liver and kidney. The *ABCC6* gene encodes for a cellular transport protein, giving rise to the concept that PXE may be a systemic metabolic disorder rather than purely a structural disorder of connective tissue. The elastic fibers are abnormal in the affected tissues. Changes include fragmentation and calcification of degenerated elastic tissue fibers in the middle and deep reticular dermis. Progressive accumulation of calcium within the elastic fibers leads to fracture and destruction.

Presentation

Cutaneous findings usually begin in the second to third decades. Calcification of elastic fibers results in yellowish discoloration of the skin. Affected skin reveals progressive yellowish coalescent papules on the lateral aspect of the neck, the flexural creases of the antecubital fossa and popliteal fossa, the axilla, and the groin. These yellow papules have been described as having a "plucked chicken skin" appearance. In severe cases, the skin appears loose and wrinkled (Figs 29-1 and 29-2).

The earliest ocular finding is diffuse mottling of the fundus. In the second to third decade, angioid streaks develop in the eye. These present as linear and branching networks of grayish discoloration radiating from the optic disc. Angioid streaks are larger in caliber than blood vessels and represent choroidal neovascularization in the elastic lamina of Bruch's membrane of the retina. Angioid streaks do not affect visual acuity. Subretinal neovascularization and hemorrhage lead to scarring and loss of vision. If the macula is involved, the loss of vision becomes permanent.

TABLE 29-1	Genetic Links to Gastrointestinal Diseases

Pseudoxanthoma elasticum: ATP-binding cassette transporter C6 (*ABCC6*)
Hereditary hemorrhagic telangiectasia 1: endoglin (*ENG*)
Hereditary hemorrhagic telangiectasia 2: activin A receptor, type II-like kinase 1 (*ACVRL1*)
Gardner's syndrome: adenomatous polyposis coli (*APC*)
Peutz–Jeghers syndrome: serine/threonine kinase (*STK11*)
Cowden's disease: phosphatase and tensin homolog (*PTEN*)
Acrodermatitis enteropathica: solute carrier family 39 (zinc transporter) member 4 (*SLC39A4*)

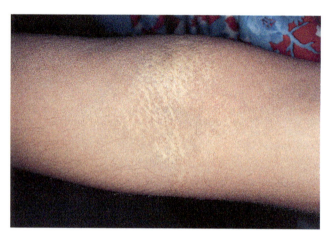

FIGURE 29-1 ■ Pseudoxanthoma elasticum.

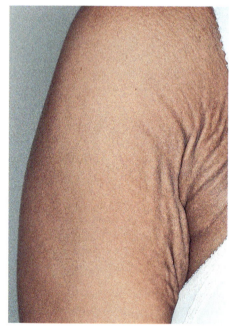

FIGURE 29-2 ■ Pseudoxanthoma elasticum with lax skin evident in the axilla.

Calcification of the elastic media of blood vessels results in hypertension, peripheral vascular disease, coronary artery disease, aneurysms, and cerebral hemorrhage. PXE affects the elastic tissue of the cardiac valves, the myocardium, and the pericardium. Gastrointestinal hemorrhage occurs in approximately 10% of patients with PXE. The most common site of bleeding is the stomach. This may develop from gastritis or peptic ulcer disease. Diffuse superficial erosions rather than focal bleeding are often found in the gastrointestinal tract. The bleeding is difficult to control due to defective vasoconstriction of the arteries. Gastric bleeding may occur early before ocular and cutaneous changes are fully developed.

Evaluation

The diagnosis is confirmed by the clinical picture and the demonstration of fragmented, calcified elastic fibers on skin biopsy that is essential for diagnosis. Skin biopsy of flexural skin or scars is warranted in both suspected cases and potentially involved family members. Examination by light microscopy demonstrates fragmentation and irregular clumping of elastic tissue in the middle to deep dermis. Staining for calcium frequently shows significant elastic tissue calcification. Although such findings are classically present in involved skin, clinically normal-appearing skin of the flexural areas may show similar findings. Biopsy may confirm a diagnosis of PXE in patients with angioid streaks and minimal cutaneous findings.

The diagnosis is suggested by angioid streaks in the second decade of life, or by a positive family history. Angioid streaks are not sufficient for the diagnosis. They are highly suggestive of the disease in patients with a positive family history. In 85% of patients with skin findings, angioid streaks are present in the eye grounds. If PXE is suspected, detailed examination by an ophthalmologist is essential. Because eye changes are seen early in life, funduscopic examination is also recommended for screening of relatives of known patients.

Recently, molecular genetic testing for the *ABCC6* gene has become available. Testing detects a mutation in one allele in almost all affected individuals and in both alleles in close to 90%. Sequence analysis detects missense mutations, nonsense mutations, frameshift mutations, as well as small deletions and insertions. Genetic testing and interpretation of results should be accompanied by genetic counseling.

Differential Diagnosis

The characteristic yellowish papules of PXE may be confused with solar elastosis. The neck is a common site for both, but PXE also occurs in the axilla, groin, and popliteal and antecubital fossae. Solar elastosis produces abnormal elastic tissue that is described histologically as dense masses in the upper dermis. The abnormal elastic tissue of solar elastosis does not stain for calcium. PXE shows fragmented clumps of elastic tissue in the mid to lower reticular dermis. Besides solar elastosis, skin lesions similar to PXE are found in conditions such as Buschke–Ollendorf syndrome, late-onset focal dermal elastosis, and cutis laxa.

Angioid streaks are valuable markers for the diagnosis of PXE, but are not pathognomonic findings. Angioid streaks may be seen in numerous disorders (Table 29-2), but are most commonly related to sickle cell anemia or

TABLE 29-2	Differential Diagnosis of Angioid Streaks

Paget's disease of the bone
Sickle cell anemia
Thalassemia
Ehlers–Danlos syndrome
Tuberous sclerosis syndrome
Sturge–Weber syndrome
Neurofibromatosis
Hemolytic anemia
Diabetes
Hemochromatosis
Hyperphosphatasemia
Hypercalcinosis
Lead poisoning
Pituitary disorders
Acromegaly
Myopia
Traumatic choroidal rupture

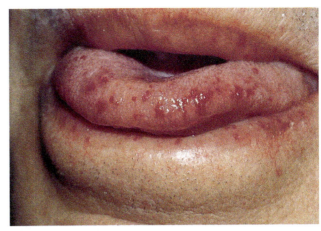

FIGURE 29-3 ■ Hereditary hemorrhagic telangiectasia. Multiple, small telangiectatic mats on the lips and tongue.

Paget's disease of the bone. No fundamental pathogenic relationship between the disorders causing angioid streaks has been established.

Treatment

There is no specific treatment for the basic defect in PXE. Weight control, avoidance of smoking, and aggressive management of hypertension and lipid disorders may reduce vascular complications. Both aspirin and nonsteroidal anti-inflammatory drugs should be avoided. Affected individuals should be discouraged from contact sports. Hemorrhage and vascular occlusive disease with PXE are managed medically.

Successful surgical removal of redundant skin for cosmetic reasons has been reported. Complications included slow healing, extrusion of calcium particles through scars, and widening of surgical scars. The majority of patients were highly satisfied with the results.

Hereditary Hemorrhagic Telangiectasia

Hereditary hemorrhagic telangiectasia (HHT) is an autosomal dominant disorder characterized by vascular dysplasia. Telangiectases are permanent dilatations of capillaries that usually blanch when pressure is applied. These telangiectases begin on the mucous membranes of the nose and mouth during childhood. Telangiectases of HHT are best demonstrated by stretching the mucosal surface of the lower lip between the thumb and the forefinger, revealing 2- to 3-mm punctate red macules that may become papular with age (Fig. 29-3). In young adults with HHT, an excess mortality has been attributed to HHT.

Pathogenesis

The prevalence of HHT is 1 per 10,000 of the population, which is much more common than previously thought. The mode of inheritance is autosomal dominant with a penetrance of approximately 97%. Two molecular subtypes of HHT are now recognized. Both HHT-1 and HHT-2 are multisystem vascular dysplasias caused by specific gene mutations found through linkage studies. The two subtypes reported have distinctions in the severity of disease and genetic markers.

HHT-1 is associated with a higher prevalence and increased severity of arteriovenous malformations. These patients have a higher risk of developing complex vascular abnormalities in the lungs and central nervous system at an early age. A mutation in the endoglin (*ENG*) gene has been described in HHT-1. Endoglin, which is a transforming growth factor-β (TGF-β)-binding protein, is expressed on capillaries, veins, and arteries. The *ENG* gene maps to chromosome 9q34.1.

HHT-2 is associated with a milder phenotype, reduced penetrance, and a later age of onset. Pulmonary arteriovenous malformations are less common in HHT-2 than in HHT-1. Activin A receptor, type II-like kinase 1 (*ACVRL1*) is the mutated gene described in HHT-2. The *ACVRL1* gene maps to chromosome 12q11-q14. *ACVRL1* is detected in highly vascularized tissues and expressed primarily on endothelial cells.

Histopathologically, irregularly dilated capillaries and venules develop in the papillary dermis. There is a lack of perivascular support, including reduced pericytes, smooth muscle, and elastic fibers. Abnormally large collagen bundles with irregular banding have also been described. Vessels with defective perivascular support are especially sensitive to insult in the gastrointestinal tract, where the epithelium is not cornified.

Presentation

Telangiectases develop on the undersurface of the tongue and floor of the mouth at puberty. Spontaneous and recurrent epistaxis is the most common presentation in childhood. Vascular abnormalities of the gastrointestinal, pulmonary, and nervous systems develop after the fourth decade of life. Telangiectatic lesions in the gastrointestinal tract cause bleeding in 20% to 30% of patients. Onset of gastrointestinal bleeding is usually in the fourth to sixth decades. Peptic ulcer disease is common in HHT patients. Bleeding is frequently from telangiectatic mucosa that has spontaneously eroded. Gastrointestinal hemorrhage tends to be progressive. With advancing age, gastrointestinal bleeding leads to severe anemia. Potential fatal problems with bleeding warrant close attention.

Elevated transaminases, γ-glutamyl transferase, and alkaline phosphatase have been reported in up to 30% of patients with HHT. Arteriovenous malformations of the liver are likely if there is hepatomegaly or a bruit over the liver. Cirrhosis of HHT is described as abnormal dilated vessels and changing stroma throughout the liver. Bleeding from hepatic arteriovenous fistulae is rare.

Pulmonary arteriovenous fistulae have been found in 15% to 33% of patients. Up to 50% of all pulmonary arteriovenous fistulae are associated with HHT. Cyanosis, clubbing, and dyspnea are late signs of arteriovenous fistulae. Most lesions are detected with a combination of chest radiography and measurement of PaO_2.

High cardiac output states secondary to severe anemia and systemic arteriovenous shunting may produce biventricular failure. Multiple arteriovenous fistulas may present with central nervous system findings, including transient ischemic attacks and cerebrovascular accidents. Cerebrovascular anomalies include arteriovenous malformation, capillary angiomas, and telangiectases. It is estimated that cerebral arteriovenous malformations occur in 5% to 10% of patients with HHT. Focal neurologic defects may result from these vascular malformations of the brain, spinal cord, and meninges. Patients with pulmonary and/or cerebral arteriovenous malformations risk early death from rupture of the diseased vessels.

Evaluation

The clinical diagnosis of HHT is based on the presence of telangiectases and on a family history of HHT. Four criteria for the diagnosis of HHT include epistaxis, telangiectases (lips, oral cavity, fingers, nose), visceral lesions, and a family history. The diagnosis is definitive with three or four criteria, but cannot be established with fewer than two. HHT lesions occur as multiple, 2- to 4-mm, usually symmetric, punctate, blanching macules, and as minimally elevated papules on the lips, face, nasal and oral mucosa, hands, feet, and upper extremities. The mode of inheritance is autosomal dominant, so a family history of bleeding is common.

If the characteristic telangiectases are present on the skin or mucous membranes, a detailed family history and history of bleeding episodes are essential. Clinical telangiectases may be few, especially in children and adolescents; therefore, close physical examination is necessary. Recurrent epistaxis at a young age may precede obvious telangiectases by many years, and this makes family history especially important. Examination of family members should focus on the wide spectrum of HHT.

Differential Diagnosis

There are a large number of diseases that can produce cutaneous vascular abnormalities. Telangiectatic mats with similar distributions appear in CREST syndrome (calcinosis, Raynaud's phenomenon, esophageal disease, sclerodactyly, and telangiectases) and scleroderma. Generalized essential telangiectasia consists of extensive, sometimes symmetric, sheets of linear telangiectases, predominantly on the limbs or trunk. Sunlight and ionizing radiation may produce localized linear telangiectases in sun-exposed areas. Traumatic lesions are usually linear, or occasionally spider-like and localized. The telangiectases of acne rosacea are linear, limited to the face and nose, and spare mucous membranes. Venous lakes are deep blue, soft papules and nodules occurring on the lips and ears that blanch only partially on diascopy, are usually few in number, and are not associated with mucosal lesions.

Treatment

Treatment should be directed at controlling complications of arteriovenous malformations before they become symptomatic. Epistaxis can be controlled with nasal packing or with electrocautery. Coagulation may only offer temporary relief. Laser therapy with a neodymium:YAG (Nd:YAG) laser is known to control bleeding. The placement of a split-thickness skin graft to protect fragile telangiectatic vessels has been successful in 25% to 64% of patients. However, telangiectatic vessels recur at the mucosal border of the graft. Prophylactic lubrication of the nasal mucosa may provide relief. There is a tendency to reduce epistaxis with estrogen therapy.

If the site can be identified, then the gastrointestinal bleeding responds to electrocautery or laser via endoscopy. If these treatments are unsuccessful, surgical resection of involved bowel segments may be necessary. Low-dose combinations of estrogen and progesterone have successfully treated severe blood loss from enteric telangiectases.

Significant arteriovenous fistulas in any location are usually controlled by resection. Embolization with both detachable balloons and coils may significantly reduce the morbidity in pulmonary arteriovenous malformations. Cerebral arteriovenous malformations have been treated with balloon and coil embolization, stereotactic surgery, or conventional neurosurgery to prevent disabling hemorrhage.

POLYPOSIS SYNDROMES

There are two recognized groups of hereditary polyposis: adenomatous polyposis syndromes and hamartomatous polyposis syndromes. Adenomatous polyposis syndromes have proven malignant potential. Hamartomatous polyposis syndromes represent malformation of the connective tissue of the intestinal mucosa. Even though they are classified as hamartomas, they still possess some risk of cancer.

Adenomatous Polyposis Syndromes

Familial adenomatous polyposis (FAP) refers to multiple adenomatous polyps numbering more than 100, and this condition predisposes to colorectal cancer with almost 100% certainty. FAP is characterized by autosomal dominant inheritance of colorectal polyposis without extracolonic manifestations. Considered to be a pathogenic variant of FAP, Gardner's syndrome is characterized by

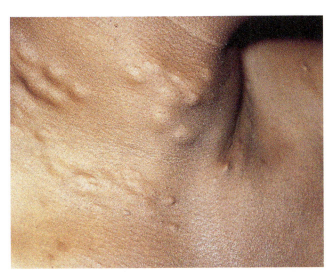

FIGURE 29-4 ■ Gardner's syndrome. Multiple epidermoid cysts are present in this patient with adenomatous colonic polyps.

an autosomal dominant inheritance with high penetrance and variable expressivity. Gardner's syndrome entails colorectal polyposis with multiple epidermoid cysts (Fig. 29-4), subcutaneous fibromas, lipomas, desmoid tumors, and osteomas of the facial bones and skull. If not treated, patients with FAP syndrome develop colon cancer beginning at ages of 20 to 30 years.

Pathogenesis

FAP and Gardner's syndrome show an autosomal dominant inheritance with a high penetrance. However, there may be considerable variation in phenotypic expression. Both sexes are equally affected. The prevalence of FAP has been estimated to be from 2 to 3:100,000.

FAP and Gardner's syndrome are caused by a highly heterogeneous spectrum of point mutations and represent a germline mutation in the adenomatous polyposis coli (*APC*) gene, located on chromosome 5q21. The *APC* gene encodes a multidomain protein that plays a role in tumor suppression by antagonizing the WNT signaling pathway. At least 70% of patients with familial polyposis coli and Gardner's syndrome have mutations in this gene. The *APC* gene acts as a tumor suppressor gene, and more than 800 mutations in the gene have been identified in families with FAP. There is growing evidence that different *APC* gene mutations correlate with specific phenotypes. Gardner's syndrome is a pathogenic variant of the APC-associated polyposis syndrome.

Presentation

The APC adenomatous polyposis syndromes are well characterized: familial polyposis coli, Gardner's syndrome, and Turcot's syndrome. Familial polyposis coli was originally separated from Gardner's syndrome solely on the basis of the absence of cutaneous findings in familial polyposis coli. Adenomatous polyps from both syndromes appear histologically, pathologically, and developmentally similar. There is great variation in the age of onset and in the number and location of polyps in both disorders. Colorectal adenomatous polyps begin to appear at 16 years of age. By 35 years of age, 95% of individuals with FAP have polyps. It may be impossible to diagnose intestinal polyposis before the age of 16, but the extracolonic manifestations of Gardner's syndrome can be recognized in infancy or early childhood.

The original description of Gardner's syndrome included significant extraintestinal manifestations: osteomas, epidermal inclusion (epidermoid) cysts, and subcutaneous fibromas in combination with intestinal polyposis. In general, osteomas precede the development of polyps. Osteomas are most commonly found in the skull and mandible. They appear in childhood prior to the development of polyps. Young children may have many small 3- to 5-mm cysts on the chest, back, and upper arms. Subcutaneous encapsulated fibromas occur on the scalp, shoulders, arms, and back.

Desmoid tumors and dental abnormalities have a significant impact on patients with Gardner's syndrome. Desmoid tumors represent benign, diffuse proliferation of soft fibrous tissue. They are abdominal wall tumors that may grow to several centimeters in size. They frequently occur at sites of trauma or surgery, but may arise de novo. Desmoid tumors are locally aggressive and have led to death. Mesenteric fibrosis occurs in a similar fashion. The dental abnormalities include odontomas, dentigenous cysts, unerupted teeth, congenital absence of teeth, and supernumerary teeth. Congenital hypertrophy of the retinal pigmented epithelium has been described in up to 90% of patients. They do not cause visual impairment.

Differentiation between Gardner's syndrome and sporadic epidermoid cysts is based primarily on the large numbers of lesions and on a positive family history in Gardner's syndrome patients. The presence of desmoid tumors should prompt consideration of the diagnosis of Gardner's syndrome.

Evaluation

The diagnosis relies primarily on clinical findings. Patients with cutaneous findings suggestive of Gardner's syndrome should undergo a detailed family history. Panoramic X-rays of the mandible may detect occult osteomas. Colonoscopy and biopsy may then confirm the diagnosis. Patients affected with both FAP and Gardner's syndrome have a lifetime risk of intestinal polyps transforming into adenocarcinoma at a rate approaching 100%.

Annual colonoscopic examination in high-risk individuals (family members) should be routine. In general, a preventive examination for the first generation of family members with Gardner's should begin during the 10th to 15th years of life. Colonoscopy is then continued every year until age 35. Molecular testing of the *APC* gene detects up to 90% of individuals with FAP syndrome. Molecular testing is most often used in the early diagnosis of at-risk family members. One benefit of molecular diagnosis is the elimination of the need for annual endoscopic screening in those who test negatively for a previously identified mutation in that family. The use of genetic testing linked to APC should be accompanied by genetic counseling to avoid adverse effects on patients and families.

Treatment

Colectomy is advised when more than 20 to 30 adenomas with advanced history have developed. Without colectomy, colon cancer is inevitable. Malignant changes in the colon have been reported as early as age 9 years. The incidence of carcinoma in preadolescent polyposis patients is about 5%, and nearly 100% by the age of 30 years. The average age of colon cancer diagnosis in untreated individuals is 39 years. If patients undergo a prophylactic colectomy with ileorectal anastomosis, there remains a risk of cancer in the remaining rectum. Close surveillance by a gastroenterologist is essential.

Desmoid tumors are surgically excised. Desmoid tumors are locally aggressive. Although they do not metastasize, they have led to death. Their infiltration into surrounding muscle and fascia may require excision, which is technically difficult because of poorly defined margins. Epidermal cysts and fibromas can be removed surgically if desired. There appears to be no increased risk of malignant degeneration in such lesions. Osteomas may be removed for cosmetic purposes.

Hamartomatous Polyposis Syndromes

Inherited hamartomatous polyposis syndromes are characterized by the presence of multiple hamartomatous polyps of the gastrointestinal tract and have an autosomal dominant mode of inheritance. Hamartomatous polyps are malformations of the intestinal mucosa that have undergone excessive growth.

Peutz–Jeghers syndrome consists of hamartomatous polyps in the gastrointestinal tract and mucocutaneous pigmentation of the lips, buccal mucosa, palms, and soles. Lentigines of the lips, buccal mucosa, and digits may appear in infancy or early childhood. Multiple hamartomatous polyps are symptomatic and are common in the small intestine. Gastrointestinal bleeding, obstruction, and intussusception are frequent complications. Uncommon cases of carcinoma affecting the entire gastrointestinal tract warrant close surveillance. Ovarian tumors and breast tumors have been reported with increasing frequency in this syndrome. Women with Peutz–Jeghers syndrome should be followed closely for associated ovarian and breast cancer. Once the diagnosis of Peutz–Jeghers syndrome is suspected, the gastrointestinal tract must be investigated with endoscopy every 2 years. Endoscopic or surgical removal of all polyps has been recommended. Screening for pancreatic cancer should be considered. Peutz–Jeghers syndrome is linked to mutations in the serine/threonine kinase *STK11* gene, mapped to chromosome 19p13.3. Molecular testing of the *STK11* gene identifies most cases. It is inherited in an autosomal dominant manner.

Phosphatase and tensin homolog (PTEN) hamartoma tumor syndrome (Cowden's syndrome) is associated with multiple colorectal polyps. It is characterized by multiple hamartomas of the skin, mucous membranes, breast, and thyroid. Facial trichilemmomas are flesh-colored, elongated, verrucous papules in a periorificial and centrofacial distribution. Papillomatosis is found on the labial, gingival, and buccal mucosae. Less common associations are palmoplantar keratoses, lipomas, hemangiomas, and neuromas. Hamartomatous polyps may be present throughout the gastrointestinal tract. The hamartomas have a potential for malignant transformation. Colon cancer is a common finding. There is a high frequency of breast cancer, therefore close surveillance for malignancy is warranted. Autosomal genome scanning using DNA markers on affected families has linked to chromosome 10q22-q23, encoding PTEN. Eighty percent of individuals with Cowden's syndrome have a detectable PTEN mutation.

The Cronkhite–Canada syndrome is characterized by generalized hamartomatous polyps, cutaneous pigmentation, hair loss, and nail atrophy. Alopecia is rapidly progressive and leads to complete hair loss. The nail dystrophy involves all nails, with a unique pattern of an inverted triangle of normal nail bordered by dystrophy and onycholysis. The pigmentation is diffuse rather than spotted as in Peutz–Jeghers syndrome. All cases have been sporadic. Prognosis is poor.

MALABSORPTION

Malabsorption may be associated with characteristic cutaneous findings, as seen in dermatitis herpetiformis and zinc deficiency. The pathognomonic cutaneous findings usually allow for diagnosis of the bowel abnormality. Less specific cutaneous signs of malabsorption are frequently present independent of the cause of the malabsorption. These include stomatitis and glossitis related to vitamin B deficiencies; angular cheilitis; corkscrew hair and purpura as a result of vitamin C deficiency; purpura associated in vitamin K deficiencies; asteatotic eczema-like eruption of uncertain cause; patchy hyperpigmentation; and slowed nail and hair growth as well as alopecia secondary to protein malnutrition.

Acrodermatitis Enteropathica

Acrodermatitis enteropathica is characterized by periorificial and acral dermatitis, diarrhea, and prominent alopecia. This is a result of intestinal malabsorption of zinc. Classic cases are genetic in origin. Acquired forms may develop in patients who are treated with total parenteral nutrition deficient in zinc, or in association with other malabsorption syndromes. The causes are summarized in Table 29-3. Oral administration with larger than normal amounts of zinc is curative but must be maintained indefinitely in the genetic form of the disease.

Pathogenesis

Acrodermatitis enteropathica is transmitted in an autosomal recessive mode mapped to gene locus 8q24.3, with evidence that the phenotype is caused by mutation in the intestinal zinc-specific transporter, solute carrier family 39 (zinc transporter) member 4 (*SLC39A4*). The *SLC39A4* gene encodes a zinc-specific transporter, which

TABLE 29-3 Causes of Zinc Deficiency
Genetic: acrodermatitis enteropathica
Dietary deficiency
Excessive alcohol ingestion
Malabsorption
Inflammatory bowel disease
Anorexia nervosa
Acquired immunodeficiency syndrome
Prolonged diarrhea
Total parenteral nutrition
Chelating agents (penicillamine)
Chronic renal disease
Pediatric "short bowel syndrome"

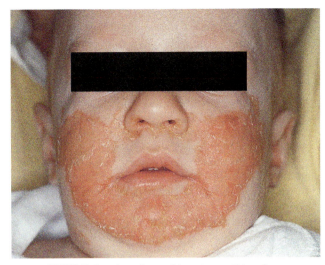

FIGURE 29-5 ■ Acrodermatitis enteropathica: face.

is highly expressed in the duodenum and jejunum. Zinc deficiency results from intestinal malabsorption. Plasma zinc levels, urinary excretion of zinc, and serum alkaline phosphatase are persistently low.

The histologic appearance of acrodermatitis enteropathica is nonspecific. The epidermis is acanthotic, with pallor and dyskeratosis of keratinocytes. Intraepidermal vesicles, subcorneal pustules, and vacuolar alteration of the dermoepidermal junction have been present in affected skin. Neutrophils may infiltrate the epidermis with extensive crusting.

Zinc is needed in various metalloenzymes for protein and DNA synthesis and for cell division. Zinc deficiency has profound effects on the immune system, including effects on T-helper cell function, T-suppressor cell function, and natural killer cell activity. Zinc also affects neutrophil chemotaxis. These abnormalities may be responsible for significant problems with intercurrent infection. Thymic hypoplasia and cortical atrophy have been reported in children. These abnormalities are reversible with zinc supplementation.

In addition to the inherited form of zinc deficiency, there are a variety of other causes (Table 29-3). Dietary zinc deficiency is prevalent in underdeveloped countries and may be present to a moderate degree in the United States, especially in infants. Meat is the best source of dietary zinc. Consumption of unrefined cereals containing high levels of phytate renders zinc unavailable for absorption. Sources of inadequate dietary intake include refusal to eat (e.g., in anorexia nervosa) and limited diet selection (e.g., vegetarian diets). Alcohol intake induces hyperzincuria by poorly understood mechanisms and produces clinical zinc deficiency states.

Zinc deficiency occurs with steatorrhea from any cause. Fat malabsorption produces an alkaline environment in the bowel. Zinc forms insoluble complexes with the fat and phosphates, resulting in an increased loss of zinc in the stool. Exudation of large amounts of zinc protein complexes into the intestinal lumen from the pancreas and intestinal mucosa contributes to the reduction in plasma zinc concentration in inflammatory bowel disease and in severe chronic diarrhea. Zinc deficiency has also been reported following intestinal bypass surgery, presumably by similar mechanisms.

Failure to include zinc in fluids for total parenteral nutrition has caused severe zinc deficiency with the clinical features seen with the autosomal recessive form of

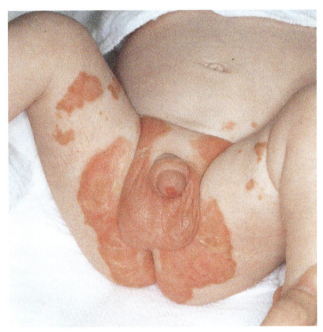

FIGURE 29-6 ■ Acrodermatitis enteropathica: groin.

acrodermatitis enteropathica. Severe zinc deficiency has also been reported following therapy with penicillamine or other chelating agents.

Presentation

Clinical findings of zinc deficiency are similar in both genetic and acquired forms. However, the cutaneous presentation of zinc deficiency is polymorphic. Findings consist of acral, periorbital, and perirectal vesiculobullous, pustular, and eczematous skin lesions (Figs. 29-5 and 29-6). Red scaly patches with crusting develop on the face, groin, flexures, and acral skin. Angular cheilitis and stomatitis accompany the acral lesions. Nail dystrophy with nail thinning may develop. Alopecia is generalized, but alopecia of the scalp, eyelashes, and eyebrows is prominent. Diarrhea, irritability, and failure to thrive develop simultaneously with the cutaneous eruptions in zinc deficiency, confirming clinical suspicion.

The onset of symptoms of genetic zinc deficiency usually occurs from 3 weeks to 18 months in infancy, after changing from breast milk to cow's milk. Low-molecular-weight binding factor transports zinc into the epithelial cells of the intestine and is present in human breast milk. Low-molecular-weight zinc-binding factor in breast milk is responsible for the superior absorption of zinc from human milk. Zinc deficiency has also been reported with the absence of zinc-binding factor in deficient breast milk. Alopecia, diarrhea, growth retardation, neuropsychiatric disorders, and recurrent infections ensue if the disorder goes unrecognized.

Evaluation

Measurement of plasma zinc concentration is diagnostic, provided the sample is not hemolyzed or contaminated. Particular care needs to be taken to ensure that test tubes and other measurement equipment are free of zinc. Lowered zinc levels in plasma may occur in the absence of true zinc deficiency. Levels fall nonspecifically in the acute phases of cardiac, hepatic, renal, pulmonary, neurologic, infectious, and malignant disorders. Zinc levels in red blood cells and hair may also be assessed to determine body zinc status, but these are generally less reliable tests. Urinary excretion of zinc is reduced as a result of zinc deficiency. Determination of 24-hour urinary zinc helps to diagnose hyperzincuria and plasma zinc deficiency caused by excessive alcohol intake and chronic renal disease. Serum alkaline phosphatase, a zinc metalloenzyme, is frequently depressed.

Differential Diagnosis

Classic acrodermatitis enteropathica is clinically characteristic when the perioral, perirectal, and digital areas are affected. Incomplete expression of these skin findings may be confused with perioral dermatitis, hand dermatitis, candidiasis, and pustular psoriasis. As the dermatitis worsens, secondary colonization and infection with bacteria and *Candida albicans* can occur.

Biotin deficiency may present as periorificial dermatitis and alopecia. It occurs in those who consume an unbalanced diet containing excessive amounts of raw egg whites. Biotin binds to avidin found in egg whites, resulting in malabsorption of biotin from the intestinal tract. The perioral and intertriginous localization of early glucagonoma syndrome may also be confused with zinc deficiency.

Zinc deficiency can be corrected easily by oral supplementation. If the intake of animal protein is adequate, 15 to 30 mg daily of zinc sulfate is adequate. If dietary protein intake is predominantly in the form of cereals, 50 to 200 mg daily may be needed. Response to therapy is dramatic. Skin lesions, diarrhea, and behavioral abnormalities reverse within days to weeks. Hair growth and growth retardation improve over the course of months.

Dermatitis Herpetiformis

Dermatitis herpetiformis (DH) is a cutaneous manifestation of celiac disease. It presents as grouped erythematous papules and vesicles over the extensor surfaces of the forearms, elbows, knees, and buttocks. Biopsy reveals a blister at the basement membrane with the accumulation of neutrophils in dermal papillary tips. The diagnosis is confirmed with a biopsy of perilesional skin revealing deposition of granular immunoglobulin A (IgA) in dermal papillary tips.

More than 85% of patients with DH demonstrate some degree of small bowel inflammation on jejunal biopsy, which is generally less severe than that in celiac disease. The attendant symptoms and signs of malabsorption are proportional to the severity of the gluten-sensitive enteropathy. DH is discussed in detail in Chapter 16. The present discussion of DH will be limited to the association with malabsorption.

Pathogenesis

More than 90% of DH patients have a characteristic *human leukocyte antigen* (HLA) genotype. Virtually all patients with DH carry either HLA DQ2 or HLA DQ8 haplotypes. This carries with it an increased frequency of atrophic gastritis, achlorhydria, intrinsic factor deficiency, and resultant systemic deficiency of vitamin B12. This clinical constellation of findings occurs in up to 10% of cases of DH. Ten percent of patients with DH have associated endocrine or connective tissue diseases. Endocrine diseases associated with DH include type 1 diabetes mellitus, thyroid disorders, and Addison's disease.

Over 90% of DH patients have some degree of gluten-sensitive enteropathy, which varies in severity from a mononuclear infiltrate in the lamina propria with minimal villous atrophy to complete flattening of the small intestinal mucosa. The enteropathy may be patchy, requiring multiple biopsy specimens for documentation. Less than 10% of DH patients have severe malabsorption. These patients represent the extreme of celiac disease, with severe mucosal flattening. The clinical signs of malabsorption in severely affected patients are directly attributable to gluten sensitivity. Symptoms of malabsorption, including steatorrhea and foul-smelling stools, are present in a minority of patients. Clinical findings of weight loss, xerosis, alopecia, and steatorrhea are found only in the most severe cases. Many more complain of cramping, abdominal pain, and bloating after eating. These milder symptoms may only be recognized by their cessation after the institution of a gluten-free diet.

The villous atrophy does not correlate with the severity of the skin disease. Many patients with histologically significant small bowel atrophy appear well nourished and even obese. In addition, the villous atrophy is not affected by dapsone therapy, which improves the skin disease. The small bowel atrophy is caused by gluten. Celiac disease and DH improve with a gluten-free diet. The enteropathy and skin disease recur with reinstitution of a regular diet.

Evaluation

The diagnosis is confirmed with the characteristic immunopathology of granular IgA deposition in perilesional skin. This IgA is directed against epidermal transglutaminase (transglutaminase 3) and the transglutaminase 3 antigen can be detected in the IgA aggregates, especially if the IgA is extensive. Serologic testing for IgA epidermal transglutaminase antibodies is positive in the vast majority of DH patients consuming a regular diet. Approximately 70% of DH patients on a regular diet have IgA tissue transglutaminase (transglutaminase 2) antibodies in their serum as a reflection of the associated celiac disease. IgA tissue transglutaminase antibodies are also positive in patients with celiac disease and no cutaneous findings. IgA endomysial antibody tests for the same tissue transglutaminase antibody by an immunofluorescent technique. These antibody tests are the most specific and sensitive serologic markers for celiac disease. The level of IgA tissue transglutaminase antibody correlates with the severity of the intestinal damage and returns to normal with adherence to a gluten-free diet. Antibody tests to gluten and gliadin are of little value in the diagnosis of DH because of a very high rate of false positives and false negatives. The final proof of gluten-sensitive enteropathy comes with improvement of symptoms on gluten-free diet therapy. It may take months to years for the skin disease to completely resolve on a gluten-free diet.

Differential Diagnosis

The differential diagnosis of DH includes pemphigus, bullous pemphigoid, linear IgA disease, bullous lupus erythematosus, bacterial folliculitis, and eczematous processes. Linear IgA disease can only be separated from DH on the basis of direct immunofluorescence.

Treatment

Both the skin and the bowel disease respond to gluten restriction, but a minimum 6-month trial should be undertaken before evaluating the effectiveness of gluten restriction. The skin disease may be treated effectively with oral dapsone. Patients should be evaluated for glucose-6-phosphate dehydrogenase deficiency to avoid catastrophic hemolytic anemia. Monitoring with complete blood count and liver function tests is necessary because of the hepatic and dose-related hematologic effects of dapsone. Maintenance on dapsone therapy is usually needed until gluten restriction has had its effect. Dapsone can then gradually be tapered and discontinued.

INFLAMMATORY BOWEL DISEASE

Inflammatory bowel disease is a general term for a group of idiopathic chronic inflammatory conditions that affect the bowel. Ulcerative colitis involves the rectum and the colon, while Crohn's disease may involve any area of the intestinal tract and is frequently discontinuous.

Presentation

Multiple extraintestinal manifestations of inflammatory bowel disease may occur (Table 29-4). Metastatic Crohn's disease is characterized by cutaneous granulomas that

TABLE 29-4 Cutaneous Associations of Inflammatory Bowel Disease

Specific Lesions
Fissures and fistulae
Metastatic Crohn's disease
Mucosal lesions

Reactive Lesions
Aphthous ulcers
Pustular vasculitis (bowel-associated dermatosis-arthritis syndrome)
Pyoderma gangrenosum
Erythema nodosum
Vasculitis
Erythema multiforme
Urticaria
Sweet's syndrome

Other Associations
Epidermolysis bullosa acquisita
Vitiligo
Alopecia areata
Fingernail clubbing

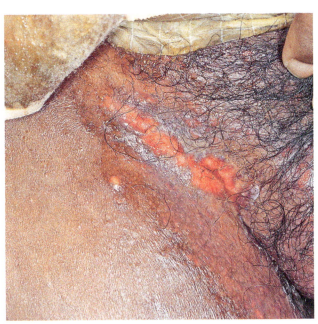

FIGURE 29-7 ■ Extraintestinal (metastatic) Crohn's disease.

occur distant from the gastrointestinal tract (Fig. 29-7). Oral aphthae occur in association with Crohn's disease and ulcerative colitis in 6% to 8% of cases. Aphthae seem to be related to actively inflamed bowel. These lesions are not specific, as up to 20% of the normal population have aphthae. Malabsorption of iron, folic acid, and vitamin B_{12} occurs with inflammatory bowel disease. Correction of these deficiencies may result in improvement of the associated aphthosis.

The incidence of pyoderma gangrenosum with inflammatory bowel disease is 1% to 5%. Inflammatory bowel disease is the single most common cause of pyoderma gangrenosum, being responsible for between 25% and 50% of cases (Figs 29-8 and 29-9). Pyoderma

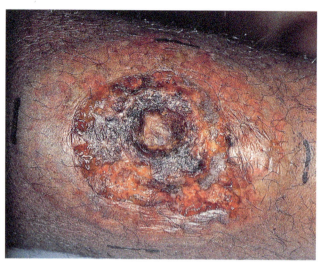

FIGURE 29-8 ■ Pyoderma gangrenosum in a patient with ulcerative colitis.

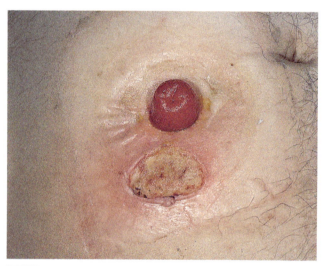

FIGURE 29-9 ■ Peristomal pyoderma gangrenosum. This patient's colon was removed for chronic ulcerative colitis more than 10 years prior to the onset of this lesion.

gangrenosum is characterized as a chronic ulceration with a violaceous undermined border. It may involve peristomal and incision sites, extremities, chest, back, abdomen, and head and neck. Rapid evolution of the ulcer is a hallmark. Exclusion of arterial/venous disease, leukocytoclastic vasculitis, and infection is crucial. Histology from the border shows endothelial injury, fibrinoid necrosis, and a prominent infiltration of neutrophils in the dermis. The activity of pyoderma gangrenosum parallels the activity of bowel disease.

Erythema nodosum may occur in 1% to 5% of patients with inflammatory bowel disease, and is frequently accompanied by peripheral arthritis in patients with Crohn's disease. The prevalence of erythema nodosum is higher in Crohn's disease than in ulcerative colitis. However, the majority of patients with erythema nodosum have underlying causes other than inflammatory bowel disease.

Additional reactive dermatoses may occur in inflammatory bowel disease. These reactive dermatoses include: Sweet's syndrome, erythema multiforme, urticaria, leukocytoclastic vasculitis, polyarteritis nodosa, and epidermolysis bullosa acquisita. Thrombophlebitis, alopecia areata, vitiligo, and digital clubbing may also occur. Many of the cutaneous changes seen in patients with inflammatory bowel disease are due to nutritional deficiencies secondary to malabsorption.

Treatment

The activity of the extraintestinal manifestations of inflammatory bowel disease often parallels the course of the intestinal disease. Medical therapy for inflammatory bowel disease improves pyoderma gangrenosum. Response to systemic immunosuppressive treatment and lack of response to conventional wound care are characteristic. Topical therapies include occlusive hydrocolloid dressings, high-potency corticosteroids, intralesional steroids, and topical tacrolimus. Therapies often include sulfasalazine, corticosteroids, azathioprine, methotrexate and cyclosporine, infliximab, and adalimumab. Colectomy may produce clinical remission of extraintestinal manifestations of ulcerative colitis. Management of erythema nodosum includes bed rest, compression stockings, nonsteroidal anti-inflammatory drugs, prednisone, colchicine, and potassium iodide. Cutaneous Crohn's disease may respond to metronidazole, prednisone, mesalamine, cyclosporine, and tumor necrosis factor inhibitors.

PANCREATIC DISEASE

The cutaneous manifestations of pancreatic disease may be secondary to pancreatitis or pancreatic carcinomas. The cutaneous findings resulting from pancreatic disease are variable. They include hemorrhage, panniculitis, thrombophlebitis, metastatic nodules, and necrolytic migratory erythema (Table 29-5).

Pancreatitis

Cutaneous disease is most often associated with acute pancreatitis. Two main types of cutaneous lesion may be seen in patients with acute pancreatitis: purpura and panniculitis. Turner's sign is an ecchymosis arising from the subcutaneous extravasation of peritoneal hemorrhagic fluid (Fig. 29-10). Purpura may be observed in as many as 5% of cases of acute pancreatitis. Anatomically, hemorrhagic fluid flows through the anterior and posterior pararenal space into the subcutaneous tissues in the flank. Hemorrhagic discoloration around the umbilicus (Cullen's sign) (Fig. 29-11) occurs as hemorrhagic fluid extends from the gastrohepatic ligament and across the falciform ligament to the periumbilical tissues.

Panniculitis is associated with both pancreatitis and pancreatic carcinoma, and has been described as subcutaneous or nodular fat necrosis. The resulting inflammatory subcutaneous nodules or plaques, 1 to 5 cm in diameter, occur especially on the thighs and lower legs, but also on the arms, buttocks, or trunk (Figs. 29-12 and 29-13).

TABLE 29-5 Nondiabetic Cutaneous Manifestations of Pancreatic Disease

Cutaneous changes related to pancreatitis
   Cutaneous hemorrhage (Cullen's, Turner's, and Fox's signs)
   Panniculitis
Cutaneous changes related to pancreatic endocrine tumors (glucagonoma syndrome)
   Necrolytic migratory erythema
Cutaneous changes related to pancreatic carcinoma
   Metastatic nodules, especially to umbilicus
   Panniculitis
   Migratory thrombophlebitis

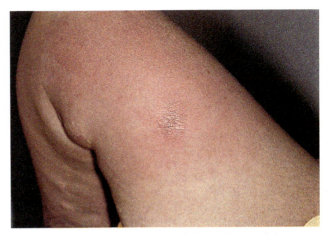

FIGURE 29-12 ■ Large erythematous indurated area of the posterior arm as a result of panniculitis.

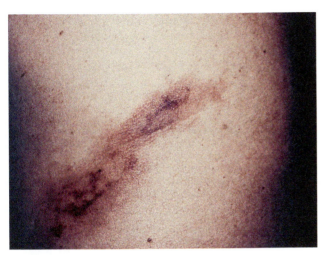

FIGURE 29-10 ■ Purpura of the left flank (Turner's sign) in a patient with acute hemorrhagic pancreatitis.

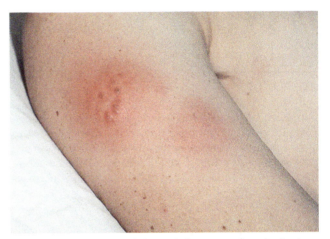

FIGURE 29-13 ■ Painful nodules and plaques as a result of subcutaneous fat necrosis.

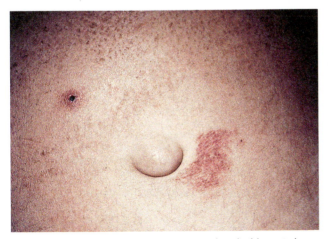

FIGURE 29-11 ■ Periumbilical purpura associated with acute hemorrhagic pancreatitis.

The lesions are frequently painful; in severe cases they rupture spontaneously, discharging a viscous, sterile material containing free and esterified cholesterol, neutral fats, soaps, and free fatty acids. Panniculitis associated with pancreatitis usually occurs in patients in their mid-30s or 40s, whereas patients with cancer are usually significantly older and are also more likely to have blood eosinophilia and only slightly elevated (or occasionally normal) levels of serum amylase and lipase. Histologically, the findings of panniculitis associated with pancreatic disease include foci of fat necrosis with "ghost-like" anucleate cells having thick "shadowy" walls and a surrounding inflammatory infiltrate of neutrophils, eosinophils, lymphocytes, histiocytes, and foreign body giant cells. The detection of these findings should prompt an exhaustive search for underlying pancreatic disease including pancreatic carcinoma. Therapy is supportive and is primarily directed at the underlying pancreatic disease.

Glucagonoma

The glucogonoma is a rare disease in which necrolytic migratory erythema is one of the presenting symptoms. Weight loss and diabetes are characteristic features of glucagonoma syndrome. Glucagonomas, which are usually malignant, occur more frequently without the typical cutaneous manifestations of the full syndrome. In addition, rare reports cite necrolytic migratory erythema occurring in patients without a pancreatic tumor or elevated levels of plasma glucagon. The majority of patients with glucagonoma syndrome have an insidious onset of symptoms, usually 1.5 to 2 years before the diagnosis is made. By the time of diagnosis, however, the majority of patients have glucagonomas with metastases to the liver and regional lymph nodes. The disease has a predilection for middle-aged persons and has been reported more frequently in women.

There is considerable similarity of patients with glucagonoma syndrome. Patients frequently have stomatitis or glossitis, diabetes, normochromic anemia, weight loss, and diarrhea. Recurrent venous thrombosis and depression have been associated with glucagonoma syndrome. Fasting plasma glucagon levels (normally 50 to 200 pg/mL) are elevated in almost all patients and may be five to 10 times the normal level.

The most distinctive feature of the syndrome is necrolytic migratory erythema, which usually occurs cyclically and has a characteristic distribution. The cutaneous eruption is widespread but is most prominent in perioral and intertriginous areas, especially the perineum. Superficial necrosis of the epidermis produces an erosive and vesiculobullous dermatosis with crusting and eventual shedding of the skin. The base of the lesions is usually remarkably erythematous, and the borders are frequently annular or serpiginous. The active inflammatory process appears to cycle every 7 to 14 days. Multiple essential nutrient and vitamin B deficiencies contribute to the dermatosis.

Biopsy is characterized by necrolysis of the upper epidermis with vacuolated keratinocytes. Marked spongiosis, pallor of the upper epidermis, frank necrolysis of the upper epidermis, vacuolization of keratinocytes, and accumulation of neutrophils in the epidermis are characteristic. The mild inflammatory infiltrate in the superficial dermis is composed primarily of mononuclear cells and is predominantly perivascular. The same changes have been described in patients with pellagra and acrodermatitis enteropathica.

After the possibility of the diagnosis of glucagonoma syndrome has been raised (based usually on the cutaneous lesions and elevated plasma glucagon levels), the search should be made for a pancreatic tumor. Chemotherapy has been used with some success to treat patients with metastatic glucagonomas.

Nonhormone-Secreting Pancreatic Carcinoma

The three most common cutaneous manifestations of nonhormone-secreting pancreatic adenocarcinomas are metastatic cutaneous nodules; migratory thrombophlebitis; and panniculitis, specifically subcutaneous or nodular fat necrosis. Panniculitis has been described in patients with adenocarcinoma of the pancreas. Cutaneous metastases, especially to the umbilicus, are not common from pancreatic carcinoma, but approximately 10% of umbilical metastases (Sister Mary Joseph's nodule) occur from pancreatic tumors. Migratory thrombophlebitis of both superficial and deep veins is also uncommon. Carcinoma of the pancreas accounts for approximately 30% of the tumors associated with thrombophlebitis. Classically, the phlebitis occurs in short segments of superficial veins and is distributed on the trunk and neck and on the extremities. The phlebitis is often resistant to anticoagulant therapy and may lead to a life-threatening embolic phenomenon. The inflammatory changes may resolve spontaneously within a few weeks, only to recur in the same or distant veins. Recurrent and migratory thrombophlebitis may be the presenting symptom of malignancy.

SUGGESTED READINGS

Dourmishev LA, Draganov PV. Paraneoplastic dermatological manifestation of gastrointestinal malignancies. World J Gastroenterol 2009;15(35):4372–9.

Fotiadis C, Tsekouras DK, Antonakis P, Sfiniadakis J, Genetzakis M, Zografos GC. Gardner's syndrome: a case report and review of the literature. World J Gastroenterol 2005;11(34):5408–11.

Huang BL, Chandra S, Shih DQ. Skin manifestations of inflammatory bowel disease. Front Physiol 2012;3:13.

Jelsig AM, Qvist N, Brusgaard K, Nielsen CB, Hansen TP, Ousager LB. Hamartomatous polyposis syndromes: a review. Orphanet J Rare Dis 2014;9:101.

Lankisch PG, Weber-Dany B, Maisonneuve P, Lowenfels AB. Skin signs in acute pancreatitis: frequency and implications for prognosis. J Intern Med 2009;265(2):299–301.

Maverakis E, Fung MA, Lynch PJ, Draznin M, Michael DJ, Ruben B, et al. Acrodermatitis enteropathica and an overview of zinc metabolism. J Am Acad Dermatol 2007;56(1):116–24.

McDonald J, Bayrak-Toydemir P, Pyeritz RE. Hereditary hemorrhagic telangiectasia: an overview of diagnosis, management, and pathogenesis. Genet Med 2011;13(7):607–16.

Patel F, Fitzmaurice S, Duong C, He Y, Fergus J, Raychaudhuri SP, et al. Effective strategies for the management of pyoderma gangrenosum: A comprehensive review. Acta Derm Venereol 2015;95(5):525–31.

Shah KR, Boland CR, Patel M, Thrash B, Menter A. Cutaneous manifestations of gastrointestinal disease: part I. J Am Acad Dermatol 2013;68(2):189. e1-21; quiz 210.

Thrash B, Patel M, Shah KR, Boland CR, Menter A. Cutaneous manifestations of gastrointestinal disease: part II. J Am Acad Dermatol 2013;68(2):211. e1-33; quiz 44–6.

Uitto J, Li Q, Jiang Q. Pseudoxanthoma elasticum: molecular genetics and putative pathomechanisms. J Invest Dermatol 2010;130(3):661–70.

van Beek AP, de Haas ER, van Vloten WA, Lips CJ, Roijers JF, Canninga-van Dijk MR. The glucagonoma syndrome and necrolytic migratory erythema: a clinical review. Eur J Endocrinol 2004;151(5):531–7.

Zone JJ. Skin manifestations of celiac disease. Gastroenterology 2005;128(4 Suppl. 1):S87–91.

CHAPTER 30

HEPATIC DISEASE AND THE SKIN

J. Mark Jackson • Jeffrey P. Callen • Kenneth E. Greer

KEY POINTS

- The cutaneous changes of hepatic disease may be related to primary diseases of the liver, cutaneous diseases with associated hepatic abnormalities, disorders with changes in many organs, including the liver and skin, and medications with direct effects on the liver or indirect effects due to hypersensitivity reactions.
- Pruritus or prurigo nodularis without an identifiable cutaneous eruption warrant an investigation for hepatic disease.
- The dermatologic stigmata of cirrhosis include jaundice, spider angiomas and other telangiectases, palmar erythema, dilated abdominal wall veins, nail changes including Terry nails, and thinning of the body hair, among others.
- Primary biliary cirrhosis, which occurs most frequently in women 40 to 60 years of age, is recognized by a combination of pruritus, jaundice, hyperpigmentation, and xanthomas.
- Hemochromatosis and Wilson's disease are autosomal recessive disorders that affect the liver and may present with skin or ocular findings, including a metallic gray or brown hyperpigmentation in the former and a pathognomonic golden-brown or green-brown pigmentation of the corneal margins in the latter.
- Both viral hepatitis and the therapies used to treat these diseases may cause a multitude of cutaneous eruptions.

A number of cutaneous stigmata are associated with hepatic disease, but none are specific. Even jaundice, classically associated with liver immaturity (neonatal jaundice) or failure, may occur with hemolysis and in the setting of perfectly normal hepatic function. The cutaneous changes of hepatic disease may be related to primary diseases of the liver; to cutaneous diseases with associated hepatic abnormalities; and to a wide variety of disorders with changes in many organs, including the liver and skin. A number of systemically administered drugs commonly used for the treatment of cutaneous disease may produce hepatic damage, including methotrexate, ketoconazole, itraconazole, terbinafine, retinoids, and vitamin A. Finally, several drugs produce hypersensitivity reactions characterized by fever, lymphadenopathy, eosinophilia, hepatitis, and cutaneous eruptions, which can result in severe liver damage. This drug reaction has been known by various terms, but most commonly is referred to as *d*rug *r*eaction with *e*osinophilia and *s*ystemic *s*ymptoms (DRESS). Drugs in this category include phenytoin, phenobarbital, carbamazepine, dapsone, minocycline, and allopurinol, among others (see Chapter 47).

Classically, cutaneous manifestations have been associated with primary hepatic diseases including alcoholic cirrhosis and hemochromatosis, but other disorders, including Wilson's disease, viral hepatitis, and primary biliary cirrhosis, have associated cutaneous findings. Porphyria cutanea tarda and erythropoietic protoporphyria, known primarily for their cutaneous manifestations, are associated with hepatic abnormalities (see Chapter 28). Patients with porphyria cutanea tarda have frequently been found to have hepatitis C virus infection. Gianotti–Crosti syndrome was originally thought to be associated with viral hepatitis, but this association may be more prevalent only in southern Europe. Lichen planus, particularly oral lichen planus, has also been associated with hepatitis C infection. Miscellaneous diseases that affect many organ systems and involve the liver and the skin include syphilis, sarcoidosis, Gaucher's disease, polyarteritis nodosa, and cytophagic histiocytic panniculitis. Many of these disorders are discussed elsewhere in this book, and others occur too infrequently to be discussed in detail here.

Cutaneous symptoms, such as pruritus and jaundice, may be important evidence for considering the diagnosis of hepatic disease, especially in conjunction with nonspecific symptoms such as fatigue, anorexia, vomiting and weight loss, diminished libido, and right upper quadrant abdominal discomfort. In addition to these symptoms, certain physical findings, especially when considered collectively, suggest the diagnosis of hepatic disease. Mucocutaneous lesions are often prominent and include scleral icterus, spider telangiectases, palmar erythema, excoriations (e.g., neurotic excoriations and prurigo nodularis), xanthelasma, alopecia, nail lesions, gynecomastia, and prominence of the cutaneous veins in the epigastrium. Any patient with symptoms of pruritus and/or findings of neurotic excoriations or prurigo nodularis (Fig. 30-1) in the absence of a primary cutaneous disease should be evaluated for liver disease.

CIRRHOSIS

Cirrhosis of the liver implies an irreversible alteration of the liver's architecture, consisting of hepatic fibrosis, areas of nodular regeneration, and a loss of a considerable number of hepatocytes. Although alcohol is one of the most common causes of cirrhosis (Laënnec's cirrhosis) in

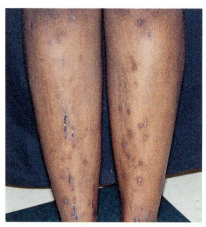

FIGURE 30-1 ■ Pruritus of hepatic disease due to sclerosing cholangitis secondary to ulcerative colitis manifesting as excoriations and eczematous dermatitis.

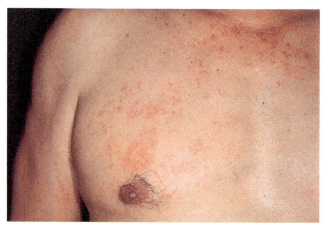

FIGURE 30-3 ■ Unilateral nevoid telangiectasia in a male patient with cirrhosis of the liver due to hepatitis C.

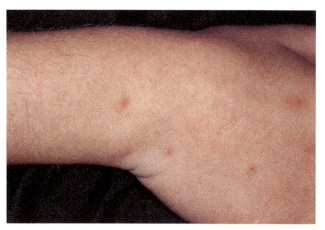

FIGURE 30-2 ■ Spider angioma on the arm and dorsal hand.

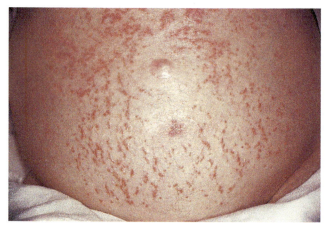

FIGURE 30-4 ■ Dilated abdominal wall veins along with xerosis and eczema associated with cirrhosis and portal hypertension. (Courtesy of Dr Neil Fenske, Tampa, FL, USA.)

the United States, cirrhosis can be caused by drugs and other toxins including acetaminophen; infections (especially hepatitis C virus); biliary obstruction (e.g., carcinoma of the pancreas or bile duct, gallstones, cystic fibrosis); metabolic diseases (e.g., hemochromatosis and Wilson's disease); chronic right-sided congestive heart failure; and a group of miscellaneous diseases such as sarcoidosis, primary biliary cirrhosis, and jejunoileal bypass. There are also a number of cases of cirrhosis that are idiopathic. Individuals with cirrhosis usually present in one of two general ways, i.e., (1) with evidence of acute hepatocellular necrosis with jaundice; or (2) with evidence of the complications of cirrhosis, brought on primarily by the rise in intrahepatic vascular resistance and subsequent portal hypertension (i.e., ascites, splenomegaly, bleeding varices, and encephalopathy). Not infrequently, patients present with a mixed picture of these two pathophysiologic pathways.

The dermatological stigmata of cirrhosis are well recognized and include changes in the skin, nails, and hair. Vascular lesions are common and include spider angiomas and other telangiectases; palmar erythema; and dilated abdominal wall veins, which occur in patients with portal hypertension and represent the development of portal systemic collaterals (Figs 30-2 to 30-4). Spider angiomas occur in a majority of patients with cirrhosis, but they are not pathognomonic of the disease because they occur commonly in young children, pregnant women, and otherwise healthy adults. They are so named because of their central pulsatile arterial punctum with radiating branching vessels. They occur almost exclusively on the upper half of the body, especially on the face, neck, and upper trunk. The spider is formed by a coiled arteriole that spirals up to a central point and then branches out into thin-walled vessels that merge with normal capillaries. The pathogenesis of these vascular lesions is unknown, but they do not appear to be related to portal hypertension, which is responsible for one of the most serious complications of cirrhosis: bleeding esophageal and gastric varices. They may be related to excess estrogen, which occurs as a result of reduced hepatic metabolism of estrogens. Palmar erythema, manifested as diffuse or splotchy erythema on the thenar and hypothenar eminences and tips of the fingers, frequently accompanies the development of the spider angiomas. Palmar erythema also occurs in healthy individuals and in association with nonhepatic diseases including human immunodeficiency virus. There may be a widespread appearance of thin, wiry telangiectases in

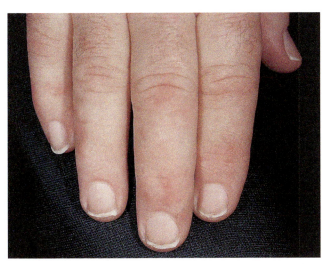

FIGURE 30-5 ■ Terry nails are represented by opaque white changes in this patient with cirrhosis.

some patients, and occasionally the lesions appear in a unilateral distribution (see Fig. 30-3).

Various forms of nail disease have been described in patients with cirrhosis, including the classic white nails described by Terry. Terry nails are characterized by a nail plate that is opaque white with the exception of the distal portion, which retains its normal pink color (Fig. 30-5). In addition, patients may develop transverse white bands (Muehrcke nails), clubbed nails, or koilonychia (spoon-shaped nails), but none of these changes is specific for hepatic disease. Changes in body hair are common and are noted primarily in men. The axillary, pubic, and pectoral hair is usually sparse, but thinning of all body hair is also common. There is often the development of a female pubic hair pattern, coinciding with other evidence of feminization, including testicular softening and gynecomastia. This is in contrast to the hypertrichosis seen in patients with porphyria cutanea tarda and liver disease.

There are a number of nonspecific systemic symptoms associated with cirrhosis of the liver, including weakness, anorexia, nausea, weight loss, and abdominal discomfort. Pruritus is less common in patients with intrahepatic cholestasis and occurs more often in diseases such as primary biliary cirrhosis, sclerosing cholangitis, and chronic extrahepatic biliary obstruction. The cirrhotic liver is usually small, firm, and nodular, and the spleen is often enlarged. Ascites may cause a remarkable distension of the abdominal cavity. Low albumin occurs in the setting of chronic hepatic dysfunction and results in edema, especially of the lower extremities. This can lead to stasis dermatitis and xerosis of the skin in areas of chronic edema. As a result of impaired hepatic function, a prothrombin deficiency may develop, resulting in cutaneous purpura, epistaxis, and gingival bleeding. This deficiency also causes difficulty in controlling the bleeding from varices. The use of intramuscular vitamin K to help reverse the prothrombin deficiency has led to rare reports of unusual annular erythematous reactions surrounding the injection site.

A review of the diagnosis, course, treatment, and prognosis of cirrhosis is beyond the scope of this book. There is, however, one additional point concerning cirrhosis that is especially important for dermatologists, and this is the potential inducement of the disease with methotrexate used to treat psoriasis or other dermatologic conditions. Methotrexate-induced hepatic changes are now believed to be more associated with obesity that is often present in patients with psoriasis. They are also more likely with increasing dosage and duration of therapy. Cirrhosis is unusual in patients treated with methotrexate who do not have other risk factors for hepatic disease. Factors that increase the propensity for cirrhosis in patients taking methotrexate include obesity, steatohepatitis, diabetes mellitus, hyperlipidemia, hepatitis A, B, or C, concomitant potentially hepatotoxic medications such as acetaminophen, statins, systemic antifungals, and/or excessive alcohol intake. It has been suggested that in the absence of other risk factors, patients on methotrexate may not need liver biopsies. Several guidelines exist for the decision to perform a liver biopsy, but recently, noninvasive techniques have been used more frequently to follow patients receiving long-term methotrexate therapy. Levels of the amino terminal peptide of type III procollagen have been used extensively in Europe, particularly the United Kingdom, for evaluation of the liver in order to detect early fibrosis, but this test is not readily available in the United States. There are two tests, known as the Fibrosure for hepatitis C and Fibrosure for steatohepatitis, which are used to follow patients with either disorder. The Fibrosure for steatohepatitis might prove useful in following patients on methotrexate, but this is not currently an FDA-approved use. There are several noninvasive methods to assess the presence of fibrosis that appear to be valid assessment tools including magnetic resonance elastography and ultrasonic elastography. These methods have not been routinely adopted for the assessment of methotrexate-induced fibrosis to date.

PRIMARY BILIARY CIRRHOSIS

Primary biliary cirrhosis, a relatively uncommon form of cirrhosis that occurs most frequently in women 40 to 60 years of age, deserves special recognition because the combination of pruritus, jaundice, hyperpigmentation, and xanthomas is specific for the disease. It is believed that the destruction of the small intrahepatic bile ducts—the primary defect in primary biliary cirrhosis—occurs on an immunologic basis. This disease is considered to be autoimmune in nature, and greater than 90% of patients have antimitochondrial antibodies. In addition, another distinct autoimmune disease is found in up to three-quarters of patients with primary biliary cirrhosis, including rheumatoid arthritis, thyroiditis, Sjögren's, and limited systemic sclerosis. The disease may also be familial. The first and often the foremost symptom of primary biliary cirrhosis is pruritus, which is the presenting complaint in one-half of patients. Patients may have multiple excoriations, and it is not unusual to see a pattern of postinflammatory hyperpigmentation in the so-called butterfly configuration on the back. This pattern results when patients have difficulty reaching the skin of the upper back but can readily scratch the periphery. The skin in the central area appears relatively normal, whereas the

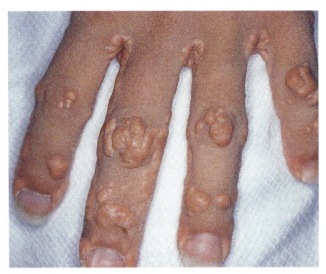

FIGURE 30-6 ■ Multiple xanthomas with hyperpigmentation in primary biliary cirrhosis.

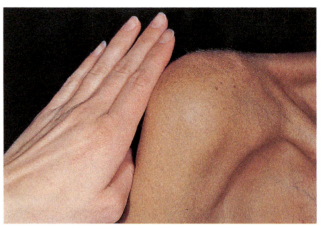

FIGURE 30-7 ■ Generalized hyperpigmentation of hemochromatosis.

border is hyperpigmented and, not infrequently, lichenified. Lichen planus may be more frequent in patients with primary biliary cirrhosis. Patients also develop jaundice, hyperpigmentation, and xanthomas, which are caused by the associated hyperlipidemia. The xanthomas may be striking and include xanthelasma, planar xanthomas in palmar creases and scars, tuberous xanthomas over the extensor aspects of joints and pressure areas, and, rarely, tendinous xanthomas (Fig. 30-6). Late in the course of the disease, patients may develop osteomalacia (secondary to diminished absorption of vitamin D), portal hypertension, and hepatic failure. Therapy for primary biliary cirrhosis includes the use of ursodeoxycholic acid and possibly fenofibrate. There are multiple drugs under investigation for primary biliary cirrhosis including oral budesonide, mycophenolate mofetil, benzafibrate, and obeticholic acid. Liver transplantation can be performed when advanced cirrhosis is present and death is imminent.

HEMOCHROMATOSIS

Hemochromatosis, also known as bronze diabetes, is an autosomal recessive disease characterized by cutaneous hyperpigmentation, diabetes mellitus, and cirrhosis of the liver. There is a basic defect in iron metabolism, resulting in increased absorption of iron from the intestine and deposition of iron in various tissues, particularly the skin, liver, heart, pancreas, and endocrine organs. There are also secondary forms of hemochromatosis that may result from excessive oral intake of iron, from repeated transfusions in patients with refractory anemia, or from a congenital transferrin deficiency. Unlike in primary biliary cirrhosis, 90% of patients with hemochromatosis are male. The disease usually becomes clinically apparent between the ages of 40 and 60 years.

The hyperpigmentation is generalized but accentuated in exposed areas (Fig. 30-7). A small percentage of patients will develop pigmentation of oral mucous membranes and on the conjunctivae, which is similar to the pattern of pigmentation seen in Addison's disease. Hyperpigmentation is the presenting manifestation in one-third of patients, and it is usually a distinctive metallic gray, although it may be brown. It results from an increase in melanin in the skin, presumably as a result of stimulation of the melanin-producing system by the excessive iron stores. The skin tends to be dry and scaly, and patients may develop other changes in the skin, hair, and nails identical to those seen with cirrhosis of the liver. Common extracutaneous features include diabetes mellitus, gonadal deficiency, cardiac disease, and a distinctive arthropathy with chondrocalcinosis. Unlike many other forms of cirrhosis, there is an effective form of therapy for some patients with hemochromatosis, namely, removal of iron stores by repeated phlebotomy.

WILSON'S DISEASE

Wilson's disease (hepatolenticular degeneration) is also a rare autosomal recessive disease associated with cirrhosis, but its clinical and pathologic manifestations result from an excessive accumulation of copper in many tissues, especially the brain, liver, corneas, and kidneys. The triad of basal ganglia degeneration, cirrhosis of the liver, and a pathognomonic pigmentation of the corneal margins (Kayser–Fleischer ring) is characteristic of the disease. The Kayser–Fleischer ring is a golden-brown or greenish-brown circle of pigment produced by the deposition of copper in Descemet's membrane at the periphery of the cornea (Fig. 30-8A). This ocular finding can be important diagnostically, but the majority of patients present with either neurologic symptoms or hepatic insufficiency. The prognosis of Wilson's disease is often grave because of a delay in early diagnosis, which allows irreparable damage to be done to the liver and nervous system. One other physical finding that might suggest the diagnosis of Wilson's disease is the presence of blue lunula, although this azure color can be seen in normal individuals and in patients taking phenolphthalein or antimalarials. Wilson's disease is often treated with D-penicillamine, which is associated with many cutaneous adverse effects, but in particular with elastosis perforans serpiginosa (Fig. 30-8B).

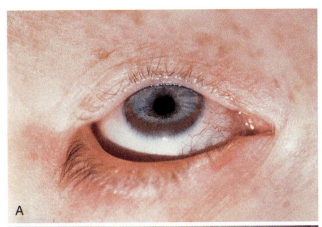

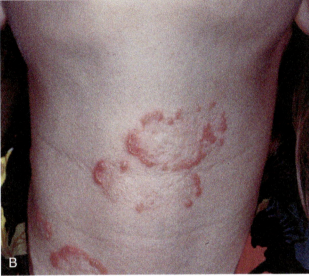

FIGURE 30-8 ■ **A**, Pigmented band (Kayser–Fleischer ring) at the periphery of the cornea in Wilson's disease. **B**, Elastosis perforans serpiginosa in a patient who had previously taken D-penicillamine.

CUTANEOUS DISEASE ASSOCIATED WITH VIRAL HEPATITIS

Viral hepatitis is caused by several agents, and the clinical course varies from subclinical and inapparent infections to severe and fulminant disease with hepatic failure and death. Some viruses preferentially attack the hepatocyte, especially hepatitis viruses A, B, and C; however, other viruses are commonly associated with acute hepatitis, including the Epstein–Barr virus (infectious mononucleosis), cytomegalovirus, rubella, herpes simplex, herpesvirus 6, and yellow fever viruses.

The hepatitis virus most frequently associated with dermatologic syndromes is hepatitis C virus, but hepatitis B virus has also been associated with some cutaneous findings. The incidence of new infections with hepatitis B has lessened with the widespread use of immunization and the testing of blood products. Hepatitis B has been associated with reactive erythemas such as urticaria and vasculitis. In Italy, hepatitis B infection has been linked to papular acrodermatitis of childhood (Gianotti–Crosti syndrome).

Hepatitis C (HCV) has become the most common cause of infectious hepatitis. HCV is spread primarily by

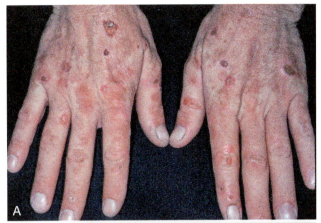

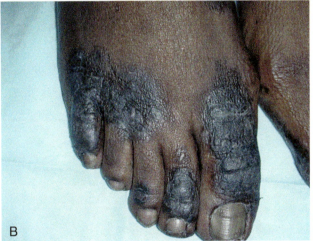

FIGURE 30-9 ■ **A**, Porphyria cutanea tarda in a patient with hepatitis C virus (HCV) infection. **B**, Necrolytic acral erythema associated with HCV infection.

parenteral routes, either by overt inoculation (e.g., transfusion or infection with a contaminated needle) or by intimate personal contact, including contact between sexual partners, and between affected patients and healthcare professionals. Patients infected with HCV usually develop a chronic infection, either in association with demonstrable hepatic disease or in otherwise seemingly healthy carriers. There are at least six serotypes of HCV and they vary in their association with progressive disease and its severity. In addition, the ingestion of alcohol is a significant cofactor that may result in more severe and more rapidly progressive liver disease. Unfortunately there is no vaccine available for this virus, as the immune response that occurs with naturally acquired infection is not protective.

Several dermatological conditions have been associated with HCV infection, including a serum sickness-like prodrome, essential mixed cryoglobulinemia, porphyria cutanea tarda (Fig. 30-9), livedo reticularis, necrolytic acral erythema (Fig. 30-9, *B*), and lichen planus. Less commonly associated findings are urticaria, vitiligo, pyoderma gangrenosum, polyarteritis nodosa, and alopecia areata. Palpable purpura or small-vessel (leukocytoclastic) vasculitis (Fig. 30-10), erythrocyanosis, and Raynaud's phenomenon may occur in patients with essential mixed cryoglobulinemia. It seems prudent to test patients with porphyria cutanea tarda, small-vessel (leukocytoclastic)

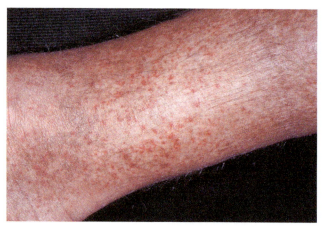

FIGURE 30-10 ■ Leukocytoclastic vasculitis (LCV) in a patient with hepatitis C virus (HCV)-induced cryoglobulinemia.

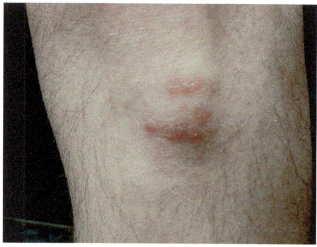

FIGURE 30-12 ■ Sarcoidal granulomas developing in scars of a patient with hepatitis C virus (HCV) on therapy with interferon.

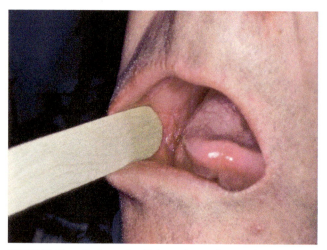

FIGURE 30-11 ■ Oral erosive lichen planus in a patient with cirrhosis and hepatitis C virus (HCV) infection.

vasculitis, polyarteritis nodosa, and possibly lichen planus for the presence of HCV. Patients with oral ulcerative lichen planus (Fig. 30-11) and those with chronic and diffuse disease are more commonly seen to have HCV in association with their cutaneous findings.

There are many other extrahepatic manifestations of HCV infection, including autoimmune thyroid disease, sialadenitis resulting in xerostomia, autoimmune thrombocytopenic purpura, aplastic anemia, neuropathy, serum sickness reactions, and non-Hodgkin's B-cell lymphoma.

Traditional therapy for HCV involved using agents such as interferon and ribavirin. Multiple new protease inhibitors have recently been developed to treat HCV. All of these agents have the potential for cutaneous reactions. Interferon has been noted to cause lichenoid tissue reactions, worsening of psoriasis, and sarcoidal-like granulomas in sites of old trauma (Fig. 30-12). Telaprevir and boceprevir are NS3/4A oral protease inhibitors specifically used to treat patients infected with HCV genotype 1. These two agents are known to cause a spongiotic papular dermatitis in as many as 50% of patients who receive them, as well as potentially causing a drug reaction with eosinophilia and systemic symptoms (Fig. 30-13). Newer protease inhibitors have a lower potential for the development of hypersensitivity reactions. These protease inhibitors have cured HCV infection in a high percentage of patients and have also been associated with a cure of the associated extrahepatic disorders including porphyria cutanea tarda and mixed cryoglobulinemia.

Screening for HCV should be performed in all patients prior to initiating therapy with any potentially hepatotoxic medication. Patients infected with HCV may have normal liver function tests, thus a routine hepatic function panel is not an adequate screening tool. Patients testing positive for HCV should have a confirmatory test via polymerase chain reaction, as false positives do occur with the routine serum screen; however, if the screen is negative, one can feel assured that there is no HCV, as few false negatives occur. Diagnosing HCV at an early stage is critical in order to prevent end-stage hepatic cirrhosis, which can progress to hepatocellular carcinoma.

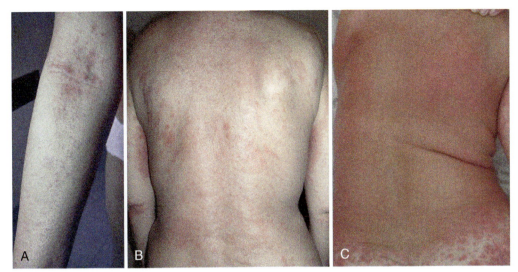

FIGURE 30-13 ■ Examples of grade 1 dermatitis (**A**), grade 2 dermatitis (**B**), and drug reaction with eosinophilia and systemic symptoms (DRESS) reactions to telaprevir-based therapy (**C**). (From Cacoub P et al. Dermatological side effects of hepatitis C and its treatment: patient management in the era of direct-acting antivirals. J Hepatol 2012;56(2):455–63. Copyright Elsevier.)

SUGGESTED READINGS

Akhter A, Said A. Cutaneous manifestations of viral hepatitis. Curr Infect Dis Rep 2015;17(2):452.

Bergasa NV. Pruritus of cholestasis. In: Carstens E, Akiyama T, editors. Itch: mechanisms and treatment. Boca Raton (FL): CRC Press; 2014. [chapter 6]. PMID: 24830019.

Ekanayake D, Roddick C, Powell LW. Recent advances in hemochromatosis: a 2015 update: a summary of proceedings of the 2014 conference held under the auspices of Hemochromatosis Australia. Hepatol Int 2015;9(2):174–82.

Jackson JM. Hepatitis C and the skin. Dermatol Clin 2002;20:449–58.

Kim YD, Ahn SH, Han KH. Emerging therapies for hepatitis C. Gut Liver 2014;8(5):471–9.

Lynch M, Higgins E, McCormick PA, Kirby B, Nolan N, Rogers S, et al. The use of transient elastography and FibroTest for monitoring hepatotoxicity in patients receiving methotrexate for psoriasis. JAMA Dermatol 2014;150(8):856–62.

Menter A, Korman NJ, Elmets CA, Feldman SR, Gelfand JM, Gordon KB, et al. Guidelines of care for the management of psoriasis and psoriatic arthritis: section 4. Guidelines of care for the management and treatment of psoriasis with traditional systemic agents. J Am Acad Dermatol 2009;61(3):451–85.

Sarkanv I. The skin-liver connection. Clin Exp Dermatol 1988;13:151–9.

CHAPTER 31

VIRAL DISEASES

Ramya Kollipara • Sheevam Shah • Stephen K. Tyring

> **KEY POINTS**
>
> - Measles is generally a benign, self-limited illness that presents with erythematous, confluent macules and papules that spread cephalocaudally and Koplik spots.
> - Hand, foot, and mouth syndrome, caused by various Coxsackie viruses, is a self-limited illness that presents with oval to linear papules and vesicles on the dorsal and lateral fingers and toes as well as painful, oral mucosal vesicles and papules.
> - Epstein–Barr virus infection can present with a variable exanthem on the trunk or upper arms, palatal petechiae, copper-colored morbilliform pruritic eruption (in patients treated with semisynthetic penicillins), or lichenoids papulovesicular exanthema on the extensor surfaces, gluteal area, and face (Gianotti–Crosti syndrome).
> - Varicella infection (chickenpox) presents with crops of vesicles that evolve to pustules and, eventually, crusts on the body and palate.
> - Herpes zoster presents with grouped vesicles, ulcers, and crust in a dermatomal distribution and can lead to secondary infection, scarring, and postherpetic neuralgia.
> - Although herpes simplex virus can result in a wide variety of clinical syndromes, herpetic lesions present with grouped vesicles on an erythematous base and occasionally chronic ulcerations of vegetative lesions in the immunocompromised patients.

Viruses produce a variety of cutaneous changes, including morbilliform, papular, and vesicular eruptions. It is often difficult to distinguish viral exanthems from morbilliform drug eruptions; however, subtle distinguishing features may enable differentiation.

MEASLES (RUBEOLA)

Measles (rubeola) is caused by a single-stranded RNA paramyxovirus. Transmission occurs via respiratory secretions. Routine administration of live attenuated vaccine is currently recommended by the Centers for Disease Control and Prevention (CDC) for all infants, college entrants, and medical personnel without serologic evidence of past infection. The incidence of measles infection has decreased dramatically with the introduction of widespread vaccination; however, a gradual increase has occurred in recent years in the United States. Some of those affected were previously vaccinated, although more parents are choosing not to vaccinate, resulting in increasing numbers of small but significant local outbreaks. However, the health benefits of vaccinations far outweigh the unfounded concerns about the potential adverse effects based on scientifically discredited concerns with no medical basis. Two distinct forms of the disease are modified measles, which occurs when an individual is infected when they have passive immunity (during breastfeeding or with remaining transplacental antibodies), and atypical measles, which largely affects persons immunized with the killed vaccine during the 1960s.

Clinical Manifestations

After a 10-day incubation period, the viral prodrome phase consists of fever (may exceed 104°F), cough, coryza, conjunctivitis, photophobia, and myalgias, and lasts about 1 week. The classic exanthem consisting of erythematous confluent macules and papules is usually apparent at 2 weeks. The cutaneous eruption spreads cephalocaudally over 3 days, and resolves with fine desquamation and a brown hyperpigmentation. Koplik spots are pathognomonic and appear on the buccal, labial, and gingival mucosae just prior to the exanthem. They are 1- to 2-mm bluish macules on an erythematous base. Measles infection is usually benign and self-limited but has the potential to be fatal in malnourished and/or immunocompromised patients.

The most common complication of measles is secondary bacterial infection. Pneumonia occurs more frequently in children and is the most common cause of death associated with the virus. Atypical measles is a characteristic clinical syndrome seen in recipients of the killed vaccine that was used in the United States from 1963 to 1967. The cutaneous eruption begins on the wrists, arms, and soles, and then spreads centrally to the extremities and trunk. The lesions are initially morbilliform and then become vesicular, purpuric, or hemorrhagic. Koplik spots are rarely present.

Diagnosis

The clinical presentation is often classic; however, in countries with low measles prevalence, confirmation should be made with viral culture or serology (anti-measles IgM). Of note, atypical measles presents with a unique antibody titer pattern. Before the onset or at the onset of the exanthema, the titer is less than 1:5 but by day 10 the titer is greater than 1:1280.

Treatment

The treatment is supportive. Immune serum globulin may be given to exposed susceptible persons who are immunocompromised. Some studies suggest the use of ribavirin in immunocompromised hosts may be beneficial.

RUBELLA

Rubella (German measles) is a self-limited childhood infection caused by a single-stranded RNA togavirus. The incidence of rubella has decreased dramatically since the introduction of a live attenuated vaccine in 1968. Transmission occurs by inhalation of infected respiratory droplets, with increased incidence during the spring months.

Clinical Manifestations

After a 2- to 3-week incubation period, illness begins with a mild prodrome consisting of malaise, anorexia, fever, headache, and coryza. The cutaneous eruption appears first on the forehead and rapidly spreads inferiorly to involve the face, trunk, and extremities. The lesions consist of pink macules and papules, which may become confluent, creating a scarlatiniform eruption (scarlet fever-like macular erythema). Pruritus may be present. The time course of the rubella exanthem is 3 days, which is a differentiating point from the usual 6-day course of the rubeola exanthem. The exanthem of rubella also does not desquamate. There may be symmetric, tender, postauricular, suboccipital, and posterior cervical lymphadenopathy. Petechiae on the soft palate, or Forschheimer spots, may also be present. Arthritis and arthralgia are common complications of infection, especially in females.

Widespread vaccination against rubella was developed largely for the prevention of congenital rubella syndrome. Maternal infection during the first 16 weeks of gestation results in a 65% risk for congenital rubella. Manifestations of congenital rubella syndrome include extramedullary hematopoiesis (blueberry muffin baby), thrombocytopenia, cataracts, deafness, and patent ductus arteriosus. The impact of maternal infection on the fetus drops precipitously after 20 weeks of gestation.

Diagnosis

The diagnosis of rubella is made clinically and confirmed serologically. The virus can be isolated by culture from the oropharynx or joint aspirate.

Treatment

Treatment is supportive care.

ERYTHEMA INFECTIOSUM

Erythema infectiosum (fifth disease) is an acute childhood exanthem caused by human parvovirus B19. Most cases develop during the winter or spring, and transmission is by respiratory droplets.

Clinical Manifestations

Most infections due to parvovirus B19 are asymptomatic; however, in school-aged children erythema infectiosum is common. A mild prodrome of low-grade fever, coryza, malaise, and headache may present initially during viremia. Soon thereafter the characteristic asymptomatic bilateral erythema of the cheeks with circumoral pallor, often referred to as a "slapped cheek," appears. This may be accompanied by pharyngitis, myalgia, diarrhea, nausea, or conjunctivitis. Within a few days the exanthem extends to the body and is described as an evanescent reticulated erythema of the trunk and extremities. Oftentimes, the exanthem recedes and recurs with high temperatures, exercise, or stress. A unique cutaneous manifestation of parvovirus B19 infection is the papular purpuric "gloves and socks" syndrome. This affects young adults and results in symmetric swelling and pain in the distal feet and hands, followed by the purpuric eruption. Complications are much more common in adults, and include arthritis, hemolytic anemia, encephalopathy, and aplastic crisis. Parvovirus infection during pregnancy can cause spontaneous abortion and hydrops fetalis.

Diagnosis

The diagnosis is usually made on clinical grounds. Serum parvovirus-specific immunoglobulin M can be measured.

Treatment

Treatment is supportive care. Joint symptoms typically respond to nonsteroidal anti-inflammatory medications. Chronic anemia and aplastic crises may require treatment with immunoglobulin or blood transfusion.

HAND, FOOT, AND MOUTH SYNDROME

Hand, foot, and mouth (HFM) syndrome is a combination of an exanthem and enanthem that primarily affects toddlers. The etiologic agent is a Coxsackie virus, most commonly A16, but also A5, A10, B1, or B3, and other enteroviruses can cause the eruption. Several recent reports document Coxsackie virus A6 (CVA6) as the cause of an atypical, often more severe HFM syndrome in adults. Coxsackie viruses are small RNA viruses of the picornavirus family. Outbreaks are characteristically limited to the summer and early fall months.

Clinical Manifestations

This syndrome is characterized by the abrupt onset of sore mouth, cutaneous eruption, and fever. Malaise, diarrhea, joint pains, and lymphadenopathy may be present. The typical acral lesions are few in number and consist of oval to linear or football-shaped red papules and vesicles located over the dorsal and lateral aspects of the fingers and toes. The palmar and plantar surfaces may also be involved (Fig. 31-1). An exanthem or red papules over the proximal extremities may also be present. Oropharyngeal lesions consist of painful papules and vesicles that become erosions scattered over the soft palate, tonsillar pillars, and posterior pharynx. In children, buttock involvement is a common finding. Of note, incomplete forms of HFM syndrome can occur, where the exanthema does not manifest at all body sites. HFM syndrome due to CVA6 can present in an atypical distribution, involving the scrotum, ear, scalp, and chin. HFM syndrome is generally a self-limited disease lasting less than 1 week.

Diagnosis

The eruption is usually characteristic. In some cases, viral culture of the stool or throat washings can be used to confirm the diagnosis. Acute and convalescent sera can also be assessed for Coxsackie viral titers.

Treatment

Treatment is supportive care.

HERPANGINA

The etiologic agent in herpangina is a Coxsackie virus: A2, A4, A5, A6, A8, and A10 are the most frequently identified culprits. It commonly occurs in children from ages 3 to 10.

Clinical Manifestations

Herpangina is characterized by the abrupt onset of fever, sore throat, anorexia, dysphagia, and vomiting. The exanthem is a morbilliform erythema with generalized pink papules, most prominent on the buttocks. Occasionally, petechiae are present. Oral lesions consist of 1- to 8-mm, painful erosions with erythematous borders located on the soft palate, uvula, posterior pharyngeal wall, tongue, or anterior tonsillar pillars. Genital ulcerations are noted occasionally. Herpangina is a mild illness, lasting only a few days. Rarely, the course is complicated by parotitis.

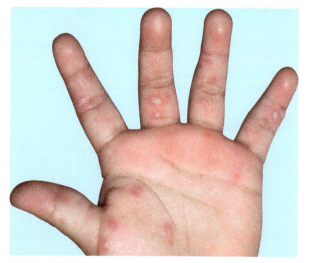

FIGURE 31-1 ■ Erythematous papules and pustules in a patient with hand, foot, and mouth syndrome.

Diagnosis

Viral culture of stool or throat washings can be used to confirm the diagnosis. Acute and convalescent sera can also be assessed.

Treatment

Treatment is supportive care.

ROSEOLA INFANTUM/EXANTHEM SUBITUM (HUMAN HERPESVIRUS 6)

Human herpesvirus 6 (HHV 6) is genetically and pathogenetically similar to cytomegalovirus. HHV 6 has been demonstrated to be the cause of exanthem subitum (also known as roseola infantum, or sixth disease). Exanthem subitum can sometimes be caused by HHV 7 as well. By age 2, nearly 100% of children are seropositive for HHV 6. HHV 7 usually causes exanthema subitum much later in life. The presumed route of transmission is by respiratory tract secretions.

Clinical Manifestations

A prodromal syndrome with a sudden high fever typically occurs 7 to 15 days after exposure to this virus. Constitutional symptoms, including malaise, coryza, sore throat, headache, anorexia, and nausea, appear with the exanthem in a few days. The exanthem consists of discrete pink macules and papules distributed primarily over the trunk, buttocks, and neck, which may coalesce to confluent erythema. A ring of pallor surrounds the individual lesions. Complete resolution occurs in 1 to 4 days. Infection is benign and self-limited with infrequent complications, the most common being febrile seizures in 10% of patients.

Diagnosis

The classic feature of an isolated high fever preceding the eruption of the exanthem is usually sufficient to make the diagnosis. Serologic studies are available for absolute confirmation.

Treatment

Treatment is supportive care.

EPSTEIN–BARR VIRUS

Epstein–Barr virus (EBV), a herpesvirus, is the primary etiologic agent in the clinical syndrome infectious mononucleosis. Infection with EBV usually occurs in childhood or adolescence and is generally mild and self-limited.

Clinical Manifestations

The incubation period of EBV is long: 3 to 7 weeks. Following this, acute infection is characterized by fever, pharyngitis, severe fatigue, and symmetric posterior cervical lymphadenopathy. Eyelid edema and hepatosplenomegaly are often prominent. Mucocutaneous manifestations are more common in younger children. There may be an exanthem on the trunk and upper arms consisting of macules, urticarial plaques, petechiae, or purpura. An enanthem consisting of palatal petechiae at the border of the soft and hard palate is common. A distinctive and pathognomonic copper-colored morbilliform pruritic eruption may develop in infected patients treated with ampicillin or other semisynthetic penicillins (Fig. 31-2). Gianotti–Crosti syndrome, often associated with EBV, manifests as symmetric lichenoid papules or papulovesicular exanthem on the extensor surfaces of the distal, extremities, gluteal areas, and face, which resolve after 1 month. EBV infection is usually self-limited. Late manifestations of EBV-related disease include lymphoproliferative disease, which might affect the skin on rare occasions.

Diagnosis

Examination of a peripheral blood smear reveals lymphocytosis with atypical lymphocytes. Mild thrombocytopenia is common, and there may be elevated liver transaminases. The presence of heterophile antibodies (monospot) or a rise in EBV-specific antibodies can confirm the diagnosis. The virus can be cultured from the oropharynx.

Treatment

Treatment is supportive care. Ampicillin should be avoided. Occasionally, systemic corticosteroids are indicated for severe complications, such as pharyngeal edema causing airway obstruction.

VARICELLA

Varicella (chicken pox) is a ubiquitous childhood infection caused by the varicella-zoster virus (VZV), a member of the herpesvirus family. Transmission occurs by airborne droplets and by direct contact.

Clinical Manifestations

The exanthem typically occurs 2 weeks after exposure, begins abruptly on the head, and spreads caudally. The primary lesion is an erythematous papule that evolves into a clear fluid-filled vesicle on an erythematous base, commonly described as a "dewdrop on a rose petal" (Fig. 31-3). The vesicles subsequently evolve into pustules and, eventually, crusts. Additional crops occur, resulting in lesions in all stages of evolution presenting simultaneously, allowing easy differentiation from smallpox, where all the lesions are in the same stage of evolution. The palms and soles are typically spared. Vesicles and erosions are often present on the palate. Mild constitutional symptoms often accompany the exanthem and are more prominent with increasing age. In children, varicella is typically a self-limited disease but may be complicated by secondary infection. Primary infection in adults or in immunocompromised hosts may be complicated by pneumonia, encephalitis, or myocarditis. Mortality in adult patients is 10% when immunocompetent and 30% in immunosuppressed patients. Maternal infection with primary VZV produces congenital varicella syndrome, which includes limb defects, cortical atrophy, low birthweight, and ocular abnormalities. The risk is greatest when infection occurs in the first trimester, with about 2% of fetuses exposed before 20 weeks' gestation being affected. Breakthrough varicella occurs in 20% of VZV immunized patients who are exposed to wild-type virus. Fifty percent of these patients have a maculopapular rash with only a few contagious blisters. Vaccination with a live attenuated virus is routinely performed now, providing a 96% seroconversion rate, and is nearly 100% effective at preventing serious disease.

Diagnosis

VZV infection is a clinical diagnosis based on clinical presentation and exposure history. In cases of uncertainty, pregnant women or immunosuppressed patients, viral culture, polymerase chain reaction (PCR), direct/indirect immunofluorescence, enzyme-linked immunosorbent

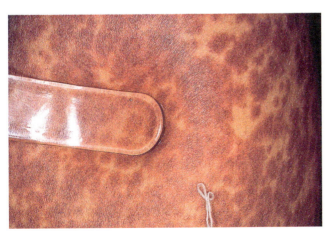

FIGURE 31-2 ∎ Ampicillin eruption in a patient with infectious mononucleosis.

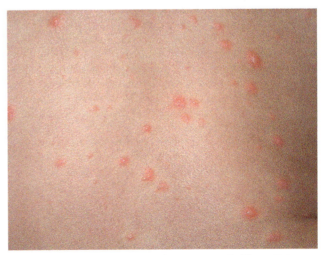

FIGURE 31-3 ∎ Small vesicular lesions surrounded by a slight erythematous hue, representative of acute varicella.

assay, or DNA-hybridization can confirm the diagnosis. Furthermore, cytologic evaluation of the fluid or the floor of a vesicle (Tzanck preparation) reveals characteristic herpesvirus-induced changes, consisting of acantholytic balloon cells with one or several nuclei. This procedure is highly interpreter-dependent, and positivity depends on the stage of the lesion, with vesicles having the highest positivity.

Treatment

In adults, oral acyclovir (or valacyclovir or famciclovir) is recommended for uncomplicated varicella and intravenous acyclovir for disseminated disease. Intravenous acyclovir is recommended for immunosuppressed children with uncomplicated or complicated varicella. Furthermore, children older than 12 years and those with chronic skin and pulmonary disease should be given acyclovir. Acyclovir is most effective when given in the first 24 hours after developing a rash but is thought to be also beneficial if started between 24 and 72 hours. In immunocompetent children less than 12 years old with uncomplicated varicella, only supportive care is recommended. Acyclovir therapy in pregnancy may benefit the mother, but may not affect fetal outcome. Varicella-zoster immunoglobulin is indicated for prophylaxis in susceptible pregnant women and in neonates whose mothers became infected shortly prior to delivery.

HERPES ZOSTER

Herpes zoster infection is also caused by VZV and represents reactivation of the latent virus from prior varicella infection.

Clinical Manifestations

A severely painful prodrome often precedes the cutaneous eruption, which is typically confined to a single dermatome (Fig. 31-4). The eruption consists of grouped vesicles that may appear purpuric and which later ulcerate and crust. The sites of predilection, in descending order, are thoracic, trigeminal, lumbosacral, and cervical dermatomes. Involvement of the ophthalmic branch of the trigeminal nerve can cause zoster keratitis or ophthalmicus, which can lead to blindness. Vesicular lesions on the nose (Hutchinson's sign) portend development of zoster ophthalmicus. Mild constitutional symptoms may be present. Immunosuppression, family history of shingles and advanced age are risk factors for herpes zoster. In patients with acquired immunodeficiency syndrome (AIDS) the eruption may be multidermatomal or disseminated and recurrent. Secondary infection of cutaneous lesions may be associated with scarring. Urinary retention and conjunctival scarring may complicate genital and periocular infections, respectively.

Diagnosis

The diagnosis may be clinically obvious because of the characteristic dermatomal distribution of clustered

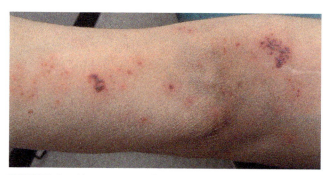

FIGURE 31-4 ■ Herpes zoster. Grouped hemorrhagic blisters in a dermatomal distribution.

vesicular lesions. Tzanck preparation reveals characteristic herpesvirus-induced changes. Viral culture can confirm the diagnosis. Immunoperoxidase studies using monoclonal antibodies and PCR detection of viral DNA can be useful for diagnosis in atypical cases.

Treatment

Herpes zoster infection is typically self-limited in immunocompetent patients. Local care to prevent secondary bacterial infection, antivirals, and analgesics for pain control are usually adequate treatment. Oral acyclovir, valacyclovir, or famciclovir for 7 days has been shown to hasten the healing time and to reduce the acute pain when initiated within 72 hours of onset of the cutaneous eruption. It is unclear whether antivirals reduce the risk or duration of postherpetic neuralgia (PHN). Patients who present with significant pain are at greatest risk for PHN. In patients presenting with a pain score of ≥4 a combination of antivirals, gabapentin, and analgesics is most effective at preventing PHN. One study demonstrated that if neuropathic pain is present at onset, treatment with gabapentin may reduce the duration and severity of PHN. Immunocompromised persons should be treated with intravenous acyclovir to prevent dissemination of the infection. Treatment of PHN is difficult. The pain often decreases with time. Topical capsaicin or lidocaine may help some patients. Oral amitriptyline, gabapentin, and pregabalin as well as low-dose opioids may also be useful. In patients who fail these measures, intrathecal injection of methylprednisolone may be beneficial.

In 2006, a vaccine for herpes zoster was approved by the Food and Drug Administration. Zostavax contains live varicella-zoster virus, is indicated in patients over 50, and has been shown to reduce the incidence of zoster by 51% and the incidence of PHN by 66%.

HERPES SIMPLEX VIRUS

Herpes simplex virus (HSV) types 1 and 2 enter the host through mucosal surfaces or breaks in the skin. The most common entry sites are oral (HSV type 1 more than type 2) and genital (HSV type 2 more than type 1) via close contact with an infected person. The hallmark of infection with HSV is its ability to establish a latent infection.

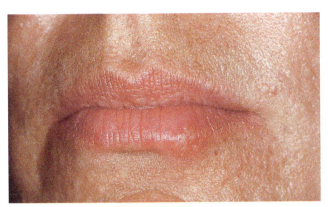

FIGURE 31-5 ■ Typical appearance of herpes labialis on the lower lip in a patient with recurrent herpes simplex infection.

Clinical Manifestations

Herpes simplex infection commonly occurs in immunocompetent persons as a recurrent painful vesicular eruption, most commonly affecting the oral and perioral (anterior soft palate, lips, or gingival) or genital regions (Fig. 31-5). Skin lesions with primary infection last 10 to 14 days and duration of recurrent lesions decreases with each recurrence. Skin-to-skin contact, such as in wrestlers, may allow for transmission of a herpes simplex viral infection known as herpes gladiatorum. Occupational exposures in medical and dental personnel can produce lesions on the hands or digits, referred to as herpetic whitlow. Recurrent eruptions are often triggered by exogenous factors, including local trauma or sunburn. The primary infection with HSV often produces a more severe systemic reaction, including high fever, regional lymphadenopathy, and malaise, which is different from the reactivated form of the disease. Neonatal herpes simplex infection is one of the most life-threatening newborn infections and is acquired by ascending infection from an infected birth canal. Neonatal HSV infection can manifest as mucocutaneous disease, encephalitis without cutaneous disease, or disseminated infection of multiple organs, most commonly the liver and adrenals. Rapid and severe progression of HSV infection may occur in patients who are immunocompromised secondary to transplant, or who have underlying diseases such as leukemia (Fig. 31-6) or HIV infection. A generalized herpetic infection of the skin may occur in persons with a preexisting cutaneous disorder, such as atopic dermatitis or psoriasis, and is termed eczema herpeticum or Kaposi's varicelliform eruption. Periocular involvement requires prompt ophthalmologic evaluation to rule out herpetic keratoconjunctivitis as herpes keratitis is the most common infectious cause of corneal blindness in the United States. HSV is the usual infectious agent to trigger recurrent erythema multiforme.

Despite the wide variation in clinical syndromes, herpetic lesions share the appearance of grouped vesicles on an erythematous base. Location is a critical feature in differentiating the various syndromes, with relatively well-localized recurrent infection producing a cluster of vesicles in the perioral or genital areas typifying infection with herpesvirus types 1 and 2. Lesions in immunocompromised patients may present as chronic ulcerations

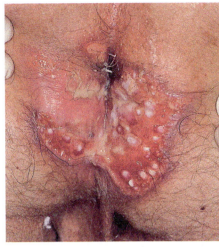

FIGURE 31-6 ■ Chronic herpetic ulceration on the buttock in a patient with chronic lymphocytic leukemia.

or hyperkeratotic or vegetative lesions resembling malignancy.

Diagnosis

Culture of the virus has been the "gold standard" of diagnosing HSV infection. The Tzanck preparation reveals characteristic herpesvirus-induced changes. Immunoperoxidase techniques using monoclonal antibodies or DNA hybridization techniques are rapid diagnostic methods. Serologic testing plays a minor role and is useful in the diagnosis of primary infection, or is helpful if the result is negative, making infection with this virus unlikely.

Treatment

In healthy individuals, herpes simplex infection is self-limited and requires only local care to prevent bacterial superinfection and to alleviate pain. Primary oral or genital infections are often associated with significant morbidity. Acyclovir, valacyclovir, or famiciclovir reduce the duration of viral shedding and pain, and speed the healing of lesions. For patients with frequent attacks, continuous suppressive therapy with acyclovir, valacyclovir, or famciclovir is highly effective without evidence of cumulative toxicity or resistance. Severe infections in immunocompromised patients or neonates require parenteral acyclovir therapy. Intravenous foscarnet is the drug of choice for HSV resistance to acyclovir in AIDS patients, but intralesional or 1% topical cidofovir is also effective.

CYTOMEGALOVIRUS

Cytomegalovirus (CMV) is another member of the herpesvirus group. This organism accounts for about 10% of mononucleosis syndrome cases, and mononucleosis is the major clinical form of acquired CMV disease. Studies of antibodies to CMV indicate that infections with this virus are ubiquitous. Congenital infection can occur by transplacental transmission of virus from an infected mother.

Clinical Manifestations

CMV mononucleosis is associated with an exanthem in about one-quarter of patients. It is characteristically a morbilliform erythema that primarily affects the face and trunk and lasts for 2 to 5 days. Occasionally, petechiae are present. There is no associated enanthem. Fever and tonsillar enlargement, malaise, and myalgia are often associated with infection, but sore throat and adenopathy are typically absent. Low-grade hepatitis is often present. The course of CMV mononucleosis is protracted, lasting weeks to months. The administration of ampicillin dramatically increases the likelihood of morbilliform eruption, as occurs with EBV mononucleosis. Congenital CMV infection presents in affected newborns as a petechial or purpuric exanthema (termed "blueberry muffin spots") with associated hepatosplenomegaly, thrombocytopenia, deafness, chorioretinitis, and growth retardation.

Diagnosis

Culture of the urine and serologic titers for CMV are the most effective means of confirming the diagnosis. Cellular inclusions can often be detected by examining the urine. Skin biopsy typically reveals a neutrophilic vascular reaction.

Treatment

In the nonimmunosuppressed host, treatment is supportive care. Retinitis in immunocompromised patients is treated with ganciclovir or cidofovir.

POLYOMAVIRUS

Polyomavirus is caused by a double-stranded DNA virus that is part of the Papoviridae virus family. The most clinically significant polyomaviruses are the JC and BK viruses. These viruses manifest in disease primarily in immunocompromised hosts, resulting in progressive multifocal leukoencephalopathy (PML) and genitourinary tract disease, respectively. Two additional important manifestations of polyomaviruses include trichodysplasia and Merkel cell carcinoma (MCC). Most studies have reported a polyomavirus incidence of 80% in MCC.

Clinical Manifestations

Although JC and BK viruses are highly prevalent, clinical manifestations are rare in immunocompetent hosts. Clinical manifestations generally occur with reactivation of the disease in immunocompromised hosts. Clinical manifestations of PML include altered mental status, motor deficits (hemiparesis or monoparesis), limb ataxia, gait ataxia, and visual symptoms including diplopia and hemianopia. BK virus commonly manifests as hemorrhagic cystitis. Trichodysplasia-associated polyomavirus results in erythematous to skin-colored spiny papules that affect the central face in addition to variable amounts of alopecia, especially affecting the eyebrows and eyelashes. MCC typically presents as a rapidly growing, painless, firm, nontender, shiny, flesh-colored or bluish-red, intracutaneous nodule. It primarily affects white, elderly persons with a mean age at diagnosis of 76 years for women and 74 years for men.

Diagnosis

Polyomavirus is most often diagnosed after the primary infection, which is usually asymptomatic in immunocompetent hosts. There are many methods of diagnosis, of which serology looking for antibodies is commonly employed. PCR and urine cytology can also be used. Viral culture is rarely used outside of a research setting.

Viral-associated trichodysplasia (VAT) is diagnosed with PCR and immunohistochemical staining. PCR identifies the presence of human polyomavirus DNA, while immunohistochemical staining identifies the middle T antigen of the human polyomavirus. It was initially thought that VAT was caused by a papillomavirus due to various features of initial stains. It was not until the identification of the middle T antigen that VAT became associated with human polyomavirus.

Biopsy with histologic examination is required to make the diagnosis of MCC. There are three histologic patterns: intermediate type (most common), trabecular type, and small-cell type.

Treatment

There are no specific treatments for the manifestations of the JC and BK polyomaviruses. PML is treated by restoring the host's adaptive immune response. In immunocompromised patients due to HIV, optimization of antiretroviral therapy is recommended. BK virus-associated hemorrhagic cystitis has been treated with intravenous cidofovir, but no controlled trials have been established to evaluate the efficacy of this treatment.

VAT has shown great clinical improvement with topical cidofovir treatment. Various antiviral therapies, including valacyclovir and valganciclovir, have also been effective in the treatment of VAT.

Surgery is the primary treatment modality for MCC. There are three approaches used. Sentinel lymph node biopsy or elective lymph node dissection is used for clinically normal regional lymph node basins. Postoperative radiation therapy is used for the primary tumor, draining lymphatics, and/or regional lymph node basins. Adjuvant chemotherapy is employed for local or regional disease.

DENGUE

Dengue is the most prevalent mosquito-borne viral disease. It is estimated that approximately 400 million dengue virus infections occur annually worldwide, with 25% of those infections producing illness. Dengue virus is a single-stranded RNA virus of the genus *Flavivirus*. The primary lifecycle of this virus occurs between humans and *Aedes* mosquitos.

Clinical Manifestations

Typical clinical manifestations of the dengue virus vary from asymptomatic infection to dengue hemorrhagic fever (DHF) with shock syndrome. Most infections are asymptomatic. Classic dengue fever is characterized by headache, retroorbital pain, and muscle and joint pains, commonly referred to as "break-bone fever." Symptoms typically develop between 4 and 7 days after the bite of an infected mosquito, after which fever can last up to 7 days. This is followed by a period of marked fatigue that can last for days to weeks. Hemorrhagic manifestations can be life-threatening. DHF can be associated with circulatory failure and shock. The World Health Organization has defined four cardinal features of DHF, including increased vascular permeability, marked thrombocytopenia ($\leq$100,000 cells/mm^3), fever lasting 2 to 7 days, and a hemorrhagic tendency or spontaneous bleeding.

Diagnosis

The diagnosis of dengue is primarily clinical. Laboratory confirmation exists in developed countries, but is often not available in developing countries. Laboratory confirmation consists of serology detection of viral RNA or NS1 antigens, which can aid in detecting dengue virus infection in its early stages. The most frequently used serologic tests include the hemagglutination inhibition assay and IgG or IgM immunoassays.

Treatment

There is no specific treatment for dengue infection. Analgesics, rest, and adequate hydration are recommended by the CDC. There is also no specific treatment for DHF. If the diagnosis is made early, fluid resuscitation and hospitalization are recommended. Although there are several vaccines under development by researchers, there are currently no approved vaccines for the treatment of dengue.

CHIKUNGUNYA

The Chikungunya virus is a single-stranded RNA virus of the genus *Alphavirus* that manifests in humans as Chikungunya fever. It is endemic in parts of West Africa, and has recently come under the spotlight due to the first acquired case in the United States in 2014. Chikungunya virus has been rapidly spreading in Asia and islands in the Indian Ocean. It is transmitted as part of a lifecycle that involves humans and species of *Aedes* mosquitoes. The major mosquito vectors are *Aedes aegypti* and *Aedes albopictus*, the same vectors involved in transmission of dengue virus.

Clinical Manifestations

Following an incubation period of 2 to 4 days, clinical manifestations include abrupt fever and malaise. Fever can be as high as 40°C. Polyarthralgia is another manifestation and most commonly is symmetrical, involving the hands, wrists, and ankles. Skin manifestations are common as well, with a macular or maculopapular rash being the most common.

Diagnosis

In endemic areas, Chikungunya infection can be diagnosed based on clinical findings. In uncommonly affected regions where laboratory facilities are available, serology is the primary tool for diagnosis. ELISA is employed looking for IgM anti-Chikungunya virus antibodies. IgG antibodies begin to appear about 2 weeks following the onset of symptoms. Viral culture and molecular techniques are used in research settings.

Treatment

Treatment of Chikungunya infection involves supportive care, including anti-inflammatory and analgesic agents. There are no vaccines approved for the prevention of Chikungunya infection; however, vaccines in early development have shown promise.

MARBURG/EBOLA

Marburg and Ebola viruses are single-stranded RNA viruses in the family *Filoviridae*. Ebola virus has gained extraordinary media attention recently due to the epidemic in West Africa. Previously, Ebola and Marburg viruses were referred to as "hemorrhagic fever viruses" due to their potential to cause bleeding, shock, and coagulation deficits. Ebola virus is no longer classified as a hemorrhagic fever virus because only a very small percentage of Ebola patients develop significant hemorrhage. The term "Ebola virus disease" is now being used instead.

Clinical Manifestations

Marburg and Ebola viruses result in similar clinical manifestations. Symptoms abruptly begin approximately 6 to 12 days after exposure. Asymptomatic patients in the incubation period are not infectious to others. Once symptomatic, however, safety precautions should be taken, as the virus is present in the blood and other bodily fluids.

Clinical manifestations include a diffuse, erythematous, nonpruritic maculopapular rash after a week of illness. Gastrointestinal symptoms are common and include watery diarrhea, nausea, and vomiting. As mentioned above, hemorrhage is not a common manifestation of Ebola virus, but is more frequently seen in Marburg virus infection. Neurologic symptoms can also develop, including altered level of consciousness, stiff neck, and/or seizures. Fatal disease is characterized by onset of more severe clinical signs early in the infection and progresses to multiorgan failure and death usually in the second week.

Diagnosis

Diagnosis of Ebola and Marburg viruses is most often initially clinical. Ebola virus becomes detectable in blood samples by reverse-transcription polymerase chain reaction (RT-PCR) within 3 days of onset of symptoms. It is imperative to have a low threshold for diagnosis, as isolation and safety measures need to be made early to prevent further transmission. Thus, the CDC has released guidelines for the evaluation of patients in the United States suspected of having Ebola virus disease. Patients confirmed to have Ebola virus disease should be transferred to specialized treatment centers. Due to the similarities in presentation of Ebola and Marburg viruses, RT-PCR can be used to distinguish between the two.

Treatment

There are no approved treatments for either Marburg or Ebola virus. Supportive care is the mainstay of treatment. Vaccines are currently under development for both viruses. For the hemorrhagic manifestations of Marburg virus, anticoagulants can be administered early to prevent disseminated intravascular coagulation and procoagulants can be administered late in the course of infection to prevent hemorrhage.

CONCLUSION

Viral infections often present with cutaneous eruptions and careful examination of these dermatologic manifestations can aid in the diagnosis of the systemic infection.

SUGGESTED READINGS

Arduino PG, Porter SR. Oral and perioral herpes simplex virus type 1 (HSV-1) infection: review of its management. Oral Dis 2006;12:254–70.

Biesbroeck L, Sidbury R. Viral exanthems: an update. Dermatol Ther 2013;26(6):433–8.

Cutts FT, Lessler J, Metcalf CJ. Measles elimination: progress, challenges and implications for rubella control. Expert Rev Vaccines 2013;12(8):917–32.

Fatahzadeh M, Schwartz RA. Human herpes simplex virus infections: epidemiology, pathogenesis, symptomatology, diagnosis and management. J Am Acad Dermatol 2007;57:737–63.

Gomez-Flores M, Mendez N, et al. New insights into HIV-1 primary skin disorders. J Int AIDS Soc 2011;14:5.

Nkoghe D, Leroy EM, Toung-mve M, Gonzalez JP. Cutaneous manifestations of filovirus infections. Int J Dermatol 2012;51(9):1037–43.

Warris A, Kroom FP. Viral exanthems. In: Cohen J, Powderly WG, Opal SM, editors. Infectous diseases: expert consult. Philadelphia: Mosby; 2010. p. 99–108.

CHAPTER 32

BACTERIAL AND RICKETTSIAL DISEASES

Dirk M. Elston

> **KEY POINTS**
>
> - Most Gram-positive skin infections can be treated with a semisynthetic penicillin or a cephalosporin.
> - Meticillin-resistant staphylococcal infections typically present as abscess or folliculitis. The primary intervention is drainage.
> - Lyme disease typically presents with erythema migrans and responds to treatment with oral doxycycline. Meningitis or cardiac involvement is treated with intravenous ceftriaxone.
> - Rickettsial diseases often present with a cutaneous eruption, fever, and headache. The treatment drug of choice is doxycycline, and in the case of Rocky Mountain spotted fever the presence of fever and headache in an endemic area should prompt treatment.

BACTERIA

Systemic diseases caused by bacteria produce a variety of cutaneous changes. Dermatologic sequelae may result from bacterial toxins, from hypersensitivity reactions, or from direct cutaneous spread of organisms. Often, the changes produced are highly characteristic and allow for a prompt diagnosis and institution of therapy.

Streptococcal Infections

Scarlet Fever

The characteristic eruption of scarlet fever typically follows infection with group A β-hemolytic streptococci that produce an erythrogenic toxin. Specific antibodies synthesized in response to the toxin confer immunity.

Clinical Manifestations. Scarlet fever occurs predominantly in children and typically follows streptococcal pharyngitis or tonsillitis. The characteristic cutaneous eruption consists of punctate erythematous papules, resulting in a sandpaper texture. The eruption begins on the neck and spreads caudally to involve the trunk and extremities. The palms and soles are generally spared. The face appears flushed, with a circumoral pallor. Petechiae may be present in creases of the elbows, groin, and axillae, a finding commonly referred to as Pastia's lines. The eruption begins to fade after 4 to 5 days with residual desquamation. A "white strawberry" tongue, consisting of prominent, swollen red papillae, appears in the first few days of the illness. This is followed by desquamation leading to the "red strawberry" tongue. Cervical adenopathy and fever are usually present.

Diagnosis. The diagnosis can be confirmed by positive culture showing infection with group A streptococci. Increases in serum levels of antistreptolysin O and anti-DNase B also help confirm recent streptococcal infection.

Treatment. Penicillin is currently the treatment of choice. Erythromycin may be used in penicillin-sensitive patients.

Rheumatic Fever

Rheumatic fever is a sequela of an upper respiratory infection with group A streptococci. The disease is characterized by inflammatory lesions affecting the joints, heart, skin, and central nervous system. The peak age incidence is 5 to 15 years and the recurrence rate in affected individuals is high.

Clinical Manifestations. The clinical manifestations of acute rheumatic fever include erythema marginatum, subcutaneous nodules, polyarthritis, carditis, and chorea. The latency period between the antecedent streptococcal pharyngitis and the onset of symptoms of acute rheumatic fever is about 3 weeks. Erythema marginatum begins as an erythematous macule or papule that extends centrifugally as the central areas clear. Adjacent lesions may coalesce and form a serpiginous pattern. The lesions are evanescent, but the overall eruption may persist for weeks. The subcutaneous nodules are firm, painless lesions varying in size from a few millimeters to a few centimeters. The overlying skin is freely movable and is not inflamed. These lesions occur in crops over bony prominences or tendons.

Diagnosis. The diagnostic criteria originally defined by Duckett Jones use major and minor criteria to support the diagnosis with a high degree of probability.

Treatment. Treatment with penicillin within 1 week of the onset of sore throat may prevent the subsequent onset of rheumatic fever. Antibiotics do not modify the course of an acute rheumatic attack. Acute rheumatic fever may be treated with systemic corticosteroids or supportively with nonsteroidal anti-inflammatory drugs. Prophylaxis with low-dose penicillin effectively prevents recurrence.

Erysipelas and Cellulitis

Erysipelas is a superficial dermal infection with group A streptococci, whereas cellulitis occurs slightly deeper in the dermis.

Clinical Manifestations. Both cellulitis and erysipelas present most commonly on a lower extremity. Facial skin can also be involved, frequently following minor trauma (Fig. 32-1). The characteristic cutaneous lesion is edematous, well demarcated, and dusky red, and may have bullae at the advancing edge. The patient may have toxemia and a high fever. Recurrent erysipelas is strongly associated with lymphedema.

Diagnosis. This diagnosis is largely made on clinical grounds, as isolation of the organism can be difficult. Bilateral disease rarely represents cellulitis and should prompt consideration of alternate diagnoses, especially lipodermatosclerosis. Streptococci cause erysipelas and the majority of cases of cellulitis, while a minority (especially bullous lesions) are caused by staphylococci. Biopsy specimens of the skin reveal dermal edema and a neutrophilic infiltrate.

Treatment. Semisynthetic penicillins or intravenous crystalline penicillin (in the case of erysipelas) are commonly used. Cephalosporins can be used in milder cases of cellulitis and clindamycin is recommended when toxin production is suspected. In penicillin-sensitive individuals, erythromycin may be used.

Impetigo

Impetigo is a superficial skin infection characterized by honey-colored crusting or subcorneal bullae. Streptococci probably initiate most cases of nonbullous impetigo, but may be rapidly outnumbered by *Staphylococcus aureus* once the skin barrier has been breached.

Clinical Manifestations. Honey-colored or dark crusts on an erythematous base are typical (Fig. 32-2). In bullous impetigo, the blisters are so superficial that they rarely remain intact and patients typically present with round denuded areas with peripheral adherent scale (Fig. 32-3).

Diagnosis. Bacterial culture from affected areas will typically yield the causative organism but most patients are treated empirically without culture.

Treatment. Limited cases may be adequately treated with topical antibiotic ointments such as mupirocin or retapamulin. Extensive lesions require systemic antibiotics. Penicillinase-resistant penicillins or cephalosporins represent good first-line therapy although other choices are sometimes appropriate based on the local antibiogram.

Furunculosis and Abscess

A furuncle represents a follicular staphylococcal abscess (Fig. 32-4). A carbuncle is formed by a coalescence of

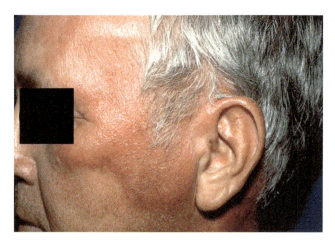

FIGURE 32-1 ■ Erysipelas is characterized by sharp circumscription and a raised border.

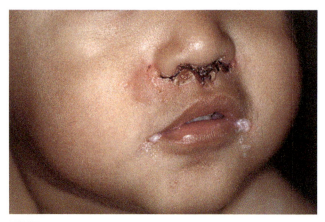

FIGURE 32-2 ■ Impetigo presents with honey-crusted to dark crusts. Nasal carriage is common.

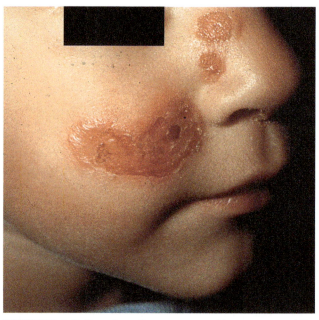

FIGURE 32-3 ■ Bullous impetigo presents with evanescent blisters that rupture quickly leaving a denuded area with a rim of scale.

furuncles. Patients with recurrent furunculosis are often nasal carriers of *S. aureus*, but skin surface carriage in moist areas such as the axilla, groin, and umbilicus may be equally important.

Treatment. Individual lesions should be drained. Widespread lesions require the addition of a penicillinase-resistant penicillin or a first-generation cephalosporin. Meticillin-resistant organisms (Fig. 32-5) should be suspected if the lesions do not respond promptly. Staphylococcal carriage may be treated with mupirocin ointment applied to the anterior nares daily for 5 days and a topical antiseptic such as chlorhexidine or bleach baths (1/4 cup per 1/2 tub) can be used to reduce skin surface carriage. Recent data also support daily oral gargles to control oropharyngeal carriage.

Staphylococcal Scalded Skin Syndrome

Staphylococcal scalded skin syndrome (SSSS) is caused by an exotoxin produced by *S. aureus*, most commonly group II phage type 71. Most patients are children, and most adults with the disorder have renal failure making them unable to eliminate the toxin.

Clinical Manifestations. The infection is heralded by the sudden onset of fever and diffuse, tender, blanchable erythema. The eruption ordinarily begins in the perioral, retroauricular, and flexural regions, with rapid spread to the remainder of the body (Fig. 32-6). Layers of adjacent epidermis may easily peel off with rubbing (Nikolsky sign). The palms, soles, and mucous membranes are spared.

Diagnosis. The diagnosis is usually made clinically. Biopsy specimens will demonstrate acantholysis within the granular layer.

Treatment. The treatment of choice is a penicillinase-resistant penicillin pending isolation of the organism, which is often not cultured from skin, as well as fluid and electrolyte management.

Toxic Shock Syndrome

Toxic shock syndrome is a multisystem illness characterized by fever >38.9°C, diffuse erythematous macules or erythroderma with acral desquamation, hypotension, and systemic involvement of three or more organ systems. It is caused by toxin-producing strains of *S. aureus*, and most reported cases have involved tampon use in menstruating women or wound infections.

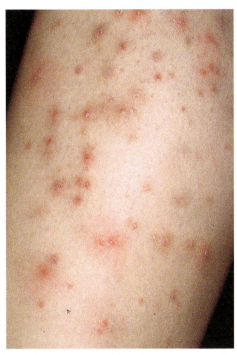

FIGURE 32-4 ■ Staphylococcal folliculitis represents discrete follicular abscesses.

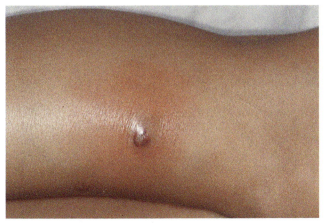

FIGURE 32-5 ■ Community-acquired MRSA infections usually present as abscesses.

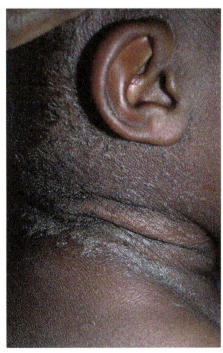

FIGURE 32-6 ■ Staphylococcal scalded skin syndrome presents with erythema and a split at the level of the granular layer.

Clinical Manifestations. The cutaneous eruption is generally a diffuse scarlatiniform erythema. Desquamation occurs about 1 week after the onset of the cutaneous eruption. Strawberry tongue and oral erosions are common.

Diagnosis. In cases related to tampon use, a positive vaginal culture for *S. aureus* can usually be obtained. Blood cultures are less commonly positive.

Treatment. Treatment consists of systemic administration of antistaphylococcal antibiotics as well as aggressive fluid and electrolyte management.

Gram-Negative Infection

Meningococcemia

Meningococcemia is caused by the Gram-negative diplococcus *Neisseria meningitidis*. The incidence has decreased because of the meningococcal vaccine, now routinely recommended for children aged 11 to 12, for those entering high school who have not been previously vaccinated, military recruits entering boot camp, college freshmen, and patients who have had a splenectomy or terminal complement deficiencies, as well as for tourists traveling to epidemic areas, including sub-Saharan Africa and areas in the Middle East, India, and Nepal. If given for travel reasons, the vaccine should be administered at least 1 week prior to departure.

Clinical Manifestations. Acral petechiae are common, but the most characteristic lesions include hemorrhagic stellate infarcts and retiform purpura. Widespread thrombi can lead to purpura fulminans.

Diagnosis. The diagnosis is confirmed by the detection of organisms on Gram stains of cutaneous lesions or blood culture. Biopsy specimens of the skin reveal leukocytoclasia with thrombi and endothelial necrosis involving large and small vessels.

Treatment. A third-generation cephalosporine such as ceftriaxone or cefotaxime is currently the treatment of choice until culture and sensitivity are established. The correction of hemodynamic instability, often in an intensive care unit, is of paramount importance.

Ecthyma Gangrenosum

Patients with ecthyma gangrenosum are typically gravely ill with pustules or hemorrhagic macules surrounded by violaceous halos. The lesions evolve to round ulcers with necrotic black centers. Common sites include intertriginous sites, the buttocks, and extremities. The diagnosis is established by Gram stain and blood culture, which typically demonstrate the Gram-negative bacillus *Pseudomonas aeruginosa*, or less commonly *Serratia marcescens*, *Klebsiella pneumoniae*, *Aeromonas hydrophilia*, *Xanthomonas maltophilia*, *Marganella morganii*, *Escherichia coli*, or *Citrobacter freundii*.

Pseudomonas aeruginosa *Folliculitis (Hot Tub Folliculitis)*

Hot tub folliculitis is characterized by pruritic follicular papules and pustules in intertriginous and covered sites following exposure to an aquatic environment with temperatures conducive to the organism's growth. Lesions typically clear spontaneously in 1 to 2 weeks if the contaminated source of water is addressed.

Cat Scratch Disease

Cat scratch disease is caused by the pleomorphic Gram-negative rod *Bartonella henselae*.

Clinical Manifestations. The initial manifestation of cat scratch disease is a transient papule, which may be followed by fever, malaise, and regional lymphadenopathy. Children may present with conjunctivitis and ipsilateral preauricular adenopathy—the oculoglandular syndrome of Parinaud. The disease may occur through contamination of existing minor wounds or the bite of a flea and does not require an actual cat scratch.

Diagnosis. Indirect fluorescence assay testing and enzyme-linked immuno sorbent assay (ELISA) are used to detect serum antibody to *B. henselae*. In tissue, the organism can best be identified with a Steiner stain or via polymerase chain reaction.

Treatment. Localized cat scratch disease is benign and self-limited. Occasionally, surgical drainage of a suppurative node is indicated. For severe disease or disease in immunocompromised hosts, both rifampin (600 to 900 mg/day) and azithromycin are effective.

Spirochetes

As the causative agent of syphilis, *Treponema pallidum* is discussed in Chapter 29. The only spirochetal organism addressed in this chapter is *Borrelia burgdorferi*.

Lyme Disease

Lyme disease is a multisystem infection caused by the spirochete *B. burgdorferi*. It is the most common tick-borne illness in the United States and is most prevalent along the northeast coast, northern Midwest, and west coast. The primary arthropod vector in the northeast and Midwest is the deer tick *Ixodes scapularis*. *I. pacificus* is the vector on the west coast.

Clinical Manifestations. Erythema migrans is the earliest manifestation and best clinical marker of this systemic disease. It occurs 1 to 2 weeks after the infectious bite and presents as an oval annular lesion that gradually expands circumferentially at a rate of about 1 cm per day. Approximately 20% of patients develop multiple annular lesions at distant sites secondary to *Borrelia* dissemination. Fever, malaise, arthralgias, cardiac and neurologic symptoms suggest more advanced disease. Acrodermatitis chronica atrophicans may be a manifestation of chronic disease characterized by erythematous atrophic lesions on the extremities.

Diagnosis. Serologic testing documents exposure, but only culture and clinical manifestations confirm active disease. ELISA is the usual method of screening, with Western blotting for confirmation. False-positive ELISA results may occur in patients with other infections, including subacute bacterial endocarditis, mononucleosis, leptospirosis, or syphilis, and in patients with systemic lupus erythematosus.

Treatment. Antibiotic management with oral doxycycline is the treatment of choice for patients with erythema migrans. Meningitis or cardiac involvement are treated with intravenous ceftriaxone. Amoxicillin is preferred for children and for pregnant or lactating women.

Rickettsia

Rickettsiae are obligate intracellular organisms with a propensity to infect vascular endothelial cells.

Rocky Mountain Spotted Fever

Rocky Mountain spotted fever (RMSF) is the most frequently reported rickettsial disease in the United States. Without treatment RMSF has a 30% mortality rate; with effective treatment this drops to 3% to 5%. The causative agent, *Rickettsia rickettsii*, is transmitted by the wood tick *Dermacentor andersoni* in western states, and in the eastern United States by the dog tick *D. variabilis*.

Clinical Manifestations. After an incubation period of about 5 to 10 days, severe headache, fever, and myalgias develop. In endemic areas, the presence of fever and headache justify treatment. Cutaneous lesions include hemorrhagic macules of the wrists, ankles, palms, and soles.

Diagnosis. Confirmation of the diagnosis can be achieved by indirect immunofluorescence assay, ELISA, immunoblot, and latex agglutination. Demonstration of *Rickettsiae* in a biopsy specimen of the skin by a direct immunofluorescence microscopic technique using a specific antibody or immunohistochemistry is also possible.

Treatment. The treatment of choice in adults and children is doxycycline; the mortality of untreated RMSF outweighs concerns for potential doxycycline-related dental adverse effects.

Endemic Typhus

Endemic typhus is caused by *R. typhi* and is transmitted by the rat flea *Xenopsylla cheopis* in western states and by *R. felis* transmitted by cat fleas in south Texas.

Clinical Manifestations. After a 12-day incubation period, a prodrome consisting of fever, chills, severe headache, and nausea develops. A few days later, a morbilliform, often petechial, cutaneous eruption appears and primarily involves the trunk. Splenomegaly and regional or widespread lymphadenopathy may be present. Systemic large-vessel vasculitis is a rare complication.

Diagnosis. The diagnosis can be made by complement fixation tests or by indirect fluorescence antibody studies using acute and convalescent sera.

Treatment. Doxycycline is the current treatment of choice.

Epidemic Typhus

Epidemic typhus is caused by *R. prowazekii* and is transmitted by the human body louse *Pediculus humanus* var. *corporis*. The primary animal reservoir is the flying squirrel, *Glaucomys volans*.

Clinical Manifestations. After a 12-day incubation period, the disease is heralded by fever, chills, headache, and weakness. A few days later a truncal macular eruption appears and spreads distally, sparing the face, palms, and soles. These macular lesions may subsequently become hemorrhagic and may lead to gangrene.

Diagnosis. Complement fixation and indirect fluorescent antibodies are available.

Treatment. The current treatment of choice is doxycycline.

Rickettsial Pox

Rickettsial pox is a mild febrile disease caused by *R. akari* and is transmitted by the housemouse mite *Allodermanyssus sanguineus*. It is common in the New York metropolitan area.

Clinical Manifestations. A primary erythematous papular lesion occurs at the site of the mite bite, which may develop an eschar, followed by fever, headache, myalgias, and a generalized varicella-like vesicular cutaneous eruption. Generalized lymphadenopathy and splenomegaly may be present.

Diagnosis. Complement fixation and indirect fluorescent antibodies or demonstration of the organism by direct fluorescent antibody or immunohistochemistry will establish the diagnosis.

Treatment. Most patients recover without treatment, but doxycycline may be required in severe cases.

Scrub Typhus

Scrub typhus, or tsutsugamushi fever, is caused by *Orientia tsutsugamushi* transmitted by trombiculid mites (chiggers). It is most common in Southeast Asia, Japan, Korea, and Australia.

Clinical Manifestations. A primary eschar develops within 1 to 2 weeks. A few days later, a truncal morbilliform cutaneous eruption, resembling roseola or rubella, develops and spreads peripherally, accompanied by high fevers and myalgia. Most deaths result from disseminated intravascular coagulation.

Diagnosis. Complement fixation and indirect fluorescent antibodies are available.

Treatment. The current treatment of choice is doxycycline.

SUGGESTED READINGS

Atanaskova N, et al. Innovative management of recurrent furunculosis. Dermatol Clin 2010;28:479.

Bangert S, et al. Bacterial resistance and impetigo treatment trends. Pediatr Dermatol 2012;29:243–8.

Berk DR, et al. MRSA, staphylococcal scalded skin syndrome, and other cutaneous bacterial emergencies. Pediatr Ann 2010;39:627–33.

Elston D. Community acquired methicillin-resistant *Staphylococcus aureus*. J Am Acad Dermatol 2007;56:1–16.

Gutierrez K, et al. Staphylococcal infections in children, California, USA, 1985–2009. Emerg Infec Dis 2013;19:10–20.

Thomas KS, et al. Penicillin to prevent recurrent leg cellulitis. N Engl J Med 2013;368:1695–703.

CHAPTER 33

FUNGAL DISEASES

Scott A. Norton

KEY POINTS

- Fungal pathogens affect the skin in many ways: superficial fungi, such as the dermatophytes, rarely cause systemic disease. Subcutaneous mycoses, such as sporotrichosis, mycetoma, and chromoblastomycosis, are typically caused by minor, inadvertent trauma that introduces environmental fungi into the skin and subcutaneous tissues. Host immunologic response toward these typically low-virulence fungi is muted.
- The classic systemic mycoses (histoplasmosis, coccidioidomycosis, blastomycosis, and paracoccidioidomycosis) are nearly always acquired via inhalation of fungal spores. Once in the lungs, the fungi adopt a pathogenic yeast-phase growth pattern. Infections are often limited to a transient pneumonitis but can disseminate hematogenously to any organ, although the skin is perhaps the most common target of a disseminated systemic mycosis.
- Immunocompromised patients are vulnerable to severe, rapidly life-threatening fungal diseases, such as aspergillosis and mucormycosis.
- Treatment for subcutaneous mycoses often requires dual therapy, e.g., oral antifungal agents with adjunctive surgical debridement.
- Treatment for inhalational mycoses is not required in cases of transient subclinical infections. For more severe cases (and especially in immunocompromised patients), treatment may consist of intravenous antifungal medications followed by prolonged oral suppressive therapy.
- There are literally tens of thousands of fungal species on earth of which less than 25 infect humans regularly—although perhaps hundreds have been isolated as rare causes of systemic disease, particularly in immunocompromised patients.

For clinical purposes, cutaneous fungal infections with systemic involvement can be divided into *subcutaneous mycoses* and *systemic mycoses*, based on the mode of acquisition and the extent of tissue involvement. The subcutaneous mycoses, of which sporotrichosis is the best known, may be considered "implantation mycoses" because they are typically acquired via traumatic percutaneous inoculation from a contaminated object.

The systemic mycoses, in contrast, may be considered "inhalational mycoses" because they are typically acquired via the respiratory route. The systemic mycoses comprise two subgroups: four diseases (histoplasmosis, coccidioidomycosis, blastomycosis, paracoccidioidomycosis) that usually cause subclinical or transient, self-limited pulmonary infections in immunocompetent individuals. Nevertheless, they may disseminate to involve the skin in both immunocompetent and immunocompromised hosts. In immunocompetent hosts, cutaneous involvement often presents with chronic crusted or granulomatous papules or plaques.

The systemic mycoses also include a subgroup of opportunistic diseases (e.g., cryptococcosis, mucormycosis, aspergillosis) that occur almost exclusively in immunocompromised hosts. These, too, may involve the skin after hematogenous dissemination. Because of the nature of the host's immunologic status, these infections often present as acute, rapidly evolving, necrotizing infections.

The most prevalent cutaneous mycoses, dermatophyte infections, are caused by keratinophilic fungi that infect epidermis, hair, and nails but rarely cause systemic disease (extremely rare instances in severely compromised hosts). These will not be discussed further. Notably, active untreated dermatophyte infections can damage the epidermal barrier and serve as a portal of entry for other infectious agents, particularly bacteria and yeasts, and complete dermatologic examination is important when searching for potential sources of infection in all hosts.

SUBCUTANEOUS MYCOSES WITH SYSTEMIC MANIFESTATIONS

The subcutaneous mycoses are caused by taxonomically diverse fungi that ordinarily subsist on decaying organic matter and have few intrinsic virulence factors. Typically people acquire these conditions through minor, often unnoticed, percutaneous trauma with dead or decaying plant materials. Mammalian immune responses to these organisms are rarely vigorous and rarely effective; therefore these mycoses usually develop into chronic, unremitting infections that are confined to skin and subcutaneous tissues. Subcutaneous mycoses are most common among people in tropical and warm temperate areas who are routinely exposed to decaying organic matter. Farmers and people who gather firewood, especially if they are barefoot, are at greatest risk.

Several other subcutaneous infections that follow minor trauma, specifically pythiosis, rhinosporidiosis, actinomycetoma, and protothecosis, are occasionally included in sections on fungal diseases, even though taxonomic tools show that the pathogens are, indeed, not fungi. These will not be discussed further.

SPOROTRICHOSIS

Sporotrichosis, caused by *Sporothrix schenckii*, has worldwide distribution, but occurs most commonly in warm, humid areas where conditions favor its saprophytic growth. The organism typically enters the skin through minor injuries with plant materials, such as rose thorns, sphagnum moss, and damp straw, on which the fungus grows. Rarely, *Sporothrix* spores may be inhaled, causing pulmonary infection with subsequent cutaneous dissemination. Currently, the largest disease clusters of any type of sporotrichosis are among children in Brazil's urban slums, where feral cats serve as the reservoir.

Clinical Manifestations

Classic sporotrichosis begins as a small painless papule at the inoculation site (Fig. 33-1). Lesions usually evolve into firm, violaceous, dermal nodules. The surface may ulcerate, forming a sporotrichotic chancre with a ragged necrotic base, surrounded by epitheliomatous hyperplasia. When primary lesions are on distal extremities, local extension, called sporotrichoid spread, may occur via cutaneous lymphatic channels. This produces an ascending chain of either smooth dermal nodules or of ulcerating subcutaneous nodules (Fig. 33-2). Lesions are most common on the hands and arms, but fixed centrofacial disease may occur in children, especially those with cat exposure (Fig. 33-3).

Disseminated sporotrichosis is rare; it requires hematogenous dissemination from either primary cutaneous infection or primary inhalational disease. The most common extracutaneous sites are lungs, bones, and meninges. Risk factors for dissemination include hematologic/lymphoreticular malignancies, alcoholism, immunosuppressive medications, and AIDS.

Diagnosis

Because *Sporothrix* organisms are usually sparse in tissue, histopathologic diagnosis of sporotrichosis has low sensitivity. Culture on standard Sabouraud's agar quickly grows a distinctive dark mold.

Treatment

Itraconazole is preferred to treat localized disease in immunocompetent adults. Oral potassium iodide solution is added in resistant cases. Disseminated disease usually requires amphotericin B followed by prolonged itraconazole therapy. In Brazil and Mexico, countries with high rates of sporotrichosis, oral terbinafine is the standard treatment.

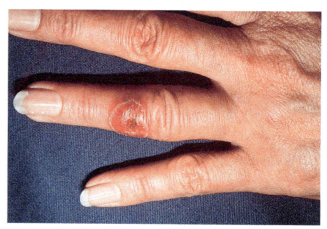

FIGURE 33-1 ■ A chancriform lesion on the digit in a patient with sporotrichosis.

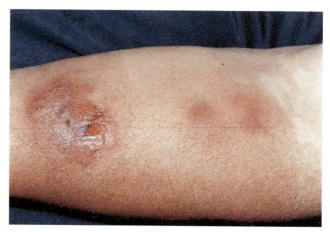

FIGURE 33-2 ■ Lymphangitic spread in a patient with sporotrichosis.

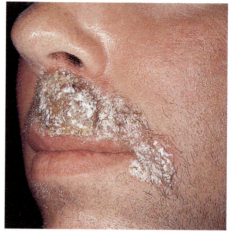

FIGURE 33-3 ■ Facial lesions of sporotrichosis.

OTHER SUBCUTANEOUS MYCOSES

Uncommon inoculation mycoses, such as chromoblastomycosis, eumycetoma, lobomycosis, and entomophthoromycosis, are generally limited to cutaneous and subcutaneous tissues. Dissemination is rare, but may occur in immunocompromised patients. These will not be discussed further.

SYSTEMIC MYCOSES

Four closely related species of fungi can cause systemic illness in immunocompetent individuals. These are *Histoplasma capsulatum* (histoplasmosis), *Blastomyces dermatitidis* (blastomycosis), *Coccidioides immitis* (coccidioidomycosis), and *Paracoccidioides brasiliensis* (paracoccidioidomycosis). The diseases are sometimes collectively called *endemic mycoses* because each was once regarded as having a restricted geographic distribution. They are also classified as *thermally dimorphic mycoses* because cultured colonies have one of two temperature-dependent morphologic appearances. At room temperature, which mimics their natural, outdoor saprophytic phase, cultures produce molds (extensive networks of hyphae that have a woolly or cottony appearance). In contrast, at body temperature, cultures form uniform, smooth colonies of yeast-like organisms. In histologic sections of diseased tissue (whether from skin, lung, or other organs), one sees only yeast, sometimes forming reproductive buds, but never hyphae. Sporotrichosis and *Penicillium marneffei* infection are also caused by thermally dimorphic fungi; these conditions are discussed elsewhere in this chapter.

People acquire these diseases mainly via inhalation of spores released by molds in nature, then lead to primary pulmonary infections. Within human tissues, the organisms assume their pathogenic yeast phase, which reproduce by forming buds with distinctive, diagnostic characteristics. In tissue, *C. immitis* forms distinctive spherical structures that produce daughter endospores internally. In histopathologic specimens, special fungal stains, such as Gomori methenamine silver or periodic acid–Schiff, greatly facilitate identification of these fungi.

A cautionary note is that dimorphic fungi should be cultured and examined in facilities with special mycologic capabilities. At room temperature, the molds, especially *C. immitis*, produce easily aerosolized propagules that create risk for accidental laboratory transmission.

Primary cutaneous involvement may occur with any of these diseases. It is rare and occurs after percutaneous inoculation of organisms.

HISTOPLASMOSIS

Histoplasmosis has been regarded as a disease primarily of the east-central United States, particularly along the Ohio River basin. In fact, *H. capsulatum* grows naturally in bird or bat guano and is found worldwide. A subspecies, *H. capsulatum* var. *duboisii*, causes disease in sub-Saharan Africa. Most histoplasmosis cases are subclinical or present as mild, self-limited pneumonitis. Disseminated histoplasmosis is a common opportunistic infection in patients with AIDS, malignancy, and other forms of immunosuppression.

Clinical Manifestations

Inhalation of spores leads to initial infection, which is asymptomatic in >80% of infected individuals. Many others have transient, self-resolving pneumonitis, often misdiagnosed as bronchitis or atypical bacterial pneumonia. Cutaneous histoplasmosis follows hematogenous dissemination from a primary pulmonary focus. Cutaneous lesions have a variety of nonspecific morphologies, including macules, papules/plaques, pustules/abscesses, ulcers, and purpuric infiltrates. Mucosal, especially oropharyngeal, ulcers are more common than lesions on keratinized skin. Erythema nodosum is a common but nonspecific reactive dermatosis, indicating a strong, successful immunologic response after primary exposure.

Diagnosis

Histoplasmosis is diagnosed by tissue or sputum cultures, serologic antibody tests, and/or urinary antigen studies. Biopsy specimens from skin or mucosa (along with lung, bone marrow, or other infected tissues) show perivascular inflammation with lymphocytes, plasma cells, and characteristic parasitized histiocytes that may contain abundant intracellular yeast, 1 to 3 µm each, which must be distinguished from several similar-sized intracellular pathogens, such as *Leishmania*. In patients with disseminated disease, bone marrow biopsy and culture may lead to the correct diagnosis. Histoplasmin skin testing is useful for population-based epidemiologic studies, not for establishing individual diagnoses.

Treatment

Patients with severe pulmonary infection or with cutaneous or mucocutaneous lesions, indicative of disseminated disease, require treatment with intravenous amphotericin. In immunocompromised patients, amphotericin is usually followed by long-term oral itraconazole therapy. Conversely, immunocompetent patients with benign, self-limited pneumonitis may be treated with supportive care alone.

COCCIDIOIDOMYCOSIS

Coccidioidomycosis, also called valley fever, is caused by infection with *C. immitis*, a soil saprophyte endemic to arid regions of southwestern United States, northern Mexico, parts of Central America, and South America. As with other respiratory mycoses, infection occurs after inhalation of spores, most commonly in people whose work exposes them to desert soil, such as farm workers, archeologists, military personnel, and construction workers. Outbreaks often occur after desert soils are stirred up by natural phenomena, such as earthquakes and dust storms. For poorly understood immunologic reasons, coccidioidomycosis is particularly virulent in African-Americans, Filipino-Americans, and in pregnant women. Immunocompromised states, including lymphoproliferative diseases and AIDS, are additional risks for dissemination.

Clinical Manifestations

Most people infected with coccidioidomycosis have asymptomatic infections. The remainder may develop primary coccidioidomycosis, a pneumonitis presenting with fever, pleuritic cough, and myalgias. Some patients have morbilliform eruptions during the acute episode. Others may develop typical erythema nodosum, a favorable sign that heralds prompt, uncomplicated resolution, seen mostly in young, healthy Caucasian/European women. Erythema multiforme may also be observed. These cutaneous reactions are nonspecific but in certain settings should prompt a suspicion of coccidioidomycosis, warranting diagnostic investigation. In normal hosts, pneumonitis clears within a month but chronic and disseminated disease occasionally occurs.

In disseminated cases, cutaneous lesions have diverse clinical morphologies, including papules, pustules, subcutaneous abscesses, granulomatous plaques, and ulcers (Fig. 33-4). Hematogenous dissemination may cause osseous coccidioidomycosis with direct cutaneous extension.

Diagnosis

Dermatologists are best able to diagnose coccidioidomycosis by finding large 30 to 60 μm spherules, with abundant endospores, in biopsy material. Other diagnostic techniques include antibody serologies and urine antigen studies. Fungal culture must be performed in specialized biosafety laboratories because at room temperature, arthroconidia are easily aerosolized, thereby risking laboratory transmission. Coccidioidin skin testing is useful for population-based epidemiologic studies, not for establishing individual diagnoses.

Treatment

In most cases, the transient primary pneumonitis resolves spontaneously; however, it is important to treat patients with immunogenetic risks, e.g., Filipino-Americans, to prevent dissemination. Amphotericin B is the treatment of choice for disseminated disease, often followed by long-term maintenance with itraconazole or fluconazole.

BLASTOMYCOSIS

Most cases of North American blastomycosis occur in states that encompass the Mississippi and Ohio River basins, where soils are rich with decaying organic matter. Cases occur in people exposed to forested areas (loggers, hunters, campers). Blastomycosis has been reported from most continents but the epidemiology outside the United States is poorly known.

Clinical Manifestations

Approximately 50% of infected patients develop symptomatic pneumonitis, presenting with cough, fevers, and myalgias. Most patients recover without antifungal treatment but some develop chronic pulmonary infection with subsequent hematogenous spread to skin, bones, or genitourinary tract. The skin is the most common extrapulmonary site. Cutaneous lesions typically start as papules or pustules on the head, neck, or extremities and evolve into indurated, verrucous plaques with actively expanding borders and central atrophic scars (Figs 33-5 and 33-6). Without treatment, the lesions continue to enlarge and may be destructive. Primary inoculation cutaneous disease has been reported in veterinarians who perform

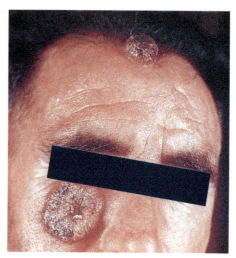

FIGURE 33-5 ■ Verrucous plaque on the cheek in a patient with North American blastomycosis.

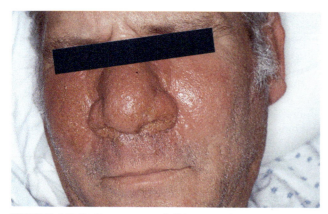

FIGURE 33-4 ■ Erythematous, cellulitic-appearing eruption on the malar skin and the nose in a man with coccidioidomycosis.

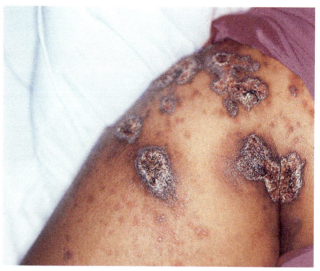

FIGURE 33-6 ■ Verrucous plaques on the arm of a patient with blastomycosis.

autopsies on dogs, as dogs have a higher incidence of pulmonary blastomycosis than do humans.

Diagnosis

Acute respiratory infection is confirmed by a sputum examination and culture. Cutaneous lesions are useful for histopathologic examination and fungal culture. The quickest way to diagnose cutaneous blastomycosis is with a potassium hydroxide preparation performed on material scraped from pustules or dark punctae that stud the lesional verrucous surfaces. One looks for yeast with a characteristic broad-based budding.

Treatment

Pulmonary disease is treated with amphotericin B. Limited cutaneous disease may be treated with oral itraconazole. Treatment duration is guided by the extent of dissemination and the patient's immune status. Blastomycosis occurs in immunocompromised patients less often than the endemic mycoses.

PARACOCCIDIOIDOMYCOSIS

Paracoccidioidomycosis, also called South American blastomycosis, is restricted to Central and South America, where it usually presents with a tuberculosis-like pulmonary syndrome accompanied by cervical adenitis and granulomatous oral lesions. Estrogen seems to suppress virulence factors, so in people aged 10 to 50 years, it is seen almost exclusively in males. AIDS patients have a particularly troublesome course.

OPPORTUNISTIC FUNGAL INFECTIONS

Opportunistic fungal infections are most commonly caused by two groups of yeasts (*Candida* and *Cryptococcus*) and two groups of molds (Mucorales and *Aspergillus*). These organisms—and hundreds of other fungal species—are found worldwide, yet cause significant disease almost exclusively in severely immunocompromised patients, especially those with AIDS, hematologic malignancies, or high-dose corticosteroid and/or cytotoxic therapy.

CRYPTOCOCCOSIS

Cryptococcosis is a systemic infection caused by closely related species, *Cryptococcus neoformans* and *Cryptococcus gattii*. The organisms are nearly ubiquitous in nature, subsisting on bird guano, and cause human disease worldwide, typically by inhalational means.

Clinical Manifestations

Cryptococcosis produces a pneumonia-like illness consisting of dyspnea and fever. Severe central nervous system manifestations are common in AIDS patients as both initial—and terminal—presentations. Cutaneous lesions are relatively common but are difficult to diagnose clinically because of diverse clinical morphology. AIDS patients with disseminated disease may have abundant, monomorphous, umbilicated, skin-colored to slightly hypopigmented, facial papules. This appearance resembles molluscum contagiosum, a poxvirus infection that is common in AIDS patients. Other opportunistic mycoses (histoplasmosis and *P. marneffei* infection) may also present with molluscum-like papules. Another common presentation in immunosuppressed patients, called cryptococcal cellulitis, consists of large, indurated, red patches and plaques (Fig. 33-7).

Diagnosis

Cryptococcal antigen tests are available for both blood and cerebrospinal fluid. In tissue, *Cryptococcus* can be identified with mucicarmine stain, which accentuates the yeast's capsule but does not stain other fungi with similar histologic morphology; bedside diagnostic tests including skin touch preps with India ink may rapidly identify this pathogen. Because skin involvement is mostly the result of dissemination, one must identify and treat other foci, particularly the central nervous system.

Treatment

The treatment of choice for cryptococcal meningoencephalitis is systemic amphotericin B combined with flucytosine. Fluconazole is a useful prophylaxis in HIV patients with prior cryptococcal meningoencephalitis. In milder, noncentral nervous system disease, prolonged fluconazole therapy may be required.

MUCORMYCOSIS

Mucormycosis is caused by opportunistic pathogens from *Rhizopus*, *Absidia*, *Mucor*, and related genera. These fungi

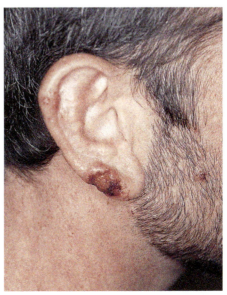

FIGURE 33-7 ■ Nodular, ulcerated lesions of disseminated cryptococcosis in an HIV-infected patient.

were formerly classified as zygomycetes, but advances in molecular taxonomy have changed the nomenclature. Mucormycetes are ubiquitous saprophytic molds found in soil and decaying matter. Infection occurs usually in patients with organ transplantation, hematologic malignancy, or uncontrolled diabetes mellitus. Mucormycetes infections are rising in frequency with the advent of antifungal prophylaxis targeting *Aspergillus* in the bone marrow transplant setting. In mammalian tissues, the fungi are angiotropic, producing extensive hyphal invasion of blood vessels, rapidly leading to widespread vascular thrombosis and tissue necrosis.

Clinical Manifestations

The most common form of mucormycosis with cutaneous involvement is rhinocerebral infection. It has a particular affinity for patients with diabetic ketoacidosis and starts acutely with midfacial and periorbital swelling, necrotic intranasal ulcers, invasion of nasal sinuses, and bloody nasal discharge. Rapid extension into deeper tissues may cause cranial nerve palsies en route to frequently fatal cerebral involvement. In addition, cutaneous lesions may follow hematogenous spread from primary pulmonary disease or from rare primary inoculation of the skin. Disseminated cutaneous lesions often produce necrotic ulcers with black eschars, resembling ecthyma gangrenosum.

Diagnosis

Possible mucormycosis must be evaluated emergently because of its high mortality, even when treated with appropriate antifungal agents. If cutaneous infection is suspected, rapid diagnosis is important, and may be augmented with frozen-section biopsies or touch-prep examinations of skin specimens in real time. In skin biopsy specimens, mucormycosis appears as extensive networks of intravascular (angioinvasive) hyphae that have variable widths, lack septae, and branch at near right angles (vs the uniform caliber of dermatophyte hyphae, which are regularly septate and have regular acute-angle bifurcations). Mucormycetes grow quickly on culture, producing cottony or woolly colonies, which require microscopic examination for speciation.

Treatment

Managing mucormycosis requires a multidisciplinary approach. Addressing the patient's immunocompromised state, if possible, is essential; often this means controlling diabetic ketoacidosis. Surgical debridement of infected tissues may be necessary, and is indicated in most cases of either limited or primary cutaneous/primary inoculation mucormycotic infections. Liposomal amphotericin B is the treatment of choice for serious infections. Newer third-generation azole agents, e.g., posaconazole, may help patients with lesser infections or who cannot tolerate amphotericin.

ASPERGILLOSIS

Aspergillosis is an opportunistic infection caused by several *Aspergillus* species, commonly *Aspergillus fumigatus* and *Aspergillus niger*. These and other *Aspergillus* species are often cultured from nails and cutaneous surfaces, yet misinterpreted as pathogens rather than recognized as benign commensal fungi. True cutaneous infections with *Aspergillus* may be primary or secondary conditions. Primary aspergillosis is caused by direct inoculation from contaminated materials, which, while rare, is more common in children than adults. More common overall is secondary cutaneous aspergillosis, which follows lymphatic or hematogenous spread from primary pulmonary foci. Patients with hematologic malignancies, those on immunosuppressive medications, and children with chronic granulomatous disease or cystic fibrosis are at risk for systemic aspergillosis.

Clinical Manifestations

Aspergillus pathogens cause several pulmonary syndromes, as well as disseminated aspergillosis, which can produce secondary cutaneous lesions, endocarditis, and endophthalmitis. Primary cutaneous aspergillosis is typically associated with contaminated adhesive dressings, intravenous lines, central venous catheters, or contaminated burns and other traumatic wounds. Cutaneous lesions are nonspecific, including macules, papules, hemorrhagic bullae, and ulcerations (Fig. 33-8). Secondary cutaneous aspergillosis may produce shallow necrotic ulcers with black eschars, essentially a type of ecthyma gangrenosum, another feared condition in individuals with hematologic malignancies.

Diagnosis

Skin biopsy specimens show septate hyphae with acute-angle branching, enmeshed in a neutrophilic dermal infiltrate, accompanied by necrosis and granuloma formation. More sophisticated molecular and serologic studies, such as assays for fungal antigens, galactomannin and β-D-glucan, have increasing roles in detecting *Aspergillus*, especially in the intensive care unit setting. While waiting for confirmatory fungal culture and serologic tests, one should initiate empiric antifungal therapy based on clinical suspicion.

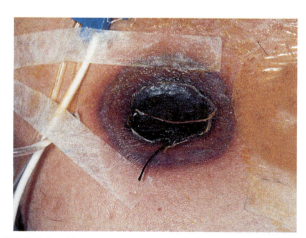

FIGURE 33-8 ■ Nodular lesions of aspergillosis following a bone marrow transplant.

Treatment

Amphotericin B is an effective empiric treatment for systemic aspergillosis, while awaiting diagnostic confirmation especially if mucormycosis, which resists voriconazole, is in the differential.

CANDIDIASIS

The genus *Candida* comprises many yeast-like fungi, some of which are an innocuous part of one's natural colonic flora. These and other *Candida* species may nevertheless cause a variety of opportunistic infections, especially in newborns, uncontrolled diabetics, and AIDS patients. Host immunologic factors account for the variability in clinical disease and determine the likelihood of life-threatening infections.

Clinical Manifestations

Localized *Candida* infections of skin and mucosa are common and include oropharyngeal candidiasis (thrush), vulvovaginitis, balanitis, intertrigo, chronic paronychia, and diaper dermatitis. Predisposing factors include heat, occlusion, moisture, impaired epithelial barrier function, and antibiotic or corticosteroid therapy. Diabetes mellitus potentiates colonization by *Candida*.

Candidiasis may affect any epithelial surface, with a predilection for moist skin folds (axillae, groin, beneath breasts, or under a pannus). The clinical appearance is usually moist and "beefy" red, often with satellite nonfollicular pustules (Fig. 33-9). Oral candidiasis usually presents as a white exudate that coats lingual and buccal mucosa (Fig. 33-10). In immunocompetent patients, natural host defenses generally limit the extent of clinical disease. Persistent, severe candidiasis may indicate malignancy or HIV infection. Oropharyngeal candidiasis, often seen in AIDS patients, causes dysphagia, leading to inanition.

Systemic candidiasis, usually resulting from a primary gastrointestinal source, is life-threatening. Most cases are caused by *Candida albicans*, followed by *Candida tropicalis*, the most common candidal species to disseminate to skin. Secondary cutaneous lesions are nonspecific and include red-to-purple macules, papules, pustules, pseudovesicles, and vasculopathic lesions.

Chronic mucocutaneous candidiasis is part of a heterogeneous group of disorders characterized by failure of T-cell lymphocytes to respond properly to *Candida*. In most chronic mucocutaneous candidiasis patients, the disease has its onset in childhood. Skin, nails, and mucous membranes are commonly affected and generally resist therapy.

Diagnosis

Local candidiasis can be diagnosed with potassium hydroxide preparations that, when performed on appropriate specimens, reveal budding yeast or pseudohyphae. Whenever candidemia is suspected, blood cultures are necessary.

Treatment

Limited cutaneous *Candida* infections can often be managed topically. In immunodeficient patients with disseminated candidiasis, systemic therapy with fluconazole or an echinocandin is indicated. Patients who have been on prolonged prophylaxis (such as after a bone marrow transplant) where resistance is an issue, or those who are infected with *Candida glabrata* or *Candida krusei*, are often treated with micafungin.

EMERGING OPPORTUNISTIC MYCOSES

P. marneffei occurs naturally in wet rice-growing areas of southeast Asia. Over the past two decades, it has been increasingly recognized as a multisystem pathogen of AIDS patients. Patients typically have a febrile illness with tuberculosis-like pulmonary disease and widespread molluscum-like papules. All patients to date have had clear epidemiologic links with Thailand or environs.

Paecilomyces lilacinus is increasingly reported as an opportunistic pathogen of bone marrow transplant patients

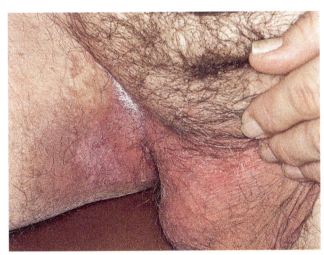

FIGURE 33-9 ■ Erythematous scaly plaque in the groin characteristic of candidal intertrigo.

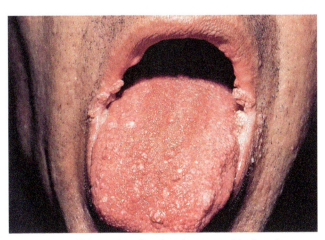

FIGURE 33-10 ■ Mucosal surface involvement with chronic mucocutaneous candidiasis.

and has a penchant for ocular infection. It often resists medical treatment and may require surgical debridement. Several members of the yeast-like genus, Trichosporon, are commonly found in nature and as commensal organisms on humans. Several species can produce mild superficial infections of the integument, e.g., concretions on hair shafts known as white piedra or *Candida*-like intertrigo, Other species, such as *T. asahii* and *T. cutaneum*, are increasingly detected as virulent invasive pathogens, particularly in patients with advanced HIV infections or who are undergoing treatment for hematologic malignancies. The dermatological manifestations of disseminated trichosporonosis vary widely, from pustules to necrotic ulcers. Invasive trichosporon infections are challenging to treat; limited therapeutic data are available but point to removal (or changing) of any medical lines and surgical devices and to courses of systemic triazole antifungal medications.

SUGGESTED READINGS

Barros MB, de Almeida Paes R, Schubach AO. *Sporothrix schenckii* and sporotrichosis. Clin Microbiol Rev 2011;24:633–54.

Norton SA. Deep fungal skin infections. In: James WD, editor. Military dermatology. Textbook of military medicine, vol. 3. Washington: Office of the Surgeon General; 1995. p. 453–92.

Ruddy BE, Mayer AP, Ko MG, Labonte HR, Borovansky JA, Boroff ES, et al. Coccidioidomycosis in African Americans. Mayo Clin Proc 2011;86:63–9.

Segal BH. Aspergillosis. N Engl J Med 2009;360:1870–84.

Smith JA, Kauffman CA. Blastomycosis. Proc Am Thorac Soc 2010;7:173–80.

Welsh O, Vera-Cabrera L, Rendon A, Gonzalez G, Bonifaz A. Coccidioidomycosis. Clin Dermatol 2012;30:573–91.

CHAPTER 34

PROTOZOAL DISEASES

Dirk M. Elston

KEY POINTS

- Trichomoniasis typically presents with vaginal pruritus and a frothy discharge, and responds well to treatment with metronidazole.
- Systemic therapy for leishmaniasis is recommended for patients who are immunosuppressed or who acquire infection in areas where mucocutaneous disease has been reported.
- Suramin remains useful to treat early Rhodesian trypanosomiasis, while melarsoprol is the drug of choice for central nervous system (CNS) disease. Pentamidine is still used for Gambian disease.
- For American trypanosomiasis, nifurtimox and benznidazole are used to reduce the severity of the acute illness.
- *Acanthamoeba* affects immunocompromised individuals, while *Balamuthia mandrillaris* causes erythema and induration of the central face and CNS invasion in previously healthy patients.

TRICHOMONIASIS

Clinical Manifestations

Trichomoniasis is caused by *Trichomonas vaginalis*, a flagellate protozoan. Trichomoniasis typically presents with vaginal pruritus, a burning sensation, and a frothy discharge. Male sexual partners may present with balanoposthitis.

Diagnosis

A wet mount typically demonstrates the motile organism, but direct fluorescent antibody and polymerase chain reaction (PCR) assays are also available.

Treatment

Treatment includes metronidazole, 2 g in a single oral dose or 500 mg twice a day for 7 days. A topical form is also available. Patients should be warned about disulfiram-type effects if alcohol is consumed. In pregnant women, topical clotrimazole may be used instead.

LEISHMANIASIS

Clinical Manifestations

The rural type of Old World leishmaniasis is characterized by moist chronic ulcers that heal within 6 months. Rodent reservoirs carry the organism, which is transmitted via a sand fly vector. Dry lesions and recurrent lesions (leishmaniasis recidivans) are associated with the urban type of disease, caused by *Leishmania tropica*. New World disease may consist of only cutaneous lesions, especially with the *mexicana* variety. The primary lesion begins as a papule that becomes crusted, verrucous, or ulcerated, with an infiltrated red border (Figs 34-1 and 34-2). Subcutaneous peripheral nodules represent a lymphangitic pattern of spread and lymphadenopathy may be present. On the Yucatan Peninsula and in Guatemala, the workers who harvest chicle for chewing gum develop chiclero ulcers on the ear. The etiologic agent is *Leishmania mexicana* and the sand fly vector *Lutzomyia flaviscutellata* (Fig. 34-3). Uta occurs in the Peruvian highlands. As with the chiclero ulcer, lesions are found on exposed sites and mucosal lesions do not occur.

Disseminated cutaneous leishmaniasis occurs with both New and Old World diseases, but the most destructive manifestations occur with mucocutaneous New World disease. Diffuse anergic leishmaniasis may resemble lepromatous leprosy or Lobo's disease.

Old World *L. tropica*, *Leishmania major*, *Leishmania aethiopica*, and *Leishmania infantum* cause cutaneous leishmaniasis. The latter also produced the Mediterranean form of visceral leishmaniasis. New World *L. mexicana* does not induce mucosal disease. *Leishmania braziliensis guyanensis*, *Leishmania braziliensis braziliensis*, and *Leishmania braziliensis panamensis* produce cutaneous lesions and the latter two are also associated with mucocutaneous disease. *Leishmania donovani* spp. *donovani*, *infantum*, and *chagasi* cause visceral leishmaniasis.

Cutaneous leishmaniasis is endemic in Southwest Asia, the Mediterranean and Latin America. In the United States, cutaneous leishmaniasis is most common in South Texas, but rare reports of cutaneous disease have occurred as far north as Pennsylvania and the Midwest.

Dogs and rodents are the natural reservoir hosts. The Old World vector is the *Phlebotomus* sand fly, whereas *Phlebotomus perniciosus* and *Lutzomyia* sand flies are the vectors for New World leishmaniasis. In humans, the aflagellare form (amastigote) is found in tissue.

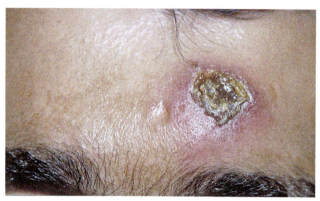

FIGURE 34-1 ■ Cutaneous leishmaniasis. Crust on an indurated base.

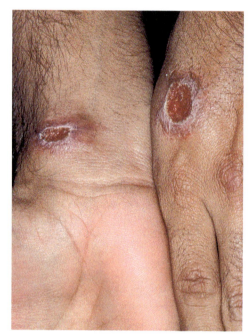

FIGURE 34-2 ■ Cutaneous leishmaniasis.

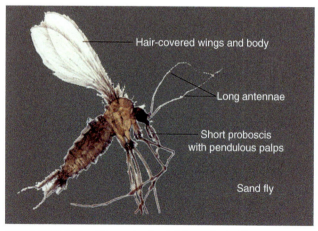

FIGURE 34-3 ■ Sand fly vector for leishmaniasis. (Courtesy of Cutis, image in the public domain.)

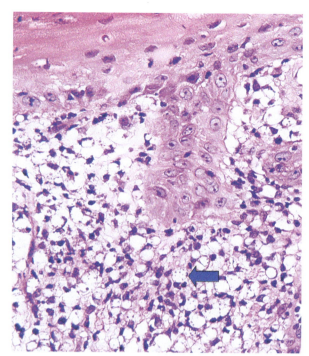

FIGURE 34-4 ■ In tissue, the amastigote form of leishmaniasis is commonly seen at the periphery of intracytoplasmic vacuoles (*movie marquee sign*).

Diagnosis

Leishmania are nonencapsulated and are seen as intracellular organisms within histiocytes, containing a nucleus and a paranucleus. Within the histiocytes the organisms often line up at the periphery of a vacuole like the bulbs surrounding an old-fashioned movie marquee (Fig. 34-4).

The diagnosis is established by demonstration of the organism in smears, biopsy, or culture. A punch biopsy from the active edge of the ulcer can be placed in Nicolle–Novy–MacNeal medium and shipped to the laboratory at room temperature. The Centers for Disease Control and Prevention (CDC) have support services available to provide media and diagnostic assistance. PCR is also available, but is not clearly superior to culture. Patients with forms capable of causing mucocutaneous disease need to be advised to monitor for signs of late sequelae/recurrence as disease can recur on the mucosal surfaces and present with nonspecific symptoms, i.e., rhinorrhea, and patients need to be followed closely if/when these types of symptoms develop.

Treatment

Spontaneous healing of primary cutaneous lesions occurs within months and can be hastened with localized hyperthermia. Other options include topical paromomycin sulfate 15% plus methylbenzethonium chloride 12%, ketoconazole cream under occlusion, cryotherapy, and photodynamic therapy. Intralesional sodium stibogluconate antimony and emetine hydrochloride are also used, and in Old World cutaneous leishmaniasis some data suggest that intramuscular meglumine antimoniate in combination with intralesional meglumine antimoniate is superior to intralesional therapy alone. Itraconazole has fewer side effects than meglumine antimoniate but results have been mixed. Oral fluconazole and zinc sulfate have been used to treat *L. major*. Intralesional meglumine therapy may be acceptable for small solitary lesions in areas with a low risk of mucosal disease.

Systemic therapy is recommended for patients who are immunosuppressed or who acquire infection in areas where mucocutaneous disease has been reported. Intravenous sodium antimony gluconate (sodium stibogluconate) is administered at a dose of 20 mg/kg/day in two divided doses for 28 days. It can be obtained from the CDC Drug Service (Atlanta, GA 30333, USA). Antimony *n*-methyl glutamine (Glucantime) is used more often in Central and South America. Second-line systemic options include fluconazole, 200 mg per day for 6 weeks, ketoconazole, dapsone, rifampicin, and allopurinol. Some of these have not been subjected to controlled clinical trials, as is true of most topical treatments. Liposomal encapsulated amphotericin B has been used effectively in antimony-resistant disease. Intramuscular pentamidine is used for *L. guyanensis* cutaneous leishmaniasis resistant to systemic antimony. Miltefosine is being used for diffuse cutaneous leishmaniasis and post-kala-azar dermal leishmaniasis, but treatment failures have occurred in the setting of *L. major* and *L. braziliensis* infections. Patients with serotypes known to be associated with mucocutaneous disease should be monitored for nasopharygeal signs and symptoms. Active mucocutaneous disease may require amphotericin B or combination therapy with an antimonial and rifampin, azithromycin, interferon-γ, or interleukin-2.

HUMAN TRYPANOSOMIASIS

Clinical Manifestations

Trypanosoma gambiense and *Trypanosoma rhodesiense* cause African trypanosomiasis, and *Trypanosoma cruzi* causes New World Chagas' disease, a disease with an expanding footprint in the New World. The organism has spread as far north as the southwestern United States.

In the early stage of African trypanosomiasis, a chancre may occur at the site of the tsetse fly bite, followed by erythema, lymphadenopathy, fever, malaise, headache, and joint pain. In the West African (Gambian) form, the illness is chronic, with progressive deterioration, whereas the East African (Rhodesian) form is an acute illness. Annular or deep erythema-nodosum-like lesions may occur and lymphadenopathy may be generalized or localized to the posterior cervical group (Winterbottom's sign).

In American trypanosomiasis (Chagas' disease), the reduviid bug (Fig. 34-5) usually bites at night. If the bite of the infected bug occurs near the eye, unilateral conjunctivitis and edema of the eyelids (Romana's sign) develop.

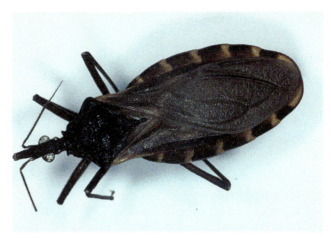

FIGURE 34-5 ■ Triatome reduviid bugs are the vector for American trypanosomiasis. (Courtesy of Cutis, image in the public domain.)

Late manifestations include myocarditis, arrhythmia, cardiac failure, megaesophagus, and megacolon.

Diagnosis

The flagellate form is noted in the blood in African trypanosomiasis, whereas intracellular amastigotes resembling leishmaniasis are noted in Chagas' disease.

Treatment

In the Rhodesian form, suramin is used to treat early disease. When the CNS is involved, melarsoprol is the drug of choice. Pentamidine isethionate is the drug of choice for the Gambian disease. Eflornithine appears to be a good alternative to melarsoprol for second-stage West African trypanosomiasis. For American trypanosomiasis, nifurtimox and benznidazole can treat the parasitemia and reduce the severity of the acute illness. Benznidazole does not prevent chronic cardiac lesions. Ruthenium complexation improves bioavailability of benznidazole and may result in better efficacy.

INTESTINAL AMEBIASIS

Clinical Manifestations

Entamoeba histolytica is the most common amebic pathogen in humans. It produces intestinal disease, but ulcerative anogenital cutaneous amebiasis may occur via direct extension. Chronic urticaria may be the presenting reactive sign of infestation.

Diagnosis

Entamoeba histolytica is 50 to 60 μm in diameter, and has basophilic cytoplasm and a single eccentric nucleus with a central nucleolus. Direct smears or biopsy may demonstrate the organism. Indirect hemagglutination test results remain elevated for years after infection, whereas the results of gel diffusion precipitation tests

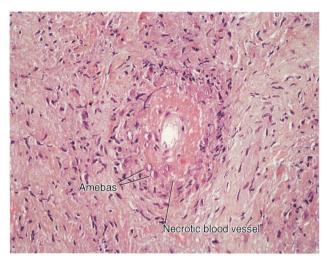

FIGURE 34-6 ■ Acanthamoeba is a vasculotropic organism resulting in vessel necrosis and ulceration.

and counterimmunoelectrophoresis become negative at 6 months.

Treatment

The treatment of choice is metronidazole (Flagyl), 750 mg orally three times a day for 10 days. Abscesses may require surgical drainage.

OTHER AMEBIC INFECTIONS

Clinical Manifestations

Acanthamoeba and *Balamuthia* are ubiquitous soil pathogens that cause granulomatous amebic encephalitis. *Acanthamoeba* affects immunocompromised individuals, especially those with acquired immunodeficiency syndrome or solid organ transplants. *Acanthamoeba* corneal infections are associated with homemade contact lens solution, and there have been iatrogenic cases associated with contaminated dental and medical equipment. Disseminated lesions present as ulcers. *B. mandrillaris* causes erythema and induration of the central face. Both organisms cause CNS disease that is typically fatal. Affected patients present with fever, nasal congestion, nasal discharge, epistaxis, cough, headaches, lethargy, altered mental status, and seizures.

Diagnosis

The organisms are visible on smears and in skin biopsy specimens (Fig. 34-6). Culture on a lawn of *Escherichia coli* will confirm the diagnosis.

Treatment

Diminazene aceturate is more active than miltefosine or pentamidine. 5-Fluorocytosine and sulfadiazine have also been used.

TOXOPLASMOSIS

Clinical Manifestations

Toxoplasmosis is caused by the zoonotic protozoan *Toxoplasma gondii*. The disease is often acquired through contact with animals, particularly cats. Congenital infection often presents with a triad of hydrocephalus, chorioretinitis, and cerebral calcification. Hepatosplenomegaly and jaundice may be present. Cutaneous lesions are typically macular and hemorrhagic, but blueberry muffin lesions, reflecting dermatoerythropoiesis, may also be seen. In acquired toxoplasmosis, cutaneous nodules, and macular hemorrhagic eruptions may occur. Other features may include scarlatiniform desquamation, eruptions mimicking roseola, erythema multiforme, dermatomyositis, or lichen planus accompanied by high fever and general malaise.

Cerebral disease has been reported in the setting of rituximab therapy and widespread disease can mimic melanoma metastases on PET scans.

Diagnosis

Toxoplasma gondii may appear as a crescent-shaped or oval protozoan and can infect any cell line. It may be identified in tissue sections, smears, or body fluids by Wright or Giemsa stain. Serologic testing is also available.

Treatment

A combination of pyrimethamine and sulfadiazine is typically used. The dosage and duration of treatment vary according to the age and immunologic competence of the patient.

SUGGESTED READING

Ahmad AF, et al. The in vitro efficacy of antimicrobial agents against the pathogenic free-living amoeba *Balamuthia mandrillaris*. J Eukaryot Microbiol September 2013;60(5):539–43.

Blum J, et al. Local or systemic treatment for New World cutaneous leishmaniasis? Re-evaluating the evidence for the risk of mucosal leishmaniasis. Int Health September 2012;4(3):153–63.

Centers for Disease Control and Prevention (CDC). Investigational drug available directly from CDC for the treatment of infections with free-living amoeba. MMWR Morb Mortal Wkly Rep August 23, 2013;62(33):666.

Hemmige V, et al. *Trypanosoma cruzi* infection: a review with emphasis on cutaneous manifestations. Int J Dermatol May 2012; 51(5):501–8.

Neitzke-Abreu HC, et al. Detection of DNA from leishmania (viannia): accuracy of polymerase chain reaction for the diagnosis of cutaneous leishmaniasis. PLoS One July 5, 2013;8(7):e62473.

Schwebke JR, et al. Intravaginal metronidazole/miconazole for the treatment of vaginal trichomoniasis. Sex Transm Dis September 2013;40(9):710–4.

CHAPTER 35

Acquired Immunodeficiency Syndrome and Sexually Transmitted Infections

Eseosa Asemota • Carrie Kovarik

KEY POINTS

- Patients with HIV/AIDS may develop cutaneous manifestations that reflect their immune-compromised state and can be grouped into infections (viral, bacterial, fungal, and parasitic/ectoparasitic), inflammatory, neoplastic, or other conditions.
- Syphilis, caused by *Treponema pallidum*, is a sexually transmitted disease that has experienced a resurgence with the HIV epidemic, and it is classically divided into four stages: primary, secondary, latent, and tertiary, with each stage potentially having cutaneous manifestations.
- Causes of sexually transmitted infectious genital ulcers include herpes simplex, syphilis, chancroid, and, less commonly, granuloma inguinale or lymphogranuloma venereum. Appropriate diagnostic testing should be performed in order to distinguish these entities and institute appropriate therapy. One should always bear in mind that all genital ulcers are not infectious, and a differential diagnosis should always be considered.
- The current Centers for Disease Control and Prevention (CDC) recommendations for treatment have been updated in 2010 and 2012 due to changes in antibiotic susceptibilities, and these are summarized and discussed.

The focus of this chapter is diseases that are sexually transmitted with dermatologic manifestations. A few disorders, e.g., mollusca contagiosa, condylomata acuminata, and scabies, are mentioned but not discussed in detail. Discussions of herpes simplex, herpes zoster, and reactive arthritis, formally referred to as Reiter's syndrome, are found in Chapters 7 and 31.

HUMAN IMMUNODEFICIENCY SYNDROME (HIV)

The acquired immunodeficiency syndrome (AIDS) is due to infection with one of two retroviruses, HIV-1 (more virulent and the cause in the majority of patients) or HIV-2. In the early 1980s, several of the initial descriptions of patients with AIDS came from dermatologists as they noted the appearance of cutaneous Kaposi's sarcoma in a new patient population. The affected individuals were not elderly men of Mediterranean or Ashkenazi Jewish descent as expected, but rather young men who had had sex with other men, and, who often had multiple partners. Over the years, additional high-risk populations were identified, including hemophiliacs who had received contaminated factor VIII concentrates, injection-drug users, and commercial sex workers and their sexual partners. In developing countries, where there is a larger burden of HIV infection, the predominant mode of transmission is heterosexual.

Sub-Saharan Africa is the most affected region, with 24.7 million people living with HIV in 2013. Also, sub-Saharan Africa accounts for almost 70% of the global total of new HIV infections. In the United States and Western Europe, the annual incidence of AIDS has reached a plateau. Public education, routine testing of pregnant women followed by antiretroviral treatment of those who are HIV-positive, and highly active antiretroviral combination therapy (HAART) have all played a role in this stabilization. With HAART therapy, however, has come a novel set of cutaneous side effects discussed below.

The majority of patients in the United States with HIV are unaware of their infection, and are responsible for the majority of new infections; many expert consensus statements recommend more widespread, or universal, screening for HIV. Dermatologists should have a low threshold to offer HIV testing in their practice.

In this section, the cutaneous manifestations of HIV infection and AIDS will be divided into infectious, inflammatory, neoplastic, and miscellaneous.

Cutaneous Manifestations: Infectious

The cutaneous manifestations of HIV infection and AIDS that are infectious in nature can be categorized into four major groups: viral, bacterial, fungal, and parasitic/ectoparasitic.

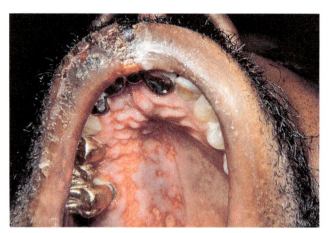

FIGURE 35-1 ■ Herpes zoster involving the palate and lip in an HIV-infected patient.

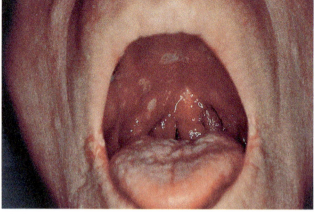

FIGURE 35-3 ■ Multiple erosions on the hard and soft palate due to herpes simplex virus in an HIV-infected patient. (Courtesy of Yale Residents' Slide Collection.)

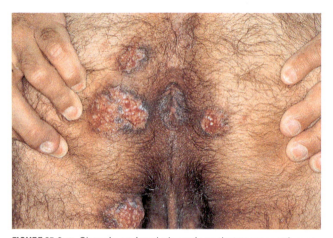

FIGURE 35-2 ■ Chronic perianal ulcerations that represent herpes simplex infection in this HIV-infected man.

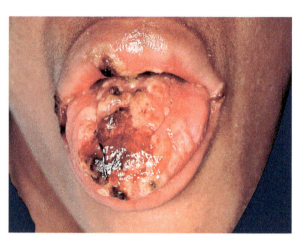

FIGURE 35-4 ■ Multiple vesicles, some of which are hemorrhagic, on the tongue and upper lip of an HIV-infected patient. Note the scalloping of the border of the lesion on the lip that is characteristic of HSV infections. (Courtesy of Yale Residents' Slide Collection.)

Viral Infections

Acute retroviral syndrome occurs approximately 2 to 4 weeks after acute HIV infection. This process is a self-limiting clinical syndrome of varying severity. It presents with "flu-like" symptoms such as fever, fatigue, weight loss, headache, myalgias, pharyngitis, lymphadenopathy, in addition to a morbilliform (measles-like) cutaneous eruption and mucosal ulcerations. Cutaneous immune responses to the HIV virus dissemination are possibly the cause of the maculopapular rash. Because the symptoms of the acute retroviral syndrome are nonspecific and anti-HIV antibodies are usually negative at this stage, the diagnosis is established by detecting plasma viral RNA (usually $>5 \times 10^4$ copies/mL, and as high as 1×10^6 copies/mL) and/or p24 antigen. The viremia is accompanied by a drop in the circulating CD4+ T-lymphocyte count and a rise in the CD8+ T-lymphocyte count.

Mucocutaneous infections due to herpes simplex virus (HSV)-1, HSV-2, and the varicella-zoster virus (VZV) are commonly seen in association with HIV infection and AIDS; the typical clinical presentations of these three viruses are reviewed in Chapter 31. Because herpes zoster (uni- or multidermatomal) can serve as one of the presenting signs of HIV infection (Fig. 35-1), this diagnosis should prompt a discussion of risk factors. In contrast to the self-limiting episodes of herpes zoster or orogenital herpes simplex that occur in immunocompetent hosts, patients with AIDS can have lesions that last for months until appropriate therapy is instituted. More recently, the development of herpes zoster or severe recurrent HSV infection has been described in the setting of immune reconstitution inflammatory syndrome (IRIS) on commencement of HAART. Chronic perianal ulcers due to HSV are sometimes misdiagnosed as decubitus ulcers (Fig. 35-2) and chronic oral ulcers as aphthous stomatitis (Fig. 35-3), until a direct immunofluorescence antibody assay, viral culture, or polymerase chain reaction (PCR) of scrapings from the ulcer edge points to the correct diagnosis. One clue to the diagnosis of HSV as the etiologic agent is scalloping of the border of the ulcer and preceding vesicles (Fig. 35-4). In patients with AIDS, chronic dermatomal and disseminated VZV lesions can become verrucous (Fig. 35-5) and the clinical diagnosis requires a high index of suspicion. For patients who are immunocompromised, including those with AIDS, antiviral

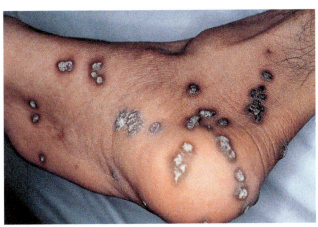

FIGURE 35-5 ■ Verrucous papules of chronic varicella-zoster virus (VZV) in a patient with AIDS. (Courtesy of Yale Residents' Slide Collection.)

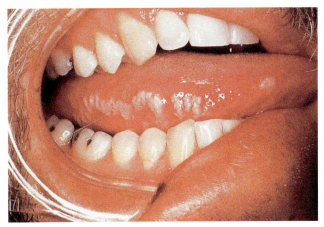

FIGURE 35-6 ■ Oral hairy leukoplakia.

therapy should be continued until there is complete clinical resolution. Hospitalization or intravenous therapy may be necessary in some cases.

When lesions of HSV or VZV fail to improve despite appropriate therapy (systemic acyclovir, famciclovir, or valacyclovir), the possibility of an acyclovir-resistant strain needs to be excluded, especially when patients have been receiving chronic suppressive therapy with oral acyclovir. Intravenous foscarnet (which does not require phosphorylation to interact with viral DNA polymerase) is the recommended treatment for acyclovir-resistant strains. However, there are reports of patients developing foscarnet-resistant strains of HSV owing to mutations in the DNA polymerase gene. An alternative treatment is topical (1% gel), intralesional, or intravenous cidofovir.

Administration of the varicella vaccine to prevent primary infection is also an important strategy to protect children and adults who do not have a prior history of varicella. The vaccine can be given to HIV-infected patients who have CD4 T-lymphocyte counts of >200 cells/µL despite the theoretical risk of live-virus vaccination in this population. Some clinicians choose to offer the zoster vaccine to HIV-infected persons who are >50 years of age and have good HIV control and CD4 counts of >200 cells/µL; however, zoster vaccination should be avoided in patients with CD4 counts of <200 cells/µL. (Note that the vaccine used to prevent reactivated VZV disease [Zostavax] contains 14 times the amount of virus as the vaccine to prevent primary infection.) If an HIV-infected adult develops a postvaccination varicella-like cutaneous eruption a prompt evaluation should be made and consideration should be given to starting antiviral therapy.

Infections with two other members of the herpes family, cytomegalovirus (CMV) and Epstein–Barr virus (EBV), are seen in HIV-infected individuals. The most common EBV-induced mucocutaneous disorder is oral hairy leukoplakia, which is characterized by filiform white plaques and papules, primarily on the lateral aspects of the tongue (Fig. 35-6). These lesions may have a somewhat corrugated appearance, and improvement is seen in the setting of HAART therapy.

Although the disorder most commonly associated with CMV is retinitis, this herpes virus can lead to gastrointestinal (GI) ulcers and, occasionally, orogenital or perianal ulcers as well as morbilliform eruptions. The detection (via specific immunohistochemical stains) of intranuclear CMV inclusions within dermal endothelial cells usually proves to be a more sensitive assay than viral cultures. In mucocutaneous ulcers, CMV often "coexists" with other viruses such as HSV or VZV, and as a result its true pathogenicity has been questioned.

Because condylomata acuminata and mollusca contagiosa (MC)—cutaneous viral infections due to human papilloma viruses (HPV) and poxvirus, respectively—can be sexually transmitted, HIV-infected patients are at increased risk for both. Because of the coexistent immunosuppression, their clinical manifestations frequently become quite exaggerated; for example, the individual lesions of MC often coalesce into broad-based plaques and may become so large as to be referred to as "giant." As expected, the condylomata involve the anogenital region, but in addition to the genitals, the most common site of involvement for MC is the face (Fig. 35-7). Even banal warts (verruca vulgaris) or flat warts can become widely distributed, as in organ transplant patients (Fig. 35-8), and often persist despite HAART.

In women, infections with certain subtypes of HPV, e.g., 16 and 18, are associated with the development of cervical cancer, and this risk increases in the setting of HIV infection. These same HPV strains also increase the risk of vulvar, penile, and anal carcinoma (Fig. 35-9). HIV-infected men who have sex with men, with high-risk HPV infection, are at greatest risk for anal cancer. Serial anal examinations in combination with anal cytology have been advocated for screening such patients, as has histologic examination of any suspicious lesion.

MC and HPV infections may prove recalcitrant to standard destructive therapies (e.g., cryotherapy, curettage, etc.), but improvement of MC has been observed after the institution of HAART. Both MC and condylomata acuminata may respond to topical imiquimod or cidofovir; occasionally, intralesional or intravenous cidofovir is administered for extensive confluent MC or condyloma. In one study of HIV-positive men who have sex with men and anal intraepithelial neoplasia, imiquimod

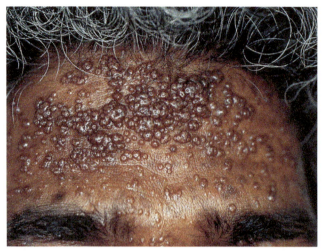

FIGURE 35-7 ■ Numerous dome-shaped papules of mollusca contagiosa on the forehead of an HIV-infected patient. Note the central dell in several of the lesions. (Courtesy of Yale Residents' Slide Collection.)

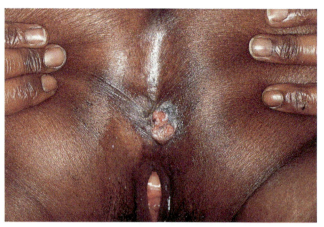

FIGURE 35-9 ■ Perianal erythematous plaque representing squamous cell carcinoma developing within condylomata acuminata. (Courtesy of Yale Residents' Slide Collection.)

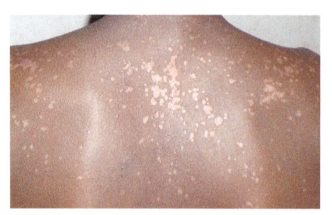

FIGURE 35-8 ■ Diffuse hypopigmented verruca plana in a patient with HIV infection.

cream (for perianal disease), and suppositories (for intra-anal disease) led to clinical and histologic clearing in 75% of those who used the medication as directed (three times per week for 16 weeks).

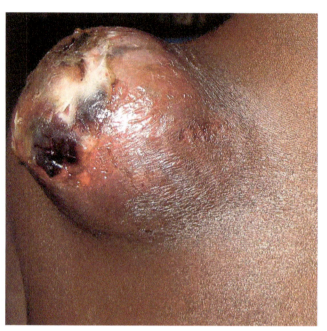

FIGURE 35-10 ■ Large vascular tumor of bacillary angiomatosis in a child with AIDS, which can mimic a tumor of Kaposi's sarcoma.

Bacterial Infections

Cutaneous bacterial infections that are seen in association with HIV infection and AIDS can be subdivided into a few major categories: soft tissue infections and folliculitis due primarily to Gram-positive cocci; bacillary angiomatosis; sexually transmitted diseases (STDs) (see below); and mycobacterial and atypical mycobacterial infections. Because HIV is often acquired via sexual contact, patients who are HIV-positive need to be screened for other STDs, and vice versa. In addition, the presence of erosions and ulcerations in the anogenital region due to bacterial diseases, such as syphilis, or viral diseases, such as HSV, can increase the transmission rate of HIV.

Soft tissue bacterial infections in patients with HIV are often due to *Staphylococcus aureus* or *Streptococcus* spp., and their clinical presentations range from folliculitis and abscesses to cellulitis and necrotizing fasciitis (Fig. 35-10). When *S. aureus* is identified as the etiology of a cutaneous infection, the possibility of nasal carriage needs to be considered as well as the possibility of meticillin-resistant *S. aureus*. The cutaneous manifestations of atypical mycobacterial infections are also protean and can vary from subtle areas of erythema to necrotic ulcers. Several species of atypical mycobacteria have been isolated from skin lesions in patients with HIV/AIDS, which may be isolated or disseminated, including *Mycobacterium haemophilum*, *M. fortuitum*, *M. malmoense*, and *M. avium intracellulare*. HIV-infected patients are also at risk for developing cutaneous tuberculosis, including disseminated miliary tuberculosis. Multidrug treatment regimens for cutaneous mycobacterial infections are the same as for systemic disease.

Bacillary angiomatosis is a bacterial infection whose diagnosis warrants the exclusion of an underlying HIV infection or immunosuppression. Only occasionally is it

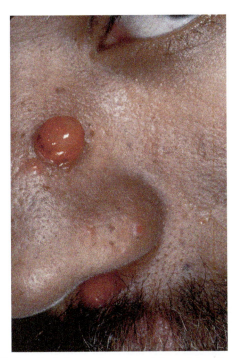

FIGURE 35-11 ■ Red dome-shaped nodules of bacillary angiomatosis in an HIV-positive patient. The lesions have an appearance similar to pyogenic granulomas. (Courtesy of NYU Slide Collection.)

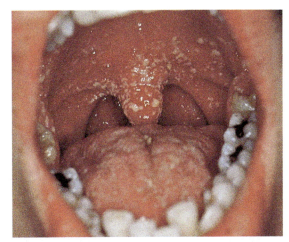

FIGURE 35-12 ■ White friable plaques of oral candidiasis in a patient with AIDS. (Courtesy of Yale Residents' Slide Collection.)

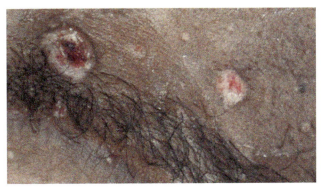

FIGURE 35-13 ■ Cutaneous cryptococcosis in a patient with AIDS manifesting as multiple dome-shaped papules, some with central umbilication reminiscent of mollusca contagiosa.

seen in normal hosts. The microorganisms responsible for the appearance of discrete proliferations of cutaneous blood vessels are *Bartonella henselae* and *B. quintana*; the former is also the etiologic agent of cat scratch disease. The characteristic skin lesion is a red to violet papule that resembles a "hemangioma," pyogenic granuloma, or a lesion of Kaposi's sarcoma (Fig. 35-11). Additional sites of involvement include the subcutis, with the formation of nodules, the liver (peliosis hepatitis), lymph nodes, bones, and heart (endocarditis). The diagnosis is established by identifying the bacteria in Warthin–Starry-stained histologic sections or by PCR-based analysis of biopsy specimens. Treatment consists primarily of first- and second-generation macrolides.

Fungal Infections

Certain fungal infections, such as oral candidiasis (thrush), can serve as presenting signs of HIV infection (Fig. 35-12), whereas others, such as cryptococcosis, are seen late in the course of the disease. HIV-infected patients are at increased risk for the development of superficial mucocutaneous fungal infections due to *Candida* spp. and dermatophytes, as well as systemic infections due to *Cryptococcus neoformans*, *Candida* spp., and dimorphic fungi (e.g., *Histoplasma capsulatum*, *Coccidioides immitis*, *Penicillium marneffei*). The cutaneous lesions of cryptococcosis and dimorphic fungal infections are often a mixture of indurated papules, plaques, and ulcerated lesions, and they sometimes resemble the dome-shaped papules of MC (Fig. 35-13). Examination of a potassium hydroxide preparation of dermal scrapings or a periodic acid–Schiff- or silver-stained histologic section allows a presumptive diagnosis, and a simultaneous tissue fungal culture provides a definitive diagnosis. Cryptococcal cutaneous infections are often a sign of disseminated disease, and should prompt thorough multisystem evaluation including a lumbar puncture.

Infections with tinea (dermatophytoses) affect three keratin-containing structures, the skin, hair, and nails. HIV-infected patients are not only prone to the more common forms of tinea, e.g., tinea pedis, tinea manuum (hand), tinea unguium (nails), and tinea corporis (Fig. 35-14), but they often have more severe or widespread lesions. These patients also develop an unusual form of tinea unguium known as proximal subungual onychomycosis. In the more common form of tinea unguium (distal subungual onychomycosis), the most pronounced dystrophic changes, e.g., thickening and yellow discoloration, are seen in the distal portions of the fingernails or toenails, whereas in the proximal form there is a white discoloration that first appears in the proximal portion of the nail. This proximal subungual form has also been observed in other immunocompromised patients, such as those who have received organ transplants.

DNA analyses have led to a reclassification of *Pneumocystis jiroveci* (*carinii*) as a fungal species. Pneumonia is the most common clinical presentation of *P. jiroveci* infection,

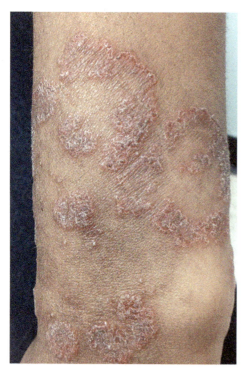

FIGURE 35-14 ■ Annular erythematous scaly plaques of tinea corporis in an immunocompromised patient.

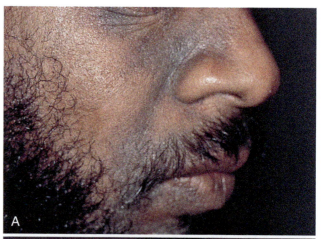
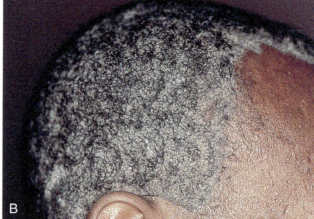

FIGURE 35-15 ■ Seborrheic dermatitis characterized by scaling in (**A**) the nasolabial groove and (**B**) the scalp in two patients with AIDS. (Courtesy of Yale Residents' Slide Collection.)

but rarely cutaneous lesions do develop, especially in the external auditory canal and nares.

Parasitic/Ectoparasitic Infections

One of the more common ectoparasitic infections in patients who have AIDS is scabies, in particular a form characterized by thick scale-crusts and numerous mites of *Sarcoptes scabiei* var. *hominis*; this is sometimes referred to as crusted or Norwegian scabies. Unlike the form of scabies seen in immunocompetent hosts, in which each person is infested with a few dozen mites, these patients have hundreds to thousands of mites and are therefore highly contagious. The thick scale is one of the explanations for the difficulty in eradicating crusted scabies with topical scabicides, such as 5% permethrin cream. One of the off-label uses of oral ivermectin is the treatment of such patients, who often require combination regimens with prolonged and repeat treatments.

HIV-infected patients frequently develop folliculitis, and its etiology can vary from *S. aureus* and herpes simplex to *Malassezia* spp., dimorphic fungi, and the *Demodex* mite. Although the latter ectoparasite is part of the normal inhabitants of the hair follicle, its presumed pathogenetic role is based upon the numerous *Demodex* mites found in the expressed follicular contents from AIDS patients with folliculitis in whom there was no other explanation for the folliculitis.

Patients with AIDS can also present with cutaneous lesions due to systemic infections with parasites such as *Toxoplasma gondii* (primarily the central nervous system [CNS]), *Acanthamoeba* spp. (primarily CNS and sinuses), *Strongyloides stercoralis* (primarily GI tract and lung), *Leishmania* spp. (primarily bone marrow), and microsporidia (primarily GI tract). Although these secondary cutaneous lesions are rather unusual and do not have unique clinical presentations, the diagnosis can be made fairly easily by identification of the responsible organisms in biopsy specimens.

Cutaneous Manifestations: Inflammatory

There are several inflammatory skin disorders that can serve as the initial clinical manifestation of HIV infection, in particular seborrheic dermatitis, psoriasis, and reactive arthritis (the disorder previously referred to as Reiter's syndrome—see Chapter 7) (Figs. 35-15 to 35-17). For some patients, this represents new-onset disease, whereas in others there is a flare of a preexisting dermatosis. In this particular clinical setting, seborrheic dermatitis, especially of the face, may be moderate to severe in intensity and the psoriasis rather extensive. Many years ago, an increased number of *Malassezia* organisms (yeasts that are part of the normal flora) were observed in HIV-infected patients with seborrheic dermatitis, and this observation contributed to the subsequent use of antifungal creams and shampoos for the treatment of this disease, both in immunocompromised and immunocompetent hosts.

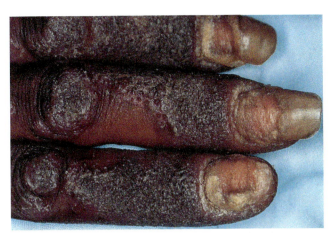

FIGURE 35-16 ■ Psoriasis of the digits in an HIV-infected patient. Note the accompanying nail dystrophy. (Courtesy of Yale Residents' Slide Collection.)

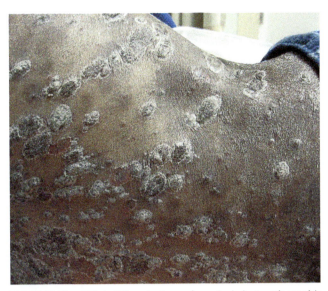

FIGURE 35-18 ■ Thick diffuse lesions of psoriasis in a patient with HIV. (Courtesy of Emily Chu.)

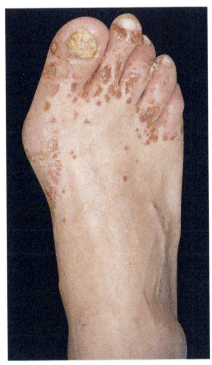

FIGURE 35-17 ■ Psoriasiform lesions of reactive arthritis (the disorder formerly referred to as Reiter's syndrome) in an HIV-infected patient.

People with advanced HIV often exhibit psoriasis (Fig. 35-18). The prevalence of psoriasis in HIV-positive individuals is comparable to that of the general population. However, psoriasis tends to be more severe in people infected with HIV. A much higher prevalence of psoriatic arthritis occurs in HIV-positive individuals with psoriasis than in those without the infection. A distinguishing hallmark feature of HIV-associated psoriasis compared with classic psoriasis is that several morphologic types can coexist in the same patient. The main postulated mechanisms of pathogenesis are a T-cell imbalance characterized by decreased CD4 T cells and a relative increase in CD8 memory T cells, a cytokine milieu predominantly mediated by interferon-γ, superantigen stimulation of autoimmunity by HIV, or other viral and bacterial infections and HLA Cw0602 status. The management of moderate and severe HIV-associated psoriasis is challenging and the risk-to-benefit ratio specific to these patients needs to be taken into account when selecting therapies such as phototherapy, acitretin, methotrexate, cyclosporine, hydroxyurea, TNF inhibitors, e.g., infliximab. Patients typically improve with early placement on highly active antiretroviral therapy.

Pruritus is a frequent complaint in patients with AIDS, and secondary lesions that simply represent chronic rubbing, e.g., lichen simplex chronicus and prurigo nodularis, can be seen admixed with more specific primary lesions. Once scabies, drug eruptions, specific dermatoses such as eczematous eruptions, arthropod bite reactions, and "systemic" causes of pruritus (e.g., cholestasis, renal failure, lymphoma, parasitic infections) are excluded, the differential diagnosis includes xerosis (see below), folliculitis, eosinophilic folliculitis, and the pruritic papular eruption of HIV/AIDS. Eosinophilic folliculitis is characterized by pruritic edematous perifollicular papules, primarily on the upper trunk and in the head and neck region (Fig. 35-19), and it is usually associated with advanced disease. In biopsy specimens, eosinophils are found within hair follicles. The skin-colored papules of the pruritic papular eruption of HIV/AIDS tend to favor the extremities, but can also involve the trunk; one hypothesis is that the eruption represents an exaggerated response to arthropod bites or other allergens. Both disorders may improve following UVB phototherapy, as well as with immune reconstitution.

Patients who are HIV-positive have an increased incidence of cutaneous drug eruptions, usually morbilliform or urticarial, but others include photolichenoid, erythrodermic, drug hypersensitivity syndrome, pigmentary changes, injection site reaction, retinoid-like reaction, or the spectrum of Stevens–Johnson syndrome/toxic

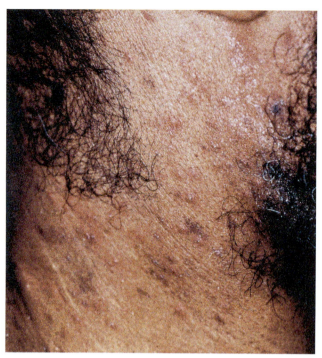

FIGURE 35-19 ■ Pruritic lesions of eosinophilic folliculitis on the neck of a man with AIDS. (Courtesy of Yale Residents' Slide Collection.)

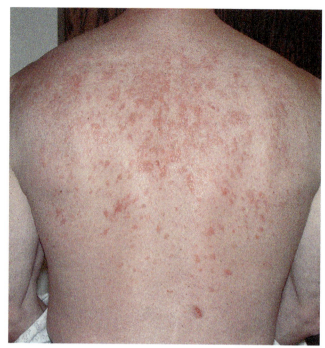

FIGURE 35-20 ■ Disseminated granuloma annulare in an HIV-infected patient. The distribution pattern is atypical. (Courtesy of Kalman Watsky, MD.)

epidermal necrolysis. This proclivity for developing allergic drug reactions (approximately 10 times greater than in the general population) became apparent when antibiotic prophylaxis became commonplace, especially the use of oral trimethoprim–sulfamethoxazole against *P. jiroveci* (*carinii*) pneumonia. Possible explanations for this phenomenon include the immune dysregulation that accompanies HIV infection, or a predisposition due to co-existing viral infections, e.g., CMV or EBV. As the name implies, photolichenoid eruptions favor sun-exposed areas, are often associated with sulfa-containing medications, and may present as areas of hyperpigmentation. However, idiopathic photosensitivity is also seen in patients with AIDS.

Lastly, cutaneous small-vessel vasculitis and erythema elevatum diutinum, a form of chronic cutaneous vasculitis often associated with streptococcal infections, are also thought to be more prevalent in HIV-infected patients. An idiopathic disorder that presents with skin-colored papules is granuloma annulare (Fig. 35-20), and in HIV-infected patients the generalized form is seen more often than the localized form (the opposite is true in immunocompetent hosts); occasionally, even oral lesions are noted.

Cutaneous Manifestations: Neoplastic

Individuals who are HIV-positive are at increased risk for the development of several neoplasms, including Kaposi's sarcoma (KS; Figs. 35-21 and 35-22), lymphoma (usually non-Hodgkin's), and cervical and anal squamous cell carcinomas (see above). Coinfection with human herpesvirus 8 is associated with the development of KS as well as body cavity lymphoma and

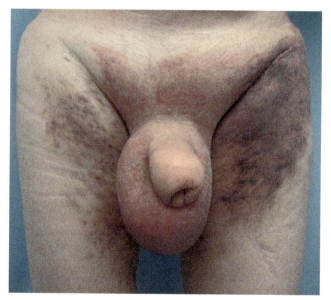

FIGURE 35-21 ■ Kaposi's sarcoma with secondary lymphedema in a patient with AIDS. Administration of liposomal doxorubicin led to improvement.

multicentric Castleman's disease; coinfection appears to be more common in men who have sex with men. Improvement of KS has been noted after the institution of HAART, as have flares as part of IRIS; some cases of KS require specific targeted therapy, which may be localized or include systemic chemotherapeutic agents. The non-Hodgkin's lymphomas seen in this setting are often extranodal, EBV-related, and involve the brain, GI tract, and/or skin. As a result, cutaneous lesions of lymphoma may occasionally be the initial

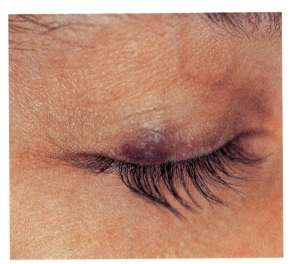

FIGURE 35-22 ■ Trichomegaly of the eyelashes plus Kaposi's sarcoma of the upper eyelid in a patient with AIDS. (Courtesy of Yale Residents' Slide Collection.)

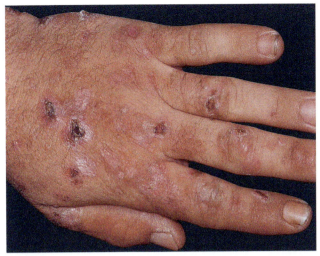

FIGURE 35-23 ■ Highly active antiretroviral combination therapy (HAART)-associated lipoatrophy of the cheeks. (Courtesy of Kalman Watsky, MD.)

clinical presentation. A HAART-associated reduction in the incidence of lymphoma has been observed. Human papillomavirus (HPV) is associated with genital and anal cancer in HIV patients, as well as oral cancer and skin cancer at other sites, such as the periungual skin.

Cutaneous Manifestations: Miscellaneous

There are several cutaneous manifestations of HIV infection that do not fit neatly into one of the previous categories of infectious, inflammatory, or neoplastic. These include xerosis (dry itchy scaly skin), which can become so pronounced as to resemble ichthyosis vulgaris; facial hyperpigmentation in the absence of systemic drugs or adrenal insufficiency; linear telangiectases of the chest; trichomegaly of the eyelashes (Fig. 35-22); changes in hair texture, e.g., thick curly hair can become fine and straight; diffuse alopecia; atopic dermatitis; telogen effluvium; and HIV-related pseudolymphoma. Complex aphthosis (multiple "canker sores") especially of the oral mucosa, can be a therapeutic challenge in patients who are HIV-positive. The ulcerations are similar in appearance to those seen in Behçet's disease, and once infectious etiologies have been excluded, systemic therapies are usually required. One of the off-label uses of oral thalidomide is the treatment of severe aphthosis in HIV-infected patients.

Lastly, lipodystrophy or the fat redistribution syndrome can be seen in patients receiving HAART. Clinical findings include a decrease of subcutaneous fat (lipoatrophy) in the face (especially of the cheeks; Fig. 35-23), extremities and buttocks, as well as a "buffalo hump," central obesity, hypertriglyceridemia, and insulin resistance. Nucleoside reverse transcriptase inhibitors such as stavudine (a thymidine analog) are associated with an increased risk of developing lipoatrophy, and protease inhibitors have been associated with abnormal fat accumulation.

SEXUALLY TRANSMITTED INFECTIONS

Syphilis

Syphilis, also known as lues, is an infectious disease primarily transmitted via sexual contact. Less often, the transmission is vertical, from mother to unborn child, resulting in congenital syphilis. The causative agent is the spirochete *Treponema pallidum*. Since World War II and the introduction of penicillin, there has been an overall decline in the incidence of syphilis in the United States. However, a resurgence of the disease did accompany the HIV epidemic, and high-risk sexual behavior that put individuals at risk for HIV infection also put them at risk for contracting syphilis.

The clinical manifestations of syphilis vary depending on the stage it presents. Classically, syphilis is divided into four stages: primary, secondary, latent, and tertiary. Except for the latent phase, specific cutaneous lesions that aid in the clinical diagnosis of this disease are often present.

Primary Syphilis

The characteristic lesion of primary syphilis is the chancre, a painless ulcer that is usually 1 to 1.5 cm in diameter. An average of 3 weeks after exposure to infectious lesions of another person, a chancre can appear at the site of penetration of the spirochetes (either via mucosa or abraded skin). The most common locations are the penis, labia, and cervix, followed by other urogenital sites, the lips, oral cavity, anus, breasts, and fingers. The majority of patients have a single ulcer (Fig. 35-24A), with multiple lesions seen in approximately one-quarter of patients. Multiple lesions are more common when coinfected with HIV (Fig. 35-24B). The base of the chancre is often moist, but not purulent, and the edges are more sharply defined than in ulcers due to *Haemophilus ducreyi*. Also, there is no scalloping of the border as is so often seen in orogenital ulcers due to herpes simplex (see Chapter 31).

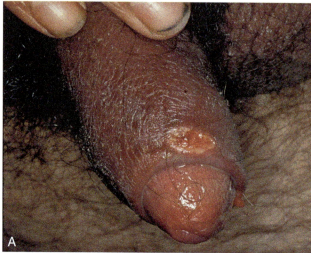

FIGURE 35-24 ■ Penile chancres: **A**, single and **B**, multiple, with characteristic clean moist bases. (Courtesy of Yale Residents' Slide Collection.)

Palpation with a gloved hand should follow visual inspection of any mucocutaneous ulcer. Unless there is a secondary bacterial infection, a chancre is not tender to palpation. More importantly, the base of the ulcer is characteristically quite firm due to the infiltration of the underlying dermis with lymphocytes, macrophages, and plasma cells. There may be regional lymphadenopathy, and because the lesions of secondary syphilis can appear prior to the spontaneous resolution of the chancre, a complete skin and oral examination is recommended. Without antibiotic therapy, the lifespan of a chancre is usually 3 to 6 weeks; with therapy (Table 35-1), the ulcer resolves within 2 weeks.

Secondary Syphilis

The secondary lesions of syphilis are a reflection of a spirochetemia, and as a result, have a widespread distribution pattern. The mucocutaneous manifestations of secondary syphilis follow the appearance of the chancre by approximately 3 to 12 weeks; however, as stated previously, there may be a temporal overlap, such that both are present in a particular patient. On the trunk and extremities cutaneous lesions are usually papulosquamous (Fig. 35-25) and less commonly macular. The papules and plaques vary in size from 2 mm to 2 cm and are pink to red-brown in color. The color is influenced by both the degree of inflammation and the melanin content of the skin. Similar-appearing lesions are seen on the palms and soles and are sometimes referred to as "copper pennies" (Fig. 35-26). Characteristically, the scale is concentrated at the edges of the thin palmoplantar papules.

TABLE 35-1 Centers for Disease Control and Prevention (CDC) Recommendations for Treatment of Various Stages of Syphilis (2010)

		First-Line	Second-Line (If Penicillin Allergic)
Primary§		Benzathine penicillin G 2.4×10^6 U IM × 1 dose	Doxycycline 100 mg po BID × 2 week*
Secondary§		Benzathine penicillin G 2.4×10^6 U IM × 1 dose	Doxycycline 100 mg po BID × 2 week*
Latent:	Early	Benzathine penicillin G 2.4×10^6 U IM × 1 dose	Doxycycline 100 mg po BID × 2 week*
	Late	Benzathine penicillin G 2.4×10^6 U IM qweek × 3 doses	Doxycycline 100 mg po BID × 4 week*
Tertiary:	CV, skin	Benzathine penicillin G 2.4×10^6 U IM qweek × 3 doses	Doxycycline 100 mg po BID × 4 week[†,‡]
	Neuro	Aqueous crystalline penicillin G $18-24 \times 10^6$ U IV in divided doses (q4h or continuous infusion) × 10–14 days OR Procaine penicillin 2.4×10^6 U IM qd plus probenecid 500 mg po q6h × 10–14 days	Desensitize; ceftriaxone 1 g IV qd × 14 days not as effective
Primary, Secondary, or Latent			
During pregnancy		Benzathine penicillin G 2.4×10^6 U IM × 1 or qweek × 3 (depending upon stage)	Desensitize
In association with HIV infection‖		Benzathine penicillin G 2.4×10^6 U IM × 1 or qweek × 3 (depending upon stage) versus qweek × 3 (all stages except neuro)	For primary and secondary, same as HIV negative; for latent, desensitize
Regimen for infants and children		**Benzathine penicillin G** 50,000 units/kg IM, up to the adult dose of 2.4 million units in a single dose OR qweek × three doses (depending upon stage)	

*Or tetracycline 500 mg po QID × 2 week. Azithromycin as a single 2-g oral dose or ceftriaxone 1 g daily either IM or IV for 10 to 14 days may also be effective in treating primary syphilis.
†Or tetracycline 500 mg po QID × 4 week.
‡HIV negative and neurosyphilis excluded.
§Without ophthalmologic or neurologic involvement.
‖Neurosyphilis excluded.
Detailed recommendations for treatment of syphilis can be found at the CDC website: www.cdc.gov/std.
Adapted from CDC; www.cdc.gov/std.

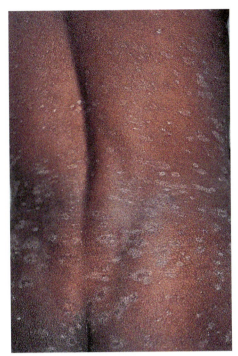

FIGURE 35-25 ■ Multiple scaly plaques on the feet of a patient with secondary syphilis.

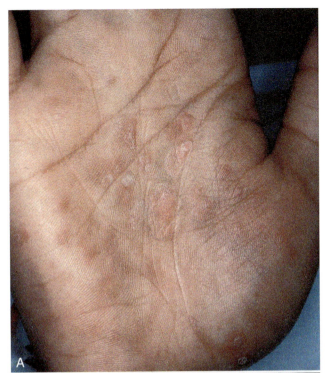

FIGURE 35-26 ■ Pink-brown to dark brown **A**, palmar and **B**, plantar lesions of secondary syphilis. Note the peripheral collarette of scale. (Courtesy of Yale Residents' Slide Collection.)

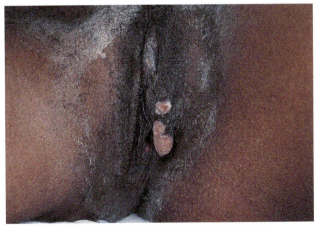

FIGURE 35-27 ■ Condyloma lata—genital lesions of secondary syphilis.

Rarely, pustules or ulcers develop within the lesions of secondary syphilis.

Additional mucocutaneous lesions of secondary syphilis include nonscarring "moth-eaten" alopecia (primarily of the scalp), mucous patches (primarily of the oral mucosa), split papules at the oral commissures, annular plaques with central hyperpigmentation (primarily of the face), granulomatous nodules, and condyloma lata, primarily in the anogenital region (Fig. 35-27). Although skin involvement is the most common manifestation of secondary syphilis, the patient may be systemically ill with symptoms such as fevers, fatigue, headache, and bone pain, as well as signs such as generalized lymphadenopathy and pharyngitis. This is in contrast to the patient with pityriasis rosea, who may have a similar-appearing rash, with a URI 6 to 10 weeks earlier, but at the time of eruption rarely has associated systemic complaints.

Other symptoms may include fever, sore throat, malaise, weight loss, and headache. Rare manifestations include hepatitis, kidney disease, arthritis, periostitis, optic neuritis, uveitis, and interstitial keratitis. Serologic evaluation is quite helpful in patients with secondary syphilis as the *rapid plasma reagin* (RPR) is positive in >99% of patients. Once the prozone phenomenon is excluded, a negative RPR would draw the diagnosis of cutaneous syphilis into question. Following appropriate treatment (Table 35-1), the titer of the RPR should decline fourfold over a period of 6 months and gradually become negative (nonreactive). The fluorescent treponemal antibody absorption (FTA-ABS) test was once said to remain positive "for life," even in treated patients, and its titer is not measured serially to monitor therapeutic response; more recently, however, a nonreactive FTA-ABS was observed in 24% of patients ($n = 882$) 3 years after treatment of primary, secondary, or early latent syphilis. Patients can also be diagnosed by histologic examination of the papulosquamous lesions, which shows dermal infiltrates of lymphocytes and plasma cells; a silver or immunohistochemical stain is required to detect the spirochetes. A dark-field examination of the serous exudate of condyloma lata can be performed, but requires exclusion of saprophytic treponemes (see below).

As with chancres, the lesions of secondary syphilis resolve spontaneously, i.e., even in the absence of appropriate therapy, after 2 to 4 months. In a minority (25%) of patients, the cutaneous eruption recurs a second or third time, but always in a transient manner. Those patients who fail to receive appropriate therapy (Table 35-1) may enter the next phase of the disease, which is referred to as latent syphilis. Although there are no clinical signs or symptoms, latent syphilis is divided into early (<1 year) and late (>1 year) stages, and treatment recommendations do differ (Table 35-1).

Tertiary Syphilis

Only about a third of patients with latent syphilis eventually develop tertiary disease. In order of frequency, the most common sites of clinically apparent involvement are the skin (15% of untreated patients), cardiovascular system (10%), and central nervous system (5%). Given the number of untreated patients and the percentage of those who develop symptomatic disease of the skin, one can see why cutaneous tertiary syphilis is quite rare, especially in developed countries. There are two major types of cutaneous disease: granulomatous (nodular or psoriasiform) and gummatous. Thick, dusky, red plaques and nodules are seen in the former and often resemble other granulomatous diseases, such as sarcoidosis. The combination of expansion plus central scar formation leads to the characteristic figurate lesions. There is more necrosis within gummas and, as a result, destruction of adjacent tissues can occur, including cartilage and bone. The RPR may be negative during tertiary syphilis.

Congenital Syphilis

Congenital syphilis is classically divided into an early phase (<2 years of age) and a late phase (>2 years of age). However, it is equally important to distinguish between clinical signs and symptoms due to active infection as opposed to stigmata that are sequelae of an in utero infection. Because congenital syphilis represents a bloodborne infection with *T. pallidum*, there is no primary phase. Many of the cutaneous manifestations of early congenital syphilis are reminiscent of secondary syphilis, except that the "papulosquamous" lesions can be bullous and tend to be more erosive. Additional clinical manifestations include "snuffles" (bloody or purulent mucinous nasal discharge), perioral and perianal fissures, hepatosplenomegaly, and osteochondritis. Manifestations of the late phase include gummas, interstitial keratitis, and neurosyphilis (usually asymptomatic).

The later in pregnancy treatment is begun, the more likely it is that the infant, although cured, may have the stigmata of an in utero infection. The most common stigmata (>50% of patients) involve either the facial bones or the dentition: frontal bossing, short maxillae, high palatal arch, saddle nose, Hutchinson's teeth (permanent upper central incisors that are widely spaced and broader at the base), and mulberry molars (multiple small cusps rather than four well-formed cusps in the first lower molar). Some of the "classic" stigmata are seen much less commonly, e.g., the complete Hutchinson's triad (Hutchinson's teeth, interstitial keratitis, and eighth-nerve deafness), rhagades (periorificial linear scars from previous fissures), saber shins, and Higouménakis' sign (unilateral thickening of the sternoclavicular portion of the clavicle).

Diagnosis

Direct Testing. A dark-field microscopy examination of a chancre's serous exudate will demonstrate the motile corkscrew-shaped treponemes. However, if the lesion is located within the oral or anal cavity, then *T. pallidum* spirochetes must be distinguished from the similar-appearing, nonpathogenic, saprophytic treponemes that reside in these areas. This requires consultation with a microbiologist and the use of species-specific immunofluorescent stains. Two other less commonly used tests can be carried out on a sample from the chancre: direct fluorescent antibody testing and nucleic acid amplification tests. Direct fluorescent testing uses antibodies tagged with fluorescein, which attach to specific syphilis proteins, while nucleic acid amplification uses techniques, such as PCR, to detect the presence of specific syphilis genes.

In addition, a skin biopsy specimen of the ulcer's edge may be obtained and a silver or immunoperoxidase staining can be performed to detect the spirochetes. Simultaneously, the biopsy specimen can be evaluated for other causes of ulcerations in the differential diagnosis.

Serology Tests. Blood tests are divided into nontreponemal and treponemal tests. Serologic assays are less sensitive in primary syphilis than in secondary syphilis, as the nontreponemal tests, e.g., venereal disease research laboratory and RPR tests, may be negative in up to 20% of patients. Nontreponemal tests are used initially in screening. However, as these tests are occasionally false-positives, confirmation is required with a treponemal test, such as *T. pallidum* particle agglutination (TPHA) or FTA-ABS. False-positives on the nontreponemal tests can occur with some viral infections, such as varicella and measles, as well as with lymphoma, tuberculosis, malaria, endocarditis, connective tissue disease, and pregnancy. False-negatives may occur in the setting of overwhelmingly high levels of *T. pallidum*, such as can be seen in HIV coinfection, termed the prozone phenomenon, which should be assessed for with serial dilutions. Treponemal antibody tests usually become positive 2 to 5 weeks after the initial infection. Serologic evaluation is quite helpful in patients with secondary syphilis as the FTA-ABS are positive in >99% of patients.

Neurosyphilis is diagnosed by finding high numbers of leukocytes (immunosorbent predominately lymphocytes) and high protein levels in the cerebrospinal fluid in the setting of a known syphilis infection.

Detection of IgM anti-*T. pallidum* antibodies in a neonate confirms the diagnosis of congenital syphilis, as IgM antibodies cannot pass from the mother to the fetus via the placenta because of their size; the Captia (IgM) enzyme-linked assay is said to have a sensitivity of 100% in this setting.

Syphilis in Association with HIV Infection and AIDS

Because HIV and *T. pallidum* share a primary mode of transmission—sexual contact—the presence of one of these infectious diseases mandates screening for the other. In addition, the ulcerated surface of a chancre provides a portal of entry for the HIV. The clinical course of early syphilis in patients with AIDS is often as described above; however, there are reports of more aggressive disease (lues maligna), an increased frequency of serologically defined treatment failures, an increased risk for the development of neurosyphilis, and a higher relapse rate of neurosyphilis following penicillin therapy. Rarely, a nonreactive RPR has been observed at the onset of the secondary phase in HIV-infected patients. Lastly, HIV infection is one of the causes of a chronic false-positive RPR. Recently, several studies documented that syphilis may also impact the course of HIV infection. These studies suggest that syphilis, like many other acute infections, causes transient increases in the viral load and decreases in the CD4 cell count that resolve after the infection is treated.

Chancroid

As with syphilis, the primary mode of transmission for chancroid is intimate contact. Therefore, those with multiple sexual partners are at highest risk for developing this infectious disease. The etiologic agent is the Gram-negative bacterium *H. ducreyi*. Cutaneous ulcers of chancroid appear in the genital region (primarily on the penis and vulva) approximately 3 to 7 days following exposure. In contrast to syphilis, there are usually multiple lesions (Fig. 35-28), including kissing lesions. The ulcers range in size from 2 mm to 3 cm and have irregular, overhanging borders that are sometimes referred to as "shaggy"; the ulcers are painful and tender to palpation, but soft. Tender prominent lymphadenopathy and abscesses (referred to as buboes) are frequently seen.

Confirmation of the clinical diagnosis of chancroid requires a bacterial culture and Gram stain of material obtained by swabbing the base of the ulcer and undersurface of the edges. Parallel linear arrays of Gram-negative rods can be seen on Gram stain, and have been likened to a school of fish. *H. ducreyi* is fastidious and requires culture on specialized media supplemented with serum and hemoglobin. PCR-based identification of organisms is now available.

The appropriate therapy is outlined in Table 35-2. As with syphilis, the differential diagnosis includes the two most common causes of genital ulcers: herpes simplex and trauma. However, when the ulcers are chronic and nonhealing, then more unusual etiologies need to be

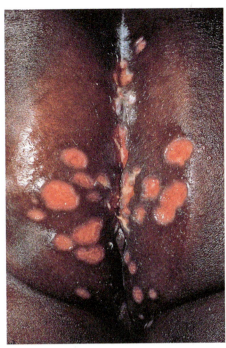

FIGURE 35-28 ■ Multiple punched-out ulcerations of chancroid. (Courtesy of N.S. Penneys, MD.)

excluded, such as squamous cell carcinoma, lymphoma, granuloma inguinale, and Behçet's disease.

Granuloma Inguinale

Granuloma inguinale is an unusual sexually transmitted disease caused by the Gram-negative bacterium *Klebsiella granulomatis*, which used to be called *Calymmatobacterium granulomatis*. The lesions are seen primarily in the genital region, and although they begin as papules, over time friable granulomatous plaques and ulcerations often attain a rather large size (Fig. 35-29). As a result, there is frequently destruction of normal tissues. The incubation period probably ranges from 2 weeks to 3 months, and the disease is much more prevalent in developing countries.

The clinical diagnosis is based on the patient's sexual history and on physical examination revealing a painless, "beefy-red ulcer" with a characteristic rolled edge of granulation tissue. In contrast to syphilitic ulcers and particularly to chancroid, inguinal lymphadenopathy is generally mild or absent.

The diagnosis of granuloma inguinale is established via crush preparations or tissue biopsy specimens in which intracellular inclusions, the responsible encapsulated rod-shaped organisms (Donovan bodies), are seen within the cytoplasm of dermal macrophages. The term "parasitized macrophages" is often used to describe this histologic finding, and it is also seen in histoplasmosis, penicilliosis, rhinoscleroma, and leishmaniasis. The distinguishing features in granuloma inguinale are the clear haloes (representing nonstaining capsules) that surround the deep-purple-staining Donovan bodies in Giemsa-stained sections and the bipolar staining of the organisms such that they resemble safety pins. Treatment options are outlined in Table 35-2.

TABLE 35-2 Therapy of Chancroid, Granuloma Inguinale, Lymphogranuloma Venereum, and Gonorrhea as Recommended by the Centers for Disease Control and Prevention (CDC) (2010/2012 Updates; www.cdc.gov/std/treatment)

	Recommended	Alternative
Chancroid	**Azithromycin** 1 g orally in a single dose—or— **Ceftriaxone** 250 mg intramuscularly (IM) in a single dose—or— **Ciprofloxacin** 500 mg orally twice a day for 3 days[a,b]—or— **Erythromycin base** 500 mg orally three times a day for 7 days[b] Sexual partners should be treated if they had sexual contact with the patient during the 10 days preceding the patient's onset of symptoms	
Granuloma inguinale	**Doxycycline** 100 mg orally twice a day for a minimum of 3 weeks[c,d]	**Azithromycin** 1 g orally once per week for a minimum of 3 weeks[c,d]—or— **Ciprofloxacin** 750 mg orally twice a day for a minimum of 3 weeks[c,d]—or— **Erythromycin base** 500 mg orally four times a day for a minimum of 3 weeks[c,d,e]—or— **Trimethoprim-sulfamethoxazole** one double-strength tablet orally twice a day for a minimum of 3 weeks[c,d]
Lymphogranuloma venereum	**Doxycycline** 100 mg orally twice a day for 21 days Sexual partners should be examined if they had sexual contact with the patient during the 60 days preceding the patient's onset of symptoms and treated if symptomatic	**Erythromycin base** 500 mg orally four times a day for 21 days[f]
Gonorrhea Uncomplicated gonococcal infections of the urethra, cervix, and rectum	**Ceftriaxone** 250 mg in a single intramuscular dose PLUS **Azithromycin** 1 g orally in a single dose or **doxycycline** 100 mg orally twice daily for 7 days	If ceftriaxone is not available: **Cefixime** 400 mg in a single oral dose PLUS **Azithromycin** 1 g orally in a single dose Or **doxycycline** 100 mg orally twice daily for 7 days PLUS Test-of-cure in 1 week If the patient has severe cephalosporin allergy: **Azithromycin** 2 g in a single oral dose PLUS Test-of-cure in 1 week
Uncomplicated gonococcal infection of the pharynx	**Ceftriaxone** 250 mg in a single intramuscular dose PLUS **Azithromycin** 1 g orally in a single dose or **doxycycline** 100 mg orally twice daily for 7 days	Desensitization to cephalosporin—or— **Azithromycin** 2 g orally only if desensitization not possible[g]
Disseminated gonococcal infection (DGI)	**Ceftriaxone** 1 g IM or IV every 24 hours All regimens should be continued for 24-48 hours After clinical improvement, at which time therapy may be switched to appropriate oral therapy to complete at least 1 week of antimicrobial treatment.	**Cefotaxime** 1 g IV every 8 hours—or— **Ceftizoxime** 1 g IV every 8 hours—or— Desensitization to cephalosporin

[a]Ciprofloxacin is contraindicated for pregnant and lactating women.
[b]Worldwide, several isolates with intermediate resistance to either ciprofloxacin or erythromycin have been reported.
[c]Therapy should be continued until all lesions have healed completely; however, relapse can occur 6–18 months later despite effective initial therapy.
[d]For any of the regimens, the addition of an aminoglycoside (gentamicin 1 mg/kg IV every 8 hours) should be considered if lesions do not respond within the first few days of therapy.
[e]Both pregnant and lactating women should be treated with the erythromycin regimen; the addition of a parenteral aminoglycoside (e.g., gentamicin) should be strongly considered.
[f]Pregnant women should be treated with the erythromycin regimen.
[g]Concern regarding emerging resistance.
Adapted from CDC; www.cdc.gov/std.

Lymphogranuloma Venereum

Lymphogranuloma venereum (LGV) is also an unusual sexually transmitted disease, the etiologic agents of which are the invasive serovars L1, L2, L2a, or L3 of *Chlamydia trachomatis*. The initial lesion is a small (<1 cm) ulcer or "button-like" papule that resolves spontaneously. This is followed by the development of inguinal and/or femoral lymphadenopathy that is often unilateral. When the enlarged coalescing lymph nodes are found both above and below Poupart's ligament, a central indentation can form, and this is commonly referred to as the "groove sign." LGV is associated with fistula formation (secondary to draining lymph nodes),

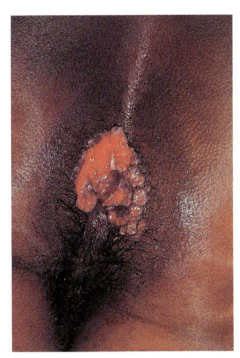

FIGURE 35-29 ■ Ulcerated plaques of granuloma inguinale.

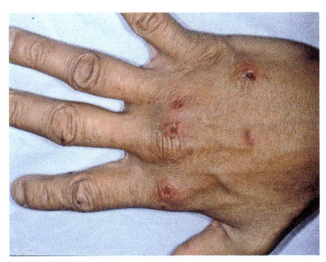

FIGURE 35-30 ■ Multiple crusted papulopustules in a patient with disseminated gonococcemia. (Courtesy of Dr. Neil A. Fenske, Tampa, FL.)

lymphedema of the genitalia, and symptomatic rectal involvement. Additional manifestations include fever, conjunctivitis, arthralgias, and a papular photoeruption. Although a definitive diagnosis requires isolation of the organism via tissue culture (requiring a special medium, cycloheximide-treated McCoy or HeLa cells), the clinician must often rely on less specific serologic assays. A high IgG titer (>1:64) and/or a fourfold increase supports the clinical diagnosis. Direct fluorescent antibody (DFA) test, and/or PCR of likely infected areas and pus, are also sometimes used. DFA test for the L-type serovar of *C. trachomatis* is the most sensitive and specific test, but is not readily available. If PCR tests on infected material are positive for *C. trachomatis*, further analysis needs to be done to determine the genotype. Recently a rapid real-time PCR has been developed to diagnose LGV.

Treatment options are outlined in Table 35-2.

Disseminated Gonococcal Infection

Bacteremia with *Neisseria gonorrhoeae* can lead to fever, tenosynovitis, arthralgias, arthritis, and a few scattered cutaneous lesions. The latter are usually in an acral location and have an erythematous to purpuric base (Fig. 35-30); a central pustule is often seen. Disseminated gonococcal infection (DGI) is seen more frequently in women (often in association with menstruation) as well as in men who have sex with men, presumably because both groups have a higher incidence of occult primary infections that remain untreated. Disseminated gonococcal infection presents in several clinical forms with a classic triad of dermatosis, tenosynovitis, and arthritis. Unusual manifestations of DGI include perihepatitis, endocarditis, and meningitis. Sites of primary infection include the cervix, urethra, rectum, and pharynx.

Treatment requires a more aggressive approach than does treatment of primary sites of infection (Table 35-2). The CDC no longer recommends the use of fluoroquinolones because of increasing resistance to this group of antibiotics in the United States. They may represent an alternative treatment, but only if antimicrobial susceptibility can be documented by culture.

SUGGESTED READINGS

Afonso JP, Tomimori J, Michalany NS, Nonogaki S, Porro AM. Pruritic papular eruption and eosinophilic folliculitis associated with human immunodeficiency virus (HIV) infection: a histopathological and immunohistochemical comparative study. J Am Acad Dermatol 2012;67(2):269–75.

Centers for Disease Control and Prevention (CDC). Sexually transmitted diseases trends in the United States. MMWR Morb Mortal Wkly Rep; 59 (No.RR-12).

Centers for Disease Control and Prevention (CDC). Update to CDC's Sexually transmitted diseases treatment guidelines, 2010: oral cephalosporins no longer a recommended treatment for gonococcal infections. MMWR Morb Mortal Wkly Rep 2012;61(31):590–4.

Chua SL, Amerson EH, Leslie KS, McCalmont TH, Leboit PE, Martin JN, Bangsberg D, Maurer TA. Factors associated with pruritic papular eruption of human immunodeficiency virus infection in the antiretroviral therapy era. Br J Dermatol 2014;170(4):832–9.

De Vries HJ. Skin as an indicator for sexually transmitted infections. Clin Dermatol 2014;32(2):196–208.

Dlova NC, Mosam A. Inflammatory noninfectious dermatoses of HIV. Dermatol Clin 2006;24:439–48.

Galarza C, Ramos W, Gutierrez EL, Ronceros G, Teran M, Uribe M, Navincopa M, Ortega-Loayza AG. Cutaneous acanthamebiasis infection in immunocompetent and immunocompromised patients. Int J Dermatol 2009;48(12):1324–9.

Gormley RH, Kovarik CL. Human papillomavirus-related genital disease in the immunocompromised host: parts I & II. J Am Acad Dermatol 2012;66(6):867–900.

Hogan MT. Cutaneous infections associated with HIV/AIDS. Dermatol Clin 2006;24:473–95.

Laurent F, Gómez-Flores M, Mendez N, Ancer-Rodríguez J, Bryant JL, Gaspari AA. Trujillo. New insights into HIV-1-primary skin disorders. J Int AIDS Soc 2011, 24;14:5.

Marin M, Güris D, Chaves SS, Schmid S, Seward JF. Advisory Committee on Immunization Practices, Centers for Disease Control and Prevention (CDC). Prevention of varicella: recommendations of the Advisory Committee on Immunization Practices (ACIP). MMWR Recomm Rep 2007; 22;56(RR-4):1–40.

Nagot N, Ouédrago A, Foulongne V, et al. Reduction of HIV-1 RNA levels with therapy to suppress herpes simplex virus. N Engl J Med 2007;356:790–9.

Palacios R, Jimenez-Onate F, Aguilar M, et al. Impact of syphilis infection on HIV viral load and CD4 cell counts in HIV-infected patients. J Acquir Immune Defic Syndr 2007;44:356–9.

Wanat KA, Gormley RH, Rosenbach M, Kovarik CL. Intralesional cidofovir for treating extensive genital verrucous herpes simplex virus infection. JAMA Dermatol 2013;149(7):881–3.

WHO fact sheet on HIV/AIDS Available from: http://www.who.int/mediacentre/factsheets/fs360/en/ [accessed 08.08.14].

CHAPTER 36

SARCOIDOSIS

Misha A. Rosenbach • Joseph C. English III • Jeffrey P. Callen

KEY POINTS

- Sarcoidosis is a multisystem granulomatous disease of unknown etiology that affects patients of all ages and ethnic groups.
- Thorough multisystem evaluation of all patients is essential, as sarcoidal inflammation may be clinically quiescent while causing significant damage.
- Cutaneous sarcoidosis is characterized by a protean array of lesion morphologies, but generally occurs as violaceous infiltrated papules clustered on the face, particularly around the nose.
- Sarcoidosis may spontaneously resolve in up to two-thirds of patients during the first few years of disease; patients with extensive skin involvement are more likely to have a chronic course.
- Mortality occurs in 5% of patients, generally those with severe pulmonary involvement, cardiac involvement, or neurosarcoidosis.
- Treatment options range from topical and intralesional steroids, to antimalarials or anti-inflammatory antibiotics, to methotrexate, to TNF-α inhibitors.

Sarcoidosis is a multisystem disorder of unknown cause characterized by the accumulation of T-cell lymphocytes, monocytes, and epithelioid macrophages from an unknown antigen(s) that induce the formation of noncaseating granulomas, leading to abnormal tissue and organ function. Sarcoidosis almost always involves the lungs; the skin, eyes, and lymph nodes are frequently involved; however, the disease can involve any organ system in the body. While there are suggestive laboratory and radiographic findings supportive of a diagnosis, there exists no gold-standard confirmatory diagnostic test. The disease is characterized by the presence of granulomatous inflammation in more than one organ. When this histopathologic change is present in tissue samples from multiple organ systems, and when appropriate tests exclude other causes of sarcoidal granulomas, the diagnosis of sarcoidosis can be confirmed.

The course of sarcoidosis is highly variable. It ranges from an acute self-healing process, to a chronic disease that primarily affects the skin, to a debilitating systemic disease that can result in blindness, progressive respiratory insufficiency, and sometimes death. Although associated with significant morbidity, sarcoidosis is rarely a primary cause of death, with fewer than 5% of patients dying of their disease, generally due to severe lung, neurologic, or cardiac involvement.

CAUSE AND PATHOGENESIS

The cause of sarcoidosis is unknown. The current understanding entails a genetically susceptible host, who is then exposed to an environmental trigger, which sets off the host immune response leading to granuloma formation and the clinical disease phenotype. Over the years many causes have been postulated, including viruses (hepatitis C, HIV, HHV-8), bacteria (*Mycobacterium*, *Propionibacterium*, *Borrelia*, *Rickettsia*, cell-wall-deficient bacteria), fungi (cryptococcus), an autoantigen or misfolded protein (amyloid A), and foreign materials (pine pollen, beryllium, talc, silica). Coexistent "autoimmune" diseases, such as autoimmune thyroiditis, alopecia areata, and vitiligo, have been reported with varying frequencies in small studies, and patients with various collagen–vascular diseases (scleroderma, lupus, or dermatomyositis) may be more prone to develop sarcoidosis.

There is no single gene that explains sarcoidosis; rather, the disease is due to a complex interaction between the host immune system and environmental triggers, with multiple genes conferring potential risk. A genetic component of sarcoidosis is recognized due to a markedly increased rate of disease in monozygotic twins compared to dizygotic twins, with a strong relative risk of 4.7 for disease in family members of affected patients. Multiple HLA alleles may play a role in conferring a predilection for developing the disease, and the genes involved may vary by ethnic group. HLA-DRB1*01 and DRB1*04 may be protective, while DRB1*03, DRB1*11, DRB1*12, DRB1*14, and DRB1*15 may confer an increased risk. One subtype of sarcoidosis, Löfgren's syndrome, characterized by hilar adenopathy, fever, arthritis, and erythema nodosum, which tends to be acute and self-resolving, may be associated with HLA-B8/DR3. African-American patients, an ethnic group with some of the highest overall incidence of sarcoidosis and a tendency toward chronic disease, may be more impacted by the HLA-DQB1 alleles. Beyond the HLA alleles, specific genes may confer disease susceptibility, including polymorphisms in the *TNF* gene and the *IL23R* gene; polymorphisms in the gene encoding angiotensin-converting enzyme have also been identified in patients with sarcoidosis. While sarcoidosis has historically been considered a Th1-predominant immune reaction, the granulomatous inflammatory cascade likely involves both the innate immune system (via Toll-like receptors) and potentially the Th17 immune system as well. The key cytokines include Th1 cytokines such as IL-2, IL-12, IL-18, and IFN-γ, granulocyte–monocyte colony stimulating factor, and TNF-α production by macrophages. The inflammatory pattern may vary by ethnicity, inciting antigenic trigger, or potentially disease phenotype, with different patterns of inflammation in patients with acute and self-resolving sarcoidosis compared to patients with chronic inflammatory or fibrotic disease. The end result is that sarcoidosis is a multifactorial combination of possible immunologic (T-cell receptor), genetic (HLA), infectious, or environmental factors (antigen[s]), and to date no single component can explain all cases of sarcoidosis.

Because of the lack of a consistent identifiable antigen(s), the polymorphic nature of the disease, and the lack of an animal model, a definitive pathogenesis is speculative at present and active research is ongoing. Sarcoidosis is believed to be a disorder of the lymphoreticular system characterized by the depression of cell-mediated immunity (delayed-type hypersensitivity), an imbalance of CD4/CD8 cells (helper-to-suppressor T-cell ratio), a hyperreactivity of B cells, and increased production of circulating immune complexes. It is believed that the interaction between T cells and antigens, antigen-presenting cells and cytokines in the correct genetic milieu affects T-cell function, which results in a secondary increase in B-cell activity. Prolonged antigenic stimulation may affect macrophages. As sarcoidal granulomas develop, enzyme secretion (in particular, secretion of angiotensin-converting enzyme—ACE) may occur. Elevation of ACE is probably the result of granuloma formation, and in some patients may reflect overall granuloma burden, although the ACE level overall lacks sensitivity, specificity, or reliability and cannot readily be utilized to either diagnose or follow disease activity over time. The precise reasons for the effects of the presumptive causative antigen(s) on patients with sarcoidosis are not understood. However, the result appears to be an overall somewhat anergic state, with a reduced reaction to recalled antigens, such as purified protein derivative, *Candida*, mumps, and the inability to sensitize an individual with sarcoidosis to an antigen such as dinitrochlorobenzene. Elevated levels of γ-globulin and nonspecific elevation of antibody titers to various viruses and fungal elements may also occur.

CLINICAL MANIFESTATIONS

Cutaneous Manifestations

The skin is involved in 25% to 30% of patients with sarcoidosis, and the cutaneous manifestations of sarcoidosis are protean. Individual skin lesions are classified as either specific or nonspecific, based on the histopathologic examination. Those cutaneous lesions represented histopathologically by noncaseating granulomas are termed "specific" cutaneous lesions of sarcoidosis. Those lesions that do not show noncaseating granulomas are termed nonspecific, and are usually applied to lesions such as erythema nodosum. The specific cutaneous lesions include papules, plaques, nodules, subcutaneous nodules ("Darrier–Roussy" sarcoidosis), scar— or tattoo—associated papules, and lupus pernio. In addition, there are multiple less common presentations of specific cutaneous lesions such as acquired ichthyosis, erythroderma, psoriasiform, ulcerative, verrucous, scarring or nonscarring alopecia, photodistributed, and angiolupoid sarcoidosis. Interestingly, nail disease has been reported both as specific and nonspecific.

The most common nonspecific manifestation of sarcoidosis is erythema nodosum (EN). These lesions are firm, slightly erythematous to red-brown subcutaneous nodules, most commonly occurring symmetrically on the anterior tibial surfaces. They are often tender to palpation. When erythema nodosum is associated with sarcoidosis, it is frequently accompanied by uveitis, fever, arthritis, and asymptomatic bilateral hilar lymphadenopathy. This four-symptom complex is referred to as Löfgren's syndrome. It is an acute form of sarcoidosis that self-resolves in 90% or more of affected individuals, although sometimes patients require transient anti-inflammatory treatment for symptom control. It is postulated that these patients have circulating immune complexes that cause erythema nodosum. Biopsies of the lungs and lymph nodes in these patients reveal sarcoidal granulomas. Biopsy is not indicated in patients who have the typical tetrad. Löfgren's syndrome is most common in patients of northern European ancestry, and is relatively rare in African-Americans. Several other sarcoidosis syndromes have been described, including Heerfordt–Waldenström syndrome (fever, parotid gland enlargement, anterior uveitis, and facial nerve palsy); Mikulicz syndrome (bilateral sarcoidosis of the lacrimal, sublingual, submandibular, and parotid glands); and sarcoidosis–lymphoma syndrome (Hodgkin or non-Hodgkin lymphoma developing in patients with chronic active sarcoidosis).

The "specific" cutaneous lesions of sarcoidosis occur in roughly 10% to 25% of patients with documented systemic sarcoidosis. The diagnosis of a cutaneous sarcoidal granuloma is made by skin biopsy. Diascopy (Fig. 36-1) may help the dermatologist consider a granulomatous disease process, revealing "apple-jelly" orange-brown colors, but is not exclusive to sarcoidosis. Certain

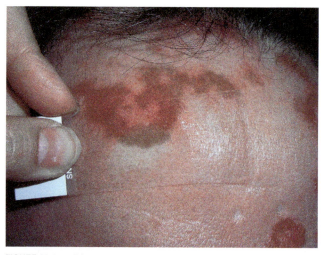

FIGURE 36-1 ■ Diascopy in a patient with sarcoidosis may aid in the clinical diagnosis.

cutaneous lesions may be highly suggestive of sarcoidosis, but none are clinically diagnostic. The cutaneous lesions of sarcoidosis can mimic many dermatoses and should frequently be included in differential diagnoses, especially the other noninfectious granulomatous diseases granuloma annulare, necrobiosis lipoidica, necrobiotic xanthogranuloma, actinic elastolytic granuloma, reactive granulomatous eruptions such as interstitial granulomatous dermatitis and palisaded neutrophilic granulomatous dermatitis, cutaneous Crohn's disease, cheilitis granulomatosis, foreign-body reactions, and the granulomatous facial dermatitidies, as well as infectious granulomatous diseases such as deep fungal infections, atypical mycobacteria, leprosy, syphilis, and cutaneous tuberculosis or cutaneous tuberculid reactions to remote tuberculosis infections. The most common cutaneous presentation of sarcoidosis is a papular lesion: small papules, erythematous-to-violaceous, 3 to 5 mm in diameter, are frequently noted on the head and neck (Fig. 36-2). The periorbital and periorificial regions are commonly involved, with lesions commonly seen around the nostrils on the nares, and around the eyes and/or mouth (Fig. 36-3). The lesions may be flesh-colored, red, violaceous, or slightly hyperpigmented. At times the papules enlarge or coalesce to form annular lesions (Fig. 36-4), nodules (Fig. 36-5), or plaques (Fig. 36-6). Papular disease at the corners of the mouth may often coalesce and split, being indistinguishable from the classic split papule of secondary syphilis.

Indurated plaque-type lesions are also common, and can involve any area of the body. Infiltrated lesions involving the face, specifically the nose and cheeks, with or without scale, are classically referred to as lupus pernio (Fig. 36-7). If extensive telangiectatic lesions are evident, this is termed angiolupoid sarcoidosis. Chronic longstanding lupus pernio and angiolupoid sarcoidosis can ulcerate, and patients with extensive nasal involvement have higher rates of sarcoidosis involving the upper respiratory tract (i.e., the sinuses), pulmonary fibrosis, and possibly bone cysts. Patients with lupus pernio or angiolupoid sarcoidosis frequently have chronic sarcoidosis, and the pulmonary involvement is often persistent. This cutaneous pattern is also often treatment refractory and requires aggressive therapeutic intervention to achieve partial or complete remission. Patients with papular, nodular, or plaque-like lesions on the face have been misrepresented innumerable times as having lupus pernio, and are not associated with

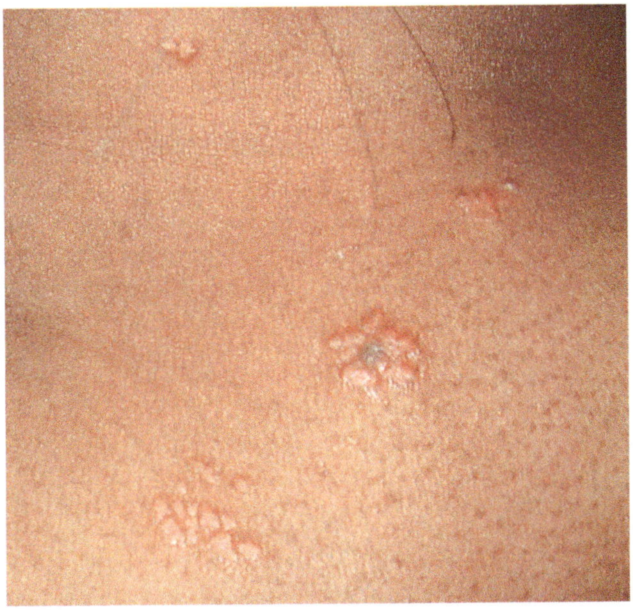

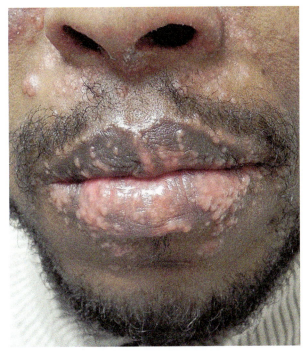

FIGURE 36-3 ■ Extensive papules of the nareas, philtrum, and lips.

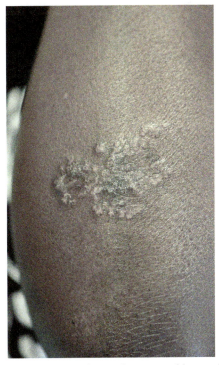

FIGURE 36-4 ■ Annular plaques in a man with sarcoidosis.

FIGURE 36-2 ■ Small papular sarcoidosis lesions on the neck; note some are forming small annular clusters or coalescing into small plaques.

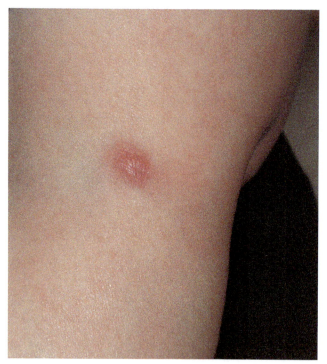

FIGURE 36-5 ■ Nodular sarcoidosis.

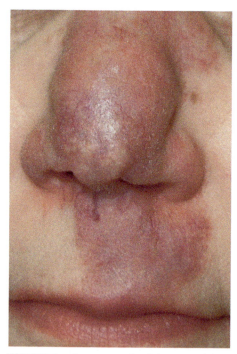

FIGURE 36-7 ■ Lupus pernio of the central face.

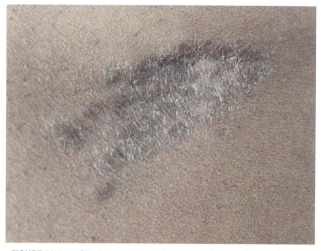

FIGURE 36-6 ■ Slightly scaly, violaceous plaque of sarcoidosis.

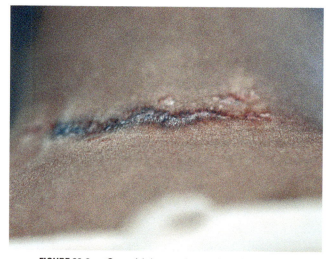

FIGURE 36-8 ■ Sarcoidal granulomas in a linear scar.

a greater risk of pulmonary disease. In fact, all cutaneous disease manifestations other than EN have yet to be convincingly proven as having prognostic implications.

Sarcoidosis often occurs in scars (Fig. 36-8), tattoos (Fig. 36-9), or on areas of skin previously damaged by infection, radiation, or prior trauma. Sometimes it becomes difficult to determine whether these lesions are indeed cutaneous sarcoidosis, or whether they are local sarcoidal reactions to a foreign substance. Pathologic analysis of biopsies from patients with systemic sarcoidosis have demonstrated that foreign material is sometimes present (approximately 25% of the time) in the skin biopsy specimens. In the absence of systemic disease, a diagnosis of sarcoidosis cannot be made with confidence, particularly when only one area of the body is involved. The subcutaneous nodular lesions are often asymptomatic, and they frequently occur on the trunk and

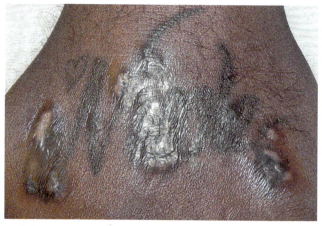

FIGURE 36-9 ■ Sarcoidal papules and plaques within a tattoo.

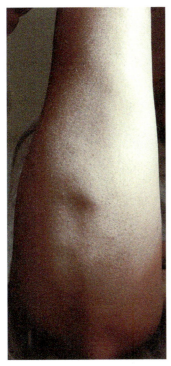

FIGURE 36-10 ■ Subcutaneous plaques and nodules in a patient with "Darrier–Roussy" variant sarcoidosis.

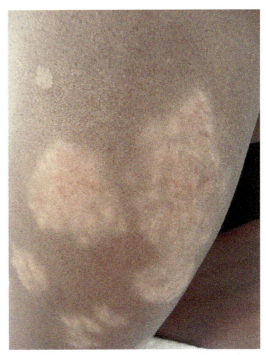

FIGURE 36-11 ■ Hypopigmentation in previously violaceous sarcoidosis during treatment; sarcoid lesions may lighten, "break up," and flatten out during therapy. The appearance of the lesions shown here is similar to how de novo hypopigmented sarcoidosis may appear.

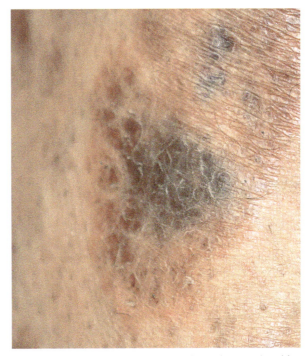

FIGURE 36-12 ■ Ichthyosiform sarcoidosis on the anterior shins.

extremities (Fig. 36-10). These lesions are rarely tender. A review of Mayo Clinic patients with subcutaneous sarcoidosis noted that such patients were more likely to be women in their fourth decade, and for there to be a strong association with bilateral hilar adenopathy, the relevance of which is uncertain given the high rates of pulmonary involvement (including hilar adenopathy) in sarcoidosis patients overall.

There are many unusual forms of sarcoidosis, as previously mentioned. Ulceration of sarcoid lesions is unusual, but can be seen on the lower extremities, where the disease may clinically and histologically mimic necrobiosis lipoidica. Verrucous lesions, although rare, occur most commonly in black females. They are reported most frequently on the lower extremities but may occur at any site. Macular hypopigmentation can rarely be seen and may be mistaken for hypopigmented mycosis fungoides or leprosy (Fig. 36-11). Ichthyosis-like lesions occur in many patients with sarcoidosis (Fig. 36-12); while there is a broad differential for causes of acquired ichthyosis, biopsies of the ichthyotic skin in patients with sarcoidosis may reveal typical granulomatous inflammation. Sarcoidosis may also affect the orogenital mucosa or the nail unit, and can cause a scarring or nonscarring alopecia (Fig. 36-13). Erythrodemic presentations of sarcoidosis are rare but have been reported. Sarcoidosis has not been reported to present with either bullae or pustules.

Intrathoracic Disease

Intrathoracic disease, including hilar adenopathy and pulmonary parenchymal disease, is the most common manifestation of systemic sarcoidosis, occurring in more than 90% of patients. Many patients are asymptomatic; symptoms may include dyspnea, a chronic, dry, nonproductive cough, or severe breathing dysfunction. Pulmonary sarcoidosis can be staged, according to chest X-ray findings, from 0 to III. Stage 0 disease consists of no changes seen on chest X-ray studies. Stage I includes bilateral hilar adenopathy in the absence of parenchymal disease. Stage II consists of hilar adenopathy with the presence of interstitial pulmonary fibrosis. Stage III consists of extensive pulmonary fibrosis in

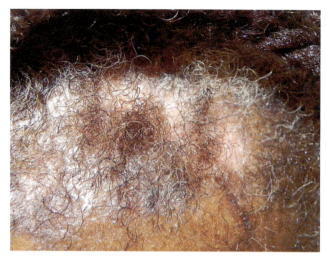

FIGURE 36-13 ■ Scarring alopecia due to chronic cutaneous sarcoidosis.

the absence of hilar adenopathy. The stages of radiographic findings do not represent chronological development. A diagnosis of sarcoidosis is often made on a "routine" chest X-ray in an entirely asymptomatic patient. Patients who have bilateral hilar adenopathy without evidence of symptoms require monitoring; often the disease resolves spontaneously in all stages of pulmonary sarcoidosis. Abnormalities may be found by careful testing with pulmonary function tests and/or with bronchoalveolar lavage or ultrasound-guided transbronchial biopsies. Techniques such as positron emission tomography and high-resolution computed tomography (CT) scanning are also used.

Bilateral hilar adenopathy is the earliest and most common intrathoracic manifestation of sarcoidosis. Patients with this finding are often asymptomatic, although erythema nodosum, uveitis, arthritis, and fever may accompany the hilar lymphadenopathy, as previously mentioned. These patients with stage I disease rarely develop progressive parenchymal disease. Biopsy is not necessary in most patients with bilateral hilar adenopathy with symptoms of Löfgren's syndrome, or in those who are asymptomatic. However, only a small proportion of patients who have either unilateral hilar adenopathy or dyspnea have sarcoidosis. The differential diagnosis of bilateral hilar adenopathy includes deep fungal infection, tuberculosis, lymphoma, and bronchogenic carcinoma. Patients with these manifestations should undergo a lung biopsy and, possibly, mediastinal nodal biopsies. Stages II and III pulmonary sarcoidosis are associated with a much higher incidence of chronic progressive disease, and resolution of the X-ray findings becomes less likely. Symptoms may be present or absent. However, abnormal pulmonary function testing correlates with more severe disease seen on chest X-ray studies, and forced vital capacity is typically followed for disease progression and in clinical trials to measure sarcoidosis response to treatment.

Ocular Manifestations

Ocular involvement occurs in approximately one-quarter of patients with sarcoidosis, and may affect any portion of the eye. Acute ocular sarcoidosis generally runs a course

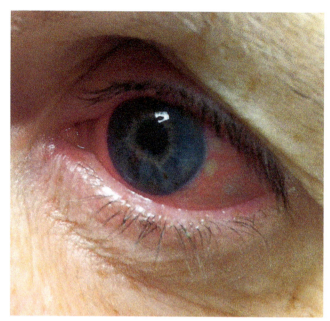

FIGURE 36-14 ■ Intense scleritis from ocular sarcoidosis.

of 2 years or less, during which time active therapy may be needed. Chronic eye disease is less common. Early aggressive intervention can prevent scarring and blindness.

The most common ocular manifestation of sarcoidosis is uveitis, which usually affects the anterior segment of the eye. Patients may be entirely asymptomatic, or they may present with a red eye, photophobia, or increased tear production (Fig. 36-14). The diagnosis is made by slit-lamp examination, which reveals "mutton fat" keratic precipitates in the anterior chamber. Less commonly, the posterior segment of the eye is involved, and its appearance correlates well with chorioretinitis and neurosarcoidosis. Uveitis must be aggressively treated to prevent adhesions, with resulting glaucoma, cataract development, or blindness. As ocular sarcoidosis may be clinically asymptomatic, up to the point of severe visual compromise, patients must undergo regular screening with at least annual ophthalmological exams.

Another common ocular finding in patients with sarcoidosis is conjunctival and lacrimal gland involvement. This may or may not produce symptoms of ocular irritation. Conjunctival granulomas occur in about one-third of patients with sarcoidosis. Conjunctival biopsy specimens may be positive even when the patient lacks clinical evidence of conjunctival involvement.

Lymph Nodes

Sarcoidal granulomas commonly infiltrate the lymph nodes. The incidence of peripheral lymphadenopathy is roughly 30% in patients with systemic sarcoidosis. Lymphadenopathy is associated with both acute and chronic disease patterns. Lymph node involvement, detected by palpation, is usually nontender, and is often not noticed by the patient. Because of the increased risk of lymphoma in patients with sarcoidosis (termed the sarcoidosis–lymphoma syndrome), extensive adenopathy or new adenopathy presenting out-of-step with a patient's

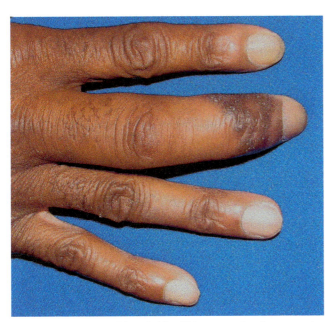

FIGURE 36-15 ■ Sarcoid arthritis. This man also has papular cutaneous lesions.

sarcoidosis should be evaluated with fine-needle aspiration or biopsy of lymph nodes, as histologically they can be easily distinguished.

Splenic involvement in sarcoidosis is detected in approximately 20% to 25% of patients. It is manifested by splenomegaly, but functional abnormalities are rare.

Musculoskeletal Manifestations

Symptomatic muscle involvement in sarcoidosis is rare, although biopsy-based detection of a sarcoidal infiltrate is not uncommon. Clinical series of large numbers of patients with sarcoidosis reveal that approximately 1% have symptoms of muscle involvement. However, when patients with sarcoidosis undergo random muscle biopsies, more than 50% have histologic evidence of granulomatous disease. At times, muscle involvement may appear as subcutaneous nodules, although this is rare.

Bone lesions occur in 10% to 15% of patients, usually correlating with chronic progressive disease. The X-ray changes are cystic lesions that usually occur in the terminal phalanges of the hands. These may be accompanied by soft tissue swelling (Fig. 36-15). Arthralgias are commonly experienced in acute sarcoidosis, particularly in patients with Löfgren's syndrome, and may be accompanied by arthritis. The wrists, knees, and ankles are the most commonly affected joints. Although chronic granulomatous arthritis has been reported, it is a rare complication of systemic sarcoidosis.

Neurosarcoidosis

Neurosarcoidosis affects 5% to 15% of patients with systemic sarcoidosis. Central nervous system involvement occurs in 50% of patients with neurosarcoidosis. The presence of neurosarcoidosis correlates with the presence of posterior uveitis and chronic cutaneous disease. The most common neurologic manifestations of sarcoidosis include cranial neuropathies such as optic nerve disease or facial nerve palsy, meningitis, and cerebral granulomas, which can lead to encephalopathy and seizures. Heerfordt–Waldenström syndrome is also frequently associated with central nervous system involvement. The detection of neurosarcoidosis can be difficult because affected tissue is not readily available for microscopic evaluation. The evaluation of a patient with suspected neurosarcoidosis can include skull X-ray studies, electroencephalography, a CT scan, and/or magnetic resonance imaging of the brain. Lumbar puncture may also be useful in patients with meningeal involvement. Small-fiber neuropathy can occur due to sarcoidosis and can present with peripheral nerve symptoms, including atypical pain.

Hepatic Sarcoidosis

Hepatic involvement in sarcoidosis is common. In a large study, hepatomegaly was detected in 20% to 50% of patients with sarcoidosis. Abnormal liver function tests are present in approximately half of patients with hepatic involvement. Liver biopsy may be useful to obtain tissue to establish a diagnosis of sarcoidosis, although care must be taken to exclude other causes of granulomatous disease of the liver, and the findings must be correlated with evidence of sarcoidal disease elsewhere in the body. Hepatic involvement rarely progresses to functional abnormalities or cirrhosis. Combined hepatosplenomegaly is associated with a poorer outcome owing to the higher overall body granuloma and fibrosis burden.

Endocrine, Metabolic, and Laboratory Abnormalities

Endocrine glands may be infiltrated by sarcoidal granulomas. Functional abnormalities are not common, although pituitary or hypothalamic infiltration can cause diabetes insipidus or, on rare occasions, panhypopituitarism. An elevated prolactin level is a useful indicator of hypothalamic sarcoidal involvement. A number of studies have indicated a potential increased risk of thyroid disease in patients with sarcoidosis, although it is not clear if that is due to direct granulomatous inflammation or shared autoimmune inflammation. Other endocrine organs, such as the parathyroid and adrenal glands and the pancreas, may be involved. However, functional impairment of these organs is unusual.

Hypercalcemia occurs in some patients with sarcoidosis. In occasional patients with widespread sarcoidosis, the serum calcium level elevation can be persistent, and can lead to urinary tract stones, nephrocalcinosis, and even renal failure. Hypercalciuria is more common than hypercalcemia and may be used as a correlate with disease activity. The granulomas in sarcoidosis are metabolically active and produce high levels of 1α-hydroxylase, converting 25-hydroxy vitamin D to its active 1,25-dihydroxy form, and leading to increased vitamin D activity and elevated serum calcium.

The serum ACE level is raised in approximately 60% of patients with systemic sarcoidosis. ACE is produced by epithelioid cells and may reflect the granuloma load in the body. ACE levels are neither sensitive nor specific to sarcoidosis, and medications and other pulmonary inflammatory processes may lead to elevations. When the ACE level is markedly elevated, two to three times the upper limit of normal, sarcoidosis may be more likely. ACE is not routinely reliable in monitoring disease activity, but may trend with granuloma burden in a subset of patients. Other blood levels, such as serum IL2 receptor or chitotriosidase, are investigational and are not widely available or clinically practical in evaluating patients with systemic sarcoidosis.

Cardiac Disease

The true incidence of cardiac involvement in sarcoidosis is not known. However, autopsy studies suggest that it is more common than clinically apparent and frequently asymptomatic. Cardiac sarcoidosis can result in symptoms of congestive heart failure, arrhythmia, or conduction defects. The most common symptom is sudden death. Appropriate screening for cardiac sarcoidosis is controversial and recommendations are rapidly changing. All patients should have a thorough review of symptoms and electrocardiography; any abnormalities (including a history of palpitations) likely warrant further testing, such as 24-hour Holter monitoring, echocardiogram, cardiac positron emission tomography, magnetic resonance imaging, or referral to a cardiologist.

Other Clinical Manifestations of Sarcoidosis

Almost any area of the body can be affected by sarcoidosis. Granulomatous renal disease has been reported on several occasions, although renal impairment is more often due to persistent hypercalcemia and hypercalcuria. Gastric granulomas, breast soft tissue granulomas, bone marrow granulomas, spinal cord lesions, and gonadal granulomas have also been reported.

Relationship of Cutaneous Disease to Systemic Disease

Many studies detail the cutaneous disease in patients with sarcoidosis. Unfortunately, none of these studies used the same methods, and many did not define the cutaneous lesions adequately. However, a few generalizations can be made. Patients with lupus pernio more frequently have sarcoidosis of the upper respiratory tract and lungs, as well as possibly more bone involvement, than do patients without lupus pernio. Those patients with EN and bilateral hilar lymphadenopathy (Löfgren's syndrome) have a self-limiting course and a good prognosis. In all cases of cutaneous sarcoidosis, patients require evaluation for systemic involvement.

HISTOPATHOLOGIC FINDINGS

Sarcoidosis is characterized by granulomas composed principally of epithelioid cells with an occasional giant cell and little or no caseation necrosis, with scant perigranulomatous lymphocytic inflammation. Inclusion bodies (Schaumann, Hamazalki–Wasserman, and asteroid bodies) may be observed in varying numbers, but these are not specific for sarcoidosis and may occur in other granulomatous conditions. The granulomas may remain seemingly unchanged for months or years, may resolve completely, or may undergo a fibrotic change. Although this is classically a dermal disease, epidermal change has been demonstrated histologically (particularly in vulvar sarcoidosis, wherein transepidermal elimination of granulomas has been reported).

The histopathologic differential diagnosis includes other granulomatous diseases, which may be excluded by special stains (infectious granulomas) and/or examination for foreign material (foreign body granulomas). Because noncaseating granulomas are not specific for sarcoidosis, other conditions must be vigorously excluded before a diagnosis of sarcoidosis can be confirmed. Thus, the diagnosis is one of exclusion. Special stains of the histopathologic specimens should include the acid-fast bacilli and Fite stain for mycobacteria, and periodic acid–Schiff stain for fungal elements. In addition, examination for a foreign body reaction with at least polarized light should be undertaken, although the presence of foreign material does not exclude the diagnosis, with refractile material reported in up to 25% of sarcoidosis skin biopsies. Various neoplasms should be excluded, particularly lymphomas, because there are occasional reports of sarcoidal tissue reactions occurring in nodes adjacent to neoplastic change.

DIAGNOSIS AND DIFFERENTIAL DIAGNOSIS

Sarcoidosis is diagnosed by a combination of clinical, radiologic, and laboratory findings plus the demonstration of noncaseating granulomas in the tissue. The differential diagnosis varies according to the organs involved. The differential mainly revolves around infectious and noninfectious granulomatous disease processes for each organ system, and has been discussed above. The only exception is the diagnosis in patients with asymptomatic bilateral hilar lymphadenopathy or in patients who have Löfgren's syndrome. These two clinical presentations are characteristic enough not to require histopathologic confirmation, but require appropriate follow-up to ensure resolution of the disease process. Tissue diagnosis through biopsies of various sites remains the main procedure to confirm the diagnosis of sarcoidosis. A prime tissue for biopsy is the skin, because it is an accessible, high-yield organ. Particular attention should be paid to changes in scars, tattoos, or to any papular, nodular, or plaque-type lesion of recent onset, particularly on the nose, around the nostrils, or around the eyes and mouth. In addition, conjunctival biopsy, even in the absence of conjunctival nodules, may be positive in up to one-third of patients with sarcoidosis. Palpable lymph nodes may be biopsied when feasible. Lung biopsy through a fiberoptic bronchoscope is also helpful in establishing a diagnosis. Mediastinoscopy may be used to approach intrathoracic nodes not accessible via bronchoscopy. Blind biopsy of the minor salivary glands on the lower lip is said to be positive in up to 60% of patients with sarcoidosis. Liver biopsy is a high-yield procedure, but its morbidity and mortality rates make it less useful than the previously mentioned techniques. Muscle biopsy may reveal sarcoidal granulomas in up to 50% of patients, particularly when a needle is used. Other less accessible sites for biopsy include the bone marrow, kidney, and spleen when involvement is suspected.

EVALUATION

After a diagnosis of sarcoidosis is made, the patient should be thoroughly evaluated to define the organ systems involved and to aid in prognostic predictions and therapeutic decisions. A team approach with the internist, ophthalmologist, pulmonologist, and dermatologist is required. A careful history and physical examination should be performed, focusing on all organ systems, but with preference given to the lungs, eyes, nervous system, heart, and skin. Laboratory blood testing for chemistries, renal function, liver enzymes, and calcium level should be done. An electrocardiogram is required, and further cardiac evaluation is indicated if there are elements of the patient's history, symptoms, or electrocardiogram abnormalities. Chest imaging studies and pulmonary function tests with diffusion studies should be ordered, and should be repeated on an annual basis. All patients should undergo ophthalmological evaluation at the time of diagnosis and annually. In patients with persistent hypercalcemia or a history of kidney stones, careful evaluation of the urine is important, which may include 24-hour urine calcium levels. Additional testing could consist of skin tests to detect anergy, purified protein derivative, or interferon-γ release assay tests, creatine kinase/aldolase for suspected muscle disease, urinalysis, quantitative immunoglobulins, and protein electrophoresis. The measurement of serum ACE levels is occasionally helpful in following patients with pulmonary sarcoidosis, but not routinely for skin disease. Vitamin D levels should be evaluated, with testing for both the 25-hydroxy and 1,25-dihydroxy forms indicated. Given the potential association of sarcoidosis with thyroid disease, screening for thyroid function testing is reasonable.

PROGNOSIS

Mortality rates in sarcoidosis vary from 3% to 6%. Cardiac disease (the most common cause in Japan), progressive pulmonary disease (the most common cause in the United States), and neurosarcoidosis have been the cause of death in some patients.

The morbidity in sarcoidosis can be severe. Blindness can result from untreated ocular disease, and pulmonary disease can cause debilitating fatigue and shortness of breath, sometimes requiring oxygen supplementation or, in severe cases, lung transplantation. Renal failure requiring dialysis has been reported from granulomatous involvement of the kidney, calcium deposits, and chronic urinary tract stones. Cosmetic deformities may occur in patients with cutaneous sarcoidosis, particularly in those with lupus pernio. Although many patients with pulmonary sarcoidosis may have resolution of their disease, the rates vary with the stage of pulmonary disease. Stage I sarcoidosis resolves in roughly 60% of patients; stage II resolves in 40% of patients; and stage III resolves in only 12%.

Despite the aberrations noted in tests of cell-mediated immunity, untreated sarcoidosis is not associated with an increased number of infections. However, it has been linked to an increase in the frequency of malignancy, although some recent meta-analyses have cast doubt on these associations and suggest there may not be an increased risk of malignancy in patients with sarcoidosis. Prior studies had suggested an increased risk of skin cancers (nonmelanoma and melanoma), and several studies have reported an increased incidence of hematologic malignancy—i.e., lymphoma, leukemia, and solid tumors (i.e., lung, testes, skin). Of note is that smoking has been associated with a reduced risk of developing pulmonary sarcoidosis because of its ability to impair the pulmonary immune function, but for obvious reasons patients should not be encouraged to smoke. It is not clear, however, from these studies whether sarcoidosis is the primary disease, or whether a local sarcoidal reaction is a response to the malignancy in this group of patients. Of interest is the induction of new-onset sarcoidosis with antineoplastic agents used to treat oncology patients with Hodgkin and non-Hodgkin lymphoma, and the biologic modifier α-interferon (IFN) in leukemia. This has also been reported in noncancer patients who have received IFN-α for chronic hepatitis C. Drug-induced sarcoidosis has also been reported in patients receiving TNF-α inhibitors for diseases such as psoriasis.

TREATMENT

Acute sarcoidosis in which bilateral hilar adenopathy exists alone or in combination with erythema nodosum, uveitis, or arthritis is usually a self-limited disease and does not require specific therapy. Symptomatic therapy for the erythema nodosum or arthritis could include nonsteroidal anti-inflammatory drugs, such as aspirin or indometacin. Acute uveitis can be treated with corticosteroid eye drops. Some patients with severe symptoms require brief courses of oral corticosteroids.

There are no Food and Drug Administration-approved treatments for cutaneous sarcoidosis, and the level of evidence supporting various off-label options is generally limited to case series and retrospective analysis. However, there exists expert opinion and consensus regarding an overall approach, starting with topical corticosteroids and progressing to immunomodulatory and immunosuppressive options. Chronic cutaneous lesions, particularly lupus pernio and indurated plaques, which can cause scarring and disfigurement, should be treated more aggressively. Topical corticosteroids and topical immunomodulators are variably effective. Topical steroids should be selected on a site-specific basis to avoid risks of atrophy and dyspigmentation. Intralesional corticosteroids are generally more effective, and in some lesions may lead to a durable response, at rates ranging from 5 to 40 mg/cc of intralesional kenalog.

Antimalarials, particularly hydroxychloroquine sulfate (200 to 400 mg/day) or chloroquine phosphate (250 mg/day), are useful in treating patients with cutaneous sarcoidosis, and should be considered first-line therapy for patients with cutaneous sarcoidosis that is not responsive or too widespread to be amenable to topical steroids. Antimalarial therapy requires ophthalmologic monitoring; however, patients with sarcoidosis should be followed routinely by ophthalmologists regardless. Antimalarials have no effect on most extracutaneous manifestations of sarcoidosis. Tetracycline class antibiotics, particularly minocycline (100 mg twice daily), may also be effective in treating cutaneous sarcoidosis.

Methotrexate (10 to 15 mg/week) is the next-line therapy to supplement or replace the use of antimalarials. Methotrexate is highly effective in treating cutaneous sarcoidosis and is furthermore frequently used to treat extracutaneous disease. Corticosteroids are another option for patients with severe cutaneous disease, but most patients will demonstrate transient disease improvement while on steroids and then relapse as the drug is tapered. Thalidomide is an alternative option to methotrexate in patients who require treatment beyond antimalarials; patients must be enrolled in a monitoring program, and the rates of side effects, particularly neuropathy, are significant.

In patients with chronic cutaneous sarcoidosis such as lupus pernio, the TNF-α inhibitors have shown promise, with excellent tolerability and response rates in patients with previously refractory disease. Adalimumab and infliximab have the most data, and etanercept was not effective in a small trial.

Other options include pentoxifylline, apremilast, azathioprine, cyclophosphamide, cyclosporine, chlorambucil, leflunomide, isotretinoin, melatonin, fumaric acid esters, and allopurinol, which have been described as beneficial in anecdotal reports or small case series for treating cutaneous sarcoidosis. Nonmedical therapies have included surgical procedures such as the use of lasers, dermabrasion, surgical excision with grafting, plastic surgery, and phototherapy (narrowband ultraviolet B phototherapy, ultraviolet A-1 phototherapy, and photodynamic therapy), but there is not enough evidence to recommend any of these as the standard of care, and destructive modalities should be used with caution as sarcoidosis may develop at sites of trauma.

Ocular sarcoidosis, which can lead to scarring and blindness, must be aggressively treated. Corticosteroid eye drops may be effective; however, patients who do not respond or who respond only partially may require intraocular corticosteroid injections or systemic corticosteroid therapy.

Progressive pulmonary disease is considered to be an indication for systemic corticosteroid therapy. Documented changes in pulmonary function tests as a result of therapy have been reported. Alternative therapies that may be effective or that reduce the corticosteroid dosage include various immunosuppressive agents, particularly methotrexate. However, too few studies are available to reliably evaluate the effects of any agent other than systemic corticosteroids.

In addition to chronic disfiguring cutaneous lesions, ocular lesions, and progressive pulmonary disease, the indications for systemic corticosteroid therapy include hypercalcemia, neurosarcoidosis, symptomatic cardiac sarcoidosis, and functional endocrinologic abnormalities.

SUGGESTED READINGS

Ahmed H, Harsdad SR. Subcutaneous sarcoidosis: Is it a specific subset of cutaneous sarcoidosis frequently associated with systemic disease? J Am Acad Dermatol 2006;54:55–60.

Baughman RP, Lower EE. Medical therapy for sarcoidosis. Semin Respir Crit Care Med 2014;35:391–406.

Callen JP. The presence of foreign bodies does not exclude the diagnosis of sarcoidosis. Arch Dermatol 2001;137:485.

Chen ES, Moller DR. Etiologic role of infectious agents. Semin Respir Crit Care Med 2014;35:285.

Chen ES, Moller DR. Sarcoidosis—scientific progress and clinical challenges. Nat Rev Rheumatol 2011;7:457.

Haimovic A, Sanchez M, Judson MA, Prystowsky S. Sarcoidosis: a comprehensive review and update for the dermatologist. Part I: cutaneous disease. J Am Acad Dermatol 2012;66:699.

Haimovic A, Sanchez M, Judson MA, Prystowsky S. Sarcoidosis: a comprehensive review and update for the dermatologist. Part II: extracutaneous disease. J Am Acad Dermatol 2012;66:719.

Judson MA. The clinical features of sarcoidosis: a comprehensive review. Clinic Rev Allerg Immunol 2014a. ePub.

Judson MA. Advances in the diagnosis and treatment of sarcoidosis. F1000 Prime Rep 2014b;6:89.

Judson MA, Costabel U, Drent M, Wells A, Koth L, et al. The WASOG Sarcoidosis organ assessment instrument: an update of a previous clinical tool. Sarcoidosis Vasc Diffuse Lung Dis 2014;31:19–27.

Moller DR. Potential etiologic agents in sarcoidosis. Proc Am Throac Soc 2007:465–8.

Rossman MD, Kreider E. Lessons learned from ACCESS (A Case Controlled Etiologic Study of Sarcoidosis). Proc Am Thorac Soc 2007;4:453–6.

Wanat KA, Rosenbach M. A practical approach to cutaneous sarcoidosis. Am J Clin Dermatol 2014;15:283–97.

CHAPTER 37

CARDIOVASCULAR DISEASES AND THE SKIN

Alisa Femia • Kathryn Schwarzenberger • Jeffrey P. Callen

KEY POINTS

- Several systemic disorders can affect both the heart and the skin.
- Cutaneous findings may serve as a diagnostic clue for many of these conditions.
- Dermatologists and cardiologists must be aware of the multisystem aspects of such disorders in order to facilitate proper diagnosis and management.
- A number of cardiac therapies may cause cutaneous complications, and awareness of such potential complications is essential for the dermatologist.
- Recognition of cutaneous findings associated with an increased occurrence of heart disease places dermatologists in a unique role to help reduce cardiovascular risk in certain patient populations.

A number of multisystem disorders can affect both the heart and the skin, and cutaneous examination often provides diagnostic clues to such entities. Recognition of the multisystem aspects of these conditions by both dermatologists and cardiologists is imperative for proper diagnosis and management. Awareness of potential cutaneous complications of cardiac therapies is also essential for the dermatologist. Therapies directed at improvement of muscle function (e.g., digoxin) rarely result in cutaneous disease, while therapies seeking to achieve fluid reduction (diuretics), afterload reduction, and control of rhythmic disturbances can affect the skin. In addition, increasingly frequent use of potent immunosuppressive agents for autoimmune cardiovascular disease and cardiac transplantation may lead to a variety of dermatologic manifestations, including an increased risk of skin cancers, again emphasizing the need for interspecialty collaboration.

This text reviews several multisystem disorders with associated cardiovascular abnormalities. Table 37-1 lists cardiac abnormalities associated with these multisystem disorders, Table 37-2 lists common dermatological findings associated with primary cardiovascular disorders, and common cutaneous side effects of cardiac medications are described in Table 37-3.

ANTIPHOSPHOLIPID ANTIBODY SYNDROME/ANTIPHOSPHOLIPID SYNDROME

Antiphospholipid antibodies (i.e., anticardiolipin, lupus anticoagulant, and anti-β2-glycoprotein-1) are associated with antiphospholipid syndrome (APS), a multisystem disorder that can affect both the heart and the skin. The disorder may be primary or secondary to an associated autoimmune disease, the most common of which is systemic lupus erythematosus. Symptoms result from antibody-driven arterial or venous thrombogenesis, and most commonly include cutaneous findings, deep vein thrombosis, pulmonary embolism, cerebrovascular accidents, and/or recurrent fetal loss. Thrombocytopenia is often seen and, importantly, does not influence the risk of thrombosis. The most common skin finding is livedo reticularis or racemosa (Fig. 37-1). Leg ulcerations, retiform purpura, livedoid vasculopathy, or superficial thrombophlebitis may also occur. Myocardial infarction and cardiac valvular disease, including nonbacterial vegetations, have been described, potentially predisposing the patient to bacterial endocarditis. Cutaneous manifestations are often the presenting feature of APS, placing the dermatologist in an important role for diagnosing this potentially morbid condition. The presence of livedo racemosa in particular in patients with APS has been associated with an increased risk for arterial thrombosis, cerebral thrombosis, and heart valve abnormalities, and should alert dermatologists to these potential complications. Recently updated diagnostic criteria require antiphospholipid antibody positivity on two serologic tests separated by 12 weeks, along with evidence of objectively confirmed thrombosis or pregnancy morbidity. Therapy is dependent upon the history of thromboembolic events, and includes anticoagulants and platelet inhibitors, as well as approaches aimed at lowering antibody levels. Hydroxychloroquine may also help prevent thrombosis, particularly in those with systemic lupus erythematosus, although a convincing body of evidence is lacking. Whether therapy has an effect on cardiac involvement remains unknown, although low-dose aspirin or anticoagulation is frequently recommended in this setting.

CARCINOID SYNDROME

Carcinoid syndrome refers to a constellation of symptoms caused by the release of neuroendocrine vasoactive

TABLE 37-1 Cardiac Manifestations in Multisystem Disorders with Prominent Cutaneous Features

Disease	Cardiac Manifestation	Cutaneous Features	Comments
Primary systemic amyloidosis	Congestive heart failure, conduction disturbances, cardiomegaly	Pinch purpura, waxy translucent papules or diffuse waxy skin infiltration, enlarged tongue, hemorrhagic bullae	Due to immunoglobulin light chains; associated with nonprogressive plasma cell dyscrasia and myeloma, as well as renal and neurologic involvement
Behçet's disease	Pericarditis, conduction abnormalities, valvular disease, coronary arteritis, myocarditis. Recurrent thromboses	Oral and genital aphthae, pathergy, pustular vasculitis, pyoderma gangrenosum-like lesions, sterile vesicopustules, erythema nodosum, superficial thrombophlebitis	Ocular involvement (leading cause of morbidity), arthritis, central nervous system (CNS) disease Inflammatory bowel disease can share many features and should be excluded
Carcinoid syndrome	Endocardial plaque—tricuspid insufficiency, pulmonary stenosis, right-sided heart failure. Left-sided cardiac manifestations exceedingly rare due to pulmonary deactivation of vasoactive substances	Flushing, telangiectases, sclerodermoid features may occur as a late manifestation	Serotonin-producing tumor, most commonly of the intestine. Usually metastatic to the liver prior to symptom onset
Cardiofaciocutaneous syndrome	Sparse, curly, woolly, or brittle hair, ichthyotic skin	Pulmonary stenosis, atrial septal defect, hypertrophic cardiomyopathy	Many other associated cutaneous findings such as keratosis pilaris, palmoplantar keratoderma, café-au-lait macules
Carney complex (including NAME and LAMB syndromes)	Atrial myxoma	Cutaneous myxomas and lentigines	Carney's includes endocrine neoplasia of the adrenal, pituitary, and/or testes. Mutations in the PRKRA1A gene have been identified in many patients with familial cardiac myxomas
Cushing's syndrome	Hypertension	Atrophy and striae, ecchymoses, acne, telangiectases	Due to overproduction of cortisol, commonly iatrogenic
Cutis laxa	Aortic dilation and rupture, pulmonary artery stenosis, right-sided heart failure	Looseness of the skin, premature aging appearance. Skin findings may be present from birth	Dominant (OMIM#123700), recessive (OMIM#219100), and X-linked (OMIM#304150) forms exist. Acquired forms also exist
Dermatomyositis	Cardiac arrhythmias, including atrial fibrillation/flutter, congestive heart failure, coronary artery disease	Gottron's papules, heliotrope rash, photodistributed poikiloderma, nail fold capillary changes	Clinically evident cardiac involvement is a poor prognostic sign
Diabetes mellitus	Coronary artery and peripheral vascular disease	See Chapter 24	—
Down syndrome	Septal defects, patent ductus arteriosus, tetralogy of Fallot	Palmoplantar hyperkeratosis, alopecia areata, cutis marmorata, fissured tongue	Characteristic dysmorphic features such as upslanting palpebral fissures, epicanthic folds, transverse palmar crease
Ehlers–Danlos syndrome	Aortic and pulmonary artery dilation, mitral and tricuspid valve prolapse, arterial rupture	Hyperelasticity of the skin, "cigarette paper" scars, ecchymoses	Cardiac diseases is limited to classic (OMIM#130000), hypermobility (OMIM#130020) and vascular (OMIM#130050) types
Endocarditis—bacterial or fungal	Vegetation and dysfunction of the valves, can lead to myocardial abscess and heart failure	Purpura, splinter hemorrhages (linear purpura in nail beds), Janeway lesions (nontender macules on palms and soles), Osler's nodules (tender subcutaneous nodules usually on distal digits)	Fever. Roth's spots (retinal hemorrhages). May simulate vasculitis
Exfoliative erythroderma	High-output cardiac failure	Exfoliative diffuse dermatitis	The eruption may be due to eczematous or atopic dermatitis, psoriasis, cutaneous T-cell lymphoma, drug eruption or other causes
Fabry's disease	Mitral valve prolapse, conduction defects, congestive heart failure, myocardial infarction, cerebrovascular accidents	Angiokeratoma corporis diffusum, which may be an early feature and lead to diagnosis	Alpha-galactosidase A deficiency, X-linked (OMIM#301500), gene map locus Xq22. Renal failure is the usual cause of death
Hemochromatosis	Congestive heart failure, supraventricular arrhythmias	Generalized bronze hyperpigmentation	Diabetes, cirrhosis

TABLE 37-1 Cardiac Manifestations in Multisystem Disorders with Prominent Cutaneous Features—cont'd

Disease	Cardiac Manifestation	Cutaneous Features	Comments
Hyperlipidemias	Coronary artery disease	Xanthomas of all types	
Kawasaki disease (mucocutaneous lymph node syndrome)	Coronary artery aneurysms are the major complication, coronary arteritis, valvular insufficiency, pericardial effusion may also occur	Glossitis and cheilitis, acral edema, desquamative erythema of the perineum, diffuse morbilliform eruption, conjunctival injection	High fever, lymphadenopathy, treatment with intravenous immune globulin can be beneficial. Infants <1 year old have highest risk of cardiac disease
Multiple lentigines (LEOPARD) syndrome	Electrocardiogram abnormalities, hypertrophic cardiomyopathy	Multiple lentigines	
Loeys–Dietz syndrome	Arterial tortuosity and aneurysm	Velvety or translucent skin in some patients	Described in 2005. Caused by heterozygous mutations in genes encoding transforming growth factor-β receptors 1 and 2; other features include hypertelorism, and bifid uvula or cleft palate. Shares features with Marfan's syndrome and vascular-type Ehlers–Danlos syndrome, but Loeys–Dietz patients lack joint hypermobility and can often be successfully treated with vascular surgery
Lyme disease	Heart block, myopericarditis	Erythema migrans, borrelial lymphocytoma in some cases in Europe	Multisystem disease divided into stages: early localized, early disseminated, and late
Multicentric reticulohistiocytosis	Pericarditis, myocarditis, congestive heart failure	Erythematous nodules of the hands and occasionally the face	Deforming arthritis is frequent
Neonatal lupus erythematosus (NLE)	Congenital heart block	Transient, photosensitive, nonscarring lesions of lupus erythematosus (SCLE-like), predilection for face and periorbital skin. May be first noted after phototherapy for neonatal jaundice. Resolve with dyspigmentation	Presumed to be due to transplacental passage of autoantibodies, most commonly Ro (SS-A). May have transient cytopenias, hepatitis. Mothers may be asymptomatic. Hydroxychloroquine may help prevent against NLE in subsequent pregnancies, but data are limited
Neurofibromatosis	Hypertension due to pheochromocytoma	Café-au-lait macules, neurofibromas, axillary freckling	—
Pseudoxanthoma elasticum	Premature atherosclerotic vascular disease, hypertension	Yellow papules on intertriginous surfaces, redundant lax skin	Upper or lower gastrointestinal hemorrhage. Angioid streaks in the eye, uterine hemorrhage. Autosomal dominant and recessive variants (OMIM#264800 and #177850)
Psoriasis	Increased risk of myocardial infarction and coronary artery disease	Well-demarcated erythematous plaques with micaceous scale, often involving knees, elbows, umbilicus, gluteal cleft, scalp	Associated with metabolic syndrome, obesity, diabetes mellitus, hyperlipidemia, smoking
Relapsing polychondritis	Aortic insufficiency, dissecting aortic aneurysm, valvular disease, arrhythmias	Beefy, red ears or other cartilaginous areas. Late cauliflower-ear deformity or other cartilaginous destruction	Arthritis, tracheal collapse. Dapsone may be helpful. Corticosteroids and/or other immunosuppressive therapies may also be beneficial
Rheumatic fever	Pancarditis in the acute phase. Late manifestations include mitral and/or aortic valve dysfunction	Erythema marginatum, subcutaneous nodules	Rare in United States. Follows pharyngitis due to group A β-hemolytic streptococcal infection. Polyarthritis, chorea, fever
Sarcoidosis	Conduction defects, congestive heart failure	Granulomatous papules, nodules, and plaques, often with a predilection for scars or tattoos. Subcutaneous nodules may also occur. Nonspecific lesions such as erythema nodosum may occur; erythema nodosum associated with better prognosis	Pulmonary disease, hypercalcemia, lymphadenopathy, hepatic, neurologic, and ocular involvement. Cardiac involvement denotes a poor prognosis and can lead to sudden death. Electrocardiogram recommended at diagnosis in all patients, echocardiogram and 24-h Holter monitor in patients with palpitations

Continued

TABLE 37-1 Cardiac Manifestations in Multisystem Disorders with Prominent Cutaneous Features—cont'd

Disease	Cardiac Manifestation	Cutaneous Features	Comments
Scleroderma	Conduction defects, pulmonary hypertension, pericarditis	Cutaneous sclerosis, Raynaud's phenomenon	Cardiac involvement denotes a poor prognosis
Syphilis	Aortitis, especially of the ascending aorta	Multiple potential skin lesions including genital chancre in primary disease, diffuse papulosquamous eruption involving the palms and soles, alopecia, condyloma lata, mucous patches in secondary disease	
Systemic lupus erythematosus	Verrucous endocarditis, pericarditis, coronary artery disease	Malar erythema, photosensitivity, lupus-specific skin lesions such as discoid and subacute cutaneous lupus	Anticardiolipin antibody may play a role in cardiac disease. Corticosteroid therapy may predispose to coronary artery disease
Tuberous sclerosis	Cardiac rhabdomyomas	Adenoma sebaceum, periungual and subungual fibromas, ash leaf macule, shagreen patch, fibrous forehead plaque	Renal and retinal hamartomas, CNS tumors, mental retardation, seizures, pulmonary lymphangioleiomyomatosis
Turner syndrome (gonadal dysgenesis)	Aortic coarctation	Alopecia of frontal scalp, webbed neck, short stature, koilonychia, numerous nevi	Despite multiple nevi, melanoma risk appears low. Increased risk of thyroid disease. May also be associated with increased incidence of alopecia areata and halo nevi
Thyroid disorders	Arrhythmias, palpitations, cardiomyopathy	Myxedema, ocular proptosis in Grave's disease, pruritus	
Vasculitis	Coronary artery vasculitis	Palpable purpura, nodules, livedo reticularis, ulcerations	Arthritis, gastrointestinal colic or bleeding, cardiac involvement is uncommon
Werner's syndrome	Premature atherosclerosis	Premature graying, alopecia, sclerodermoid changes, loss of subcutaneous fat, ankle ulcerations	Myocardial infarction is usually responsible for death by the fifth decade. Autosomal recessive (OMIM#277700, gene map locus 8p12-p11.2). Other features include cataracts, malignancy

TABLE 37-2 Cutaneous Findings Observed in Association with Primary Cardiac Abnormalities

Cutaneous Changes	Cardiac Disorders
Diagonal earlobe crease, androgenetic alopecia, thoracic hairiness	Coronary artery disease/atherosclerosis
Dependent edema, ascites	Congestive heart failure
Increased risk of skin cancers (some data suggest higher risk than renal transplant) Increased risk of herpes simplex and varicella zoster	Cardiac transplantation from any cause
Stasis dermatitis, peripheral edema, lipodermatosclerosis, lower leg ulcerations (often adjacent to the medial malleolus)	Hypertension—venous
Palpable purpura, livedo reticularis, ulcerations	Embolic phenomenon (i.e., due to cholesterol emboli [often follows an invasive procedure, such as catheterization or angiography], left atrial myxoma, subacute bacterial endocarditis)
Osler's nodes, Janeway's lesions, petechiae, purpuric pustules, splinter hemorrhages, leukocytoclastic vasculitis	Endocarditis—bacterial, fungal, or vegetative
Xanthelasma, plane xanthomas, tendon xanthomas	Hyperlipidemia
Eruptive xanthomas, tuberous xanthomas	Hypertriglyceridemia
Cyanosis	Cyanotic heart disease, circulating methemoglobin or sulfhemoglobin, arterial or venous obstruction, arteriolar vasoconstriction (i.e., Raynaud's phenomenon)
Clubbing	Cyanotic heart disease, pulmonary disease may also be associated with clubbing

TABLE 37-3 Common Cutaneous Side Effects of Cardiac Medications

Cutaneous Changes	Medication/Procedure
Photosensitivity, resultant slate blue-gray pigmentation	Amiodarone
Angioedema, drug-induced subacute cutaneous lupus erythematosus	ACE inhibitors
Flare of psoriasis, worsening of Raynaud's	β-Adrenergic blockers
Hypertrichosis	Minoxidil
Petechiae (thrombocytopenia), photosensitivity	Quinidine
Drug-induced systemic lupus erythematosus	Procainamide hydrochloride
Photosensitivity, drug-induced subacute cutaneous lupus erythematosus	Thiazide diuretics, calcium channel blockers, ACE inhibitors
Gynecomastia	Spironolactone
Xerosis	Statins
Pedal edema	Calcium channel blockers
Petechiae from heparin-induced thrombocytopenia, retiform purpura or noninflammatory necrosis from heparin-induced necrosis	Heparin
Painful, well-demarcated erythema that rapidly becomes necrotic due to warfarin necrosis, more common in fatty areas	Warfarin
Radiation burns	Prolonged angioplasty and radiation exposure

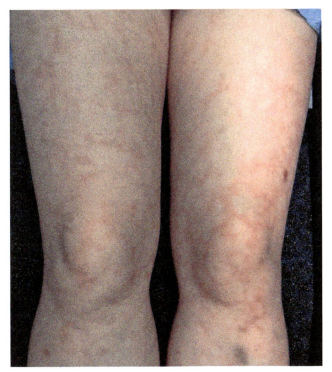

FIGURE 37-1 ■ Reticulated erythematous–violaceous erythema involving the bilateral lower extremities, representative of livedo racemosa in a patient with antiphospholipid syndrome.

substances, primarily serotonin, from a carcinoid tumor. Paroxysmal flushing of the face, neck, and chest, along with intermittent diarrhea, bronchospasm, and hypotension, are the characteristic findings. Symptoms typically occur with liver metastasis or with tumors originating in the stomach or lung. Telangiectases and sclerodermoid changes may occur with continued disease. Right-sided heart failure, tricuspid insufficiency, and pulmonic stenosis are the most common cardiac manifestations. Cardiac involvement is present in approximately 50% of symptomatic patients and contributes to a poor prognosis, emphasizing the need for early diagnosis and intervention. Dermatologists may facilitate diagnosis by suspecting carcinoid syndrome in patients with unexplained paroxysmal flushing. Other causes of similar flushing include physiologic events, pheochromocytoma, VIPoma, systemic mast cell disease, rosacea, alcohol, and certain medications (i.e., niacin).

MALIGNANT ATROPHIC PAPULOSIS (DEGOS DISEASE)

Malignant atrophic papulosis is a rare, idiopathic arteriopathy characterized by pale-red papules with central necrosis that evolve into atrophic, ivory-porcelain white scars with telangiectatic rims. Similar lesions may occur in the gastrointestinal tract or central nervous system (CNS), and, less commonly, the ophthalmologic, pulmonary, or cardiovascular systems. Pericarditis and/or pericardial effusions are the typical cardiac manifestations. Systemic involvement may result in death from ischemic complications or uncontrolled hemorrhage; intestinal perforation is the most common cause of death. Skin lesions may precede systemic involvement by months to years, placing the dermatologist in a unique role to identify early systemic disease.

EARLOBE CREASES

An increased prevalence of the diagonal earlobe crease occurs with age. The cutaneous change is characterized by a crease extending from the tragus to the posterior pinna, involving at least one-third of the distance. While data have been somewhat conflicting, most studies correlate a diagonal earlobe crease with an increased risk of coronary artery disease (CAD), and limited data have linked the diagonal earlobe crease to carotid artery atherosclerosis. Moreover, incorporating the diagonal earlobe crease into a CAD risk algorithm (the Diamond–Forrester algorithm) was recently shown to improve predictive ability for CAD. As such, thorough cardiac risk assessment has been suggested in patients with a diagonal earlobe crease. Two hypotheses link the diagonal earlobe crease to CAD: (1) end arteries with little collateral circulation supply both sites; and (2) a generalized loss of elastin and elastic fibers produces both conditions.

ANDROGENETIC ALOPECIA

Early androgenetic alopecia has been linked to insulin resistance and indirectly to an increased risk for CAD, particularly in men under 60 years of age. Recent data also associate female androgenetic alopecia with CAD in women under the age of 55 years.

HEMOCHROMATOSIS

Hemochromatosis is a common inherited disorder leading to excessive iron deposition, especially in the liver, heart, pancreas, joints, and pituitary. Hyperpigmentation of the skin, particularly in photoexposed areas, is thought to be due to enhanced melanin production resulting from excessive cutaneous iron deposits. The skin is involved in the majority of patients, providing a diagnostic clue to this multisystem condition. Advanced cardiac disease is a leading cause of death in this population. Cardiac involvement is initially characterized by diastolic dysfunction and arrhythmias, and, in later stages, dilated cardiomyopathy and heart failure. With early detection and therapy, cardiac involvement may be preventable, and early cardiac disease reversible. Repeated phlebotomy is the treatment of choice.

RELAPSING POLYCHONDRITIS

Relapsing polychondritis is a rare disorder characterized by recurrent inflammation of cartilaginous tissue, most commonly affecting the ears, nose, joints, and respiratory tract. An associated autoimmune disease or myelodysplastic syndrome is present in roughly 30% of patients. Sudden-onset, tender erythema and edema of the external ear, sparing the earlobe (Fig. 37-2), is present at disease onset in roughly 20%, and is the most common manifestation. Inflammation subsides spontaneously over 1 to 2 weeks, and then recurs, potentially resulting in cartilage deformity and destruction. Small-vessel vasculitis, livedo reticularis, and erythema nodosum may also occur, more commonly in patients with associated myelodysplastic syndrome. Cardiac involvement, including aortic insufficiency, aortic aneurysms, valvular disease, and/or arrhythmias occurs in approximately 30% of patients. Given that heart disease may develop insidiously, routine echocardiograms have been suggested. The most severe complication in relapsing polychondritis is potentially fatal asphyxia as a result of tracheal collapse. Autoantibodies against type II collagen and matrilin-1 have been linked to the disorder, but are neither sensitive nor specific. Ear cartilage biopsy may support the diagnosis, but ultimately, diagnosis rests on clinical findings. Therapy is directed at blocking the neutrophilic inflammatory reaction, and systemic corticosteroids, immunosuppressive agents, colchicine, and dapsone have been used.

EMBOLIC PHENOMENA

Emboli may originate from many causes, including thrombi, infections, oxalate crystals, or crystallized paraproteins. Cholesterol emboli can occur due to dislodging

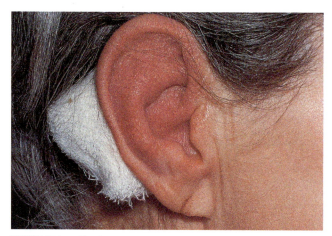

FIGURE 37-2 ■ Erythematous eruption of the earlobe representative of relapsing polychondritis.

of atheromatous plaques during angiography, causing a syndrome associated with prominent livedo reticularis, retiform purpura, and peripheral eosinophilia. Myxomas, typically of the atrium, are another cause of emboli, as seen in "Carney complex" (myxomas of skin, heart, and/or breast, endocrine disorders, and lentigines) and its variants LAMB (lentigines, atrial myxoma, mucocutaneous myxoma, and blue nevi) and NAME (nevi, atrial myxoma, myxoid neurofibromata, and ephelides) syndromes. Cutaneous lesions resulting from emboli, most commonly splinter hemorrhages, petechiae, purpura, digital necrosis, and livedo reticularis, are caused by upstream medium- or small-vessel obstruction. Emboli may also affect internal organs, such as the CNS, eyes, and kidneys. Treatment is supportive and directed at the underlying cause.

EHLERS–DANLOS SYNDROME

Ehlers–Danlos syndrome includes a heterogeneous group of inherited collagen defect disorders characterized by joint hypermobility, hyperextensible skin, and variable organ involvement (Fig. 37-3). Easy bruising and "cigarette paper" scars are common cutaneous manifestations. Cardiac manifestations include mitral and tricuspid valve prolapse, aortic dilatation with insufficiency, and arterial rupture, occurring most commonly in the classic, hypermobility, and vascular types.

MULTIPLE LENTIGINES (LEOPARD) AND NOONAN SYNDROMES

LEOPARD and Noonan syndromes fall within a group of autosomal dominant disorders caused by defects in the RAS–MAPK pathway. LEOPARD syndrome is characterized by lentigines, electrocardiographic abnormalities, ocular hypertelorism, pulmonary stenosis, genital abnormalities, retardation of growth, and deafness (sensorineural). The lentigines are concentrated on the trunk and present at birth or early childhood, darkening with age and potentially serving as a diagnostic clue (Fig. 37-4). Noonan syndrome, allelic with LEOPARD syndrome, is characterized by short stature, characteristic facies,

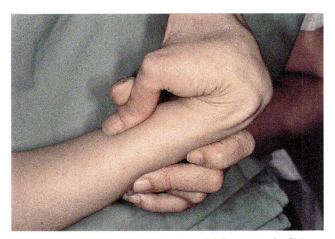

FIGURE 37-3 ■ Hyperextensible skin and joints seen in Ehlers–Danlos syndrome.

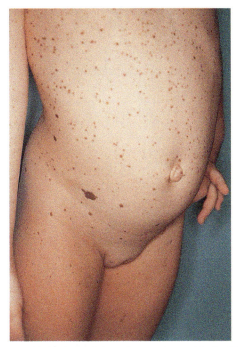

FIGURE 37-4 ■ Multiple lentigines in a patient with the LEOPARD syndrome. (Courtesy of Paul Lucky, MD, Cincinnati, Ohio. Reprinted with permission from Color Atlas of Dermatology. Philadelphia: WB Saunders, 2000.)

cubitus valgus, undescended testes, and cardiovascular abnormalities. Skin findings include lymphedema, nevi, and keratosis pilaris atrophicans. An array of cardiac findings can occur in both syndromes. Hypertrophic cardiomyopathy is the most common cardiac anomaly in LEOPARD syndrome, whereas pulmonic stenosis is the most common in Noonan syndrome. Mutations in the *PTPN11* gene have been identified in some patients with both syndromes.

PSEUDOXANTHOMA ELASTICUM

Pseudoxanthoma elasticum is a heritable disorder characterized by abnormal calcification of elastic fibers. The skin, eyes, and cardiovascular system are most commonly affected. Yellowish papules and skin laxity, particularly affecting the intertriginous surfaces (including the neck), are often the presenting features. Skin biopsy reveals calcified and fragmented elastic fibers. Intermittent claudication, stroke, abdominal angina, hypertension, ischemic cardiac disease, and eventual congestive heart failure may occur, impacting prognosis. Cardiovascular evaluation should occur in all patients with pseudoxanthoma elasticum.

PSORIASIS AND HEART DISEASE

A convincing body of evidence, including meta-analyses and population-based studies, associates moderate–severe psoriasis with an increased risk of cardiovascular disease and of death from cardiovascular disease. Specific cardiovascular risk factors, such as obesity, hypertriglyceridemia, and metabolic syndrome, have been linked with psoriasis, and recent meta-analyses confirmed associations with diabetes and hypertension as well. Furthermore, a recent population-based study linked psoriasis with chronic kidney disease, and a recent meta-analysis associated mild psoriasis with increased risk of stroke and myocardial infarction. The precise mechanisms responsible for these associations are still being evaluated, but shared pathways between skin inflammation and atherosclerosis, particularly involving T cells and neutrophils, have been proposed. The impact of psoriasis therapy on cardiovascular risk remains unclear, but recent epidemiologic data support a protective effect, particularly with tumor necrosis factor (TNF) inhibitors. In fact, a large retrospective study suggests that TNF inhibitors, oral medications (i.e., methotrexate, cyclosporine, acitretin), and phototherapy may confer a decreased cardiovascular risk, with the strongest association seen with TNF inhibitors. Additionally, in a large Danish population-based study, TNF inhibitors and methotrexate were associated with a decreased risk for cardiovascular events and all-cause mortality. Recent expert group consensus has advocated for cardiovascular risk assessment in all patients with moderate–severe psoriasis, including annual blood pressure, body mass index, waist circumference, lipids, fasting glucose, HbA1c, and smoking status inquiries.

MYOSITIS

Cardiac involvement in idiopathic inflammatory myopathies has been well described, including in patients with dermatomyositis. Subclinical involvement in the form of conduction abnormalities and arrhythmias frequently occurs. Symptomatic CAD or heart failure is less common, but can occur, with a recent meta-analysis reporting a pooled risk ratio of 2.24 for CAD in idiopathic inflammatory myopathies. Overt cardiac disease portends a poor prognosis, and an increased death rate from myocardial infarction has been reported. It has been suggested that systemic immunomodulatory therapy may improve cardiac manifestations in some patients. In the juvenile population, diabetes mellitus has been associated with lipodystrophy, dyslipidemia, diabetes, and cardiac involvement, and recently, limited data suggest that sustained early skin activity may predict cardiac systolic dysfunction in this population.

SUGGESTED READINGS

Abdelmalek NF, Gerber TL, Menter A. Cardiocutaneous syndromes and associations. J Am Acad Dermatol 2002;46:161–83.

Ahlehoff O, Skov L, Gislason G, et al. Cardiovascular outcomes and systemic anti-inflammatory drugs in patients with severe psoriasis: 5-year follow-up of a Danish nationwide cohort. J Eur Acad Dermatol Venereol 2015;29(6):1128–34.

Gelfand JM, Neimann AL, Shin DB, et al. Risk of myocardial infarction in patients with psoriasis. JAMA 2006;296:1735–41.

Kremers HM, McEvoy MT, Dann FJ, et al. Heart disease in psoriasis. J Am Acad Dermatol 2007;57:347–54.

Lundberg IE. The heart in dermatomyositis and polymyositis. Rheumatology 2006;45:iv18–21.

Miric D, Fabijanic D, Giunio L, et al. Dermatological indicators of coronary risk: a case-control study. Int J Cardiol 1998;67:251–5.

Mosca S, Gargiulo P, Balato N, et al. Ischemic cardiovascular involvement in psoriasis: a systemic review. Int J Cardiol 2014;178C:191–9.

Motamed M, Pelekoudas N. The predictive value of diagonal ear-lobe crease sign. Int J Clin Pract 1998;52:305–6.

Pupo RA, Wiss K, Solomon AR. Disorders affecting the skin and the heart. Dermatol Clin 1989;7:517–29.

Ungpraser P, Suksaranjit P, Spanuchart I, et al. Risk of coronary artery disease in patients with idiopathic inflammatory myopathies: A systematic review and meta-analysis of observational studies. Sem Arthitis Rheum 2014;44:63–7.

CHAPTER 38

RENAL DISEASE AND THE SKIN

Mary P. Maiberger • Julia R. Nunley

KEY POINTS

- Skin manifestations of chronic kidney disease (CKD) are commonly encountered and can be due to (1) the cause of the underlying renal disease, either acquired or heritable; (2) conditions unique to uremia; or (3) immunosuppressive therapies and/or immunosuppression itself in renal transplant recipients.
- Diabetes and hypertension account for most cases of end-stage renal disease (ESRD) in the United States; however, many diseases, such as amyloidosis, connective tissue diseases, hepatitis C and B viral infections, and numerous genetic diseases may also cause ESRD. These conditions often possess characteristic cutaneous findings, which may be the first clue to an underlying kidney disease.
- Skin findings such as alopecia, nail changes, pigmentary alteration, pruritus, and xerosis are not specific to uremia per se, but are frequently observed in patients with impaired renal function and impact quality of life.
- Calciphylaxis is a rare but severe syndrome with high morbidity and mortality that involves calcium deposition in small vessels within the dermis and subcutaneous tissue, leading to exquisitely tender, retiform purpuric plaques that frequently ulcerate.
- Acquired perforating dermatoses represent a spectrum of disorders with transepidermal elimination of material from the dermis with little damage to surrounding tissue, clinically presenting as keratotic lesions most commonly on the trunk and extremities.
- Nephrogenic systemic fibrosis is characterized by thickened collagen in the skin and other organs, hyperpigmented, brawny plaques and papules most frequently starting on the extremities, and an association with exposure to gadolinium-based contrast agents in patients with renal compromise.
- Bullous diseases in CKD include porphyria cutanea tarda (PCT), pseudoporphyria, and bullous disease of dialysis.
- Renal transplant recipients are at risk for medication-related cutaneous changes, infections, and cutaneous malignancies secondary to immunosuppression.

INTRODUCTION

Chronic kidney disease (CKD) has numerous deleterious systemic effects including impaired function of the heart, brain, and nervous system, altered hormonal balance and bone metabolism, and increased susceptibility to infections. Cutaneous disorders are common in patients with CKD and can be due to various genetic or acquired conditions or metabolic abnormalities. These dermatologic manifestations can be summarized in three categories: (1) dermatologic signs of diseases causing renal failure (Table 38-1); (2) dermatologic conditions relatively unique to uremia (Table 38-2); and (3) cutaneous disorders in renal transplant recipients (RTR) related to immunosuppression and/or drugs used to immunosuppress (Table 38-3). This chapter will focus on dermatologic conditions unique to uremia, while disorders in categories 1 and 3 are summarized in table format only. Given that mortality from CKD is decreasing, the prevalence of this disease is increasing. Therefore, dermatologists will continue to encounter cutaneous manifestations of CKD and may be the first to identify and treat many of these conditions.

DERMATOLOGIC MANIFESTATIONS OF SYSTEMIC AND GENETIC DISORDERS CAUSING CHRONIC RENAL DISEASE

A number of systemic and heritable disorders have both cutaneous and renal manifestations, summarized in Table 38-1.

DERMATOLOGIC MANIFESTATIONS OF UREMIA

Many patients with end-stage renal disease (ESRD) are maintained by hemodialysis or peritoneal dialysis; however, these modalities cannot fully compensate. As such, most patients develop significant metabolic abnormalities including: anemia, metabolic acidosis, altered calcium-phosphate homeostasis, hyperparathyroidism, and glucose intolerance. These derangements are responsible for the uremic condition and significantly impact many organ systems. Whereas some dermatologic manifestations are relatively unique to patients undergoing dialysis, such as calciphylaxis; others, such as xerosis and pruritus, are not specific to uremia, but have a high prevalence in patients with ESRD (Table 38-2).

TABLE 38-1 Dermatologic Conditions in Diseases Causing Chronic Kidney Disease

Disease	Dermatologic Manifestations	Renal Features
Metabolic Disorders		
Diabetes mellitus	Acanthosis nigricans Eruptive xanthomas Necrobiosis lipoidica Diabetic dermopathy Bullous diabeticorum	Diabetic nephropathy Nephrotic syndrome
Amyloidosis	Macroglossia Purpura (most classically in the periorbital region)	Nephrotic syndrome
Atherosclerosis/cholesterol emboli	Blue toes Cutaneous necrosis Retiform purpura Splinter hemorrhage	Renal emboli with hematuria and eosinophiluria
Connective Tissue Diseases		
Systemic sclerosis	Calcinosis cutis Cutaneous sclerosis Distal digital infarcts Nailfold capillary changes Sclerodactyly Mat telangiectases Salt-and-pepper depigmentation	Malignant hypertension Renal crisis
Polyarteritis nodosa	Palpable purpura Nodules Ulcers	Glomerulonephritis Vasculitis
Systemic lupus erythematosus	Acute cutaneous lupus erythematosus (butterfly rash) Chronic cutaneous lupus (discoid lupus) Livedo reticularis Subacute cutaneous lupus erythematosus	Glomerulonephritis Nephrotic syndrome
Granulomatosis with polyangiitis (GPA; formerly Wegener's granulomatosis)	Palpable purpura Petechiae Saddle nose deformity Strawberry gums	Glomerulonephritis Vasculitis
Hepatitis Viruses		

Hepatitis C	Lichen planus
	Porphyria cutanea tarda:
	    Photodistributed
	    Milia
	    Sclerodermatous changes
	    Vesicles/bullae
	    Hypertrichosis (on temples)
	Necrolytic acral erythema
	Mixed cryoglobulinemia:
	    Digital infarcts
	    Livedo reticularis
	    Palpable purpura
		Glomerulonephritis

Hepatitis B	Polyarteritis nodosa	Glomerulonephritis
Genetic Disorders		
Fabry's disease *Inheritance: X-linked recessive* *Defect: α-galactosidase-A deficiency*	Angiokeratomas of lower abdomen, hip, and inguinal region	Varying degrees of proteinuria Urinary globotriaosylceramide Cortical and parapelvic cysts Renal failure is more common in men
Birt–Hogg–Dubé *Inheritance: autosomal dominant* *Defect: folliculin gene (FLCN) mutation*	Trichodiscomas Fibrofolliculomas Acrochordons (see Chapter 17)	Renal cancers of variable histology
Tuberous sclerosis *Inheritance: genetically heterogeneous; autosomal dominant transmission with high spontaneous mutation rate* *Defect: genes TSC1/TSC2 with protein products hamartin and tuberin*	Facial angiofibromas Connective tissue nevi Hypopigmented macules ("ash-leaf macules") Shagreen patch Periungual fibromas (see Chapter 17)	Angiomyolipomas Renal cysts Polycystic kidneys Renal cell carcinoma
Nail–patella syndrome *Inheritance: autosomal dominant*	Nail dysplasia: Triangular lunulae	Varying degrees of proteinuria Renal tubular defects

TABLE 38-1 **Dermatologic Conditions in Diseases Causing Chronic Kidney Disease—cont'd**

Disease	Dermatologic Manifestations	Renal Features
Defect: LIM-homeodomain protein LMX1B	Hypoplastic nails Lack of creases over distal interphalangeal joints	
Hereditary multiple leiomyomas of skin Inheritance: autosomal dominant Defect: mutation in gene encoding fumarate hydratase	Multiple cutaneous leiomyomas, typically regionally grouped (see Chapter 17)	Renal cell carcinoma

TABLE 38-2 **Dermatologic Diseases Associated with Uremia**

Alopecia
Calcinosis cutis
Calciphylaxis
Kyrle disease (acquired perforating dermatosis)
Nail changes:
    Beau's lines
    Half-and-half nails (Lindsay's nails)
    Nailfold capillary abnormalities
Nephrogenic systemic fibrosis
Pruritus-related skin changes
Pigmentary alteration
Porphyria cutanea tarda
Pseudoporphyria
Xerosis
Uremic frost

Alopecia

While common in patients with ESRD, alopecia has not been studied specifically in this patient population. Conditions associated with alopecia include systemic lupus erythematosus (SLE), malnutrition, or a chronic telogen effluvium, possibly due to other comorbidities or medications commonly used in this population including antihypertensives, lipid-lowering agents, or anticoagulants.

Calcinosis Cutis

Initially described by Virchow in 1855, calcinosis cutis results from calcification of the skin due to local or systemic factors. Four major types of calcinosis cutis exist: dystrophic, metastatic, iatrogenic, and idiopathic. The metastatic type, which occurs in association with an elevated calcium/phosphate ratio, is most common in ESRD. Reported in 1% of ESRD patients on hemodialysis, metastatic calcinosis cutis is generally a late complication. Clinically, patients develop rock-hard papules, nodules, or plaques, which may exude a chalky discharge through the epidermis (Fig. 38-1); periarticular sites or fingertips are most commonly affected. While generally asymptomatic, mobility can be compromised and lesions are occasionally tender. Histology reveals homogeneous blue material in the dermis, occasionally with foreign body giant cells; calcium deposition can be confirmed by special staining. There is no gold-standard treatment; however, normalization of calcium and phosphate levels may result in lesion regression. For refractory cases in the setting of hyperparathyroidism, parathyroidectomy may be beneficial.

Calciphylaxis

Calciphylaxis, also termed calcific uremic arteriolopathy, represents a cutaneous, ischemic, small-vessel vasculopathy associated with extreme pain, morbidity, and mortality, most classically in patients with CKD. First associated with uremia in 1898 by White, it was not until 1962 that Selye constructed an experimental model in nephrectomized rats in which he precipitated systemic calcification similar to the human syndrome. Between 1% and 4% of dialysis patients develop calciphylaxis. Reports of calciphylaxis in nonuremic settings also exist, often in association with malignancy, alcoholic liver disease, primary hyperparathyroidism, diabetes mellitus, Crohn's disease, or connective tissue diseases. Although the pathogenesis remains obscure, hypercoagulable states, including protein C and protein S abnormalities as well as the presence of antiphospholipid antibodies, have been detected in patients with calciphylaxis; it is plausible that intrinsic coagulation may contribute to tissue necrosis. Risk factors for calciphylaxis include hypercalcemia, use of calcium-containing phosphate binders, vitamin D therapy, hyperphosphatemia, elevated calcium-phosphate product, hyperparathyroidism, female gender, diabetes mellitus, obesity, systemic corticosteroid use, immunosuppression, hypercoagulable conditions, and trauma.

Calciphylaxis develops as exquisitely painful, often symmetric, retiform purpuric plaques that frequently ulcerate; anatomic areas with significant subcutaneous fat are more often affected (Fig. 38-2). Early lesions may appear as nonspecific violaceous mottling, livedo reticularis, or erythematous papules, nodules, or plaques. Later-stage lesions typically have stellate purpura with central necrosis; lesions in variable stages of development may be present in the same patient. Laboratory abnormalities may include hypercalcemia and hyperphosphatemia with an elevated calcium-phosphate product, generally greater than 60 to 70 mg^2/dL^2.

Skin biopsy specimens reveal calcification within the media of small- and medium-sized arterioles with extensive intimal hyperplasia and fibrosis commonly with a mixed inflammatory infiltrate (Fig. 38-3). Subcutaneous calcium deposits with panniculitis and fat necrosis, as well as vascular microthrombi, are occasionally seen. Notably, a deep incisional or wedge biopsy is often more helpful than a punch biopsy in confirming a diagnosis of

TABLE 38-3 Diseases Associated with Renal Transplantation

Disease	Notable Features
Medication-Related Disorders	
Cushingoid Changes • Moon facies • Cervical fat pad (buffalo hump) • Striae distensae • Cutaneous atrophy • Telangiectases • Senile purpura	• Develop in 50–90% of patients • Associated with systemic corticosteroid use; may improve with corticosteroid dose reduction
Gingivial hyperplasia	• Occurs in one-third of patients on cyclosporine • Occurs early and improves with time
Disorders of the Pilosebaceous Unit • Acne vulgaris/steroid acne • Folliculitis • Hypertrichosis • Keratosis pilaris • Sebaceous gland hyperplasia	• Steroid acne is seen in 15% of patients, mainly on chest and back, improves with corticosteroid dose reduction • Acne vulgaris may occasionally be seen secondary to cyclosporine use • Hypertrichosis is seen in 60% of patients; known to be associated with cyclosporine; may be associated with keratosis pilaris
Immunosuppression-Related Disorders	
Infections • Bacterial • Fungal • Mycobacterial • Parasitic • Viral	• Often related to degree of immunosuppression • Heightened risk during first 6 months following transplantation • Fungal infections are more common overall, seen in 7–75% of patients; pityrosporum is the most common fungal infection • Viral infections, mainly from herpes viruses, are typically most severe in the first year following transplantation; diseases related to human papilloma viruses develop later
Malignancies • Actinic keratosis (precancerous) • Basal cell carcinoma (BCC) • Kaposi sarcoma (KS) • Melanoma • Merkel cell carcinoma • Squamous cell carcinoma (SCC)	• Risk varies according to the degree of immunosuppression, time after transplantation, geographic location, amount of ultraviolet light exposure, and predominant skin type • Nonmelanoma skin cancer incidence is 20–40 times that of the general population • Nonmelanoma skin cancers are more aggressive, have a higher recurrence rate, and a greater metastatic potential than in the general population • Of the immunosuppressive medications used in the transplant population, sirolimus is the least likely to cause an increase in the risk for skin cancer • SCC is the most common cutaneous malignancy following transplantation, with a risk of 50–250 times that of the general population • BCC occurs 6–10 times more frequently than in the general population • KS incidence is 400–500 times higher than in the general population; the greatest risk is in the first year following transplantation • Melanoma is seen 2–9 times more frequently than in the general population

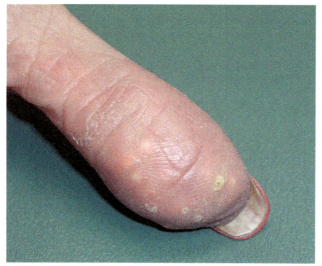

FIGURE 38-1 ■ Calcinosis cutis: painful lesions on the distal fingertips of a patient with metastatic calcinosis cutis attributed to renal disease.

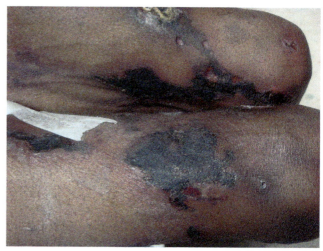

FIGURE 38-2 ■ Calciphylaxis: exquisitely tender stellate purpura with overlying necrosis on the lower extremity of a patient with renal failure.

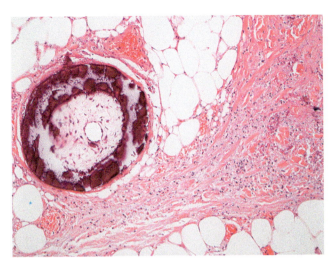

FIGURE 38-3 ■ Histopathology of calciphylaxis typically demonstrates calcification within the media of small- and medium-sized arterioles with extensive intimal hyperplasia and fibrosis. (Courtesy of Jyoti Kapil, MD.)

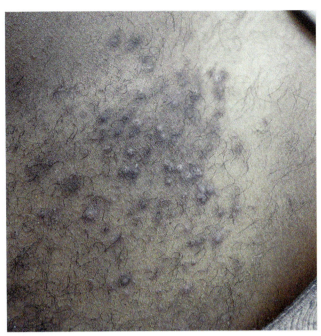

FIGURE 38-4 ■ Kyrle disease: note the lichenified, hyperkeratotic papules in a patient on hemodialysis with intractable pruritus.

calciphylaxis. In addition, a high level of clinical suspicion is warranted, particularly in a susceptible individual, as biopsy location, depth, and timing may lead to false reassurance that calciphylaxis is not present.

Treatment for calciphylaxis is multimodal, encompassing both medical and surgical intervention. Precipitating factors should be eliminated including iron, calcium, and vitamin D supplementation. If the calcium-phosphate product is elevated, it should be normalized safely with conservative therapy including dietary changes, low-calcium bath dialysis, and nonaluminum phosphate binders. Calcimimetics may be beneficial, as they increase the sensitivity of calcium receptors, thus decreasing parathyroid secretion; bisphosphonates, which increase osteoprotegerin production and inhibit arterial calcification, may also be of benefit. Although controversial, parathyroidectomy may be considered if hyperparathyroidism is present and conservative therapy fails.

Over the past decade, intravenous sodium thiosulfate (STS) has increasingly been used in the treatment of both uremic and nonuremic cases of calciphylaxis, acting as a potent antioxidant and increasing the solubility of calcium deposits. Rapid pain relief has been reported, along with disease stabilization and/or improvement. Doses range from 5 to 25 g administered intravenously three times weekly (after dialysis in the hemodialysis population). Although generally well tolerated, a notable side effect is the risk of an anion gap metabolic acidosis due to thiosulfuric acid, which can be managed by altering the bicarbonate level of the dialyzate. While decreased pain and disease stabilization are often noted with STS, wound healing can be prolonged, usually requiring the use of advanced wound care modalities, careful debridement of necrotic tissue, as well as hyperbaric oxygen in some cases. The mortality rate for calciphylaxis is between 60% and 80% in patients with ulcerative disease, and the impact of STS on mortality has not been investigated. Current 1- and 5-year survival rates in patients with calciphylaxis are 45% and 33%, respectively.

Kyrle Disease (Acquired Perforating Dermatoses)

Acquired perforating dermatoses (APD) represent a spectrum of disorders with transepidermal elimination of material with little damage to surrounding tissue, often associated with ESRD and/or diabetes mellitus. The perforating disorders seen in ESRD can show classic clinical and histologic features of Kyrle disease, perforating folliculitis, or reactive perforating collagenosis. Approximately 4% to 10% of patients on hemodialysis are affected and develop pruritic, keratotic papules, nodules, or verrucous plaques, most often on the extremities and trunk although the face and scalp may rarely be involved (Fig. 38-4). Papules are generally umbilicated with a central plug and have a predilection for the extensor surfaces. The etiology of APD remains unknown. Treatment is challenging and is often aimed at improving the underlying pruritus. Therapeutic options reported include potent topical corticosteroids, often under occlusion, intralesional corticosteroids, topical or oral retinoids, cryotherapy, and ultraviolet B (UVB) phototherapy, all with variable success. In some cases, spontaneous resolution has been observed.

Nail Changes

Lindsay's nails, or half-and-half nails, represent the most common nail change associated with CKD, and are seen in nearly 40% of patients on dialysis, disappearing within months following renal transplantation. They are characterized by a white color proximally and a nonblanching red to brown color distally (Fig. 38-5). The white color is attributed to nail bed edema. Other common nail changes observed in patients with CKD include Beau's lines, onycholysis, and nailfold capillary abnormalities.

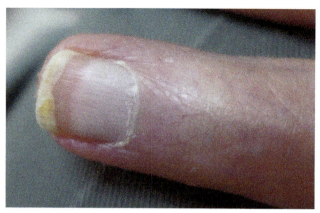

FIGURE 38-5 ■ Lindsay's nails or half-and-half nails in a patient with chronic renal failure with the characteristic proximal white portion and distal pink/brown portion of the nail.

Nephrogenic Systemic Fibrosis

Nephrogenic systemic fibrosis (NSF), initially referred to as nephrogenic fibrosing dermopathy, was first described by Cowper et al. in 1997 as a scleroderma-like fibrosing disease of the skin associated with renal insufficiency and hemodialysis. It has no age or gender bias and was eventually recognized to have both skin and systemic involvement. Although initially unclear, the etiology of NSF has been linked to gadolinium exposure from imaging studies in patients with renal insufficiency. In 2010, in addition to a black box warning, the Food and Drug Administration stated that three contrast agents—gadopentetate dimeglumine (Magnevist™), gadodiamide (Omniscan™), and gadoversetamide (OptiMARK™)—were contraindicated in patients with either acute or CKD. While the specific mechanism is unknown, disease development is thought to be related to a specific cell type, a circulating fibrocyte, stimulated by gadolinium.

NSF presents as rapidly progressive, symmetrically distributed, thickened, indurated papules and plaques, often on the extremities and trunk; early lesions may be pruritic (Fig. 38-6). As fibrosis progresses, the skin becomes tethered with brawny hyperpigmentation, often resulting in pain and joint contractures. Later, patients may develop epidermal atrophy, hair loss, and follicular dimpling or a peau d'orange appearance. Fibrosis may also affect skeletal muscle, the diaphragm, lymph nodes, heart, lungs, pleura, liver, thyroid, and genitourinary tract. In addition, patients with NSF can have yellow plaques on the sclera of their eyes with accompanying conjunctival injection. While NSF can be mistaken for other cutaneous sclerosing disorders, it lacks the facial involvement of systemic sclerosis or scleromyxedema. In addition, in patients with systemic sclerosis, the cutaneous sclerosis tends to start more distally than in patients with NSF, involving even the distal fingers. Furthermore, Raynaud's phenomenon and nailfold capillary changes are also absent in patients with NSF. Laboratory testing generally demonstrates the absence of antibodies or a paraprotein often seen in connective tissue disorders or scleromyxedema, respectively. A deep biopsy is essential for diagnosis, revealing thickened collagen bundles with few inflammatory cells and increased dermal fibroblast-like cells that stain positively for CD34 and procollagen I. Particles of gadolinium can be detected in some tissue specimens.

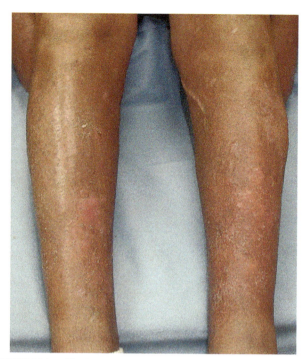

FIGURE 38-6 ■ Nephrogenic systemic fibrosis: symmetric, indurated, hyperpigmented plaques on the bilateral legs of a patient with chronic kidney disease.

NSF results in increased morbidity and mortality, and patients may suffer from debilitating contractures and decreased mobility. Treatment options are limited, with reports of benefit with imatinib, rapamycin, UVA1 phototherapy, intravenous immunoglobulin, plasmapheresis, extracorporeal photopheresis, intravenous sodium thiosulfate, and renal transplantation. The implementation of restrictive guidelines and avoidance of gadolinium-based contrast agents in patients with CKD have greatly reduced the incidence of NSF. Although not fully eradicated, NSF may soon hopefully be a disease of the past.

Pruritus-Related Skin Changes

Intractable and severe pruritus commonly occurs in patients with ESRD and has no association with age, sex, race, or precipitating disease. It can be constant or intermittent, generalized or localized, and can intensify on the patient's back and forearms. Between 50% and 90% of patients on dialysis experience pruritus, often beginning 6 months or more after initiating dialysis. In some patients, pruritus is alleviated during dialysis while others suffer constantly. Excoriations, prurigo nodules, and lichenification develop as a result of chronic scratching. Knowledge regarding the mechanism of uremic pruritus is limited. Possible etiologies include generalized xerosis, metabolic and endocrine abnormalities, a uremia-induced neuropathy, and a decreased clearance of pruritus-causing substances called "middle molecules," which are thought to be poorly dialyzable substances due to their larger molecular size.

Treatment of pruritus in patients with renal disease is challenging. Neither normalization of calcium-phosphate homeostasis nor removal of the parathyroid glands provides uniform relief. Treatment options include emollients, antihistamines, topical corticosteroids, and UVB phototherapy; UVB phototherapy is generally the most effective, often in conjunction with sedating antihistamines. Recent studies suggest that opiate-receptor antagonists, such as naloxone and naltrexone, or medications such as gabapentin or pregabalin, may be beneficial in some patients; however, no treatment is universally successful. Pruritus typically resolves after transplantation.

Pigmentary Alteration

Occurring in 25% to 75% of the dialysis population, pigmentary changes increase over time and are thought to be primarily due to uremia. A yellowish hue, possibly from cutaneous deposition of retained urochromes and carotene, occurs over time. In addition, a brownish, photo-distributed, hyperpigmentation may occur, which is due to excess melanin production stimulated by an elevation in poorly dialyzed beta-melanocyte stimulating hormone. Furthermore, deposition of hemosiderin, from iron overload, can transform this hyperpigmentation to a more brown-to-gray discoloration.

Bullous Disease (Porphyria and Pseudoporphyria)

Various blistering disorders can be seen in patients with renal disease and include porphyria cutanea tarda (PCT), pseudoporphyria, and the poorly understood bullous disease of dialysis. The development of PCT in patients with ESRD is likely multifactorial: plasma porphyrins are poorly dialyzed and elevated in many dialysis patients; iron overload from blood transfusions; and an increased incidence of hepatitis C in the dialysis population may be related factors. Pseudoporphyria and the bullous disease of dialysis are clinically similar to PCT, but lack the associated elevated porphyrin levels (Fig. 38-7). Many of these cases may be medication-related. These conditions are further summarized in Chapter 28.

Uremic Frost

First described in 1865 by Hirschsprung, uremic frost is rarely encountered today due to the widespread availability of dialysis. When the blood urea nitrogen (BUN) level rises, urea concentrates in the sweat and deposits on the skin following evaporation. The crystals are visible, giving rise to uremic frost, only when the BUN is extremely high, usually greater than 250 to 300 mg/dL. This condition is typically first seen in the beard area, or on other areas of the face, neck, or trunk, as fine white-to-yellow crystals. It represents a grave prognostic sign, unless therapy is emergently initiated.

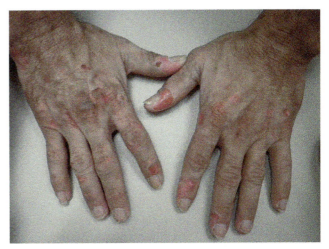

FIGURE 38-7 ■ Pseudoporphyria or bullous disease of dialysis arising in a hemodialysis patient, clinically indistinguishable from porphyria cutanea tarda, presenting with numerous erosions and bullae on the dorsal hands and fingers.

Xerosis

For unclear reasons, between 50% and 90% of patients on dialysis have significant xerosis. Some suggest that the water content of the skin may be decreased, perhaps in association with a reduction in sweat volume and/or atrophy of sebaceous glands, while others speculate a role for hypervitaminosis A; however, when directly measured these levels are typically normal in ESRD patients. Treatment includes emollients, with or without keratolytic agents.

DERMATOLOGIC CONDITIONS ASSOCIATED WITH RENAL TRANSPLANTATION

Although many patients with ESRD benefit from dialysis, it cannot fully compensate for kidney function, and the best option for many is renal allograft transplantation. This, too, can result in numerous cutaneous complications, both from the immunosuppressive medications essential for allograft survival and from the state of immunosuppression. These conditions are summarized in Table 38-3.

SUGGESTED READINGS

Bernstein EJ, Schmidt-Lauber C, Kay J. Nephrogenic systemic fibrosis: a systemic fibrosing disease resulting from gadolinium exposure. Best Pract Res Clin Rheumatol 2012;26:489–503.
Giardi M, Kay J, Elston D, LeBoit P, Abu-Alfa A, Cowper S. Nephrogenic systemic fibrosis: clinicopathological definition and workup recommendations. J Am Acad Dermatol 2011;65:1095–106.
Kurban MS, Boueiz A, Kibbi AG. Cutaneous manifestations of chronic kidney disease. Clin Dermatol 2008;26:255–64.
Vedvyas C, Winterfield L, Vleugels RA. Calciphylaxis: a systemic review of existing and emerging therapies. J Am Acad Dermatol 2012;67:e254–260.

CHAPTER 39

CUTANEOUS MANIFESTATIONS OBSERVED IN TRANSPLANT RECIPIENTS

Fiona Zwald • Manisha J. Loss • Dennis L. Cooper • Jean L. Bolognia

> **KEY POINTS**
>
> - Skin infections occur at a great frequency in solid organ and bone marrow transplant recipients largely as a consequence of immunosuppression.
> - Neoplasms, particularly squamous cell carcinomas, occur at greater frequency, are more difficult to manage, and are more likely to metastasize than in the nontransplant population.
> - Graft-versus-host disease, particularly the chronic variant, remains a problem, particularly among patients with bone marrow or stem cell transplantation.
> - The drugs used for immune suppression have potential mucocutaneous adverse reactions, which must be managed.

The use of immunosuppressive medications has allowed the long-term survival of transplanted solid organs. As a direct result of the required immunosuppression, there is an increase in the incidence and prevalence of both skin infections and neoplasms. Furthermore, the immunosuppressive agents themselves can produce a wide range of cutaneous side effects.

The clinical diagnosis of cutaneous disorders in transplant recipients can prove challenging because the clinical presentation, including the morphology of the lesions, is often altered by the ongoing immunosuppression. This immunosuppression can lead to an exaggeration of clinical findings, as in the case of verrucae vulgaris, or more aggressive behavior, as in the case of cutaneous squamous cell carcinoma or the attenuation of clinical findings such as the diminished inflammatory response seen in deep fungal infections.

INFECTIONS

The early years of renal transplantation were marked by frequent life-threatening infections, with over half of patients dying of infections during the first 3 years after transplantation. Although much progress has been made in the past decade with regard to prophylaxis (antibacterial, antifungal, and antiviral), early diagnosis, and effective treatment, infections remain a major cause of morbidity and mortality in transplant recipients.

Organ transplant recipients are susceptible to bacterial, viral, and fungal skin infections. Infections during the first month after transplantation are usually caused by nosocomial pathogens or reactivation of latent disease. Up to 6 months after transplantation, reactivation of latent disease or opportunistic infections predominate. Continuation or initiation of moderate- to high-dose corticosteroids increases the risk of developing the latter. Late infections may be caused by opportunistic or conventional pathogens, with the former seen more commonly in those with heightened immunosuppression because of the need to treat graft rejection or active graft-versus-host disease (GVHD).

Antiviral

Infections with herpesviruses (in particular herpes simplex virus-1 [HSV-1], HSV-2, varicella-zoster virus [VZV], and cytomegalovirus [CMV]) were once a common cause of morbidity and mortality during the first year following transplantation. For example, in one series, 97% of patients had one or more herpesvirus infections. However, with the routine use of prophylactic antivirals and the preemptive use of valganciclovir or ganciclovir (e.g., based on weekly blood CMV antigen or polymerase chain reaction [PCR] assays in allogeneic hematopoietic stem cell transplant patients), this situation has improved dramatically. Chronic human papillomavirus infections, however, still remain a significant problem in patients who have received solid organ transplants, because of their need for lifelong immunosuppression. In contrast, an attempt is made to taper and then discontinue immunosuppressive therapy in allogeneic hematopoietic stem cell transplant patients over 12 to 18 months—that is, unless there is active GVHD.

Herpes Simplex Virus (HSV-1, HSV-2)

Herpes simplex virus (HSV) was a common cause of infection in transplant recipients until the use of prophylactic acyclovir became commonplace. Although active infections with this virus can occur at any time, they were observed most frequently during the first month after transplantation. In the absence of antiviral therapy, viral shedding rates were found to be as high as 70% in renal transplant patients, 20% in heart–lung recipients, and 60% in bone marrow recipients. The vast majority of HSV infections represent reactivation of a latent infection; occasionally, transplant patients can develop primary disease, and rarely, HSV transmission via transplanted organs has been reported. Reactivation of HSV appears

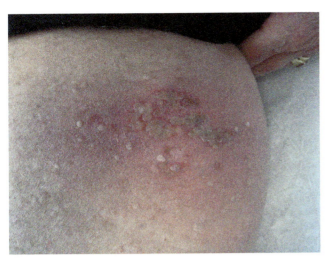

FIGURE 39-1 ■ Classic reactivation of herpes simplex virus-2 in a heart lung transplant recipient.

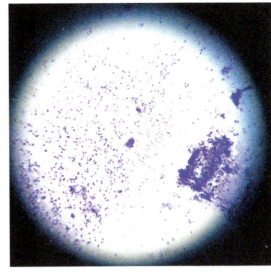

FIGURE 39-2 ■ Tzanck smear demonstrating a multinucleated giant cell centrally.

to be a consequence of impaired cellular immunity, as it occurs despite high titers of antibodies directed against the virus.

In mucocutaneous sites, the initial primary lesions of HSV are similar to those seen in immunocompetent hosts, i.e., grouped vesicles, crusts, or erosions on an erythematous base. However, in addition to sites such as the nasal mucosa, vermilion border of the lip, oral mucosa that overlies bone, fingers, buttocks, and genitalia, HSV infections in immunocompromised hosts often involve the "soft" oral mucosa, the perianal region, and the esophagus. In addition, rather than being self-limited infections that last for 7 to 10 days even in the absence of antiviral therapy (as in immunocompetent hosts), these herpetic ulcers tend to be chronic and expansive (Fig. 39-1).

In transplant patients, systemic HSV infections are rather uncommon and are often not accompanied by cutaneous lesions. As a result, the clinical diagnosis requires a high index of suspicion. Reported sites of systemic involvement include the central nervous system (CNS), lungs and liver, as well as the gastrointestinal tract. Occasionally, in the setting of immunosuppression, cutaneous lesions of HSV are "disseminated" on the trunk or extremities.

Because of its accuracy and rapid turnaround time of a few hours, the most helpful diagnostic procedure for HSV infections is the PCR assay. In the case of mucocutaneous lesions, it is important to provide the laboratory with an ample supply of keratinocytes. A viral culture should also be done on any tissue sample, including skin, submitted for the PCR assay. Dermatologists still do an office-based test known as a Tzanck preparation (Fig. 39-2) to look for virally infected multinucleated giant cells (seen in HSV-1, HSV-2, VZV, and occasionally CMV infections), but this test is less sensitive than the PCR assay and requires more expertise to interpret.

Depending on the severity, treatment options for active HSV infection in an immunocompromised host include oral agents with enhanced bioavailability (e.g., famciclovir, valacyclovir), or intravenous acyclovir. The antivirals should be continued until there is complete clinical clearing (rather than for a preset number of days), and treatment is usually successful if the diagnosis is made promptly. As in patients with HIV infection who have received multiple or prolonged courses of acyclovir, acyclovir-resistant strains of HSV have been reported, and in these patients intravenous foscarnet (and less often intravenous cidofovir) is employed; topical cidofovir (1% gel) may be tried in milder cases.

Varicella-Zoster Virus

Herpes zoster is a common infection in transplant recipients, occurring in up to 15% of cases. As in immunocompetent hosts, it is a result of the reactivation of the varicella-zoster virus (VZV) that resides in dorsal root or cranial nerve ganglia. Clinical disease is usually characterized by a unilateral distribution of grouped vesicles or crusts on an erythematous base, with lesions usually being confined to one or a few adjacent dermatomes (Fig. 39-3A). However, both chronic VZV and cutaneous dissemination of VZV can occur in this patient population (Fig. 39-3B); in the latter situation, at least 20 lesions reminiscent of varicella are widely scattered on the trunk and extremities. Less often there is associated meningoencephalitis, pneumonitis, or hepatitis. Prolonged infection is associated with reduced specific cellular immune responsiveness.

As is the case with HSV infections, the diagnosis of herpes zoster is established via the PCR assay, Tzanck smears, and/or PCR; viral cultures of VZV require a longer incubation period than those of HSV. In patients with severe disease, cutaneous dissemination, or suspected systemic involvement, the treatment of choice is intravenous acyclovir. If the disease is mild and there is no evidence of cutaneous dissemination, then oral agents with greater bioavailability (e.g., famciclovir, valacyclovir) can be prescribed.

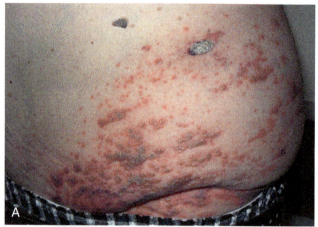
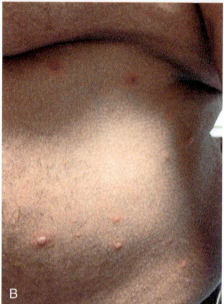

FIGURE 39-3 ■ **A,** Multiple vesicles on an erythematous base that resemble varicella in a renal transplant patient with disseminated zoster. **B,** Dermatomal herpes zoster in a renal transplant recipient.

Cytomegalovirus

Cytomegalovirus (CMV) is one of the more common opportunistic infections in transplant recipients and is potentially a major source of morbidity and mortality. Until the development of more effective anti-CMV medications, this virus accounted for up to 25% of deaths, 20% of graft failures, 30% of febrile episodes, and 35% of leukopenic episodes in renal transplant patients. One of the major advances, especially in allogeneic hematopoietic stem cell transplant patients, has been the use of weekly antibody staining of circulating neutrophils or weekly PCR-based assays of peripheral blood as a means of detecting CMV antigen or CMV DNA, respectively, and hence early infections. The latter assays are particularly helpful in neutropenic patients. In the setting of positive results, "preemptive" oral valganciclovir or intravenous ganciclovir therapy can be instituted prior to the development of clinical symptoms such as fever, pneumonitis, or enterocolitis.

Infections in transplant recipients may be primary, i.e., due to the presence of CMV in the transplanted organ or cells, or they may represent reactivation of a latent infection. In the past, clinical infections were most common during the first 6 months after transplantation; e.g., in one series of kidney transplant patients the median time of onset was 46 days after transplantation. However, with more solid organ transplant patients receiving prophylactic therapy during the first 3 months after transplantation, the time of onset is often delayed until after discontinuation of antiviral therapy.

Clinical manifestations of CMV infection include leukopenia, pneumonitis, gastroenteritis, retinitis, hepatitis, and encephalitis, as well as a mononucleosis-type syndrome. Skin involvement is present in a small percentage of patients with systemic CMV infection; cutaneous presentations include morbilliform eruptions, verrucous plaques, petechiae and purpura, and ulcerations. It can also be seen incidentally in cutaneous biopsies in patients with no active eruption. In mucocutaneous ulcers CMV often coexists with other viruses such as HSV or VZV, and as a result its true pathogenicity has been questioned.

The diagnosis of CMV infection is suggested histopathologically by the presence of intranuclear inclusions surrounded by a halo within endothelial cells. Viral culture or a PCR-based assay of involved tissues, including the skin, is required for confirmation. It is important not to confuse active infection with viral shedding, as is commonly seen in the urine or throat washings of transplant patients.

Human Herpesvirus 6

In addition to causing exanthema subitum (roseola infantum) in healthy young children, human herpesvirus 6 (HHV-6) has been associated with fever, pancytopenia, pneumonitis, gastroenteritis, and encephalitis in transplant patients. There are also a few scattered reports of an associated morbilliform eruption at the time of reactivation. Viral DNA can be detected in the skin as well as peripheral blood mononuclear cells.

Epstein–Barr Virus and Human Herpesvirus 8

Infections with two other herpesviruses, Epstein–Barr virus (EBV) and human herpesvirus 8 (HHV-8), are associated with the development of neoplasms in transplant patients: post-transplant lymphoproliferative disorder and Kaposi's sarcoma (KS), respectively. The term post-transplant lymphoproliferative disorder is used rather than lymphoma because the histologic findings range from a polyclonal B-cell infiltrate to a monoclonal B-cell lymphoma. Rarely, T-cell lymphomas are seen.

Because this lymphoproliferative disorder is reflective of "over"-immunosuppression, a reduction in immunosuppressive therapy is a component of the initial therapy. Clearly, the extent to which the immunosuppressive agents can be reduced depends on the type of transplant. Renal transplant patients have the option of being placed back on dialysis, but patients with heart, lung, or liver transplants cannot afford graft rejection. For localized

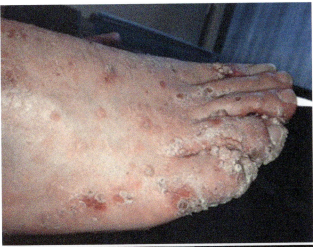

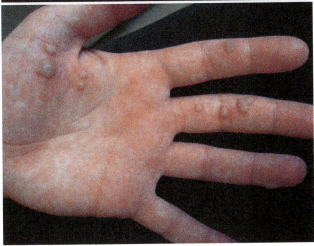

FIGURE 39-4 ■ Multiple verrucae vulgares in a patient who had received a lung transplant.

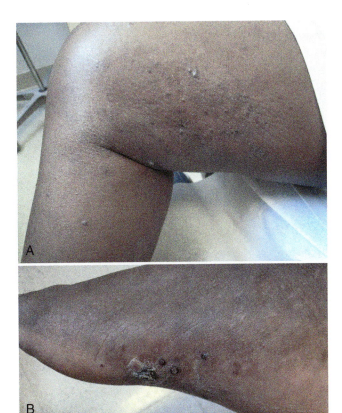

FIGURE 39-5 ■ **A,** Kaposi sarcoma with woody induration of leg in a renal transplant recipient. **B,** Kaposi sarcoma of the foot in the same renal transplant recipient.

disease, surgical excision or radiation therapy combined with a reduction in immunosuppression may prove sufficient. However, extensive or rapidly progressive disease requires systemic therapy with rituximab, often in combination with multidrug chemotherapy. Discontinuation of standard immunosuppression in conjunction with administration of chemotherapy usually does not lead to graft rejection, given the immunosuppressive effects of the chemotherapy.

The association between HHV-8 and KS is seen in both immunocompetent and immunosuppressed patients (see Chapters 23 and 35). In solid organ transplant recipients, the prevalence of KS is 50 times that of the general population in endemic areas, and increases to 400 to 500 times in nonendemic areas. Regression of the mucocutaneous lesions of KS has been observed in transplant patients following a reduction in the level of immunosuppression or a switch from a systemic calcineurin inhibitor to mTOR inhibitor therapies such as sirolimus (rapamycin).

Human Papillomavirus

Verrucae vulgaris (viral warts) are very common in patients who have received solid organ transplants and reflect their requirement for lifelong immunosuppression. The prevalence of warts increases with the duration of graft survival, such that the majority of renal transplant recipients with graft durations of more than 5 years have verrucae. There are over 90 different types of human papillomavirus (HPV), and specific types or groupings are associated with particular clinical forms of the disease. For example, HPV types 1, 2, and 4 are associated with banal warts, often on the hands and feet (Fig. 39-4); HPV types 3 and 10 are associated with flat warts (verruca plana); and HPV types 6 and 11 (nononcogenic) as well as 16 and 18 (oncogenic) are associated with condylomata acuminata (venereal warts) (Fig. 39-5).

Not only can transplant patients have all of the HPV types just mentioned, but they have been found to harbor unusual types that were once thought to be uniquely associated with a rare disease known as epidermodysplasia verruciformis (e.g., HPV 5, 8, 19 to 25). In addition, the warts are frequently extensive and even more difficult to treat than in the general population. The oncogenic potential of some of these HPV types combined with the chronic immunosuppression creates a difficult situation in a number of patients. The potential for developing squamous cell carcinomas of the cervix, vulva, and anus in addition to the skin (see below) represents a real threat to these patients, and an ongoing screening program that includes close inspection and biopsy of any suspicious lesion is required. Treatment of HPV infections is discussed in Chapters 33 and 35.

Molluscum Contagiosum

Mollusca contagiosum (MC) are 2- to 10-mm dome-shaped skin-colored to pink papules that have a central umbilication. They are caused by a poxvirus. Infections with MC are more common in patients with atopic dermatitis and in immunocompromised hosts (see Chapters 33 and 35). In the latter group, lesions can prove difficult to treat. Cutaneous lesions of cryptococcosis and systemic dimorphic fungal infections can resemble MC, and therefore dermal scrapings or a skin biopsy specimen should be examined if the diagnosis is uncertain.

Bacterial

Pyogenic Bacteria

Staphylococcus aureus causes the majority of all pyodermas and soft-tissue infections seen in transplant recipients. The incidence of *S. aureus* nasal carriage is higher in transplant recipients and the spectrum of pyodermas includes folliculitis, furuncles, abscesses, impetigo, and ecthyma. Their clinical presentations may be atypical owing to the concomitant immunosuppression (Fig. 39-6); in the case of cellulitis, there may be less erythema than is observed in normal hosts. Meticillin-resistant *S. aureus* is a problem in transplant patients as it is in immunocompetent hosts therefore cultures must always be taken in soft tissue infections.

Incision and drainage of abscesses is a key component of treatment, and for severe infections empiric intravenous vancomycin or linezolid is recommended until antimicrobial susceptibility results become available. *Streptococcus pyogenes* commonly colonizes the upper respiratory tract and secondarily infects (impetiginizes) minor skin lesions from which invasive infection can arise. Other streptococci, such as Group B streptococci, commonly colonize the perineum causing soft tissue infection. Immunosuppressed patients are particularly prone to necrotizing fasciitis, a severe form of soft tissue infection extending into the subcutaneous fat and deep fascia. Treatment includes broad antibiotic coverage, often supplemented with clindamycin and possibly intravenous immunoglobulin, in addition to intensive care monitoring and surgical debridement as appropriate.

A condition dubbed "transplant elbow," consisting of recurrent staphylococcal infections in the skin overlying the extensor elbows, has been described in transplant recipients. The cause is related to skin atrophy secondary to the use of systemic corticosteroids, and is linked to repeated trauma produced when the patients use their elbows to rise from sitting because of the corticosteroid-induced myopathy affecting the hip girdle.

In transplant patients the cause of cutaneous infections cannot be assumed to be Gram-positive cocci: additional organisms need to be considered, such as Gram-negative rods (Fig. 39-7), Gram-positive rods (e.g., *Bacillus cereus*), atypical mycobacteria, herpesviruses, and opportunistic fungi and parasites. In immunocompromised hosts there are multiple infectious etiologies for lesions that resemble ecthyma gangrenosum (see below), i.e., the list extends beyond *Pseudomonas aeruginosa*.

Nocardia. Both cutaneous and systemic nocardiosis have been reported in transplant patients. Hematogenous dissemination from a pulmonary focus can lead to secondary sites of infection in the skin, as well as in other organs such as the brain. Primary cutaneous infection can present as abscesses, ulcers, granulomas, soft-tissue infection, mycetoma, or sporotrichoid infection. If cutaneous nocardiosis is diagnosed in a transplant patient, it is important to look for additional sites of involvement to determine if it is primary versus secondary due to dissemination.

A presumptive diagnosis can be made by identifying fine-branching filaments in a Gram stain of dermal scrapings or a biopsy specimen; a modified acid-fast stain can also be used to identify the organisms. Both *Nocardia asteroides* and *N. brasiliensis* are slow-growing bacteria and culture plates need to be held for longer periods than in the case of other more common bacteria. For isolated lesions, surgical excision is an option, but treatment with antibiotics, in particular trimethoprim–sulfamethoxazole, is usually successful. Long-term therapy is important to prevent reactivation of quiescent disease.

Mycobacteria

In endemic areas the incidence of tuberculosis is significantly greater in renal transplant patients than in the general population. Infection may represent reactivation of

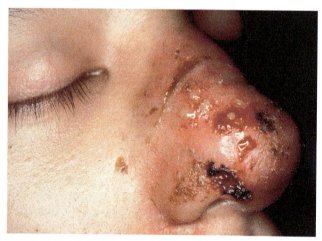

FIGURE 39-6 ■ Soft tissue infection of the nose due to *Staphylococcus aureus* in a patient with leukemia and neutropenia prior to allogeneic hematopoietic stem cell transplant. (Courtesy of Yale Residents' Slide Collection.)

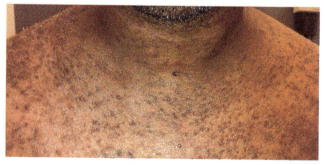

FIGURE 39-7 ■ Monomorphic papules and pustules on the chest of a renal transplant recipient with Gram-negative folliculitis.

latent disease, community-acquired disease, or very rarely transmission by the donor kidney. Cutaneous lesions due to *Mycobacterium tuberculosis* range from scrofuloderma (spread of a tuberculous process from the underlying tissue) and lupus vulgaris as manifestations of reactivation to periorificial ulcers and widespread papulovesicles in patients with overwhelming disease.

Atypical mycobacterial infections of the skin can either be primary, e.g., due to inoculation of organisms at a site of trauma, or secondary as a reflection of systemic disease. The former are seen in both immunocompetent and immunocompromised hosts, and a classic example of an associated organism would be *M. marinum*. A lymphocutaneous pattern, also referred to as sporotrichoid, is commonly observed with the initial papule or nodule at the site of inoculation and the subsequent development of nodules along the path of lymphatic drainage. In immunocompromised hosts, the clinical appearance of atypical mycobacterial infections can be muted due to the suppression of inflammation, or exaggerated due to the suppression of host defenses, i.e., they can vary from subtle erythema to large, nonhealing ulcers.

The diagnosis of cutaneous mycobacterial infections depends on the identification of acid-fast bacilli in biopsy specimens and isolation of the responsible organisms by specialized culture techniques. If available, PCR can also be performed for more rapid results. In the case of tuberculosis, the QuantiFERON-TB Gold test, in which the amount of interferon (IFN)-γ is measured following incubation of the patient's blood with two synthetic peptides from *M. tuberculosis* (but absent in BCG vaccine strains), is increasingly being utilized. However, indeterminate results (i.e., failure of the internal positive control) are more common in immunocompromised individuals. Lastly, a search should be undertaken for additional sites of involvement, e.g., pulmonary. Specific multidrug treatment regimens are dictated by the species isolated and the antibiotic sensitivities (www.cdc.gov/mmwr/preview/mmwrhtml/rr5211a1.htm).

The treatment of cutaneous mycobacterial infections is complex and is dependent on the extent of the disease, the species, and the degree of immunosuppression. The treatment of infections with typical mycobacteria requires three of the following agents: isoniazid, rifampicin, pyrazinamide, and ethambutol. In the case of multidrug resistance, a combination with quinolones or clarithromycin is considered. These medications can impact blood levels and efficacy of concomitant immunosuppressive agents and should be carefully monitored. For deep cutaneous infections, surgical excision may be essential in order to reduce large collections of mycobacterial infection. Additionally, revision of immunosuppression to bolster the immune response may be essential for successful treatment of any mycobacterial infection in the immunosuppressed patient.

Fungal

Superficial Fungi

Superficial fungal infections are due primarily to yeasts, in particular *Candida* spp., and dermatophytes, especially *Trichophyton rubrum* and *T. mentagrophytes*. Cutaneous candidiasis is exacerbated by oral corticosteroids and broad-spectrum antibiotics as well as hyperglycemia, a confounding problem in many renal transplant patients. The clinical presentations include oral thrush, perlèche, onycholysis, chronic paronychia, onychomycosis of the fingernails, intertrigo, balanitis, and vulvovaginitis. Another yeast that can cause clinical disease in transplant patients is *Malassezia furfur* (previously known as *Pityrosporum*). The primary manifestations are pityriasis (tinea) versicolor and pityrosporum folliculitis (Fig. 39-8). Diagnoses of these yeast infections can be accomplished by examination of a potassium hydroxide (KOH) preparation and, in the case of candidiasis, fungal culture.

In addition to the very common dermatophyte infections such as tinea pedis (feet), tinea manuum (hands), and tinea unguium (nails), transplant patients can develop extensive lesions of tinea corporis and tinea facei (Fig. 39-9). The immunosuppression also increases the

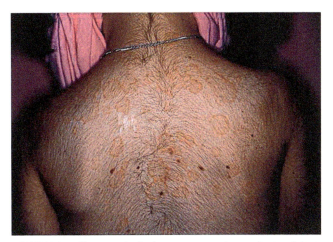

FIGURE 39-8 ■ Tinea versicolor in a young renal transplant recipient.

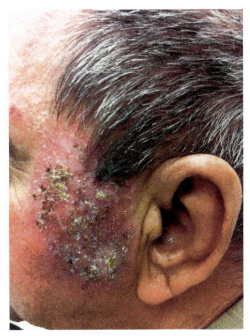

FIGURE 39-9 ■ Tinea faciei (Majocchi's granuloma) on the face of a lung transplant patient.

risk of developing Majocchi's granuloma (a tinea infection of the hair follicles, which is characterized by follicular papules and papulopustules; Fig. 39-9) as well as a particular type of nail infection known as proximal subungual onychomycosis (see Chapters 33 and 35). Deep or invasive dermatophytosis, where the fungi are actually found in the dermis, is quite rare but is usually seen in immunocompromised hosts. Oral candidiasis, or thrush, is the most common fungal infection in transplant recipients, usually more prominent in the first year post transplant. For classical fungal skin infections, diagnosis rests on the KOH examination and fungal culture. Cutaneous infections due to *Candida* and *Malassezia* spp. are best treated with topical imidazoles or oral fluconazole, whereas cutaneous dermatophyte infections are best treated with topical or oral allylamines (e.g., terbinafine).

Deep Fungal Infections

In patients who require more profound immunosuppression, systemic infections due to opportunistic pathogens such as *Cryptococcus*, *Candida*, *Aspergillus*, and saprophytes can occur. Systemic infections due to dimorphic fungi can also become widely disseminated in transplant patients.

Candida. Disseminated candidiasis was classically the most common systemic mycosis, but a significant reduction in incidence and mortality has occurred with the use of prophylactic fluconazole. The replacement of bone marrow transplants (average time to engraftment, 21 days) with peripheral blood stem cell transplants (average time to engraftment, 14 days) has also reduced the incidence of disseminated candidiasis in the immediate post-transplant period.

Neutropenia, systemic corticosteroids, hyperglycemia, placement of central intravenous catheters, and the use of broad-spectrum antibiotics are predisposing factors. Fever, myalgias, and cutaneous lesions are the classic triad, but cutaneous lesions are present in only 10% to 15% of patients. Most commonly, multiple firm pink papules with central pallor are observed (Fig. 39-10*A*); additional skin findings include purpuric macules and papules (Fig. 39-10*B*), pustules and subcutaneous nodules. The pustules may initially be misdiagnosed as simple folliculitis. Whereas myalgias are classically associated with systemic candidiasis, muscle pain and tenderness due to septic emboli can be seen with other opportunistic infections (see below).

Although disseminated candidiasis is associated with positive blood cultures more often than are other systemic fungal infections, blood cultures may be negative. However, a biopsy specimen from a purpuric lesion is usually diagnostic, with yeast forms and pseudohyphae present in the dermis (Fig. 39-10*C*) and vascular spaces. A tissue fungal culture should be performed using sterile technique, i.e., the culture should be representative of organisms growing in the dermis, not the surface stratum corneum. *Candida* spp. that have been isolated from patients with disseminated candidiasis include *C. albicans*, *C. tropicalis*, *C. krusei*, *C. parapsilosis*, and *C. glabrata*.

Treatment of disseminated candidiasis depends on the severity of the illness as well as the specific isolate and its

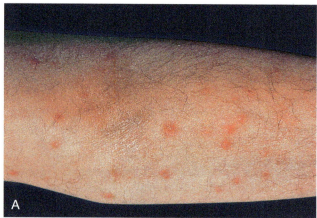
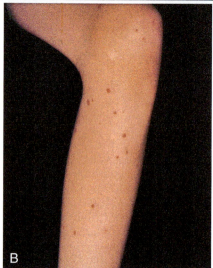
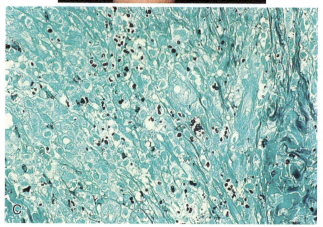

FIGURE 39-10 ■ **A** and **B,** Disseminated candidiasis in two patients with leukemia and neutropenia due to the preparative regimen prior to transplant. **C,** A silver stain of the skin biopsy specimen demonstrates the numerous yeast forms and pseudohyphae in the dermis. (Courtesy of Yale Residents' Slide Collection.)

sensitivities. The use of prophylactic fluconazole has led to a greater incidence of non-*C. albicans* species, which may be resistant to fluconazole: e.g., *C. krusei* is well known to be resistant to fluconazole. Therapeutic options include intravenous and oral azoles/triazoles (e.g., fluconazole [unless disease developed while on this drug], voriconazole) or echinocandins (e.g., caspofungin, micafungin, anidulafungin), which inhibit glycan synthase.

Intravenous amphotericin (including the liposomal forms) is also effective, but its use has declined owing to its toxicity, as well as the availability of other equally effective drugs with fewer side effects.

Aspergillus. Immunocompromised hosts are also at risk for the development of infections with the opportunistic fungus *Aspergillus*, in particular *A. flavus* and *A. fumigatus*. Invasive infections with *Aspergillus* spp., a ubiquitous dimorphic fungus, are the second most frequent opportunistic infections in transplant recipients, particularly in the early period post transplantation, and in some settings have overtaken *Candida* spp. as the most common opportunistic fungal infection if the patient is not on an *Aspergillus*-active azole as prophylaxis. The major risk factors remain systemic corticosteroid therapy and prolonged neutropenia. As is the case with disseminated candidiasis, shorter engraftment times after peripheral blood stem cell transplants (compared to bone marrow transplants) have reduced the number of early *Aspergillus* infections. Later infections in hematopoietic stem cell transplant patients are usually associated with the use of corticosteroid therapy for GVHD. Voriconazole is frequently used as prophylaxis in high-risk patients; however, due to the recently reported risk of skin cancer associated with the use of voriconazole, alternative agents, e.g., posaconazole, are recommended in certain transplant recipients who are particularly susceptible to skin cancer (see below).

Primary cutaneous infections develop at sites of trauma, including those from intravenous catheter use. Both occlusive adhesive tape and arm boards have been associated with primary *Aspergillus* infections, but fortunately their use has decreased as the use of indwelling central venous catheters has increased. Secondary cutaneous lesions of *Aspergillus* represent septic emboli due to systemic infection. The primary source is often pulmonary, and the cutaneous lesions vary from erythematous papules to ecthyma gangrenosum-like lesions (Fig. 39-11*A*). Biopsy specimens demonstrate septate, acute-branching fungi in the dermis and invading the walls of blood vessels (Fig. 39-11*B*).

If the primary lesions of aspergillosis are fairly well circumscribed, treatment consists of surgical excision and oral antifungal agents. Voriconazole is widely prescribed for use as a prophylactic agent and treatment of invasive fungal infections in transplant recipients. Voriconazole has now been established as an independent risk factor for the development of cutaneous malignancy in transplant recipients. Several series have reported skin cancer, particularly cutaneous squamous cell carcinoma, among hematopoietic stem cell and solid organ transplant patients receiving long-term voriconazole (12 months). Though the mechanism of voriconazole-induced skin cancer is unknown, it may induce phototoxicity due to its primary metabolite, voriconazole N-oxide. The FDA has altered its labeling to state that voriconazole should be used carefully, for durations of less than 6 to 9 months, particularly among patients with risk factors for skin cancer. In patients requiring prolonged voriconazole, diligent skin cancer screening examinations, sun protection, and liberal use of UV protectants is advisable.

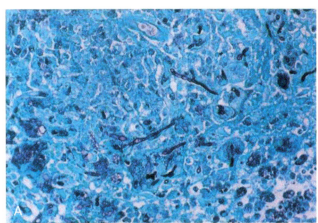
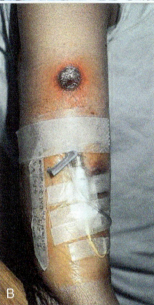

FIGURE 39-11 ■ **A,** Erythematous plaque with large central necrotic eschar located proximal to IV catheter due to *Aspergillus* in a neutropenic patient with leukemia. **B,** *Aspergillus* skin biopsy specimen showing septate hyphae branching at acute angles.

Currently, however, systemic disease is treated with voriconazole, which has been shown to be more effective than amphotericin for documented *Aspergillus* infections. Echinocandins represent second-line therapy. An attempt has also been made to reduce the dose of oral corticosteroids, but despite all these measures the mortality rate for systemic aspergillosis remains quite high.

Cryptococcus. Immunocompromised hosts, from those with AIDS to those who have undergone renal transplantation, are prone to infections with the yeast *Cryptococcus neoformans*. Both primary and secondary skin lesions are seen in transplant patients, and the latter represent systemic dissemination, usually from a primary focus in the lungs. In addition, a very common site of involvement is the CNS. Cutaneous manifestations vary from nondescript papules and ulcers to cellulitis and lesions that resemble molluscum contagiosum (see Chapter 33). Biopsy specimens of involved skin demonstrate multiple yeast forms within the dermis, and in the majority of patients the characteristic capsules are also seen. Depending on the severity of the infection and the sites of involvement, treatment consists of fluconazole, and, if necessary, amphotericin B; in the setting of CNS infection, flucytosine is added to amphotericin B.

Dimorphic Fungi

In the United States, the three major dimorphic fungi are *Histoplasma capsulatum*, *Coccidioides immitis*, and *Blastomyces dermatitidis*. Each is associated with a particular region of the country: the Ohio Valley (histoplasmosis), the southwest and California (coccidiomycosis), and the southeast and Midwest river valleys (blastomycosis). The primary route of infection is inhalation, and individuals in endemic regions often have asymptomatic infections or flu-like syndromes. With immunosuppression, reactivation and dissemination can occur.

All three dimorphic fungi can produce a wide range of mucocutaneous lesions, including papulonodules, pustules, expanding plaques with peripheral pustules, abscesses, and ulcerations; in the case of histoplasmosis, oral ulcers are characteristic. Biopsy specimens demonstrate both granulomatous and neutrophilic infiltrates, and yeast forms of *H. capsulatum* and *B. dermatitidis* can be found within macrophages and giant cells. In the case of coccidiomycosis, large spherules full of endospores are seen rather than yeast forms.

Additional sites of involvement vary depending on the specific fungus, with *H. capsulatum* favoring the reticuloendothelial system (liver, spleen, and bone marrow), *C. immitis* favoring the bones, joints, and CNS, and *B. dermatitidis* favoring the skin and bones. For all three fungal infections, treatment options include itraconazole and amphotericin B, and in the case of coccidiomycosis, fluconazole is an additional option.

Other Opportunistic Mycoses and Parasites

Immunocompromised hosts develop infections secondary to saprophytic fungi, which in normal hosts are often disregarded as contaminants. The genera include *Alternaria*, *Dreschlera*, *Fusarium*, *Mucor*, *Rhizopus*, and *Absidia*. The cutaneous lesions often represent septic emboli, and their clinical appearances are similar to emboli due to Gram-negative rods or other fungi such as *Aspergillus* (Fig. 39-11). In addition, cutaneous extension of underlying fungal sinus infections can present initially as unilateral facial edema. Recognition of this subtle presentation allows earlier diagnosis and treatment. Soft tissue extension and systemic spread can also occur in immunocompromised hosts with saprophytic onychomycosis (Fig. 39-12). Unfortunately, even with proper therapy consisting of surgical debridement (if possible) and institution of systemic medications such as voriconazole (*Fusarium*) or amphotericin B, treatment failure is common (Fig. 39-13).

In addition to saprophytic fungi, immunocompromised patients can also develop folliculitis due to *Demodex* mites (demodicidosis; see Chapter 33) as well as systemic infections with parasites such as *Strongyloides stercoralis* and *Acanthamoeba* spp. In disseminated strongyloidiasis

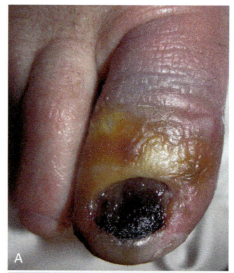
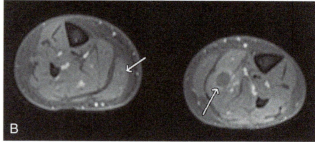

FIGURE 39-12 ■ **A**, Soft tissue infection with necrosis in a patient who had received an allogeneic hematopoietic stem cell transplant and in whom the primary focus was saprophytic onychomyocosis due to *Fusarium*. **B**, Magnetic resonance imaging scan of the lower extremities demonstrating multiple septic emboli of *Fusarium* within muscles (*white arrows*). (**A**, Courtesy of Yale Residents' Slide Collection.)

purpuric macules and patches are seen, especially on the abdomen, in addition to pulmonary and gastrointestinal involvement; the mortality rate is quite high. Infections with *Acanthamoeba* spp. often originate in the paranasal sinuses or lungs, and systemic dissemination can involve the CNS as well as the skin (Fig. 39-14).

NEOPLASMS

Patients who have received transplants are at increased risk for the development of several different neoplasms, including Kaposi's sarcoma (see Chapter 23) and nonmelanoma skin cancers. This is particularly true of solid organ transplant patients, because they require lifelong immunosuppression, and the incidence of cutaneous tumors increases with the duration of immunosuppression.

Squamous Cell and Basal Cell Carcinoma

The two major forms of nonmelanoma skin cancer (NMSC) are basal cell carcinoma (BCC) (Figs 39-15 to 39-19) and squamous cell carcinoma (SCC) (Fig. 39-16). In the general population, the usual ratio of BCC to SCC is approximately 4:1, but this ratio is nearly reversed in

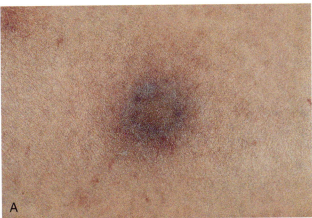
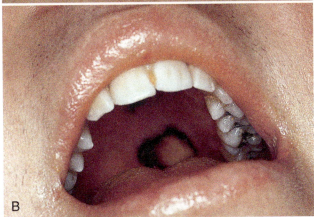
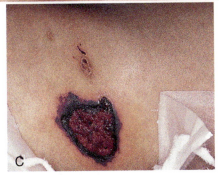

FIGURE 39-13 ■ Septic emboli due to *Fusarium* (**A**) and *Dreschlera* (**B** and **C**) in two allogeneic bone marrow transplant patients. Note the similarity of the clinical appearance of these lesions to those seen in Figs 39-8 and 39-11. (**A**, Courtesy of Yale Residents' Slide Collection.)

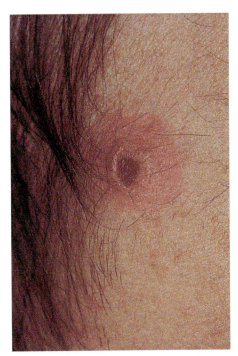

FIGURE 39-14 ■ Septic embolus due to *Acanthamoeba* in a patient who received a haploidentical stem cell transplant and subsequently died of this amebic infection. (Courtesy of Yale Residents' Slide Collection.)

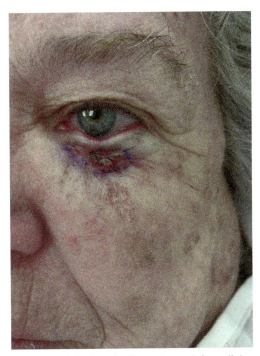

FIGURE 39-15 ■ Nodular basal cell carcinoma left medial canthus.

solid organ transplant patients. Compared to the general population, there is a 65-fold and a 10-fold increase in the incidence of cutaneous SCCs and BCCs, respectively, in solid organ transplant recipients. In two studies from the United States and Australia, the incidence of NMSCs was 35% 10 years post transplant (heart transplant recipients) and 44% 9 years post transplant (renal transplant recipients), respectively. A striking statistic derived from an investigation of Australian heart transplant recipients was that metastatic NMSC accounted for 27% of the deaths that occurred more than 4 years post transplant. High-risk SCC constitutes tumors that are recurrent, large size (>2 cm), eye, ear or lip location, with perineural invasion and/or poor differentiation on histology (Fig. 39-17).

The clinical appearance of these tumors is the same as in normal hosts. The BCCs are pearly to pink-colored papules that often have telangiectases within them; some of the lesions develop a central hemorrhagic crust (scab), and others have central ulceration (Fig. 39-15). The SCCs are usually pink to red papules, nodules, or plaques that have associated scale, such that they may resemble a common wart, psoriasis, or

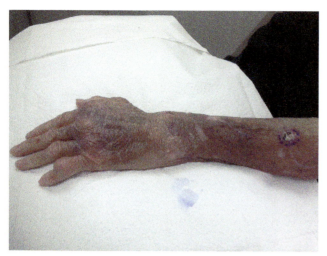

FIGURE 39-16 ■ Squamous cell carcinoma of the helix-keratoacanthoma type.

eczema. This is especially true of the in situ form of SCC known as Bowen's disease. SCC of the keratoacanthoma type is an exophytic lesion with a central crateriform ulcer (Fig. 39-16).

In general, these tumors develop in sun-exposed sites as in normal hosts, and are seen most commonly in fair-skinned individuals who have received a significant amount of cumulative sun exposure. Clues to the latter include wrinkles, yellow discoloration of the posterior neck and lateral forehead (solar elastosis), mottled pigmentation, and actinic (solar) keratoses. Actinic keratoses (AKs) are often referred to as precancers because they can develop into SCCs (but not BCCs); they have a characteristic hard scale and are best appreciated by palpation (Fig. 39-18).

Sun exposure is not the only factor involved in pathogenesis. Infection with HPV also plays a role, especially in SCCs that develop in association with condylomata acuminata due to oncogenic types of HPV. The role of

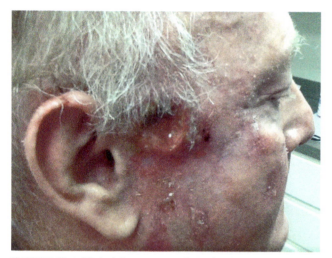

FIGURE 39-17 ■ High-risk recurrent, ulcerative squamous cell carcinoma left temple in a renal transplant recipient.

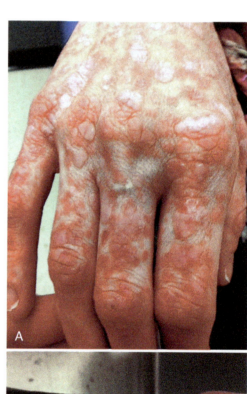

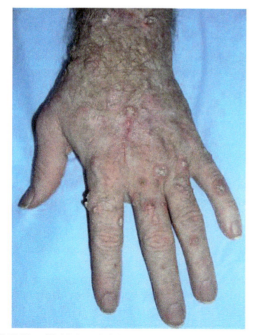

FIGURE 39-18 ■ Multiple actinic keratoses and areas of dyspigmentation on the dorsum of the hand in a renal transplant patient.

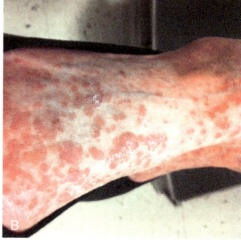

FIGURE 39-19 ■ Scaly, guttate, polymorphic, pinkish macules and thin plaques of epidermodysplasia verruciformis. **A,** Dorsal and **B,** dorsal foot.

infection with HPV in the development of cutaneous squamous cell carcinoma is still unclear. An extremely diverse group of HPV types, mainly consisting of epidermodysplasia-verruciformis (EV)-associated HPV types, can be detected in benign, premalignant, and malignant skin lesions of organ transplant recipients (Fig. 39-19). Frequently, there are multiple HPV types present in single skin biopsies. Typically, the prevalence of viral warts rises steadily after transplantation and a strong association exists between the number of HPV-induced warts and the development of skin cancer. The hair follicle region might be the reservoir of EV-HPV. The E6 protein from a range of cutaneous HPV types effectively inhibits apoptosis in response to UV light-induced damage. It is therefore conceivable that individuals who are infected by EV-HPV are at an increased risk of developing actinic keratoses and squamous cell carcinomas, possibly by chronically preventing UV light-induced apoptosis.

The frequency of total body skin examinations is determined according to the degree and duration of immunosuppression, type of organ transplant received, skin pigmentation, amount of cumulative sun exposure, presence or absence of condylomata acuminata, and number of previous actinic keratoses and nonmelanoma skin cancers. At one end of the spectrum are those individuals who develop multiple tumors every few months, and in this group reduction of immunosuppression as well as prophylactic therapies such as oral retinoids need to be considered. Acitretin has been shown to reduce the number of new SCCs that develop in transplant patients, but a rebound effect occurs if the medication is discontinued. The side effects of the oral retinoids, e.g., birth defects, hypertriglyceridemia, must of course be weighed against the benefits.

Prompt diagnosis and treatment of cutaneous SCCs is indicated in transplant patients, given the aggressive nature of these tumors. Therapeutic options include electrodesiccation and curettage for in situ lesions, routine surgical excision, microscopically controlled excision (Mohs' technique) for large, rapidly growing, ill-defined or recurrent lesions, and, occasionally, postoperative adjuvant radiation therapy (e.g., if there is neurotropism). Topical 5-fluorouracil or imiquimod and photodynamic therapy have been used in individuals with numerous AKs and significant actinic damage. In solid organ transplant recipients who continue to develop multiple NMSCs, immunosuppression with sirolimus (rapamycin), rather than cyclosporine or tacrolimus, or minimization of immunosuppression in consultation with the transplant team can be considered.

Miscellaneous

Follicular dystrophy of immunosuppression (trichodysplasia spinulosa) is an entity that has been described over the past decade in patients (including transplant recipients) who are immunocompromised. Various theories have been proposed with regard to etiology, from being virally induced ("viral-associated trichodysplasia of immunosuppression") to a side effect of cyclosporine ("cyclosporine-induced follicular dystrophy"). Patients develop follicular papules, especially on the central face, as well as loss of the eyebrows and eyelashes.

GRAFT-VERSUS-HOST DISEASE

Graft-versus-host disease (GVHD) is the most common cause of morbidity and mortality in allogeneic hematopoietic stem cell transplant recipients. It is caused by an immunologic reaction of immunocompetent donor T lymphocytes in a recipient who is incapable of rejecting the graft. T-cell depletion of the allograft reduces the risk of GVHD but is associated with a higher incidence of tumor recurrence and graft failure. The reason for the higher risk of recurrence is the lack of a graft-versus-tumor effect. As a result, most transplants are still carried out with unmodified (i.e., T-cell replete) grafts and are associated with a significant risk of acute and chronic GVHD.

Treatment of recurrent lymphomas and leukemias after allogeneic transplant includes a rapid reduction in immunosuppression and infusions of donor T lymphocytes. The major risk of these strategies is GVHD, and as a result the clinician is constantly trying to balance tumor control on the one hand with GVHD on the other.

Acute GVHD

GVHD is classically divided into acute (<100 days post transplant) and chronic (>100 days post transplant), but this division has become less distinct with currently employed protocols. Significant acute GVHD occurs in 25% to 40% of allogeneic hematopoietic stem cell transplant patients. Risk factors include an unrelated (but matched) donor, a related donor but with a mismatch at one or more human leukocyte antigens, an unmodified graft, an older age of the donor or the recipient, and a female donor with a male recipient.

In acute GVHD the major sites of involvement are the skin, liver (hepatitis), and gastrointestinal tract (diarrhea). The cutaneous eruption is reminiscent of the common maculopapular (morbilliform) drug eruption. The initial lesions often appear on the hands and feet (Fig. 39-20). There is a grading system for acute cutaneous GVHD,

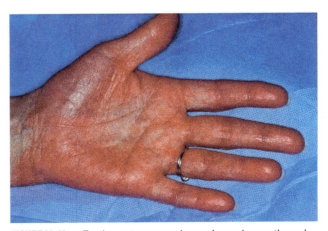

FIGURE 39-20 ■ Erythematous macules and papules on the palm of a patient 30 days post-allogeneic bone marrow transplant.

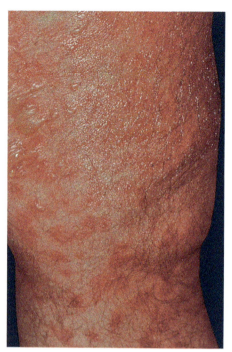

FIGURE 39-21 ■ Edematous plaques and bullae in a patient with acute graft-versus-host disease following an allogeneic bone marrow transplant. (Courtesy of Yale Residents' Slide Collection.)

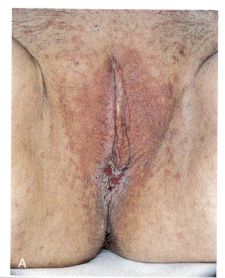

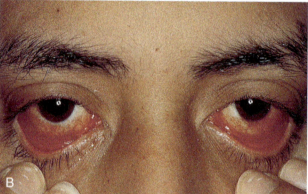

FIGURE 39-22 ■ Acute graft-versus-host-disease involving the mucous membranes of the genitalia (**A**) and the conjunctivae (**B**) in two patients following allogeneic bone marrow transplants. (B, Courtesy of Yale Residents' Slide Collection.)

which takes into account the percentage of body surface area involved when the eruption is maculopapular (stage I, <25%; stage II, 25% to 50%; stage III, >50%). Erythroderma with bulla formation (Fig. 39-21) and/or desquamation represents stage IV. Additional sites of involvement include mucosal surfaces such as the conjunctivae (Fig. 39-22).

Histologic features of acute cutaneous GVHD include necrotic keratinocytes and lymphocytes within the epidermis as well as in the upper papillary dermis. When the lymphocytes are adjacent to necrotic keratinocytes, this is termed satellite cell necrosis. Unfortunately, the histologic findings in early GVHD may be rather nonspecific, and the differential diagnosis includes drug eruptions and viral exanthems, the same as the clinical differential diagnosis of the morbilliform eruption. One study suggested that the decision to treat suspected acute GVHD depended not on skin biopsy findings, but rather on the clinical severity of the presumed acute GVHD (at the time of the biopsy). However, this study did not address the subsequent taper of immunosuppressants, which could be influenced by the biopsy findings.

Classically, prophylactic treatment for acute GVHD consists of cyclosporine (CsA) or tacrolimus in conjunction with methotrexate. However, methotrexate is increasingly being replaced by mycophenolate mofetil or sirolimus (rapamycin), because these two drugs result in a reduced incidence of mucositis. The CsA or tacrolimus is continued for approximately 180 days post transplant and then tapered. Treatment of acute GVHD, which develops during prophylactic therapy, consists initially of systemic corticosteroids. In patients who do not respond to the addition of corticosteroids, there is no standard treatment protocol, but options include extracorporeal photopheresis (ECP), infliximab, daclizumab, basiliximab, and mycophenolate mofetil, with most unresponsive patients developing chronic GVHD.

Chronic GVHD

Chronic GVHD is more common in allogeneic hematopoietic stem cell transplant patients who have had acute GVHD. It may occur as a progression of acute GVHD, as a recurrence following a disease-free interval, or in the absence of a history of acute GVHD (i.e., de novo). Chronic GVHD occurs in approximately 50% to 80% of patients who have received such transplants. In addition to the skin, gut and liver, chronic GVHD can affect the eyes and salivary glands (a Sjögren's-like syndrome), the lung (bronchiolitis obliterans), and the esophagus (a scleroderma-like process). Chronic cutaneous GVHD is classically divided into two major forms, lichenoid and sclerodermoid.

Lichenoid GVHD shares clinical and histologic features with lichen planus and is characterized by flat-topped, pink to violet scaly papules (Fig. 39-23A) and white lacy plaques on the oral mucosa. Occasionally, there is scalp involvement that results in scarring alopecia. Biopsy specimens demonstrate a lichenoid infiltrate (lymphocytes abutting

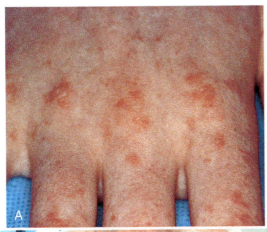

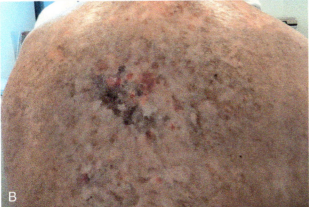

FIGURE 39-23 ■ **A**, Flat-topped pink scaly papules of chronic graft-versus-host-disease (GVHD) on the dorsal aspect of the hand. **B**, Chronic GVHD with an atypical melanocytic proliferation. (A, Courtesy of Yale Residents' Slide Collection.)

TABLE 39-1	Characteristic Mucocutaneous Side Effects
Medication	**Mucocutaneous Side Effects***
Corticosteroids	Folliculitis, acne, abnormal fat distribution, atrophy, striae, purpura, acanthosis nigricans
Cyclosporine	Hypertrichosis, gingival hyperplasia, sebaceous hyperplasia, epidermal cysts, folliculitis, alopecia
Tacrolimus	Pruritus, peripheral edema, ecchymoses, alopecia, photosensitivity, folliculitis
Azathioprine	Morbilliform eruption, urticaria, hypersensitivity reaction, rare Sweet's-like reaction
Mycophenolate mofetil	Peripheral edema, acne, thrombophlebitis, hypersensitivity reaction
Sirolimus (rapamycin)	Acne, peripheral and facial edema, aphthae, gingival hyperplasia

*In addition to cutaneous infections and neoplasms.

the dermoepidermal junction) with vacuolar degeneration of the basal layer and necrotic keratinocytes, similar to the histologic findings of lichen planus.

The name sclerodermoid GVHD comes from the more diffuse cutaneous sclerosis that is seen in late-stage, severe chronic GVHD. However, the early and potentially reversible form of this disease would more appropriately be termed morpheaform. This is because these earlier lesions are circumscribed firm plaques measuring several centimeters in diameter and thus have a clinical appearance very similar to that of morphea. Early lesions frequently involve the girdle area as well as the extensor aspects of the extremities. In addition, patients often have plaques—especially on the neck, upper trunk, and previous intravenous catheter sites—that resemble lichen sclerosus, i.e., shiny, hypopigmented plaques with scale and/or follicular plugging. With progression, the morpheaform plaques coalesce and may encase the trunk circumferentially; the clinical picture is then more reminiscent of diffuse scleroderma with dyspigmentation (Fig. 39-23B). Histologically, there is thickening and sclerosis of the dermis, with replacement of subcutaneous fat and entrapment of eccrine glands (similar findings are seen in morphea and scleroderma).

In addition to the morpheaform and sclerodermoid forms of chronic GVHD, an occasional patient will have a clinical presentation that resembles eosinophilic fasciitis. This should come as no surprise, given the overlap between deep morphea and eosinophilic fasciitis. Similarities between several autoimmune connective tissue diseases and chronic GVHD may reflect a failure to either delete autoreactive T cells or produce immunoregulatory T cells.

Treatment of chronic GVHD is similar to that of acute GVHD and includes prednisone, CsA, tacrolimus, mycophenolate mofetil, and ECP. For chronic GVHD limited to the skin, topical corticosteroids, hydroxychloroquine, psoralens plus UVA (PUVA), UVA-I, or extracorporeal photopheresis can be employed. Recently, rituximab was shown to be effective for the cutaneous and musculoskeletal manifestations of chronic GVHD and imatinib mesylate improved cutaneous sclerosis, but the mechanisms of action of these agents are unclear. None of these modalities, however, are predictably effective.

DRUG EFFECTS

The cutaneous side effects of the primary medications prescribed for transplant patients are outlined in Table 39-1. In recent years there has been a movement away from CsA and toward tacrolimus, as well as a movement away from azathioprine and toward mycophenolate mofetil and sirolimus (rapamycin). In the future, agents that have specific anti-inflammatory effects will probably play a larger role in the treatment of GVHD and organ rejection.

SUGGESTED READINGS

Bavinck JN, Tieben LM, Van der Woude FJ, et al. Prevention of skin cancer and reduction of keratotic skin lesions during acitretin therapy in renal transplant recipients: a double-blind, placebo-controlled study. J Clin Oncol 1995;13:1933–8.

Bouwes Bavinck JN, Feltkamp M, Struijk L, ter Schegget J. Human papillomavirus and skin cancer risk in organ transplant recipients. J Investig Dermatol Symp Proc 2001;6(3):207–11.

Chakrabarti S, Pillay D, Ratcliffe D, et al. Resistance to antiviral drugs in herpes simplex virus infections among allogeneic stem cell transplant recipients: risk factors and prognostic significance. J Infect Dis 2000;181:2055–8.

Cowen EW, Nguyen JC, Miller DD, et al. Chronic phototoxicity and aggressive squamous cell carcinoma of the skin in children and adults during treatment with voriconazole. J Am Acad Dermatol 2010;62(1):31–7.

Herbrecht R, Denning DW, Patterson TF, et al. Voriconazole versus amphotericin B for primary therapy of invasive aspergillosis. N Engl J Med 2002;347:408–15.

Horn TD, Zahurak ML, Atkins D, et al. Lichen planus-like histopathologic characteristics in the cutaneous graft-vs-host reaction. Prognostic significance independent of time course after allogeneic bone marrow transplantation. Arch Dermatol 1997;133:961–5.

Nichols WG. Management of infectious complications in the hematopoietic stem cell transplant recipient. J Intens Care Med 2003;18:295–312.

Sable CA, Strohmaier KM, Chodakewitz JA. Advances in antifungal therapy. Ann Rev Med 2008;59:361–79.

Schaffer JV, McNiff JM, Seropian S, et al. Lichen sclerosus and eosinophilic fasciitis as manifestations of chronic graft-versus-host disease: expanding the sclerodermoid spectrum. J Am Acad Dermatol 2005;53:591–601.

Venkatesan P, Perfect JR, Myers SA. Evaluation and management of fungal infections in immunocompromised patients. Dermatol Ther 2005;18:44–57.

Williams K, Mansh M, Chin-Hong P, Singer J, Arron S. Voriconazole-associated cutaneous malignancy: a literature review on photocarcinogenesis in organ transplant recipients. Clin Infect Dis 2014;58(7):997–1002.

Wolfson JS, Sober AJ, Rubin RH. Dermatologic manifestations of infections in immunocompromised patients. Medicine 1985;64:115–33.

Zwald FO, Brown M. Skin cancer in organ transplant recipients: advance in therapy and management: part I. Epidemiology of skin cancer in solid organ transplant recipients. J Am Acad Dermatol 2011;65(2):253–61.

Zwald FO, Brown M. Skin cancer in organ transplant recipients: advances in therapy and management: part II. Management of skin cancer in solid organ transplant recipients. J Am Acad Dermatol 2011;65(2):263–79.

Zwald FO, Spratt M, Lemos BD, et al. Duration of voriconazole exposure: an independent risk factor for skin cancer after lung transplantation. Dermatol Surg 2012;38(8):1369–74.

CHAPTER 40

NEUROCUTANEOUS DISEASE

Sarah D. Cipriano • John J. Zone

KEY POINTS

- Neurofibromatosis is an autosomal dominant disorder characterized by cutaneous neurofibromas, café-au-lait macules, and myriad systemic features with marked variability of expression.
- Patients with neurofibromatosis are at risk for the development of a malignant peripheral nerve sheath tumor.
- Increasing or constant pain, change in consistency, or rapid growth of a nodule within an existing plexiform neurofibroma are concerning signs of malignant transformation.
- Tuberous sclerosis complex (TSC) is an autosomal dominant, multisystem disorder characterized by the development of hamartomas in multiple organ systems, including the brain, eyes, heart, lung, liver, kidneys, and skin.
- Dermatologic features of TSC can be easily recognizable and are present in >90% of patients with TSC.
- Knowledge of the functional relationship between TSC1/TSC2 and mTORC1 has led to important clinical advances in the use of mTOR inhibitors for the treatment of several clinical manifestations of TSC.
- Sturge–Weber syndrome (SWS) is a sporadic congenital condition characterized by a facial capillary malformation (port-wine stain [PWS]) in association with leptomeningeal angiomatosis and glaucoma.
- The neurologic features of SWS may be progressive and include seizures, focal neurologic impairment, and cognitive deficits.
- Ataxia–telangiectasia (AT) is an autosomal recessive disorder consisting of progressive cerebellar ataxia, ocular and cutaneous telangiectasia, and variable immune deficiency.
- Approximately 10–25% of patients with AT develop a malignancy, the majority of which are lymphoproliferative disorders.

Discussions of neurocutaneous disease are frequently limited to descriptions of the four "phakomatoses." These conditions were grouped together because they all involved central nervous system (CNS) and retinal tumors (phakomas). The phakomatoses include neurofibromatosis, tuberous sclerosis complex, Sturge-Weber syndrome, and von Hippel–Lindau syndrome (VHL), the first three of which have striking cutaneous manifestations. Knowledge of the pathogenesis of these disorders had been static for many years. However, advances in gene identification have led to the discovery of the genes responsible for these neurocutaneous disorders. Identification of the genes, their products and role in pathogenesis has led to significant clinical advances in treatment. This discussion provides a broad overview of the most important neurocutaneous disorders as well as a variety of other conditions in which cutaneous and nervous system findings are shared.

CLASSIFICATION

The relationship between the skin and the nervous system may be based on: (1) a developmental abnormality, frequently a result of a shared embryogenesis; or (2) the systemic effect on both organ systems of a metabolic disorder, infection, or immune response. The developmental and metabolic disorders are primarily of genetic origin, whereas the infectious and immune abnormalities represent the response of the skin and nervous system to a common insult. The neural crest is a transient embryonic structure that gives rise to dorsal root ganglion cells, Schwann cells, autonomic ganglion cells, as well as melanocytes. Abnormalities of the neural crest cells lead to a myriad of clinical findings. Unfortunately, the resulting disease entities can seldom be distilled to a pattern that can be totally explained by deductive reasoning. Disorders involving both the skin and the nervous system can be briefly categorized if one includes only the phakomatoses, but the list becomes very extensive if less common syndromes and systemic diseases involving both organ systems are included. The classifications in Table 40-1 include the classic neurocutaneous disorders and representative examples of various syndromes.

The term "phakomatosis" is derived from the Greek word "phakos" meaning "mother spot or mole." Although originally used to describe the retinal lesions of tuberous sclerosis, it has come to refer to a group of disorders including: (1) tuberous sclerosis complex; (2) neurofibromatosis; (3) Sturge–Weber disease; and (4) VHL syndrome. These disorders, as well as other vascular abnormalities, will be discussed in detail. The remainder of the developmental disorders represents disorders of epidermal cells and their appendages that share an ectodermal origin with the nervous system. The syndromes mentioned in Table 40-1 are rare but represent examples of probable neural crest abnormalities as well as poorly understood but well-documented disorders involving both the skin and the nervous system.

TABLE 40-1	Classification of Neurocutaneous Disease

1. Dysplasia of neural crest cells
   a. Neurofibromatosis
   b. Tuberous sclerosis
2. Vascular malformations
   a. Sturge–Weber syndrome
   b. Cobb syndrome
   c. Ataxia-telangiectasia
   d. von Hippel–Lindau syndrome
3. Pigmentary abnormalities
   a. Waardenburg syndrome
   b. Incontinentia pigmenti
   c. Hypomelanosis of Ito
   d. Vogt–Koyanagi–Harada syndrome
4. Epidermal nevus syndrome
5. Ichthyosis-associated syndromes

NEUROFIBROMATOSIS (VON RECKLINGHAUSEN DISEASE)

Neurofibromas may occur in several clinical settings. Sporadic solitary cutaneous tumors can arise in adulthood and are not associated with café-au-lait spots. There are three major clinically and genetically distinguishable forms of neurofibromatosis: neurofibromatosis type 1, neurofibromatosis type 2, and schwannomatosis. Classic neurofibromatosis (type 1 or NF1—OMIM #162200) as described by von Recklinghausen is characterized by multiple café-au-lait macules, cutaneous neurofibromas, and myriad systemic involvement with marked variability of expression. Acoustic neurofibromatosis (type 2 or NF2—OMIM #101000) presents with bilateral acoustic neuromas as well as café-au-lait macules and cutaneous neurofibromas. The gene for NF2 is localized on chromosome 22 and encodes a negative growth regulator called MERLIN. Schwannomatosis (neurilemmomatosis—OMIM #162091) is characterized by multiple noncutaneous schwannomas in the absence of acoustic tumors. Mutations in the tumor suppressor genes SMARCB1 and LZTR1 are thought to be responsible for the majority of cases. Segmental (dermatomal) neurofibromatosis is a syndrome where café-au-lait macules, cutaneous neurofibromas, and sometimes visceral neurofibromas are limited to a sharply defined unilateral body segment. Watson's syndrome, a variant of NF1, has multiple café-au-lait macules, short stature, and pulmonary valvular stenosis, but only a small number of neurofibromas. This discussion will be limited to NF1 and the term "neurofibromatosis" is used to refer to only that disorder.

Pathogenesis

Neurofibromatosis is an autosomal dominant disorder affecting approximately 1 in 3000 live births. De novo mutations represent around 50% of patients with neurofibromatosis. Penetrance approaches 100% by age 20, but the expressivity is highly variable. With an estimated mutation rate of 1 in 10,000 per gamete per generation, the NF1 gene has one of the highest mutation rates of any genetic disorder. Currently over 1000 pathogenic variants in NF1 have been identified. About 90% of new mutations occur on the paternally derived chromosome with the majority causing truncation of the gene product.

The NF1 gene has been localized to chromosome 17q11.2. The basic defect lies in the abnormal expression of a tumor suppressor gene called neurofibromin. This gene product has functional and structural homology with a guanosine triphosphatase-activation protein (GTPase) that downregulates $p21^{ras}$ proto-oncogene activity. In its active (GTP) state, the $p21^{ras}$ protein binds guanine nucleotides with high affinity, acting as a signal transducer for cellular proliferation. Neurofibromin switches off this signaling by hydrolyzing GTP to guanosine diphosphate (Fig. 40-1). A defect in neurofibromin would result in a constitutively active $p21^{ras}$ protein leading to cell growth and possible tumor formation. Interestingly, neurofibromin is found in the skin, brain, spleen, liver, and muscle, not just in the neural crest cells. The abnormal proliferation seen in neurofibromatosis is focused on the neural crest for reasons that are not yet clear at the molecular level.

It is generally believed that a somatic "second hit" mutation with loss of heterozygosity results in the progression of malignant tumors and possibly in the formation of benign neurofibromas. However, given the wide clinical phenotypes found even among close relatives, a defect in the neurofibromin protein cannot in itself explain this variability. Other studies point to evidence that modifying genes (genes that are unlinked to the NF1 gene, but play a phenotypical role in neurofibromatosis) may be behind these differences. Clinical outcomes would depend on where the second mutation at another gene occurs. Finally, recent research has shown that the environment, especially trauma, may lead to the formation of benign neurofibromas. Since neurofibromin is involved in the healing process, defective neurofibromin in conjunction with a traumatic event may lead to abnormal cellular proliferation and tumor formation.

Clinical Manifestations

Café-au-Lait Macules

Present in virtually all patients, these hyperpigmented macules are the earliest clinical features found in neurofibromatosis (Table 40-2). Up to 15% of the normal population have one to three café-au-lait spots. The current criterion for the disease is the presence of six or more café-au-lait macules larger than 1.5 cm for adults and 0.5 cm for prepubertal individuals (Fig. 40-2). Café-au-lait spots are usually present at birth, or shortly thereafter, and progressively increase in number and size. The macular hyperpigmentation is usually homogeneous with sharply defined edges. Distribution is random, sparing the scalp, palms, and soles They tend to darken in response to sunlight and will fade with time and become less noticeable.

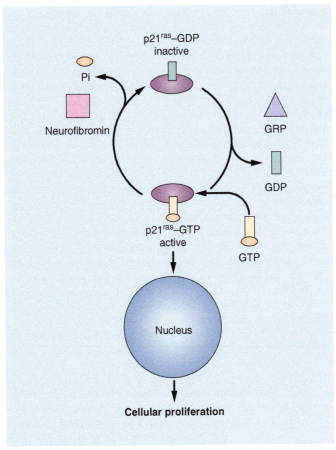

FIGURE 40-1 ■ Neurofibromin is involved in inactivating the p21ras/GTP complex.

TABLE 40-2	Order of Appearance of the Clinical Features Listed in the National Institutes of Health (NIH) Criteria for Neurofibromatosis

Café-au-lait macules
Axillary freckling
Lisch nodules
Neurofibromas

Skin Fold Freckling

The freckle-like pathognomonic lesions (Crowe's sign) (Fig. 40-2) generally occur between 3 and 5 years of age in the axillae and/or groin. Around 90% of adults have the freckling. These freckles are typically small, distinguishing them from café-au-lait macules. Other involved areas include the area above the eyelids, around the neck, and submammary region in females.

Neurofibromas

Neurofibromas may be subdivided according to their appearance and location into the following groups: cutaneous, nodular (subcutaneous), and plexiform. All are composed of various combinations of Schwann cells,

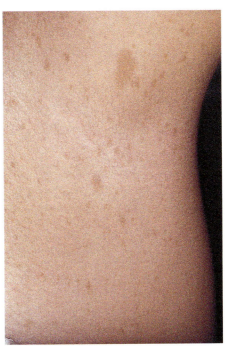

FIGURE 40-2 ■ A café-au-lait spot and multiple freckles (Crowe's sign) in the axillary vault is seen in this patient with neurofibromatosis.

fibroblasts, perineural cells, vascular elements, and mast cells. Cutaneous neurofibromas are rarely present in infancy; more often they begin to appear in late childhood and adolescence and gradually increase in size and number. Clinically, they are soft, fleshy, sessile, or pedunculated tumors that can be invaginated (buttonhole sign) (Fig. 40-3). Subcutaneous, or nodular, neurofibromas tend to become apparent in late childhood or early adulthood. Subcutaneous lesions can be noted on palpation of the skin and may present with tenderness or tingling distributed along the affected nerve. Both pregnancy and puberty are known to increase the number and size of neurofibromas. Plexiform neurofibromas may be superficial, deep, or a combination of both. These tumors arise from multiple nerve fascicles, tend to grow along the length of a nerve, and can feel like a "bag of worms." They can extend into surrounding structures, including the skin, fascia, muscle, bone, and internal organs. They can be painful and affect the growth and function of the affected area.

Patients with neurofibromatosis are at risk for the development of a malignant peripheral nerve sheath tumor (MPNST). Patients with NF1 have a 10% lifetime risk of developing this highly aggressive spindle cell tumor. MPNSTs typically arise from plexiform neurofibromas. Significant and constant pain, change in consistency, or rapid growth of a nodule within an existing plexiform neurofibroma are concerning signs of malignant transformation.

Lisch Nodules

These pigmented iris hamartomas are present in >90% of adults with neurofibromatosis. They are asymptomatic and are not correlated with other manifestations or with severity of the disease. Clinically they appear as randomly distributed cream-colored to brownish nodules on the iris. While most are easy to visualize, a slit-lamp evaluation by an experienced ophthalmologist is often needed to rule out the presence of single "salt grain" lesions. Histologically, they represent melanocytic hamartomas.

Central Nervous System Involvement

CNS tumors develop in 3% to 10% of patients and include benign neoplasms such as optic nerve gliomas, acoustic neuromas, neurolemmomas, meningiomas, ependymomas, astrocytomas, and neurofibromas. Such growths present clinically with signs and symptoms of CNS mass lesions. Spinal tumors often present with localizing peripheral signs. Optic pathway glioma (OPG), the most common of these tumors, involves some combination of the optic nerves, chiasm, or optic tract. They may result in papilledema, retrobulbar neuritis, and eventually optic atrophy. Some may manifest as precocious puberty due to hypothalamic encroachment. Most OPGs develop within the first 6 years of life and the majority of cases run a benign course and do not require intervention. For those whose tumors do progress, chemotherapy is the treatment of choice. Malignant tumors, most commonly low-grade astrocytomas, may also occur. They affect the brainstem and may present with symptoms of mass effect such as cranial neuropathies and hydrocephalus. However, these lesions tend to have a less aggressive course when compared to pontine tumors that are not associated with neurofibromatosis.

A more recent issue is the presence of high-intensity signals on T2 magnetic resonance imaging (MRI). These NF-associated bright spots (also called unidentified bright objects) are often found within the basal ganglia, cerebellum, and brainstem in up to 70% to 80% of patients with neurofibromatosis. What these images represent remains unclear. Current speculation includes harmatomas, dysplasia, demyelination, vacuolar changes, or low-grade tumors. The clinical significance of these findings is also in dispute. Some studies have shown that the presence of bright spots is associated with lower IQ scores, but this conclusion has remained controversial. Some practitioners believe that the findings of bright spots should be included as a criterion for the diagnosis of neurofibromatosis and may be diagnostic in 30% of the cases of children who do not meet the current criteria. However, consideration must be taken in regard to children who may need anesthesia in order to have an MRI performed.

Learning disabilities occur in 50% to 75% of patients. Frank intellectual disability is seen in about 5% of patients. The learning problems associated with neurofibromatosis persist into adulthood. There is a higher incidence of attention-deficit disorder, autism spectrum disorders, behavioral abnormalities, and psychosocial issues. Headaches occur with increased frequency even in the absence of CNS tumors. Mild speech impediments are present in 30% to 40% of cases, and cerebrovascular compromise as a result of involvement of cerebral arteries with neurofibromas does occur. Major and minor motor seizures occur in less than 5% of cases in the absence

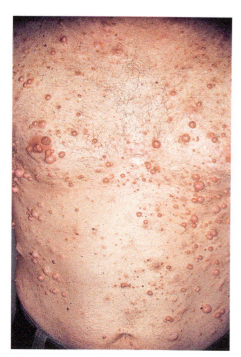

FIGURE 40-3 ■ Multiple neurofibromas are present in this individual.

of identifiable mass lesions or cerebral vascular involvement. An additional 26% of patients will have abnormal or borderline findings on electroencephalogram.

Macrocephaly is present in at least 27% of patients. This manifestation is more common after 6 years of age. There is no correlation between macrocephaly and impaired intellectual performance, seizures, or electroencephalographic abnormalities.

Musculoskeletal Disorders

Sphenoid wing dysplasia is a distinctive osteopathy of neurofibromatosis. It presents as a unilateral defect affecting the orbital plate and frontal bone. Dysplasia of a long bone occurs in nearly 14% of patients with neurofibromatosis and usually presents in the first year of life. The most commonly affected bone is the tibia, which will bow in an anterolateral direction. Repeated fracture and failure to heal can result in a pseudoarthrosis, which is a false joint. Scoliosis has been reported to occur in up to 10% of patients with neurofibromatosis and usually becomes apparent by age 10 years. Dystrophic scoliosis is a rapidly progressive form with the potential to cause a variety of neurologic complications. Radiographic bone abnormalities may also result from pressure by intraosseous or paraosseous neurofibromas. No consensus on treatment is available and severe cases have led to amputation. Short stature is also another feature more prominent in individuals with neurofibromatosis. Growth curves comparing nonaffected and affected children show similar growth profiles until preadolescence at which point the growth rate for children with neurofibromatosis decreases significantly. In addition, they are at increased risk of osteoporosis and osteopenia later in life.

Vascular Disorders

Hypertension is more prevalent in patients with NF1 and can develop at any age. The hypertension is usually essential, but may occur secondary to renal artery stenosis, coarctation of the aorta, or pheochromocytoma. Vasculopathy may involve arteries of the heart and brain. Congenital heart defects and valvar pulmonic stenosis are more common in individuals with neurofibromatosis.

Gastrointestinal Disorders

Visceral tumors arise from intra-abdominal neural tissue and include neurofibromas, leiomyomas, and miscellaneous tumors. The most common complications are obstruction, intussusception, and hemorrhage caused by erosions or necrosis of pedunculated tumors. Persistent constipation occurs in 10% of cases and is due to disorganization of the tunica muscularis and Auerbach's plexus of the colon.

Endocrine Disorders

Aberrant endocrine function is not a regular finding in neurofibromatosis and although frequently mentioned is probably present in less than 1% of cases. Pheochromocytoma, often benign and unilateral, is the most common endocrine abnormality. It predominantly produces norepinephrine. Medullary carcinoma of the thyroid and hyperparathyroidism are even less common. In addition, it has been reported that optic gliomas in children with hypothalamic involvement may present with either premature or delayed puberty.

Miscellaneous Disorders

Miscellaneous malignancies, including Wilms' tumor, rhabdomyosarcoma, and leukemia, and a variety of tumors of neural crest origin, including malignant melanomas, are more common in patients with neurofibromatosis than in the population at large. An association with juvenile xanthogranuloma and juvenile myelomonocytic leukemia has been found in children with neurofibromatosis. It is felt that the loss of the tumor suppression function of the NF1 gene predisposes those with neurofibromatosis to myeloid disorders.

Differential Diagnosis

The diagnostic criteria outlined by the US National Institutes of Health are based upon specific clinical features of NF1. Two or more of the following criteria are needed:
1. Six or more café-au-lait spots greater than 1.5 cm in adults and 0.5 cm in prepubertal children.
2. Two or more neurofibromas of any type or one plexiform neurofibroma.
3. Axillary or inguinal freckling.
4. Optic glioma.
5. Two or more Lisch nodules.
6. A distinctive bony lesion, such as sphenoid dysplasia or thickening of a long bone cortex with or without pseudoarthrosis.
7. A first-degree relative with NF1.

These diagnostic criteria are both highly sensitive and specific for adults with neurofibromatosis. They are less sensitive in children, especially those under 8 years of age, because some of the criteria do not manifest at a young age. Other minor features that may assist in the diagnosis include macrocephaly, hypertelorism, short stature, and thorax abnormalities.

Legius syndrome (OMIM #611431), an autosomal dominant NF1-like disorder, is a genetically distinct disorder with a similar phenotype to NF1. It results from germline loss-of-function mutations in SPRED1. The SPRED1 gene encodes a negative regulator of the RAS-MAPK pathway, similar to neurofibromin. This disorder is characterized by multiple CALMs, axillary freckling, and macrocephaly. These individuals do not have neurofibromas, Lisch nodules, or NF1 gene abnormalities.

Patient Evaluation

Given the myriad of clinical features in neurofibromatosis, the utility of extensive screening tests remains controversial. In general, clinical evaluation tends to be more helpful to detect complications than are screening investigations in asymptomatic patients. Annual visits should include a thorough physical exam, a formal ophthalmologic exam, assessment for precocious puberty, developmental assessment, review of school performance, and monitoring of plexiform neurofibromas.

Genetic Testing

With the current methodologies available approximately 85% to 95% of the currently known mutations can be identified. In familial cases of neurofibromatosis, indirect linkage studies can be performed. Genes are said to be linked when markers close to the NF1 locus segregate together during recombination. Through the extensive evaluation of multiple family members, analysis of the markers associated with the abnormal NF1 gene can be identified and used for genetic counseling. In addition, in utero diagnosis studies are currently available. However, genetic testing in neurofibromatosis remains problematic. The large variability in phenotypic expression of neurofibromatosis does not correlate with specific genetic mutations. Positive genetic results do not predict the presence, age of onset, or the severity of disease. There are two exceptions. Patients with whole gene deletions, which occur in 4% to 5% of patients with NF1, present with a large tumor burden, more severe cognitive impairment, large hands and feet, dysmorphic facial features, and have a higher lifetime risk of developing MPNSTs. A three-base-pair in-frame deletion in exon 17 of the NF1 gene is the second exception. Patients with this genetic mutation have an absence of cutaneous neurofibromas and appear to have a lower incidence of serious complications.

Negative genetic analysis does not exclude the disease. As a result the demand for prenatal testing remains limited. Genetic testing may offer benefit as a diagnostic tool in suspected patients who do not meet criteria. However, as the cost and the prognostic capabilities of these tests improve, genetic testing may play a more significant role in the future.

Treatment

Neurofibromatosis is a multisystem disorder requiring management by multiple disciplines. Current management focuses on genetic counseling and symptomatic treatment of specific complications. Patients with NF1 have an estimated lifespan that is 15 years lower than the general population with malignant degeneration being the major cause of early death. There is no overall treatment for neurofibromatosis. Individual manifestations and complications are treated as they arise. Regular follow-up and surgical removal of rapidly enlarging lesions should be undertaken. In addition, removal of disfiguring or functionally compromising lesions is recommended. The removal of subcutaneous neurofibromas may result in neurologic deficit and should be performed by a skilled surgeon. Various medical treatments for plexiform neurofibromas are being evaluated in ongoing clinical trials.

The cosmetic, medical, behavioral, and social features of this disease may diminish the quality of life in patients with neurofibromatosis. Awareness of the various complications and methods of coping with them are essential to decrease long-term morbidity rate.

TUBEROUS SCLEROSIS COMPLEX (BOURNEVILLE'S DISEASE)

TSC (OMIM #191100 and #613254) is an autosomal dominant, multisystem disorder characterized by the development of hamartomas in multiple organ systems, including the brain, eyes, heart, lung, liver, kidneys, and skin. The classic triad of TSC included seizures, cognitive impairment, and angiofibromas. However, this triad only occurs in 29% of patients and 6% can lack all three symptoms.

Pathogenesis

Tuberous sclerosis shows no racial, ethnic, or sexual predilection. The incidence is estimated at 1 in 6000–10,000 live births. The true incidence is unknown because of a number of undiagnosed cases among mildly affected or asymptomatic individuals. It is inherited in an autosomal dominant pattern, with almost complete penetrance, but the majority of cases (~80%) are attributed to sporadic new mutations. The effective fertility is reduced by the frequent severe mental retardation. The phenotype of tuberous sclerosis is highly variable.

Two genes, TSC1 and TSC2, are identified as the genetic defects in tuberous sclerosis. TSC2 mutations are four times as common as TSC1 mutations among de novo cases. The prevalence of TSC1 and TSC2 mutations is approximately equal among familial cases. TSC1 is found on chromosome 9q34 and encodes a 130-kDa protein called hamartin. TSC2 is found on chromosome 16p13 and encodes a 180-kDa protein called tuberin. It is believed that loss of heterozygosity through a somatic "second hit" mutation leads to the unmasking of the disease process. Patients with TSC2 mutations have more severe disease than patients with TSC1 mutations.

Evidence supports the belief that tuberin and hamartin form an intracellular heterodimer that functions as a tumor suppressor and senses various intra- and extracellular signals including growth factor stimulation, hypoxia, and energy levels. This complex also targets a Ras homolog enriched in the brain (Rheb), which in turn inhibits mammalian target of rapamycin (mTOR), a serine/threonine kinase involved in cell growth and proliferation. This tuberin/hamartin complex contains a region with homology to the catalytic domain of rap1 GTPase-activation protein. This heterodimer protein induces the inactive state by stimulating GTPase-activation protein (GAP) and functions by downregulating Rheb. Rheb in its active states induces mTOR, which in turn phosphorylates 4E binding protein (4e-BP1), ribosomal protein S6 kinase b (S6K1), and eukaryotic translation factor 2; all are involved in ribosomal biosynthesis recruitment and translation initiation. It is a mutation within the GAP domain of the protein that results in most cases of TSC. Better understanding of the role of the hamartin/tuberin complex in mTOR signaling led to the development of the mTOR inhibitor everolimus.

Clinical Manifestations

Facial Angiofibromas

The hamartomas, previously called adenoma sebaceum, are erythematous, smooth papules involving the nasolabial folds, cheeks, and chin in a symmetrical distribution (Fig. 40-4). They are found in 70% to 90% of patients with tuberous sclerosis older than 5 years when the clinician closely examines the patient. They progressively increase in size and number during puberty. They are commonly associated with facial telangiectasia and facial flushing. When found, they are virtually pathognomonic of tuberous sclerosis. The main histologic findings are those of a fibrovascular hamartomatous proliferation with concomitant atrophy and compression of adnexal structures in the skin.

Hypomelanotic Macules (Ash Leaf Macules)

These macules are one of the most common and earliest manifestations of TSC. Ash leaf spots are asymmetrically distributed, hypopigmented macules most commonly found on the trunk and buttocks (Fig. 40-5). They vary in size from a few millimeters to many centimeters in diameter and range in number from three to 100. Their configuration is usually leaf-like ("ash leaf macule") or polygonal. They have been reported in >90% of cases of tuberous sclerosis and persist throughout life. Ash leaf macules are probably present at birth in the vast majority of patients with tuberous sclerosis (based on studies in which neonates were closely examined using a Wood's light). A Wood's light, through accentuation of areas of depigmentation, may be needed to detect subtle macules on light-skinned individuals. Examination of biopsy specimens reveals a normal number of melanocytes but a decreased intensity of melanization with a decrease in the size and degree of melanization of the melanosomes with electron microscopy. A second type of hypopigmented macule found in TSC is the confetti-like macule. These tiny 1- to 3-mm hypopigmented macules are symmetrically distributed over the extremities. They are more common in the second decade of life.

Ungual Fibromas (Koenen's Tumors)

These are pink to flesh-colored papules ranging in size from 1 to 10 mm that arise from the toenail bed or the fingernail bed (Fig. 40-6). They can be located in the lateral nail groove, under the nail plate, or along the proximal

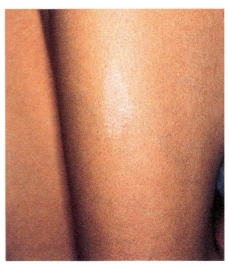

FIGURE 40-5 ■ A hypopigmented spot on the thigh in the shape of an ash leaf is present in this patient with tuberous sclerosis.

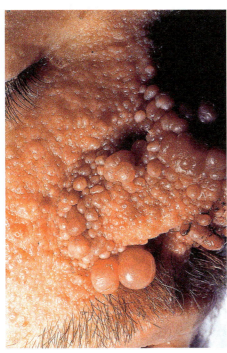

FIGURE 40-4 ■ Multiple facial angiofibromas in a patient with tuberous sclerosis.

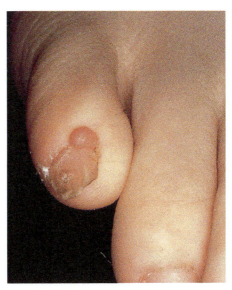

FIGURE 40-6 ■ A periungual fibroma is present in this patient with tuberous sclerosis.

nail groove. They usually appear at puberty and are present in about 20% of cases overall. They may cause pain and have a tendency to recur after surgical removal. Histologically, they resemble facial angiofibromas, with fibrosis and capillary dilatation. Older lesions may contain large, stellate fibroblasts with a "glial appearance."

Shagreen Patch

These connective tissue hamartomas are plaques (Fig. 40-7), usually found on the trunk, particularly in the lumbosacral area. They vary in size from a few millimeters to >10 cm. They are yellowish-brown to pink in color and have a firm consistency, resembling an orange peel. The lesions are rarely found in infancy and become more common after puberty, reaching a peak prevalence of 70% to 80% of cases of tuberous sclerosis. The Shagreen patch, however, differs neither clinically nor histopathologically from other connective tissue nevi that may occur as isolated developmental defects in otherwise normal individuals.

Miscellaneous Nevoid Lesions

Café-au-lait spots may occur as an isolated finding in 10% to 20% of tuberous sclerosis patients. Patches of gray or white have also been noted in up to 20% of patients with tuberous sclerosis. Fibromas of various sizes and shapes may occur in other locations. These include: (1) large, asymmetrical fibromas of the face and scalp, called fibrous cephalic plaque; (2) soft, pedunculated growths on the neck, trunk, or extremities (molluscum fibrosum pendulum); (3) grouped, firm papules of the neck, trunk, and extremities; and (4) pedunculated or sessile nodules of the buccal or gingival mucosa. The forehead plaque is observed in about 25% of patients and may be the most specific skin finding for TSC. Multiple gingival fibromas are a minor feature in the clinical criteria of TSC.

Central Nervous System Involvement

Focal or generalized seizures occur in up to 90% of patients with tuberous sclerosis and may be the first symptom to suggest the diagnosis. Infantile spasms, which are generalized myoclonic seizures, are a common presenting symptom of TSC. These are largely related to glioneuronal hamartomas, called cortical tubers, and subependymal nodules. Cortical glioneuronal hamartomas and subependymal nodules are identified by brain MRI in over 80% of patients with TSC. Most lesions are multiple and involve the frontal or parietal lobe. These tumors calcify in about 50% of patients and produce characteristic roentgenographic changes. A characteristic brain tumor, called subependymal giant cell tumors (SGCTs), are found in 5% to 20% of patients. Also called subependymal giant cell astrocytomas, these tumors may enlarge and obstruct the flow of cerebrospinal fluid and result in hydrocephalus. It is thought that SGCTs arise from preexisting subependymal nodules. The number of tubers correlates with the extent of seizure status and cognitive function. Sixty to 70% of patients demonstrate both seizures and cognitive impairment by 3 years of age. Cerebral white matter radial migration lines are another form of cortical dysplasia, which is associated with epilepsy and learning difficulties. Intellectual disability has a prevalence of 40% to 50% in TSC. Autism and behavioral problems are common in children with TSC.

Retinal hamartomas are observed in 30% to 50% of patients with TSC. Retinal gliomas may appear as peripheral, noncalcified lesions that are flat, white to salmon-colored, and circular (phakoma—"white spot"). On funduscopic exam, they can be difficult to identify before calcification has occurred, but after calcification they are easily identified as pearly white tumors near the disc margin. They are frequently located superficial to a retinal vessel. The second type of retinal lesion is the classic nodular lesion resembling a mulberry, with clusters of small, glistening granules. Generally, the retinal lesions do not grow significantly and blindness is rare. Treatment is not necessary. Retinal hypopigmentation, called a retinal achromic patch, can be found in 39% of patients with TSC and is considered a minor feature. Hypopigmented macules of the iris, white eyelashes, and hamartomatous tumors of the eyelids and conjunctivae may also occur.

Renal Involvement

Two characteristic renal lesions occur in tuberous sclerosis: angiomyolipomas and renal cysts. The prevalence of angiomyolipomas increases with age (present in over 90% of patients above the age of 10 years). They can be the sole manifestation of TSC. Angiomyolipomas are usually multiple, bilateral, and innocuous. When they are symptomatic, the patient may experience pain and/or hematuria. They range in size from a few millimeters to 20 cm, and the mass effect of the tumor is usually responsible for symptoms. Tumors greater than 4 cm are at an increased risk for bleeding. Renal failure is very rare. There are multiple reports of malignant transformation of angiomyolipomas without associated metastases.

Renal cysts may be small and asymptomatic or large and result in renal impairment. Interestingly, the

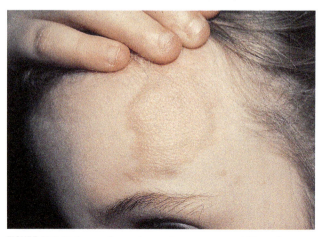

FIGURE 40-7 ■ An erythematous plaque representative of a connective tissue nevus is present in this paients with tuberous sclerosis.

TSC2 gene is located next to the gene responsible for autosomal dominant polycystic kidney disease (PKD1). Mutation involving both TSC2 and PKD1 has been associated with severe forms of renal cysts. Smaller cysts are found in those with mutations involving only the TSC2 or TSC1 gene. Rare cases of renal cell carcinoma have been seen.

Cardiac and Pulmonary Involvement

Cardiac involvement in tuberous sclerosis includes multiple, discrete rhabdomyomas, which occur in 30% to 50% of patients. Cardiac rhabdomyomas typically develop in utero and are often detected on prenatal ultrasound. Up to 80% of children with cardiac rhabdomyomas have tuberous sclerosis. These tumors are usually benign and regress over time. However, the deaths that do occur are related to outflow obstruction or conduction defects. They are associated with cardiac arrhythmias including Wolff–Parkinson–White syndrome.

Pulmonary involvement is rare and usually consists of diffuse interstitial fibrosis, called lymphangiomyomatosis (LAM). This condition is a cystic lung disease, which can result in significant limitation of pulmonary function. Pneumothorax, progressive exertional dyspnea, and cor pulmonale may occur. This condition may worsen during pregnancy and can be a life-threatening complication of TSC. LAM is also diagnosed in patients without TSC. Other pulmonary manifestations of TSC include multifocal micronodular pneumocyte hyperplasia and clear cell tumor of the lung.

Miscellaneous Systemic Findings

A number of variable and nonspecific findings have been reported. These include goiter, hypothyroidism, Cushing's syndrome, abnormal glucose tolerance tests, precocious puberty, adrenal hyperplasia, splenic hamartomas, cystic radiographic lesions of the metacarpals and phalanges, sclerotic lesions of the skull, and pitted defects of dental enamel. Dental pitting has a high prevalence in TSC and is a minor feature in the clinical criteria of TSC.

Differential Diagnosis

Diagnosis may be difficult as there is no single symptom present in all patients. The characteristic skin ash leaf macules in children with seizures and/or mental retardation are sufficient to establish the diagnosis. However, the early stages of the disease and the forme fruste may give trouble in diagnosis. Some features of TSC remain asymptomatic; whereas others appear, grow, and regress with time, which reduces the likelihood of detection and diagnosis. Many patients with TSC are not diagnosed until adulthood.

Multiple facial angiofibromas and collagenomas have been observed in Birt–Hogg–Dubé (BHD) syndrome and multiple endocrine neoplasia type 1 (MEN1). In these conditions, the development of facial angiofibromas occurs later than in TSC. When angiofibromas occur in adulthood, they should be considered a minor feature and the differential diagnosis should be expanded to include BHD and MEN1.

Patient Evaluation

A detailed family history with examination of family members is required. However, 80% of cases represent de novo mutations and a negative family history should not be used to rule out tuberous sclerosis. Dermatologic features can be easily recognizable and are present in >90% of patients with TSC. A skin biopsy of an appropriate skin lesion may support the diagnosis. Early recognition of TSC is vital because the implementation of recommended evaluation studies (e.g., neuroimaging studies) may prevent serious clinical consequences. A recent International Tuberous Sclerosis Complex Consensus Conference has revised the diagnostic criteria for tuberous sclerosis (Table 40-3) and provided recommended guidelines for surveillance and management. A detailed skin and oral exam should be performed. Patients should have a detailed ophthalmologic examination, looking for hamartomas; brain MRI to evaluate the severity of CNS involvement; high-resolution chest computed tomography (CT) and pulmonary function tests for females 18 years and older to detect pulmonary involvement; echocardiogram for pediatric patients to evaluate intracardiac tumors; and radiographic evaluation for renal masses. It is recommended that all pediatric patients have a baseline electroencephalograph, even in the absence of clinical seizures.

TABLE 40-3 Revised Diagnostic Criteria for Tuberous Sclerosis Complex (TSC)

A. Genetic diagnostic criteria
  The identification of either a TSC1 or TSC2 pathogenic mutation in DNA from normal tissue
B. Clinical diagnostic criteria
Major features
  Angiofibromas (≥3) or fibrous cephalic plaque
  Ungual fibromas (≥2)
  Hypomelanotic macules (≥3, at least 5 mm in diameter)
  Shagreen patch
  Multiple retinal hamartomas
  Cortical dysplasias*
  Subependymal nodules
  Subependymal giant cell astrocytoma
  Cardiac rhabdomyoma
  Lymphangiomyomatosis[†]
  Angiomyolipoma[†]
Minor features
  Dental enamel pits (≥3)
  Intraoral fibromas
  Nonrenal hamartomas
  Retinal achromic patch
  "Confetti" skin lesions
  Multiple renal cysts

Definite TSC: either two major features or one major feature with two minor features.
Possible TSC: either one major feature or two or more minor features.
*Includes tubers and cerebral white matter radial migration lines.
[†]When both lymphangiomyomatosis and renal angiomyolipomas are present, other features of TSC should be present before a definitive diagnosis is assigned.
Adapted from Northrup et al. (2012).

During the TSC Consensus Conference, the panel recommended that cranial imaging with MRI be performed every 1 to 3 years until age 25 years to monitor for the development of SCGTs. Women should have a chest CT at least once during adulthood to evaluate the rare risk of developing lymphangioleiomyomatosis. Screening for TSC-associated neuropsychiatric disorders should occur with each follow-up visit. Other periodic studies should be based on the history and clinical findings.

Genetic Testing

Molecular genetic testing is currently available for detection of 75% to 80% of the mutations found in TSC1 or TSC2. Identification of a pathogenic mutation in TSC1 or TSC2 is an independent diagnostic criterion, sufficient for the diagnosis of TSC. Gene testing is recommended for genetic counseling purposes or when the diagnosis of TSC is suspected or in question but cannot be clinically confirmed. Genetic counseling is essential for adults with even minimal involvement from tuberous sclerosis, since their children may be severely affected. There is a 50% risk of an affected parent transmitting the disorder to their offspring. Prenatal testing can be performed in families with a known TSC mutation. A normal result does not exclude TSC as a significant fraction (10% to 25%) of TSC patients have no mutation identified by conventional genetic testing.

Treatment

TSC is a multisystem disorder requiring management by multiple disciplines. TSC is a progressive disorder with individual features emerging at different times. Neurologic manifestations of TSC represent the leading cause of associated morbidity and mortality. Knowledge of the functional relationship between TSC1/TSC2 and mTORC1 has led to important clinical advances in the use of mTOR inhibitors for the treatment of several clinical manifestations of TSC, including cerebral subependymal giant cell astrocytoma, renal angiolipomas, and pulmonary lymphangioleiomyomatosis.

Seizures in TSC are difficult to treat with conventional antiepileptic medications. At least one-third of patients develop refractory epilepsy. Vigabatrin and adrenocorticotropin hormone have been recommended as first-line therapies for infantile spasms. The exact mechanism of vigabatrin is unclear. Studies show that vigabatrin inhibits the mTOR pathway in mouse models. Simple partial or complex partial seizures are often treated with anticonvulsants. Sirolimus (rapamycin) and everolimus (a rapamycin analog) have successfully been used to treat renal angiomyolipomas and SCGTs in studies in patients with TSC. Sirolimus has also reduced the growth of LAM in some, but not all, treated patients. Inhibition of the mTOR pathway with rapamycin or rapamycin analogs has been shown to be effective in murine models of TSC and has promising results regarding seizure control in patients with TSC. Ongoing clinical trials are studying the effects of these medications on other neurological complications.

Surgical and medical therapy with mTOR inhibitors are the two main treatment options for extracutaneous hamartomas. Indications for surgery vary and the choice between surgical resection and medical therapy depends on individual circumstances.

Patients may request treatment of cutaneous lesions for cosmetic reasons. Facial angiofibromas respond to electrocautery and laser ablation with excellent cosmetic results, but regrowth is common. Topical rapamycin has also been used with success to treat facial angiofibromas.

STURGE–WEBER SYNDROME

SWS (OMIM #185300) is a sporadic congenital condition characterized by a facial capillary malformation (PWS) in association with leptomeningeal angiomatosis and glaucoma. The PWS in SWS is characteristically present on the forehead and upper eyelid, in the area of the ophthalmic branch of the trigeminal nerve (Fig. 40-8). This may occur alone or in combination with the V2 and V3 distributions. The neurologic features of SWS may be progressive and include seizures, focal neurologic impairment, and cognitive deficits. Ocular features include glaucoma and capillary-venous vascular malformations of the conjunctiva, episclera, choroid, and retina.

Pathogenesis

SWS is caused by a somatic mosaic mutation in the GNAQ gene, which encodes a nucleotide-binding protein, G-alpha-q, that functions to regulate intracellular signaling pathways. Somatic mutations in GNAQ occurring at a later stage in embryogenesis may affect only precursors of vascular endothelial cells and lead to nonsyndromic PWSs, while mutations occurring earlier may affect a greater variety of precursor cells and lead to SWS.

The vascular abnormalities of Sturge–Weber disease probably represent a mesodermal defect that occurs in

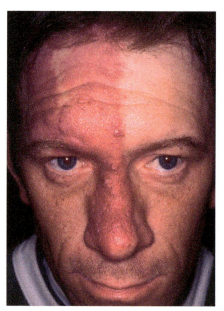

FIGURE 40-8 ■ A unilateral port-wine stain is present in this man with Sturge–Weber syndrome.

the fourth to eighth weeks of embryonic development. At this point, the ectoderm, which will form the skin, overlies the tissue that will eventually become the ipsilateral cerebrum. Subsequently, the leptomeningeal vessels develop into venous angiomas with a network of thin-walled ectatic venules filling the subarachnoid space. At birth, the PWS is flat and grows in proportion to the growth of the child. The cerebral angiomas develop progressive loss of venous drainage with subsequent venous stasis and calcification. Calcification is believed to be the result of deposition of colloid fibers on a matrix of reticulin fibers with precipitation of calcium salts on reticulin fibers. This calcification increases throughout life. The combination of vascular ectasia and calcification then produces ischemia of underlying cerebral tissue with resultant diffuse cortical atrophy and the resultant nervous system abnormalities.

Clinical Manifestations

PWSs are a common type of vascular malformation, occurring in 0.3% of newborn infants. They appear as flat, vascular lesions ranging in color from pink to deep purple. The lesion consists of dilated and excessively numerous but well-defined capillaries in the dermis. As PWSs age, the vessel walls become progressively more ectatic, producing exophytic blueberry-like ectasias in mid-adult life. By the fifth decade, over 50% of patients with a facial PWS have hypertrophy and nodularity within the lesion. In SWS, the PWS is most commonly present in the distribution of the first or second division of the trigeminal nerve.

Leptomeningeal vascular malformations, also called leptomeningeal angiomatosis, occur in 8% to 20% of cases when a typical facial PWS is present. Although any part of the cerebrum can be involved, the parietal and occipital areas are most commonly affected. When there is a unilateral PWS, the leptomeningeal angiomatosis tends to be ipsilateral. Seizures are the most common CNS feature. Epilepsy develops in 75% to 80% of patients with SWS. Seizures may begin shortly after birth but usually occur in late infancy or early childhood. Seizures frequently begin with febrile episodes that precipitate contralateral focal motor seizures. Generalized seizures develop later. Stroke-like episodes occur in patients with SWS, presenting as transient hemiparesis or visual field defects. Hemiparesis, hemiplegia, hemisensory defects, homonymous hemianopsia, and limb atrophy may occur. Headaches are also a common symptom in patients with SWS.

Cognitive impairment may be minimal in early childhood but is progressive after the onset of seizures. Factors associated with developmental delay include bilateral cerebral lesions, the extent of cerebral atrophy, the presence of refractory epilepsy, and the presence of multiple types of seizures. Some evidence points to the possibility that seizures may inhibit blood flow resulting in increased neurological impairment. Control of seizures by medical or surgical means may slow the progression of the mental defect. Behavioral problems also occur in patients with SWS. Lower cognitive function, epilepsy, and greater frequency of seizures are associated with more psychological problems.

Ocular involvement occurs in about 60% of patients with SWS. Glaucoma is the most serious ocular problem and occurs in 30% to 70% of cases. The risk of glaucoma is highest in the first decade of life. Involvement of the PWS of both lids of the affected eye is usually associated with glaucoma. Capillary-venous malformations of the choroid may produce glaucoma or retinal detachment that may be congenital or may occur later in life. Angioid streaks of the retina and enlargement of the globe may occur. Heterochromia of the iris may occur, which is caused by aggregated melanocytic hamartomas on the anterior surface of the iris.

Neuroendocrine abnormalities of growth hormone deficiency and central hypothyroidism occur more frequently in patients with SWS.

The characteristic cerebral angiomas, calcification, and atrophy may occur in the absence of skin lesions in 5% to 14% of cases. Such cases are still termed Sturge–Weber disease but obviously do not fulfill the traditional criteria for the syndrome. Occasionally, individuals with SWS also have extensive cutaneous malformations, limb hypertrophy, and vascular and lymphatic malformations, which are consistent with Klippel–Trenaunay syndrome. These children have been classified as having Klippel–Trenaunay–Weber syndrome.

Evaluation and Treatment

The diagnosis of SWS can be straightforward in a patient with a PWS, glaucoma, clinical evidence of cerebral involvement, and neuroimaging confirmation. The diagnosis becomes more challenging in an infant with a facial PSW without neurologic symptoms. Radiologic calcifications are seldom present at birth, but are in early childhood. MRI with gadolinium is the preferred neuroimaging technique. Newer MRI sequences are under study to increase the ability to make the early diagnosis of brain involvement in some patients. SWS cannot be ruled out with a normal brain MRI within the first few months of life. An MRI is typically performed in infancy only if specific ocular or neurologic abnormalities are present. In older symptomatic children, the typical MRI findings include leptomeningeal enhancement, dilated deep draining vessels, and a glomus malformation. The CT findings of intracranial calcification are highly characteristic, showing double lines of curvilinear densities that parallel the cerebral convolutions, producing a "tramline" pattern. Electroencephalographic evidence of brain involvement usually occurs in early childhood.

There is tremendous variation in the extent of neurological involvement and in the severity of symptoms. The site and extent of brain involvement influence the neurological manifestations. Seizures can be difficult to control with anticonvulsants and surgical therapy may become necessary. Visually guided lobectomy with excision of the angiomatous cortex is a surgical approach in the patient with focal lesions. Hemispherectomy is considered in the patient with intractable seizures and unihemispheric involvement. Periodic lifelong assessment of visual function and eye pressure is crucial to recognize and treat glaucoma before it results in loss of vision.

Improvement of the appearance of cutaneous lesions may be accomplished with cosmetics (e.g., Covermark™ or Dermablend™). Laser technology has greatly improved the cosmetic results of therapy. The pulsed dye laser (PDL) is specifically designed for cutaneous vascular lesions. PDL allows for short bursts of energy at intravascular hemoglobin within the lesional vessels, while sparing other tissue components. These modalities have proven to be particularly effective in the treatment of PWSs in young children. Greater than 75% lightening may eventually be achieved. Laser treatments are also effective for shrinking oral lesions or for the papular ectatic lesions that develop later in life.

COBB SYNDROME

Cobb syndrome is the association of a PWS or cavernous hemangioma with a vascular malformation involving the same metamere of the spinal cord. Neurological symptoms are related to the spinal cord vascular malformation and may include pain, motor dysfunction, paresthesias, and paraplegia. Treatment options include surgery and endovascular embolization.

ATAXIA–TELANGIECTASIA (LOUIS–BAR SYNDROME)

Ataxia-telangiectasia (AT) (OMIM #208900) is an autosomal recessive disorder consisting of progressive cerebellar ataxia, ocular and cutaneous telangiectasia, and variable immune deficiency. The immune deficiency predisposes the patient to recurrent sinopulmonary infections and to an increased incidence of neoplasia. Patients have a defect in cell growth and chromosomal integrity that is associated with increased sensitivity to ionizing radiation. Recent advancements in the understanding of diseases with similar radiosensitive phenotypes have led to elucidations and better understanding of various AT-like disorders. The discussion here will be limited to the classical AT phenotype.

Pathogenesis

AT occurs in 1 in 40,000 to 100,000 live births, with the incidence of asymptomatic heterozygotes being as high as 1 in 100. The gene responsible for AT is located on chromosome 11q22.3 and is designated ATM (for ataxia telangiectasia mutation). This gene encompasses 150 kb of DNA and encodes a phosphoprotein. This protein has significant homology to a subunit of phosphatidylinositol 3-kinase, which is involved in cell cycle regulation, maintenance of genomic stability, and response to DNA damage.

Fibroblasts and lymphoblasts are extremely sensitive to X-rays and chemotherapeutic killing. These cells have defective DNA repair following radiation and fail to slow their rate of DNA synthesis. These defects are due to the inability to arrest the cell cycle at the G1 and G2 phases in response to DNA damage, instead progressing to the S phase and mitosis, respectively. It is believed that the ATM protein activates the p53 protein, triggering the p53 signaling pathway involved in checkpoint regulation in the DNA cell cycle. In addition, there is evidence that ATM is involved in the activation of proteins involved in DNA strand repair and recombination regulation.

Clinical Manifestations

Ataxia is the earliest clinical manifestation, which typically appears when affected children begin to walk. Eye movements are often normal in preschoolers, but children later develop oculomotor difficulties. Choreoathetosis, dysarthric speech, and myotonic jerks become prominent during childhood. Patients are often confined to a wheelchair by adolescence. Telangiectases develop between 2 and 8 years of age and occur first as wire-like vessels on the bulbar conjunctiva and later on the exposed areas of the auricle, the neck, and the flexor folds of the extremities. Other skin abnormalities may include premature graying of hair, loss of subcutaneous fat, vitiligo, café-au-lait spots, and noninfectious granulomas. Endocrine abnormalities frequently develop with time and include hyperinsulinism with insulin resistance, hypogonadism with delayed sexual development, and growth retardation. Recurrent sinopulmonary infections occur in most patients, with eventual bronchiectasis and respiratory failure as the most common cause of death. Mild to moderate cognitive impairment is frequently present early in the course of AT.

Defects in both cellular and humoral immunity are seen. Cellular defects are to be expected, in view of the consistent finding of an absent or hypoplastic thymus. Cellular defects include impaired skin test responses to recall antigens, reduced lymphocyte numbers, and decreased percentages of T cells. Two-thirds of the patients have reduced in vitro proliferative response to mitogens and to specific antigens. Antigen challenge with foreign protein or with virus produces a poor antibody response related to abnormal antibody levels. Seventy percent of patients are IgA-deficient, 80% are IgE-deficient, and 60% are IgG-deficient. These defects are caused primarily by defective antibody synthesis. It is hypothesized that genetic recombination, required for normal humoral and cellular immune function, is impaired with deficiency of the ATM gene. There is persistent production of fetal proteins, as evidenced by the nearly constant finding of elevated serum alpha-fetoprotein levels. Measuring alpha-fetoprotein can aid in establishing the diagnosis in individuals older than 2 years of age.

Approximately 10% to 25% of patients develop malignancy. Eighty-five percent of these neoplasms are lymphoproliferative disorders. In addition, those who are heterozygous for the ATM gene are at an increased risk for malignancy, particularly breast cancer in women. There is an approximately twofold increase in the risk of breast cancer associated with heterozygosity for ATM mutations that cause AT in biallelic carriers. These striking abnormalities are believed to be due to compromised immune surveillance, chromosomal instability, and tumor suppressor function of the ATM gene.

Treatment

Therapy is limited to treatment of infections, early detection of malignancy, and genetic counseling. Most patients die of infection or malignancy in childhood. Currently over 400 known mutations have been found on the ATM gene and genotype/phenotype relationships remain poorly understood. The diagnosis may be suspected antenatally by the in utero elevation of alpha-fetoprotein concentration.

OTHER NEUROCUTANEOUS DISEASES

von Hippel–Lindau Syndrome (OMIM #193300)

von Hippel-Lindau syndrome (VHL) is a dominantly inherited familial cancer syndrome affecting 1 in 36,000 individuals. VHL predisposes patients to various malignant and benign tumors. The VHL gene is located on chromosome 3 and functions as a tumor suppressor. The most frequent neoplasms are cerebellar, spinal hemangioblastoma, renal cell carcinoma, pheochromocytoma, and pancreatic tumors. A PWS may occur over the head and neck in some patients, but most patients do not have cutaneous lesions.

Waardenburg Syndrome (OMIM #193500)

Waardenburg syndrome (WS) is a genetically heterogeneous, inherited pigmentary disorder characterized by achromia of the hair, skin, and eyes; congenital hearing loss; and dystopia canthorum (increase in distance between the inner canthi). It is categorized into four types based on phenotype. WS1 is the classic form, distinguished by the presence of dystopia canthorum. WS2 lacks dystopia canthorum and is associated with increased frequency of deafness. WS3 has associated limb abnormalities and WS4 has features of Hirschsprung disease. WS1 and WS3 are caused by mutations in the PAX3 gene, whereas WS2 is caused by mutations in the transcription factor MITF gene and SNAI2 gene. WS4 is a result of mutation in the genes for endothelin-B receptor (EDNRB) or its ligand (EDN3), or mutation in the SOX10 gene. There is no specific treatment available.

Incontinentia Pigmenti (OMIM #308300)

Incontinentia pigmenti (IP) is an X-linked dominant, multisystem disorder that is usually lethal antenatally in males. It is caused by a mutation in the NEMO gene at Xq28. In affected females, it presents perinatally as scattered erythema and vesicles. Within months, these lesions progress to verrucous linear plaques (Fig. 40-9), which are then eventually replaced by hyperpigmented macules and patches. Hyperpigmented swirls develop on the trunk and extremities along the lines of Blaschko (lines of ectodermal embryologic development). With time, these swirls become hypopigmented. Noncutaneous findings occur in a high percentage of patients, which include anomalies of the CNS, eyes, teeth, hair, nails, and bones. CNS abnormalities occur in 20% to 30% of patients and include seizures, developmental delay, and spastic abnormalities. Patients require baseline and longitudinal follow-up with neurology and ophthalmology. The skin lesions do not require a specific therapy.

Hypomelanosis of Ito (Incontinentia Pigmenti Achromians OMIM #300337)

Hypomelanosis of Ito (HI) is a form of pigment mosaicism, characterized by a clone of skin cells with a decreased ability to make pigment. HI presents with hypopigmented streaks and whorls along the lines of Blaschko (Fig. 40-10). Nervous system abnormalities occur in about 30% of the patients and may include seizures, electroencephalogram abnormalities, strabismus, and language impairment. Hypopigmentation tends to fade with age.

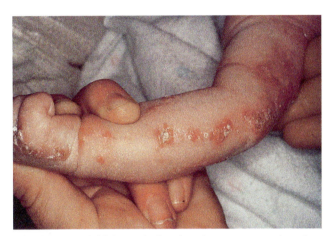

FIGURE 40-9 ■ Multiple vesiculated and verrucous and vesiculated lesions in a Blaschkoid distribution in this patient with incontinentia pigmenti.

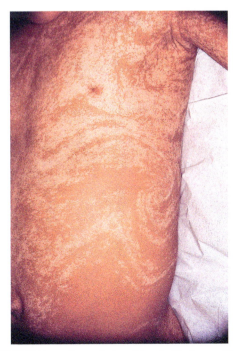

FIGURE 40-10 ■ Hypopigmented swirls of skin in a patient with incontinentia pigmenti achromians.

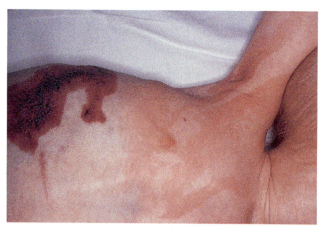

FIGURE 40-11 ■ The patient shown has epidermal nevus syndrome with multiple anomalies, hemangiomas, and epidermal nevi, as represented by the fine, slightly pigmented skin.

Vogt–Koyanagi–Harada Syndrome

This syndrome features depigmentation of the skin (especially of the eyebrows and eyelashes), headache, sterile meningitis, uveitis, and occasionally optic neuritis. Onset is associated with a febrile illness and is not known to be inherited or related to a preexistent neural crest defect.

Epidermal Nevus Syndrome

Epidermal nevus syndrome is a group of disorders in which epidermal nevi are associated with musculoskeletal, ocular, and/or neurologic abnormalities. The manifestations of epidermal nevus syndrome represent genomic mosaicism with varying clinical involvement depending on the genetic defect and timing of the mutation during development. The epidermal nevi are often extensive with unilateral or occasionally bilateral verrucous papules or scaling plaques that are arranged in continuous or interrupted streaks (Fig. 40-11). The lesions vary in color from yellow to brown and are usually asymptomatic. Noncutaneous abnormalities include hemimegalencephaly, seizures, hemiparesis, developmental delay, ocular lipodermoids, coloboma, choristoma, abnormal skull shape, kyphoscoliosis, and limb hypertrophy. Hypophosphatemic vitamin D-resistant rickets has been observed in patients with extensive epidermal nevi.

Ichthyosis-Associated Syndromes

There have been multiple cases of congenital abnormalities of the nervous system associated with ichthyosis. An example includes Sjögren–Larsson syndrome, which is an autosomal recessive disorder resulting from mutations in the fatty aldehyde dehydrogenase gene FALDH. Clinical features include lamellar ichthyosis with pruritus, thickened palms and soles (palmoplantar keratoderma), macular degeneration with retinal crystals, mental retardation, seizures, and spastic diplegia or quadriplegia. No therapy to date has been found to slow the progressive neurologic deterioration.

SUGGESTED READINGS

De Bella K, Szudek J, Friedman JM, et al. Use of the National Institutes of Health criteria for diagnosis of neurofibromatosis 1 in children. Pediatrics 2000;105:608–14.
Friedman JM, Gutmann DH, MacCollin M, Riccardi VM, et al. Neurofibromatosis: phenotype, natural history, and pathogenesis. 3rd ed. Baltimore: Johns Hopkins University Press; 1999.
Gatti RA, Becker-Catania S, Chun HH, et al. The pathogenesis of ataxia-telangiectasia. Learning from a Rosetta Stone. Clin Rev Allergy Immunol 2001;20(1):87–108.
Krueger DA, Northrup H. Tuberous sclerosis complex surveillance and management: recommendations of the 2012 International Tuberous Sclerosis Complex Consensus Conference. Pedatr Neurol 2013;49:255–65.
Lo W, Marchuk DA, Ball K, et al. Updates and future horizons on the understanding, diagnosis, and treatment of Sturge-Weber syndrome brain involvement. Dev Med Child Neurol 2012;54:214–23.
Meyn MS. Ataxia-telangiectasia, cancer and the pathobiology of the ATM gene. Clin Genet 1999;55:289–304.
Northrup H, Krueger DA. Tuberous sclerosis complex diagnostic criteria update: recommendations of the 2012 International Tuberous Sclerosis Complex Consensus Group. Pediatr Neurol 2013;49:243–54.
Williams VC, Lucas J, Babcock MA, et al. Neurofibromatosis type 1 revisited. Pediatrics 2009;123:124–33.

CHAPTER 41

PREGNANCY

Bethanee J. Schlosser

KEY POINTS

- Physiologic changes associated with pregnancy have effects on the skin including pigmentary changes such as linea nigra and melasma; vascular changes such as telangiectasia, varicosities, and spider angiomata; connective tissue changes such as striae distensae; and changes on glandular structures, hair, nails, and mucosal surfaces.
- Pregnancy can also impact neoplasms both benign and malignant.
- There is a variable and often unpredictable effect of pregnancy on preexisting chronic skin diseases including psoriasis, atopic dermatitis, dermatomyositis, lupus erythematosus, and infections including viral, fungal, and mycobacterial in nature.
- Pruritus is a prominent feature of pregnancy that might be related to a preexisting condition, to cholestasis, or occur in association with a "specific" dermatosis of pregnancy.
- There are two major "specific" pregnancy dermatoses: polymorphic eruption of pregnancy (formerly known as pruritic urticarial papules and plaques of pregnancy) and pemphigoid gestationis.

Myriad cutaneous changes, both physiologic and pathologic, occur in the context of pregnancy. Pregnancy-related alterations of the skin may be classified as: (1) physiologic changes; (2) changes to cutaneous neoplasms; (3) preexisting skin disease or internal disease with skin manifestations affected by pregnancy; (4) pruritus in pregnancy; and (5) dermatoses specific to pregnancy. This chapter reviews the nonspecific and specific dermatologic changes observed in pregnancy, emphasizing the need for accurate diagnosis and prompt recognition of any associated maternal or fetal risks.

PHYSIOLOGIC SKIN CHANGES

Pregnancy causes physiologic changes to the skin, hair, nails, and mucous membranes. Observed changes in skin during pregnancy result from alterations in pigmentation, vasculature, connective tissue, and glands. Although sometimes striking, such physiologic changes have no impact on maternal or fetal health.

Pigmentary Changes

Hyperpigmentation

Up to 90% of pregnant women demonstrate some degree of hyperpigmentation, which most often is localized and discrete. Generalized hyperpigmentation rarely occurs in pregnancy. When observed, additional etiologies (i.e., adrenal insufficiency, thyrotoxicosis) should be considered. Hyperpigmentation during pregnancy most commonly manifests as linea nigra, a darkening of the linea alba (the tendinous median line on the anterior abdominal wall spanning from the pubic symphysis to the xiphoid process), which appears in the first trimester of pregnancy and is more pronounced in women with darker skin types. Physiologic hyperpigmentation also affects the nipples, areolae, neck, axillae, genitalia, perineum, perianal skin, and medial thighs. Hyperpigmentation resolves gradually postpartum over several months.

Pigmentary demarcation lines, sharp delineations between areas of more and less pigmented skin, occurring most commonly on the lower extremities (type B Futcher lines), have been reported to darken or appear de novo during pregnancy. Uncommon pigmentary patterns that can be encountered in pregnancy include pseudoacanthosis nigricans, dermal melanocytosis, and vulvar melanosis.

Melasma (chloasma, "mask of pregnancy") presents as symmetric, irregular hyperpigmented patches involving sun-exposed areas of the cheeks and nose (malar pattern); the forehead, nose, cheeks, upper cutaneous lip, and chin (centrofacial pattern); or the ramus of the mandible (mandibular pattern). Prevalence of melasma in pregnancy ranges from 5% to 46%, varying greatly by demographic population and geography. Risk factors for melasma include intermediate skin phototypes (Fitzpatrick III–IV), ultraviolet (UV) radiation exposure, family history of melasma, oral contraceptive pill use, and thyroid dysfunction, as well as number of pregnancies and age at first pregnancy. Approximately half of women report onset of melasma in the context of pregnancy or oral contraceptive pill use. The pathogenesis of melasma is poorly understood; elevated levels of estrogen, progesterone, and melanocyte-stimulating hormone during pregnancy may play a role.

Melasma usually resolves with treatment within 1 year postpartum; spontaneous remission rates are low (6%). Pigmentary abnormalities persist in up to 30% of patients; risk factors include previous oral contraceptive pill use and more severe melasma pigmentation. Melasma may recur with subsequent pregnancies or oral contraceptive pill use. Avoidance of UV exposure and regular use of broad-spectrum sunscreen (≥SPF30) have preventive and therapeutic benefit. Patients should be advised to avoid potentially irritating and sensitizing cosmetics and to consider nonhormonal methods of contraception. Melasma can be treated postpartum with hydroquinone, azelaic acid, topical retinoids, or combinations thereof. Additional postpartum treatment modalities include laser treatment and chemical peels.

Jaundice

The serum bilirubin level may increase in 2% to 6% of uncomplicated pregnancies but is almost always less than 2 mg/dL. Severe hepatic dysfunction during pregnancy is rare. The most common cause of jaundice in pregnant women is viral hepatitis. Jaundice can develop in severe cases of intrahepatic cholestasis of pregnancy (ICP) (see "Pruritus in Pregnancy" section).

Vascular Changes

Elevated estrogen levels and increased blood volume during pregnancy result in proliferation of blood vessels, vascular distention, vasomotor instability, and increased cutaneous blood flow. Cutaneous vascular changes typically regress postpartum.

Palmar Erythema

Approximately two-thirds of white women and one-third of black women develop palmar erythema in pregnancy with onset in the first trimester. Palmar erythema tends to be symmetric and may be diffuse or limited to the thenar and hypothenar eminences, metocarpophalangeal joints, and finger pulps. Patients may report intermittent burning sensation. In pregnancy, there is no association between palmary erythema and hepatic or thyroid dysfunction. Palmar erythema resolves postpartum.

Spider Angioma

Spider angiomas (arterial spiders, nevi araneus, spider nevi, vascular spiders) occur in about two-thirds of white women and 11% of black women with onset between the second and fifth months of pregnancy. Spider angioma presents as a central erythematous papule (dilated arteriole) with radiating telangiectactic branches, often surrounded by a 3- to 4-mm anemic halo. Spider angiomas of pregnancy develop most commonly in areas drained by the superior vena cava (i.e., head, neck, upper chest, upper extremities). The majority resolve within 3 months of delivery. Cosmetic treatment modalities for persistent angiomas include electrodesiccation, intense pulsed light, and vascular laser.

Edema

Nonpitting edema of the eyelids, face, and lower extremities may develop later in pregnancy and is seen in one-third of women by week 38. Eyelid edema occurs in approximately 50% of pregnant women, whereas benign lower-extremity edema develops in about 70%. The presence of edema in a pregnant woman should alert the physician to the possibility of pregnancy-induced hypertension, which carries a significant risk to mother and fetus, and appropriate further evaluation should be undertaken.

Varicosities

Compression of the pelvic and femoral vessels by the gravid uterus results in the formation of lower-extremity (saphenous), vulvar, and hemorrhoidal varicosities. Genetic predisposition poses additional risk. Lower-extremity varicosities occur in 40% of pregnant women. Rest, lower-extremity elevation, avoidance of prolonged standing or sitting, use of gradient compression/elastic stockings and sleeping in a left lateral decubitus position may improve lower body circulation and reduce varicosity-associated symptoms. Varicosities may improve postpartum but generally do not regress completely. Postpartum treatment options include sclerotherapy, laser, and phlebectomy. Varicosities are likely to recur in subsequent pregnancies.

Cutis Marmorata

Cutis marmorata presents as transient, bluish, mottled patches on the lower extremities with cold exposure. Attributed to vasomotor instability secondary to increased estrogen levels, cutis marmorata is not unique to pregnancy and has no impact on maternal or fetal health.

Connective Tissue Changes

Striae Gravidarum

Striae gravidarum (striae distensae, stretch marks) are a common though poorly understood phenomenon. Prevalence ranges from 50% to 90%, and all races are susceptible. Onset of striae formation in pregnancy occurs prior to 24 weeks gestation in 43% of women. The etiology of striae gravidarum is unknown. Hormonal and physical factors are believed to result in a reduced number and altered orientation of dermal elastic fibers and fibrillin microfibrils. Risk factors for striae gravidarum include family history of striae gravidarum, personal history of breast or thigh striae, younger maternal age, and greater weight gain during pregnancy. Striae gravidarum initially present as pink to violaceous linear or arcuate patches, which gradually transform into hypopigmented atrophic, finely wrinkled plaques. The most common locations are the abdomen, breasts, and thighs; additional sites include the buttocks, hips, lower back, and upper arms. Striae may become less apparent over time but do not fully disappear. To date, no successful preventive treatments for striae gravidarum formation have been identified. Vascular laser and intense pulsed light improve the erythema of early striae. Topical retinoids (with or without glycolic acid) and laser and light treatment modalities may improve striae appearance.

Glandular Changes

Eccrine gland function increases during pregnancy, which may explain the increased prevalence of miliaria, dyshidrosis, and hyperhidrosis. Reduced palmar sweating, however, has been reported. Apocrine gland activity may decrease during pregnancy, contributing to the reduced prevalence of Fox–Fordyce disease in pregnancy. Pregnancy has varying effects on hidradenitis suppurativa; a minority of pregnant women report improvement in hidradenitis suppurativa during pregnancy. Variable changes in sebaceous gland activity have been reported, and the course of acne during gestation is unpredictable. One study showed that acne was affected by pregnancy in 70% of patients, with 41% experiencing improvement and 29% worsening. Montgomery tubercles form as small brown papules on the areolae in 30% to 50% of women during the first trimester as the result of sebaceous gland hypertrophy; these regress postpartum.

Hair Changes

Hirsutism in pregnancy results from increased activity of ovarian and placental androgens on the pilosebaceous unit and is more prominent in women with abundant body hair or dark hair at baseline. Hirsutism occurs most often on the face but may involve the arms, legs, back, and lower abdomen. While lanugo hair regresses within 6 months postpartum, terminal hair growth is typically permanent. If hirsutism is severe or is accompanied by other signs of virilization, androgen-secreting tumor of the ovary or adrenal gland, luteoma, theca lutein cyst, and polycystic ovary disease should be excluded.

Telogen effluvium refers to hair loss that occurs when a significant proportion of hairs synchronously enter the telogen phase. In the later stages of pregnancy as much as 95% of scalp hair is in anagen phase, which then abruptly cycles into telogen phase after delivery. Postpartum telogen hair counts of 24% at 6 weeks and 65% at 2 months have been reported. Causes for the shift from anagen to telogen may include the stress of delivery and changes in endocrine balance, including prolactin secretion with lactation. Increased hair shedding of variable severity becomes apparent 1 to 5 months postpartum. Hair regrowth occurs spontaneously within 6 to 12 months, but complete resolution may require up to 15 months. Scalp hair density may never return to baseline prepregnancy density, especially in women with concomitant female pattern hair loss.

Frontoparietal hair recession reminiscent of male pattern androgenic alopecia has been reported late in pregnancy; this typically resolves postpartum.

Nail Changes

Nail growth increases during pregnancy. Additional changes include brittleness, distal onycholysis, leukonychia, melanonychia, softening, subungual hyperkeratosis, and transverse grooves. Nail changes may occur as early as the sixth week of gestation. The etiology of these changes remains unclear, but some may also be seen in nonpregnant women taking oral contraceptives. Nail changes generally improve postpartum, and no specific treatment is required. Patients should be evaluated for dermatoses that affect the nail unit (i.e., psoriasis, lichen planus) and infections. External sensitizers (nail polish and polish removers) should be eliminated. Nails should be trimmed short, and the use of a nail moisturizer may provide benefit.

Mucous Membrane Changes

Pregnancy gingivitis affects 30% to 75% of pregnant women. Clinically, it presents in the first trimester as hyperplasia and blunting of the gingival interdental papillae with erythema, edema, ulceration, and bleeding of variable severity. Patients typically have preexisting gingivitis, and pregnancy merely exacerbates the baseline condition. Treatment consists of rigorous dental hygiene, professional debridement/scaling, and occasionally oral antibiotics. Oral pyogenic granulomas develop in 2% of pregnant women (see "Cutaneous Neoplasms Affected By Pregnancy"). Additional mucosal changes in pregnancy include hyperemia and congestion of the nasal mucosa, and a bluish-purple discoloration of the vaginal mucosa (Chadwick's sign) and the cervix (Goodell's sign).

CUTANEOUS NEOPLASMS AFFECTED BY PREGNANCY

Various cutaneous neoplasms are affected by pregnancy (Table 41-1).

Melanocytic Nevus

Preexisting melanocytic nevi may enlarge and/or darken, and new nevi may appear during pregnancy. Prospective studies, however, utilizing dermoscopy and spectrophotometric intracutaneous analysis have not demonstrated significant changes in melanocytic nevi during pregnancy. Women with dysplastic nevus syndrome may exhibit higher rates of clinical changes in their melanocytic nevi during pregnancy compared to nonpregnancy time periods. A changing pigmented lesion in a pregnant woman should not be attributed to pregnancy alone and should be evaluated just as for nonpregnant patients. There is no evidence that gestation induces dysplastic/malignant transformation of preexisting nevi.

TABLE 41-1 Cutaneous Neoplasms Affected by Pregnancy

Dermatofibroma
Dermatofibrosarcoma protuberans
Desmoid tumor
Glomangioma
Glomus tumor
Hemangioendothelioma
Hemangioma
Keloid
Leiomyoma
Melanocytic nevus
Melanoma
Molluscum fibrosum gravidarum (acrochordon)
Neurofibroma
Pyogenic granuloma of pregnancy (granuloma gravidarum)

Melanoma

Melanoma is the most common cancer for reproductive-age women. Estimated incidence of melanoma complicating pregnancy ranges from 0.1 to 2.8 per 1000 pregnancies. Despite initial concerns about adverse effects of pregnancy on malignant melanoma, most recent studies consistently demonstrate that pregnancy does not adversely affect the survival of women diagnosed with localized melanoma before, during, or after pregnancy. Melanoma prognosis for the pregnant woman should be based on the same established criteria, including Breslow depth and ulceration, utilized for nonpregnant patients. Transplacental metastasis of maternal malignancy is rare; malignant melanoma, however, is the most common malignancy to metastasize to the placenta (20 cases). In the setting of placental melanoma metastasis, fetal metastasis occurs in only 25%, and the most common sites are the skin and liver. For pregnant women with metastatic melanoma, the risks and benefits of adjuvant systemic therapy should be discussed; the option of termination of pregnancy should be considered early enough to provide adequate time for decision-making.

Molluscum Fibrosum Gravidarum

Molluscum fibrosum gravidarum (acrochordons, skin tags) are soft tissue fibromas that typically occur in the latter half of pregnancy on the skin of the face, neck, chest, axillae, inframammary folds, and groin. Papules may regress postpartum. Residual lesions may be removed via snipping, cryotherapy, or electrocautery.

Neurofibroma

More than half of women with neurofibromatosis type 1 note an increase in the growth of new or existing neurofibromas during pregnancy; one-third of neurofibromas decrease in size after delivery. Large neurofibromas may be complicated by intralesional hemorrhage. It is unclear whether women with neurofibromatosis are at increased risk of hypertension, preterm delivery, growth restriction, or other maternal/fetal complications; close monitoring is recommended.

Pyogenic Granuloma

Pyogenic granuloma of pregnancy (epulis gravidarum, granuloma gravidarum, pregnancy epulis, pregnancy tumor) is a common, benign neoplasm resulting from hyperplasia of capillaries and fibroblasts (lobular capillary hemangioma). Pyogenic granulomas present as red, friable, sessile, or pedunculated papules. Lesions are typically painless but bleed with minimal trauma. Oral pyogenic granulomas, located on the labial, gingival, lingual, palatal, or buccal mucosa, develop in 2% of pregnant women; dental plaque deposits or pregnancy gingivitis may incite their formation. Additional common sites include the face and hands/fingers. Pyogenic granulomas may occur at any time during pregnancy, may recur after removal, and tend to regress postpartum.

PREEXISTING SKIN DISEASES AND INTERNAL DISEASES WITH SKIN MANIFESTATIONS AFFECTED BY PREGNANCY

Pregnancy may exert variable, and often unpredictable, effects on both systemic and cutaneous inflammatory diseases due to the altered immunologic profile designed to prevent fetal rejection (Table 41-2). Diseases associated primarily with a Th1-immune response typically improve during pregnancy while Th2-associated disorders tend to deteriorate during gestation. Diseases that are more likely to improve during gestation include chronic plaque psoriasis, linear IgA bullous dermatosis, rheumatoid arthritis, and sarcoidosis.

Atopic Dermatitis

Atopic dermatitis (AD) is the most common dermatosis in pregnancy, accounting for 36% to 50% of all dermatoses in large studies. Most affected women have new-onset AD; only 27% report a personal history of atopy (asthma, eczema, hay fever) and/or infantile AD. For women with preexisting AD, 52% deteriorate and 24% improve during

TABLE 41-2 Skin Diseases and Internal Diseases with Cutaneous Manifestations Aggravated by Pregnancy

Infections
Herpes simplex virus infection
Human immunodeficiency virus infection and acquired immunodeficiency syndrome
Human papillomavirus infection (bowenoid papulosis, condyloma acuminata, verruca vulgaris)
Leprosy
Pityrosporum folliculitis
Trichomoniasis
Varicella-zoster virus infection
Vulvovaginal candidiasis

Autoimmune Diseases
Dermatomyositis
Lupus erythematosus
Pemphigus foliaceus
Pemphigus vulgaris/vegetans
Systemic sclerosis

Metabolic Diseases
Acrodermatitis enteropathica
Porphyria cutanea tarda

Connective Tissue Diseases
Ehlers–Danlos syndrome
Pseudoxanthoma elasticum

Miscellaneous Disorders
Acanthosis nigricans
Erythema multiforme
Erythema nodosum
Erythrokeratoderma variabilis
Hereditary hemorrhagic telangiectasia
Mycosis fungoides
Tuberous sclerosis

gestation. Family history of atopy (50%) and a history of infantile eczema in offspring (19%) are additional risk factors for AD in pregnancy. Onset of cutaneous lesions occurs prior to the third trimester in 75%, and one-third of patients recall similar eruption in previous pregnancies. There is no association with parity or gestation. AD presents most commonly with pruritic, erythematous scaling patches affecting the face, neck, flexures of the extremities, and trunk. Less common manifestations include follicular truncal eczema, papular eczema, and dyshidrosis. Superinfection (bacteria, viral) is not uncommon, and prurigo papules may develop from chronic manipulation.

Diagnosis is clinical. Histopathology is nonspecific, and immunofluorescence (IF) studies are negative. Serum IgE levels are elevated in 20% to 70% of patients but have no diagnostic or prognostic significance. Treatment is similar to nonpregnant individuals and focuses on improvement in skin barrier function with emollient use, reduction in cutaneous inflammation via topical corticosteroids, reduction in pruritus using oral antihistamines, and treating secondary microbial infections. UVB phototherapy can be used safely during pregnancy. Even moderate topical steroid use in pregnancy should be discussed with the patient's obstetrician, as studies have shown there is potential for absorption, which can lead to intrauterine growth restriction, small-for-gestational age fetuses, and/or low birth weight.

AD affects neither maternal nor fetal prognosis. The influence of breastfeeding and maternal food antigen avoidance during pregnancy and lactation on the risk of AD in offspring is debatable. AD typically improves after delivery but may persist for several months. Recurrence with subsequent pregnancy is common.

Autoimmune Progesterone Dermatitis

Autoimmune progesterone dermatitis (APD) is a rare, poorly characterized, cyclical pruritic eruption believed to be related to fluctuations in serum progesterone levels. APD is caused by hypersensitivity to progesterone, endogenous or exogenous, and progesterone autoantibodies are involved in pathogenesis. The heterogeneous clinical presentation includes features of urticaria, eczema, erythema multiforme, or vesiculobullous eruption posing considerable diagnostic challenge. Oral stomatitis and aphthous ulcers may occur. Anaphylaxis is rare. Catamenial flares 3 to 10 days prior to menses and subsequent resolution within a few days of menstruation are typical. Diagnosis hinges on the presence of cyclical premenstrual flares, reproducibility of cutaneous eruption upon intramuscular challenge with progesterone, and response to inhibition of ovulation. Rare cases of new-onset, spontaneous resolution and worsening of APD have each been reported in pregnancy.

Impetigo Herpetiformis

Impetigo herpetiformis (IH, pustular psoriasis of pregnancy) represents an acute pustular phase of psoriasis precipitated by endocrinologic changes in pregnancy; some debate whether IH is a rare form of generalized pustular psoriasis unique to pregnancy. Pathogenesis remains unclear but is believed to relate to high levels of progesterone seen late in pregnancy and low serum levels of calcium. IH has also been reported in the setting of hypoparathyroidism or status post-thyroidectomy.

IH most frequently develops in the third trimester but has been reported at any stage of gestation and postpartum. There is no association with either parity or gestation. Although familial clustering has been reported, personal or family history of psoriasis is often absent.

Epidermal, pinhead-sized, pustules are arranged in groups or concentric rings at the periphery of erythematous, sometimes polycyclic, plaques. Over time, lesions evolve to yellow crusted plaques. IH initially affects the flexures and intertriginous areas with subsequent centrifugal spread and generalization. The face, hands, and feet are typically spared. Pruritus is not usually prominent. Oral mucosa may demonstrate circinate plaques or erosions. Subungual pustules may cause onycholysis and/or onychomadesis. Eruption onset is often accompanied by fever, chills, malaise, diarrhea, and vomiting, with potential dehydration. Complications secondary to hypocalcemia, including tetany, convulsions, and delirium, occur less frequently.

Cutaneous histopathology shows features of pustular psoriasis; parakeratosis and psoriasiform hyperplasia may be observed. IF studies are negative. Laboratory abnormalities include leukocytosis with neutrophilia, elevated erythrocyte sedimentation rate, hypocalcemia, low serum vitamin D levels, and/or hypoparathyroidism. Blood and skin cultures are negative except in cases of bacterial superinfection.

Systemic corticosteroids have historically been first-line treatment and are utilized at varying doses (initial prednisolone or prednisone 15 to 30 mg/day with increase to 60 to 80 mg/day if needed); potential risks include macrosomia, gestational diabetes, and premature rupture of membranes. In 2012, the Medical Board of the National Psoriasis Foundation recommended cyclosporine (2 to 3 mg/kg/day) and infliximab as additional first-line agents for IH. Hypocalcemia must be promptly identified and corrected given the associated morbidities. Fluid management, vitamin D supplementation and treatment of bacterial superinfection should be undertaken. In severe cases, induction of labor or delivery via Cesarean may be considered. Additional treatments for recalcitrant IH postpartum include oral retinoids, methotrexate, or PUVA (psoralen combined with ultraviolet A), either as single agent or combination therapy; individual medications should be evaluated for penetration to breast milk in patients who are breastfeeding.

Historical case reports of IH indicated increased perinatal mortality from cardiac or renal failure or septicemia. Such risks are currently uncommon, and maternal prognosis has improved dramatically with early diagnosis, supportive care, and aggressive treatment. Fetal risks including intrauterine growth retardation, stillbirth, premature birth, and fetal abnormalities are attributed to placental insufficiency and have been reported even when the disease was well controlled mandating intensive fetal monitoring. IH typically resolves postpartum, but lesions may persist for weeks. IH tends to recur in subsequent pregnancy, often with earlier onset and greater severity; it may also recur with menses and hormonal contraceptive use.

Mucocutaneous Infections

Pregnancy adversely influences the frequency and/or severity of a number of mucocutaneous infections (Table 41-2). Similarly, mucocutaneous infections may have significant prognostic implications for pregnant women and their offspring.

Condylomata Acuminata

Condylomata acuminata (genital warts) are caused by the human papillomavirus (HPV), most commonly types 6 and 11. Condylomata have been reported to grow more rapidly during pregnancy and may enlarge such that they interfere with vaginal delivery. Condylomata acuminata in pregnant women have been associated with laryngeal papillomas (recurrent respiratory papillomatosis) in infants although the route of transmission (transplacental, perinatal, postnatal) is not completely understood. It is not clear whether Cesarean delivery prevents HPV transmission to the newborn. Cesarean delivery may, however, be indicated when the pelvic outlet is obstructed by genital warts or when vaginal delivery would result in excessive bleeding. Ablative or destructive therapies for condylomata are acceptable in pregnancy. Topical imiquimod appears to be low risk, but data are limited. The use of podophyllin, podofilox (podophyllotoxin), or sinecatechins is contraindicated during pregnancy.

Herpes Simplex Virus Infection

Maternal herpes simplex virus (HSV) infections associated with fetal risks include: (1) localized primary or recurrent genital HSV infection and (2) disseminated mucocutaneous and/or visceral HSV infection. Localized maternal genital HSV infection occurs either as primary or recurrent infection. Although transmission of HSV to the fetus may occur from either primary or recurrent maternal infection, primary maternal genital infection poses a much higher risk to the fetus. Neonates born to mothers with a history of recurrent genital HSV infections but no active lesions at the time of delivery rarely become infected (<1%). Women without symptoms or signs of genital HSV infection can deliver vaginally. Prematurity, spontaneous abortion, intrauterine growth retardation and neonatal herpes may occur in 40% of neonates born to women who contract primary HSV infection during pregnancy. Neonatal herpes is often a mild illness localized to skin, eyes, and mouth but may progress to encephalitis (15% mortality) or disseminated disease (57% mortality). The fetus that acquires HSV in the second or third trimesters may sustain severe neonatal morbidity and death. Maternal disseminated mucocutaneous HSV infection may occur during the third trimester. Sequelae from dissemination can be severe and increase maternal and fetal mortality rates to approximately 40%. Oral acyclovir can be used safely in all stages of pregnancy and during lactation. A smaller body of evidence supports the use valacyclovir and famciclovir, both believed to pose low risk in pregnant women.

Leprosy

Leprosy reactions are triggered by pregnancy and the associated altered immunity: type 1 (reversal) reaction peaks postpartum and type 2 reaction (erythema nodosum leprosum) occurs throughout pregnancy and lactation; the latter has been associated with "silent neuritis," with resultant early loss of nerve function. These reactions should be treated with oral corticosteroids. Thalidomide is contraindicated in pregnancy. Fetal risk associated with maternal leprosy includes low birth weight. Twenty percent of children born to mothers with leprosy will develop leprosy by adolescence.

Varicella-Zoster Virus Infection

Maternal primary varicella infection occurs in less than 0.4 to 0.7 per 1000 pregnant women with potential negative sequelae for maternal, fetal, and neonatal health. Approximately 10% to 20% of pregnant women with varicella will develop pneumonia with up to 40% maternal mortality. Premature labor occurs in 10%. Transplacental transmission of varicella infection can result in congenital varicella syndrome or neonatal varicella infection depending on the timing of virus exposure. The risk of congenital varicella syndrome is low and occurs only with varicella infection exposure in the first (0.4%) and second trimesters (2%). Features include skin scarring, limb hypoplasia, chorioretinitis, and microcephaly. Neonatal varicella infection occurs when maternal disease develops from 5 days before delivery to 2 days after delivery. Neonatal varicella infection may manifest as disseminated mucocutaneous infection, visceral infection, or pneumonia and carries significant fetal mortality (up to 30%). Women of reproductive age who are susceptible to varicella should be offered varicella vaccination; vaccination should be performed at least 30 days prior to conceiving and can be given immediately after delivery and during lactation.

Vulvovaginal Candidiasis

Vulvovaginal candidiasis (VVC) occurs more frequently during pregnancy (up to 50% of pregnant women, of whom 10 to 40% are asymptomatic). *Candida albicans* accounts for 80% to 90% of all cases of VVC, with nonalbicans species (*Candida glabrata*, *Candida tropicalis*, etc.) comprising the remainder. VVC presents with vulvovaginal erythema, edema, fissuring, and pruritus with or without abnormal vaginal discharge. The Centers for Disease Control an Prevention recommends treatment of uncomplicated VVC in pregnant women using an azole antifungal intravaginally for 7 days. Nystatin (100,000 U per vagina daily for 14 days) is a safe alternative. Oral fluconazole (400 mg/day) has been associated with major fetal malformations limiting its use in pregnancy. VVC can be associated with intraamniotic infection and may increase the risk of preterm premature rupture of membranes. Congenital candidiasis results from ascending infection in utero and presents with generalized erythematous papules and pustules that appear within 12 hours of delivery. Neonatal candidiasis can develop from passage of the infant through an infected birth canal and manifests as an erythematous, erosive eruption with satellite pustules involving the diaper area and/or oral thrush appearing several days after delivery.

Autoimmune Diseases

Dermatomyositis

Dermatomyositis often worsens during gestation and may occur for the first time in pregnancy. An exacerbation of cutaneous manifestations and/or proximal muscle weakness has been reported in about half of affected women. Spontaneous abortions, stillbirths, and neonatal deaths may occur in more than 50% of women with active disease.

Lupus Erythematosus

Chronic cutaneous lupus erythematosus is not affected by pregnancy. Pregnant women with systemic lupus erythematosus (SLE) without renal or cardiac disease, or who have been in remission for at least 3 months prior to conception, typically do not experience worsening of their disease during pregnancy. Risk factors for worsening of SLE during pregnancy and fetal complications include SLE activity at pregnancy onset, thrombocytopenia, lupus nephritis, arterial hypertension, antiphospholipid syndromes and preeclampsia. Half of patients with active disease at the time of conception will worsen during gestation. Overall disease flares are common during pregnancy (up to 65% of affected women). Most flares are mild to moderate; only 15% to 30% of patients experience a moderate to severe flare during pregnancy. When SLE presents initially during pregnancy, a high rate of severe manifestations, including nephritis, cardiac disease, hepatitis, pancreatitis, fever, and lymphadenopathy, is observed. Maternal and fetal risks associated with SLE, particularly in the setting of lupus nephritis, include preeclampsia (30% to 40%), intrauterine growth restriction (13%), fetal loss (6%), and preterm delivery (39%).

Neonatal lupus erythematosus develops secondary to transplacental transfer of maternal anti-Ro/SS-A, or less commonly anti-La/SS-B or anti-U_1RNP, antibodies. Neonatal lupus erythematosus manifests as a self-limited papulosquamous or annular–polycyclic eruption. Systemic complications include pericarditis/myocarditis, cytopenias, and hepatosplenomegaly. Congenital heart block occurs in 1% to 2% of babies exposed to anti-Ro/SS-A and/or anti-La/SS-B antibodies, but this risk increases to up to 20% if the mother has previously delivered an infant with neonatal lupus erythematosus. Although many mothers are asymptomatic and unaware of their autoantibody status, a significant percentage (26% to 57%) eventually develops a connective tissue disease. Recurrent fetal loss typifies antiphospholipid antibody syndrome; patients may also have thrombotic venous or arterial disease, thrombocytopenia, and/or cardiac valve disease.

Pemphigus

Pemphigus vulgaris, vegetans, or foliaceus may develop or worsen (more than 50%) during pregnancy; postpartum flare occurs frequently. In pemphigus vulgaris, fetal and neonatal skin lesions can develop secondary to transplacental transfer of maternal IgG antibody but resolve spontaneously within 2 to 3 weeks postpartum. Pemphigus has been associated with spontaneous abortion, preterm labor, and stillbirth.

Systemic Sclerosis

Systemic sclerosis remains stable in most patients during pregnancy. Raynaud's phenomenon may improve. Only women with systemic involvement are at increased risk of maternal (8% to 12% pulmonary hypertension with 17% to 33% maternal mortality; renal crises) and obstetrical (fetal growth restriction 6%, preterm delivery 25%) complications. Women with recent-onset and rapidly progressive skin disease are at particular risk of renal crisis.

Additional Skin Diseases

Acrodermatitis Enteropathica

Acrodermatitis enteropathica (AE) is a rare autosomal recessive metabolic disorder caused by a mutation in the zinc transporter protein hZIP4 that results in partial deficiency in the gastrointestinal absorption of zinc. AE manifests with alopecia, diarrhea, and a periorificial, genital, and acral dermatitis consisting of erythematous, eroded patches. Mild disease may remit at puberty. Early in gestation, serum zinc levels decrease, due to increased consumption and/or the influence of estrogens, and AE often flares. Dermatitis may progressively worsen until delivery, after which rapid clearing is the rule. Oral zinc supplementation can normalize plasma zinc levels and prevent/resolve cutaneous flares. AE poses no risk to the fetus. Oral contraceptive use may exacerbate AE.

Ehlers–Danlos Syndrome

Ehlers–Danlos syndrome (EDS) is a heterogeneous hereditary disease characterized by alterations of collagen. Overall incidence is approximately 1:5000. Principal manifestations include skin hyperextensibility, joint hypermobility, and connective tissue fragility. Abnormal type 3 collagen production results in increased fragility and potential rupture of arteries, intestines, and the uterus, and women with EDS type IV (vascular) are at significant risk for obstetric complications. Maternal mortality for EDS type IV is 11.5% and is greatest in the peripartum and immediate postpartum period; causes of maternal death include uterine rupture and great vessel rupture. Additional risks include preterm premature rupture of membranes, severe postpartum hemorrhage, delayed wound healing, and increased wound dehiscence.

Erythema Nodosum

Erythema nodosum (EN) is a common panniculitis with a female predominance (three- to fivefold). Two to six percent of EN cases are attributed to pregnancy. EN most often occurs in the second trimester and persists until delivery. It characteristically presents with acute onset, erythematous, tender nodules on the pretibia. Ulceration and scarring do not occur, but hyperpigmentation (erythema contusiforme) is common. Pregnant women should be fully evaluated for infectious (*Streptococcus*, Epstein–Barr virus) and inflammatory (sarcoidosis) causes before the eruption is attributed solely to pregnancy. Treatment is generally supportive and may include bed rest, elastic bandages, analgesics, as well as intralesional corticosteroids. EN does not adversely impact maternal or fetal health.

Hereditary Hemorrhagic Telangiectasia, Marfan Syndrome, Tuberous Sclerosis

The serious and potentially fatal maternal risks associated with the vascular complications of hereditary hemorrhagic telangiectasia (arteriovenous malformations of the brain, gastrointestinal tract, and lungs), Marfan syndrome (aortic aneurysm and dissection), and tuberous sclerosis (renal artery angiomyolipoma and aneurysm) should be promptly recognized and managed.

Porphyrias

Acute intermittent porphyria, porphyria cutanea tarda (PCT), and variegate porphyria can worsen in pregnancy because they are adversely affected by estrogen; exacerbation due to oral contraceptives has also been reported. Exacerbation of PCT has been reported during the first trimester with improvement later in pregnancy. Activity parallels an increase in serum estrogen levels and urinary porphyrins in the first trimester and a fall in levels later in gestation. A population-based cohort study from the Norwegian Porphyria Register demonstrated an increased risk of perinatal death among first-time mothers with active acute porphyria and mothers with heritable PCT. First-time mothers with sporadic PCT had an excess risk of low birth weight and premature delivery.

Pseudoxanthoma Elasticum

Pseudoxanthoma elasticum (PXE), a rare inherited connective tissue disorder caused by mutations in the ATP-binding cassette transporter C6 (ABCC6), results in progressive degeneration of elastic fibers within the skin, retina, and cardiovascular system. Prevalence varies from 1/70,000 to 1/160,000. There is a female predominance of 2:1. Small yellow papules arise symmetrically on the lateral neck, antecubital and popliteal fossae, axillae, and inguinal and periumbilical skin. Oral and anogenital mucosae may also be affected. Angioid streaks of the retina result from calcification of elastic fibers in Bruch's membrane. Progressive calcification of the elastic media and intima of blood vessels may manifest as decreased peripheral pulses, gastrointestinal hemorrhage, renal artery stenosis with hypertension, and coronary artery disease/myocardial infarction. Pregnancy may accelerate the vascular complications of PXE and is associated with an increased risk of gastrointestinal hemorrhage. Additional risks include arterial hypertension and thromboembolism. Placental insufficiency may cause intrauterine growth retardation and increased spontaneous abortion. No increased rates of delivery complications have been reported.

PRURITUS IN PREGNANCY

Pruritus has been reported in 18% of pregnancies in the absence of any cutaneous or systemic pathology and most commonly affects the scalp, genitalia, perianal skin, and abdomen especially in the third trimester. Before pruritus is attributed solely to pregnancy, pruritic dermatoses (i.e., AD, drug eruption, pityriasis rosea), cutaneous infections (i.e., pediculosis, scabies, dermatophytosis), and systemic causes of generalized pruritus (i.e., lymphoma, HIV infection, hepatitis C virus infection, as well as hepatobiliary or renal dysfunction) should be excluded. ICP should also be considered in the setting of pruritus without primary cutaneous lesions.

Intrahepatic Cholestasis of Pregnancy

Intrahepatic cholestasis of pregnancy (ICP, icterus gravidarum, obstetric cholestasis, prurigo gravidarum) is the most common pregnancy-specific liver disorder and the second most common cause of jaundice in pregnancy. Incidence varies by geography and is much higher in South America (9.2% to 15.6%) than in Scandinavia (1.5%) or Europe (0.1% to 0.2%). Risk factors include advanced maternal age (>35 years), multiparity, history of intrahepatic cholestasis in previous pregnancy, history of oral contraceptive use, and family history of intrahepatic cholestasis. Genetic, hormonal, and environmental (seasonal, geographic) factors have been implicated in the pathogenesis. Patients with ICP have mutations in the hepatic phospholipid transporter MDR3/ABCB4, aminophospholipid transporter (ATP8B1/FIC1), and bile salt export protein (BSEP/ABCB11). Clinical presentation varies from mild pruritus without jaundice to cholestatic jaundice. Pruritus typically develops after 30 weeks gestation; it is often initially acral, worsens at nighttime, and may precede laboratory abnormalities. Cutaneous findings are limited to excoriations and prurigo papules/nodules. Nonspecific symptoms include anorexia, epigastric discomfort, fatigue, insomnia, and malaise. Half of patients may notice darker urine and acholic stools; jaundice is uncommon (14% to 25%). Patients may develop steatorrhea with subsequent increased risk of hemorrhage secondary to vitamin K malabsorption.

Elevation of serum total bile acids (>11 µmol/L, up to 10- to 25-fold) is the most sensitive biochemical marker of ICP and correlates with severity of pruritus. Mild increases in hepatic transaminases (typically less than twofold the upper limits of normal pregnancy) occur in up to 60% of patients. Elevations in gamma-glutamyltransferase and bilirubin are less common (<33% and 10% to 25%, respectively).

ICP poses significant risk to the fetus including preterm delivery/prematurity (44%), meconium staining (25% to 45%), intrapartum fetal distress (22%), and intrauterine fetal death/stillbirth (1% to 2%). Risk of fetal complications increases when the maternal serum bile acid level exceeds 40 µmol/L. Malabsorption of vitamin K is associated with an increased risk of intracranial hemorrhage; prophylactic administration of vitamin K has been advocated. The identified fetal risks mandate close fetal surveillance.

Ursodeoxycholic acid (15 mg/kg/day, 500 mg twice a day) is first-line treatment for moderate to severe cholestasis and reduces bile acid levels in cord blood, colostrum, and amniotic fluid. Increasing evidence shows that ursodeoxycholic acid reduces fetal risks associated with ICP. Cholestyramine (8 to 16 g/day) can improve pruritus, but it does not improve the biochemical aberrations or fetal complications of ICP. Furthermore, patients may experience rebound of pruritus after the first week of treatment. Cholestyramine, which can precipitate vitamin K deficiency, should be administered with weekly vitamin K supplementation. Limited benefits have been seen with epomediol, silymarin, S-adenosyl-1-methionine, activated charcoal, dexamethasone, and phenobarbital. Effective pruritus control with UVB phototherapy has also been reported.

Following delivery, pruritus typically resolves within 48 hours, and laboratory abnormalities resolve within 2 to 4 weeks. Patients should be advised that ICP may recur in subsequent pregnancies (45% to 70%) or with oral contraceptive use. Women with a history of ICP are at greater risk for developing hepatobiliary disease (i.e., cholelithiasis, pancreatitis) later in life.

SPECIFIC DERMATOSES OF PREGNANCY

The classification of specific dermatoses of pregnancy has evolved over time. Pemphigoid gestationis (PG) and polymorphic eruption of pregnancy (PEP) are well-defined entities, but the etiopathogenesis of prurigo of pregnancy (PP) and pruritic folliculitis of pregnancy (PFP) is not well understood. Discourse regarding the classification of prurigo of pregnancy and pruritic folliculitis of pregnancy under the umbrella term "atopic eruption of pregnancy" continues.

Pemphigoid Gestationis

Pemphigoid gestationis (PG, herpes gestationis) is a rare, pruritic, autoimmune skin disease of pregnancy and the puerperium and is immunopathologically similar to bullous pemphigoid. PG incidence ranges from 1:2000 to 1:50,000 pregnancies depending on the frequency of HLA-haplotypes DR3 and DR4. PG has also occurred in the setting of trophoblastic tumors (hydatidiform mole, choriocarcinoma). Pathogenic IgG_1 autoantibodies target an epitope (NC16A2 or MCW-1) in the noncollagenous domain of the bullous pemphigoid 180-kDa hemidesmosomal glycoprotein (BP180) of the dermal–epidermal junction leading to tissue disruption and blister formation; these autoantibodies have been shown to cross-react with chorionic and amniotic epithelia.

Onset of PG predominantly occurs in the second and third trimesters although first trimester onset has also been reported. Ten to 16% of cases begin early postpartum. Pruritus is prominent and often intense. Urticarial papules/plaques may evolve to tense bullae; lesions may assume an annular configuration (Figs 41-1 and 41-2). Characteristically, lesions initially involve the periumbilical abdomen and subsequently generalize to the trunk and extremities. Acral involvement of palms and soles is typical. The face and mucous membranes are usually spared. Scarring only occurs in the setting of excoriation or superinfection.

Diagnosis requires immunologic testing in addition to routine histopathology. Direct IF of perilesional skin shows linear C3 deposition along the basement membrane zone, with demonstrable IgG in only 25% of cases. Nevertheless, IgG is positive when indirect complement-added IF is performed. In salt-split testing, the antibody binds to the roof of the specimen. Linear deposition of C3 and IgG_1 has also been demonstrated in the skin of neonates of affected mothers and in the basement membrane zone of amniotic epithelium. Enzyme-linked immunosorbent assay for detection of IgG autoantibodies against the BP180 NC16A domain demonstrate high sensitivity and specificity; titers correlate with disease activity. Cutaneous histopathology of urticarial lesions demonstrates a spongiotic epidermis, marked papillary dermal edema, and eosinophilic inflammatory infiltrate. Vacuolar degeneration of keratinocytes, occasionally accompanied by individual basal cell necrosis and subepidermal blister formation, may be seen in early urticarial lesions but is more prominent in fully developed bullae.

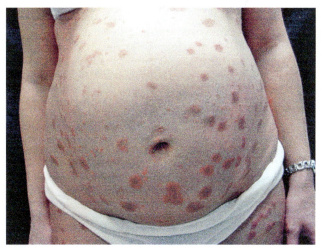

FIGURE 41-1 ■ Pemphigoid gestationis presenting with multiple urticarial plaques, many with small vesicles at the periphery. Note involvement of the immediate periumbilical skin.

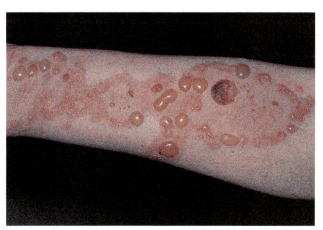

FIGURE 41-2 ■ Grouped tense bullae on an urticarial base in a woman with pemphigoid gestationis.

Peripheral blood eosinophilia may be present but has no prognostic significance.

Treatment depends on the severity and extent of disease and aims to relieve pruritus and prevent blister formation. Very mild disease may be adequately treated with topical corticosteroids (superpotent if needed) and oral antihistamines. Most patients will require systemic therapy, the most common of which is oral corticosteroids (prednisolone/prednisone, 0.5 to 1.0 mg/kg/day). Once new blisters cease to form, tapering may commence. Corticosteroids can be increased at the time of delivery in anticipation of the characteristic immediate postpartum disease exacerbation. Plasmapheresis, intravenous immunoglobulin, and cyclosporine, in various combinations, may also be utilized during pregnancy. Postpartum treatment reports utilizing methotrexate, azathioprine, gold, cyclosporine, cyclophosphamide, intravenous immunoglobulin, and minocycline with niacinamide demonstrate inconsistent results. Successful treatment of recalcitrant PG with goserelin-induced chemical oophorectomy or ritodrine has been reported.

Though PG improves late in pregnancy, the disease characteristically flares at delivery or early postpartum in up to 75% of patients. The duration of PG postpartum widely varies, ranging from 5 weeks to 18 months. Patients who develop prolonged disease tend to have greater age, higher parity, more generalized lesions, and a history of PG in previous pregnancies. Breastfeeding may shorten duration of active lesions. PG recurs in 95% of subsequent pregnancies and may be earlier in onset and more severe during recurrences. PG also recurs with menses and oral contraceptive use in 12% to 64% and 20% to 50%, respectively.

PG is associated with increased maternal risk of Graves' disease (~14%). Small cohorts have shown an association with low birth weight and preterm delivery, which correlated with severity of PG and not corticosteroid use. Fetal complications are thought to be due to low-grade placental insufficiency. No increase in fetal mortality has been documented, with the exception of one case of fetal cerebral hemorrhage. Transient vesiculobullous lesions occur in 5% to 10% of neonates secondary to passive transplacental transfer of maternal PG antibodies.

Polymorphic Eruption of Pregnancy

Polymorphic eruption of pregnancy (PEP, pruritic urticarial papules and plaques of pregnancy [PUPPP], late-onset prurigo of pregnancy, toxic erythema of pregnancy, toxemic rash of pregnancy) is the most common specific dermatosis of pregnancy, occurring in 1:160 to 1:200 pregnancies. PEP classically affects primigravids (73%) with onset in the third trimester. Onset in other trimesters or postpartum has also been reported. Additional risk factors for polymorphic eruption include multiple gestations (10-fold increase), increased maternal weight gain and male fetus (2:1 risk, 55% of cases).

The pathogenesis of PEP is unclear. Association with increased maternal weight gain and multiple gestations lends support to the proposed theory that rapid distension of the abdominal wall (and/or a reaction to the distension) may incite the inflammatory process of PEP. Fetal DNA has been detected in PEP lesions raising questions about potential relevance of microchimerism to pathogenesis.

Characteristically, PEP begins as pruritic, erythematous urticarial papules within the abdominal striae distensae (two-thirds of patients); there is clear sparing of the immediate periumbilical skin (in contrast to PG) (Fig. 41-3). Over time, the distribution may evolve to

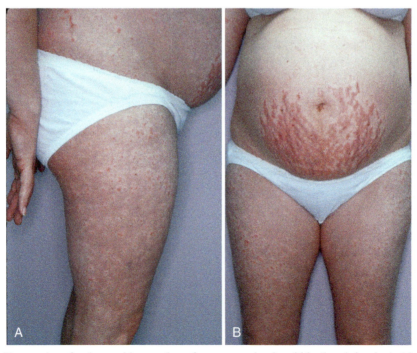

FIGURE 41-3 ■ **A, B,** Pruritic papules of polymorphic eruption of pregnancy begin within the abdominal striae distensae. Note clear sparing of the periumbilical area.

include the trunk and extremities; the face, palms, soles, and mucous membranes are typically spared. The eruption is often polymorphous and may assume annular, polycyclic, and targetoid configurations. Bullous lesions, especially on the lower extremities, and eczematous changes are not infrequent (50%).

Histopathology is nonspecific and may demonstrate spongiosis, parakeratosis, mild acanthosis, and exocytosis as well as a superficial and mid-dermal perivascular lymphohistiocytic infiltrate with variable numbers of eosinophils. IF studies are negative. Laboratory evaluation is normal.

Treatment is symptomatic, with topical antipruritic medications, topical corticosteroids, and oral antihistamines. Patients with severe and/or generalized disease may require systemic corticosteroids (prednisolone 0.5 mg/kg/day) of variable duration. Anecdotal reports demonstrate utility for UVB phototherapy.

PEP does not impact maternal or fetal prognosis. Increased rate of Cesarean delivery in women with PEP has been reported, but PEP itself is not itself an indication for Cesarean delivery or early induction of labor. PEP remits spontaneously within 7 to 10 days of delivery and generally does not recur in subsequent pregnancies.

Prurigo of Pregnancy

Prurigo of pregnancy (PP, Besnier's prurigo gestationis, Nurse's early prurigo of pregnancy) affects approximately 1:300 to 1:450 pregnancies. The etiology of PP remains unknown. Some authors have recently classified PP under "atopic eruption of pregnancy," based on serum IgE elevation and a personal or family history of AD in a significant percentage of patients with PP. Many PP patients may fulfill only minor criteria of atopy.

PP typically begins in the second or third trimester of pregnancy (weeks 25 to 30) with pruritic, erythematous papules and nodules on the extensors of the proximal extremities and trunk. Over time, lesions exhibit variable excoriation and crusting; eczematous changes may also occur. Histopathology is nonspecific, and IF studies are negative. Serum IgE levels may be elevated in some patients. Treatment of PP is symptomatic and includes topical antipruritic medications, moderately potent topical corticosteroids, and oral antihistamines. UVB phototherapy may provide benefit. The disease persists through gestation and typically resolves after delivery, although some cases may persist for up to 3 months postpartum. PP does not impact maternal or fetal outcomes. Recurrence with subsequent pregnancies is variable.

Pruritic Folliculitis of Pregnancy

Pruritic folliculitis of pregnancy (PFP) is a rare, benign sterile folliculitis. The etiology is unclear, and its investigation and classification have been hindered by its nonspecific clinical and histological features. Previously noted associations with increased serum androgens or ICP were shown to be coincidental. PFP lacks comedones arguing against its status as a form of hormonally induced acne.

Onset of the eruption occurs between the fourth and ninth months of gestation. Patients develop 3- to 5-mm erythematous follicular papules and pustules on the upper trunk; lesions may become generalized, but the face is typically spared. Patients characteristically note pruritus but may be asymptomatic. Skin histopathology demonstrates features of a sterile folliculitis with negative stains for microorganisms. IF and serologic tests are negative. Pustule microbial cultures are negative.

PFP has been treated with topical corticosteroids, benzoyl peroxide, and narrowband UVB phototherapy. Oral antihistamines may control pruritus. PFP has no impact on maternal or fetal outcomes. The eruption resolves spontaneously within weeks after delivery and rarely recurs in subsequent pregnancies.

SUGGESTED READINGS

ACOG Committee on Practice Bulletins. ACOG Practice Bulletin. Clinical management guidelines for obstetricians-gynecologists. No. 82 June 2007. Management of herpes in pregnancy. Obstet Gynecol 2007;109:1489–98.

Ambros-Rudolph CM, Müllegger RR, Vaughan-Jones SA, et al. The specific dermatoses of pregnancy revisited and reclassified: results of a retrospective two-center study on 505 pregnant patients. J Am Acad Dermatol 2006;54:395–404.

American College of Obstetricians and Gynecologists. Practice bulletin no. 151: Cytomegalovirus, parvovirus B19, varicella zoster, and toxoplasmosis in pregnancy. Obstet Gynecol 2015;125:1510–25.

Cohen LM, Kroumpouzos G. Pruritic dermatoses of pregnancy: to lump or to split? J Am Acad Dermatol 2007;56:708–9.

Driscoll MS, Grant-Kells JM. Nevi and melanoma in the pregnant woman. Clin Dermatol 2009;27:116–21.

Geraghty LN, Pomeranz MK. Physiologic changes and dermatoses of pregnancy. Int J Dermatol 2011;50:771–82.

Ostensen M, Andreoli L, Brucato A, et al. State of the art: reproduction and pregnancy in rheumatic diseases. Autoimmun Rev 2015;14:376–86.

Ozkan S, Ceylan Y, Ozkan OV, et al. Review of a challenging clinical issue: intrahepatic cholestasis of pregnancy. World J Gastroenterol 2015;21:7134–41.

Regnier S, Fermand V, Levy P, et al. A case–control study of polymorphic eruption of pregnancy. J Am Acad Dermatol 2008;58:63–7.

Roth MM. Pregnancy dermatoses: diagnosis, management, and controversies. Am J Clin Dermatol 2011;12:25–41.

CHAPTER 42

Mast Cell Disease

Michael D. Tharp

KEY POINTS

- Mastocytosis is a disease of both children and adults.
- Most children have skin-limited disease and an excellent prognosis.
- Many adults have either cutaneous only or indolent systemic mastocytosis, and a very good prognosis.
- Patients with more advanced disease have a worse prognosis, which may include the development of a second hematologic malignancy.
- The diagnosis is established by demonstrating increased mast cells in the skin or other organs.
- Treatment is limited to controlling the symptoms of released mast cell mediators.

Mast cell disease, or mastocytosis, represents a spectrum of clinical disorders that results from an abnormal proliferation of mast cells (MCs). The onset ranges from the time of birth to late adulthood. In a report of 101 children with mastocytosis, disease onset occurred in 73% of patients within 6 months of age and 97% of patients by age 2 years. The prevalence of mastocytosis among infants and children ranges from 5.4 cases per 1000 in a Spanish population to 1 case per 500 in a Mexican cohort. The prevalence of mastocytosis in adults is unknown but believed to be even more rare. This disorder is equally distributed between males and females; it has been reported in all races, and most patients have no familial association; however, there have been over 40 cases of familial mast cell disease, some of which have involved several generations.

PATHOGENESIS

MCs are derived from CD34+ precursor cells arising in the bone marrow and circulate as monocytic cells. Circulating mast cell precursors in the blood express CD34, the tyrosine kinase KIT (CD117), and FcγRII, but not high-affinity IgE receptors (FcεRI). KIT is a type III tyrosine kinase that is expressed on MCs, melanocytes, primitive hematopoietic stem cells, primordial germ cells, and interstitial cells of Cajal. Activation of KIT induces cellular growth and extends cell survival by preventing apoptosis. The ligand for KIT is stem cell factor (SCF), which is important for mast cell growth. SCF is produced by bone marrow stromal cells, fibroblasts, keratinocytes, endothelial cells, and reproductive Sertoli and granulosa cells. Under normal conditions, once mast cell precursors enter tissues they become KIT+/CD34-/FcγRII-/FcεRI+ and develop characteristic cytoplasmic granules.

Alterations in *c-KIT* structure have been implicated in the pathogenesis of mast cell disease. Specifically, somatic mutations in codon 816 of the *c-KIT* proto-oncogene have been identified in adults and children with mastocytosis. The result is a substitution of the amino acid aspartic acid (D) with valine (V) or another amino acid; examples include D816V, D816Y, D816F, D816I, and D816H. This mutation causes constitutive activation of KIT, thereby leading to continued mast cell development. Additional mutations in *c-KIT* (del419, K509I, F522C, V533D, A533D, V559A, V560G, R815K, I817V, D820G, E839K) also have been reported in adults and children with mastocytosis, but are more rare. Frequently these mutations are detected in mRNA not DNA. In a recent study of 50 children with mastocytosis, ranging in age from 0 to 16 years, activating mutations were detected in 86% of the patients. Forty-two percent were in codon 816 and the remainder were within the gene that encodes the proximal extracellular region (fifth immunoglobulin-like domain). All the *c-KIT* mutations except M541L found in these children were associated with constitutive KIT activation. Interestingly, an inactivating mutation (e.g., E839K) also has been described in a child with mastocytosis, In the extremely rare familial mast cell disease, *c-KIT* mutation detection has been variable, ranging from none to the expression of K509I and A533D mutations. The finding of inactivating or no *c-KIT* mutations in some patients and families with mastocytosis suggests that factors beyond an abnormal KIT receptor play a role in this disease. In fact, additional gene mutations have been identified in some adult patients with more advanced mastocytosis and include the tumor suppressor gene *TET2* as well as *ASCL1*, *JAK2*, *SRSF2*, *DNMT3A*, *RUNX1*, and *CBL*. Taken together, these observations suggest that mutations in *c-KIT* lead to the development of mastocytosis but that additional gene mutations occur and may be necessary for life-long disease.

CLASSIFICATION OF MAST CELL DISEASE

The classification of mast cell disease has been defined by the World Health Organization (WHO) with the following disease categories: cutaneous mastocytosis (CM), indolent systemic mastocytosis (ISM), smoldering systemic mastocytosis (SSM), isolated bone marrow mastocytosis (IBMM), systemic mastocytosis with an associated clonal hematologic nonmast cell lineage disease (SM-AHNMD),

TABLE 42-1	Classification of Mast Cell Disease

Cutaneous mastocytosis (CM)
    Macular and papular CM
    Diffuse CM
    Mastocytoma
Indolent systemic mastocytosis (ISM)
    Smoldering systemic mastocytosis (SSM)
    Isolated bone marrow mastocytosis (IBMM)
Systemic mastocytosis with an associated clonal hematologic nonmast cell lineage disease (SM-AHNMD)
    SM–myelodysplastic syndrome
    SM–myeloproliferative disorder
    SM–chronic eosinophilic leukemia
    SM–non-Hodgkin's lymphoma
Aggressive systemic mastocytosis (ASM)
    With eosinophilia (SM-eo)
Mast cell leukemia (MCL)
Mast cell sarcoma
Extracutaneous mastocytoma

TABLE 42-2	Criteria for Diagnosing Systemic Mast Cell Disease

Major
Multifocal dense mast cell infiltrates (>15 MCs/aggregate) in the bone marrow or extracutaneous organs

Minor
25% MCs are spindle-shaped or atypical in a bone marrow aspirate smear or tissue sections
c-KIT mutation at codon 816 in blood, bone marrow, or extracutaneous tissue
Expression of CD2 and/or CD25 by CD117$^+$ MCs
Total serum tryptase persistently >20 ng/mL (in the absence of another nonmast cell hematologic disorder)

TABLE 42-3	Mast Cell Mediators

Preformed Mediators	Cytokines
Histamine	TNF-α
Heparin	IL-1
	IL-3
	IL-4
Chemotactic factors for	IL-5
polymorphonuclear neutrophils	IL-6
and eosinophils	IL-8
Tryptase	IL-9
Chymase	IL-10
	IL-13
	IL-16
	IL-18
	SCF
	GM-CSF

Newly Formed Mediators
PGD$_2$,
LTC$_4$, LTD$_4$, LTE$_4$
PAF

aggressive systemic mastocytosis (ASM), mast cell leukemia (MCL), mast cell sarcoma, and extracutaneous mastocytoma (Table 42-1). Patients with CM and ISM represent the largest groups, and include most children with CM and many adults with CM or ISM. All CM patients and many ISM patients have cutaneous lesions. Cutaneous involvement in mast cell disease is defined by typical lesions of mastocytosis (see "Clinical Manifestations"), and pathological changes that demonstrate either monomorphic mast cell clusters (>15 MCs/cluster) or scattered MCs at more than 20 MCs/high-power field (hpf). Systemic mast cell disease is defined by major and minor criteria in which the major criteria are represented by multifocal dense mast cell infiltrates (15 MCs/aggregate) in the bone marrow or other extracutaneous organs, and the minor criteria include the presence of >25% spindle-shaped or atypical-appearing MCs in tissue sections or a bone marrow aspirate smear, the presence of a c-KIT mutation at codon 816, the expression of CD2 and/or CD25 by MCs and a persistent total serum tryptase level of >20 ng/mL (Table 42-2). The diagnosis of SM is established in patients having the major and one minor criteria or three minor criteria. Whereas most patients with SM have indolent disease, a smaller subset has been recognized as SSM because of greater disease burden, e.g., hepatosplenomegaly, lymphadenopathy, serum tryptase levels >200 ng/mL. Another recognized group of SM patients is one with an associated clonal hematologic nonmast cell disorder. Hematologic diseases associated with this SM group include: polycythemia rubra vera, myelodysplastic syndrome, chronic eosinophilic leukemia, chronic myeloid leukemia, chronic myelomonocytic leukemia, lymphocytic leukemia, acute erythroblastic leukemia, megaloblastic leukemia, and non-Hodgkin's lymphoma. Patients with SM-AHNMD may or may not have skin lesions, but frequently have liver, spleen, and/or lymph node involvement. They often are older adults, and many have constitutional symptoms such as fever, anorexia, weight loss, and generalized malaise. Aggressive systemic mast cell disease is characterized by lymphadenopathy with or without peripheral blood eosinophilia. Patients with this rare disorder often lack cutaneous lesions, but frequently have mast cell infiltrates involving the bone marrow, gastrointestinal tract, liver, spleen, and lymph nodes. MCL is an extremely rare condition, and the diagnosis is established by demonstrating MCs in the peripheral blood and/or >20% MCs in a bone marrow aspirate smear. Most MCL patients do not have cutaneous lesions, but frequently experience fever, weight loss, abdominal pain, diarrhea, nausea, and vomiting. These patients also have detectable hepatosplenomegaly and lymphadenopathy resulting from extensive mast cell infiltration of these organs. Bone marrow biopsies from MCL patients demonstrate increased MCs, which are often spindle-shaped or morphologically atypical. Mast cell sarcomas and extracutaneous mastocytomas are extremely rare, with only a few isolated case reports.

CLINICAL MANIFESTATIONS

Symptoms

Symptoms associated with mast cell disease are attributable in great part to the release of mast cell mediators, such as histamine, eicosanoids, and cytokines (Table 42-3). These symptoms may range from pruritus and flushing to abdominal pain and diarrhea, to palpitations, dizziness, and syncope (Table 42-4). In many instances the symptoms can

TABLE 42-4	Symptoms and Signs of Mastocytosis
Cardiopulmonary	**Gastrointestinal**
Chest pain	Abdominal cramps
Dizziness	Diarrhea
Dyspnea	Epigastric pain*
Palpitations	Nausea
Syncope	Vomiting
Skin	**Neurologic**
Bullae (children)	Cognitive disorganization*
Flushing	Headaches
Pruritus	**Constitutional**
Urticaria	Fatigue*
Skeletal	Fever*
Bone pain*	Malaise*
	Weight loss*

*Suggests the possibility of systemic mastocytosis.

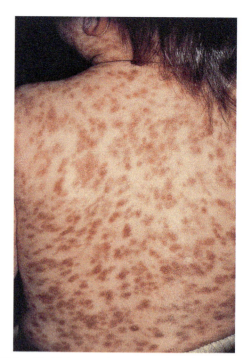

FIGURE 42-2 ■ Multiple tan to brown papules of urticaria pigmentosa.

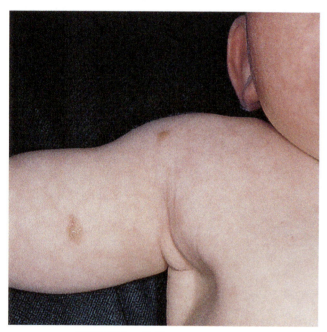

FIGURE 42-1 ■ Solitary mastocytoma.

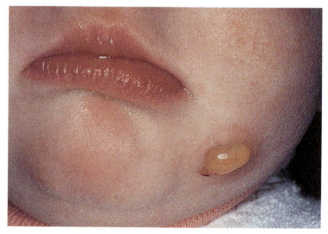

FIGURE 42-3 ■ Bullous mastocytoma.

be reduced or suppressed by antihistamines, suggesting mast cell-derived histamine as a cause. Many patients with CM or ISM have few, if any, symptoms, and may experience only intermittent bouts of pruritus. Of interest is the relative lack of pulmonary symptoms in SM patients. Complaints of fever, night sweats, malaise, weight loss, bone pain, epigastric distress, and problems with mentation (cognitive disorganization) often signal the presence of SM. Symptoms of mast cell disease can be exacerbated by exercise, heat, local trauma to skin lesions, as well as the ingestion of alcohol, narcotics, salicylates, and anticholinergic agents. Some systemic anesthetic agents (e.g., opiates) also may precipitate anaphylaxis.

Cutaneous Lesions

Most children have CM, which is frequently manifest by either a solitary tan or yellow-tan plaque or nodule (mastocytoma) (Fig. 42-1) or variable numbers of tan to brown papules (urticaria pigmentosa, UP) (Fig. 42-2). Mastocytomas often occur on the distal extremities, but may arise in any anatomical location. Urticaria pigmentosa usually presents early in childhood and often spares the face, scalp, palms, and soles. Whereas telangiectatic macules (telangiectasia macularis eruptiva perstans, TMEP) are a rare manifestation of CM in young patients, at least three children have been reported with TMEP. Some children develop diffuse cutaneous mastocytosis (DCM), which appears as numerous erythematous, yellow-tan papules and plaques. Infants and children with UP and DCM also may experience nonscarring vesicles or bullae (Fig. 42-3). Blistering reactions in CM lesions usually resolve by 3 to 5 years of age. Despite the widespread involvement, children with DCM rarely progress to SM. In a study of 10 children with DCM, none progressed to SM in an 8-year follow-up. The skin manifestations of adult mastocytosis differ significantly from those in children, and appear as reddish-brown macules and papules several millimeters in diameter (Fig. 42-4). These lesions are most

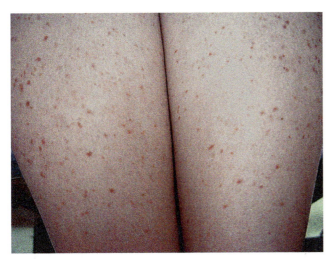

FIGURE 42-4 ■ Typical reddish-brown skin lesions of adult mastocytosis.

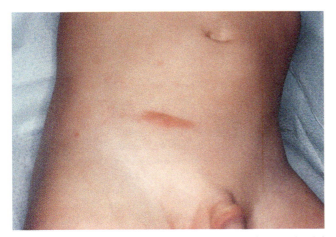

FIGURE 42-5 ■ Darier sign: note the formation of an urticarial wheal at the site of stroking the skin.

numerous on the trunk and proximal extremities, and appear less frequently on the face, distal extremities, palms, or soles. While individual lesions do resolve in these patients, over time the total lesion number usually increases. Mastocytomas and DCM in adults are extremely rare.

The presence of increased mast cell numbers in the skin of patients with mast cell disease can be demonstrated clinically by firmly rubbing a characteristic lesion. The formation of an urticarial wheal (Darier's sign) (Fig. 42-5) at the lesion site is indicative of mast cell mediator release. Darier's sign is readily demonstrated in mastocytomas and childhood UP lesions, whereas it may be barely detectable in common adult mast cell disease lesions and TMEP. This can be explained by the fact that mast cell concentrations in mastocytomas and childhood UP are approximately 150 and 40 times, respectively, higher than in normal skin. The mast cell content in adult mast cell disease lesions is only eight to nine times greater than in normal skin.

Systemic Manifestations

Skeletal involvement is common in adult patients with SM, with a reported incidence of approximately 70%. On X-ray these changes appear as radio-opacities, radiolucencies, or a mixture of the two, with the skull, spine, and pelvis being most commonly involved. Osteoporosis is the most common change in patients with diffuse skeletal disease, followed by osteosclerosis and mixed lesions of osteosclerosis and osteoporosis. These bony changes are believed to result from the local release of mast cell mediators. Children with mastocytosis rarely have bone involvement.

Bone marrow involvement frequently (70% to 90%) occurs in adult SM patients but is rarely seen in children. The diagnosis of mast cell disease in the bone marrow is established by identifying clusters of MCs (>15 tryptase-positive staining MCs/cluster) that express CD25 and/or CD2, which are not routinely detected on normal MCs. The diagnosis of SM on bone marrow biopsy may be difficult in patients with SM-AHNMD because of the coexistence of the hematologic disorder. The presence of >5% MCs on a bone marrow aspirate smear in SM patients suggests an unfavorable prognosis, and the identification of >20% MCs on a bone marrow smear is diagnostic of MCL.

Splenomegaly has been reported in approximately 50% of adult SM patients; however, in two recent larger studies, each with over 140 adult mastocytosis patients, splenomegaly was observed in only 8% to 9% of individuals. Splenomegaly is most common in ASM and MCL. Lymph node enlargement is uncommon in ISM patients, but occurs in patients with ASM and MCL. Among 58 patients, with systemic involvement, 26% had peripheral lymphadenopathy, whereas 19% had central nodal disease. Patients with SM also may experience gastrointestinal symptoms such as abdominal pain, diarrhea, nausea, and vomiting. Diarrhea is usually episodic and can result from malabsorption, increased motility, and/or acid hypersecretion. Gastrointestinal hemorrhage has been reported in some patients with SM, and is often secondary to gastritis or peptic ulcers. Radiographic changes in the gastrointestinal tract of SM patients include urticaria-like lesions, thickened gastric, duodenal or jejunal folds, as well as mucosal nodules and/or peptic ulcers. Biopsies of mucosal nodules often show numerous MCs with varying numbers of eosinophils. Hepatomegaly also is detectable in approximately 40% of adult SM patients, but most of these have normal liver function tests.

A mixed organic brain syndrome manifested by irritability, fatigue, headache, poor attention span and motivation, limited short-term memory, inability to work effectively, and difficulty in interacting with other people has been described in SM patients. It has been hypothesized that these symptoms are secondary to released mast cell mediators. Electroencephalographic studies in these patients have ranged from normal to changes consistent with a toxic or metabolic process.

DIAGNOSIS

The diagnosis of mastocytosis is established by demonstrating increased MCs in one or more organs (Table 42-5). In patients with skin lesions, increased MCs can be established in a biopsy of lesional skin. Nodular,

TABLE 42-5	Diagnostic Tests for Patients with Mastocytosis

Direct Tests
Biopsy of the skin
Biopsy of the gastrointestinal tract
Biopsy of the bone marrow

Indirect Tests
Serum tryptase (total or α) levels
24-h urinary histamine metabolite levels (methylimidazole acetic acid)
Urinary prostaglandin D2 (PGD_2) levels
Bone X-rays or bone scan

papular, and macular lesions of mast cell disease have been reported to have respectively 150-, 40-, and eight- to ninefold increases in mast cell content compared to normal skin. Special stains, such as toluidine blue, Giemsa, and Leder, or monoclonal antibodies that recognize tryptase or CD117 (KIT) are helpful for identifying tissue MCs. The proposed pathologic criteria for skin involvement in mastocytosis patients include either the presence of >15 monomorphic MCs/cluster or >20 scattered MCs/hpf on microscopic evaluation of a lesional skin biopsy specimen and the presence of a *c-KIT* mutation at the 816 codon. Normal-appearing skin from patients with mast cell disease has normal numbers of MCs, and skin biopsies of normal-appearing skin in patients with suspected mast cell disease are not helpful in establishing the diagnosis. Biopsies from either the bone marrow or the gastrointestinal tract may be indicated for patients in whom the diagnosis of SM is expected, but who lack skin lesions.

Detection of circulating mast cell mediators and/or their metabolites can offer indirect evidence of mastocytosis (Table 42-5). Two forms (α and β) of mast cell-derived tryptase have been identified. α-Tryptase is persistently elevated in patients with SM, and thus may be useful for assessing total body mast cell burden. β-Tryptase, on the other hand, is often detected in mast cell disease patients as well as in other hematologic disorders and normal patients experiencing anaphylactic symptoms. In one study, 50% of patients with total serum tryptase levels between 20 and 75 ng/mL had evidence of SM, whereas all patients with levels >75 ng/mL had proven systemic involvement. Of note, a total serum tryptase level >20 ng/mL represents one of the minor criteria for SM.[38] Elevations in urinary histamine metabolites also have been documented in some SM patients. In many instances, unmetabolized urinary histamine levels may be normal in asymptomatic SM patients, whereas the major metabolite of histamine, 1,4-methylimidazole acetic acid (MeImAA), is often persistently elevated. Certain foods with high histamine content, such as spinach, eggplant (aubergine), cheeses (Parmesan, blue, and Roquefort), and red wines, can artificially elevate the levels of urinary histamine and its metabolites. The major urinary metabolite of prostaglandin D2 (PGD_2), 9α,11β-dihydroxy-15-oxo-2,3,18,19-tetranorprost-5-ene-1,20-dioic acid (PGD_2M), has also been reported to be increased in some SM patients.

PROGNOSIS

Most children have CM and thus an excellent prognosis with a limited disease course. Approximately 50% of these patients are expected to have their disease resolved by adolescence, with the remainder noting a marked reduction in lesion numbers by adulthood. The overall prognosis of patients having ISM appears good. In a study of 145 adults with ISM, the cumulative probabilities of disease progression to ASM at 10 and 25 years were 1.7% and 8.4%, respectively. Prognosis for patients with SM-AHNMD appears to be directly related to the severity of the associated hematologic disorder. ASM patients have an unfavorable prognosis, with a mean survival of only a few years, and the prognosis for MCL is also extremely poor, with an expected survival of a year or less from the time of diagnosis.

TREATMENT

At present there is no cure for mastocytosis; treatment is therefore directed at alleviating symptoms. Patients with CMs and ISM often have few, if any, symptoms, and therefore require little or no therapy. Patients should be cautioned to avoid potential mast cell-degranulating agents such as ingested alcohol, anticholinergic preparations, aspirin, nonsteroidal agents, narcotics, and polymyxin B sulfate. In addition, heat and friction can induce local or systemic symptoms, and therefore should be avoided whenever possible. A number of systemic anesthetic agents, including lidocaine (lignocaine), morphine, codeine, D-tubocurarine, metocurine, etomidate, thiopental, succinylcholine, enflurane, and isoflurane, have been directly or indirectly implicated in precipitating anaphylactoid reactions in mastocytosis patients. Although observations are limited, it appears that propofol, vecuronium, and fentanyl are safe alternative systemic anesthetics for patients with mast cell disease. Because anaphylaxis has been observed hours after general anesthesia, it has been recommended that mastocytosis patients be monitored postoperatively for at least 24 hours. In contrast to its systemic administration, local injections of lidocaine can be used safely in mastocytosis patients.

Histamine (H_1) or combined H_1 and H_2 antagonists are often helpful in controlling many of the symptoms associated with mast cell disease. The second-generation antihistamines, cetirizine, loratadine, and fexofenadine, have distinct advantages over first-generation antihistamines because they have longer half-lives and are more specific H_1 antagonists. Often higher than recommended doses of combined H_1 antihistamines are required for symptom control. For example, some patients may require fexofenadine 360 mg in the morning and up to 40 mg of cetirizine at night for control of histamine-related symptoms. In some instances the addition of an H_2 antagonist (cimetidine, ranitidine, famotidine, or nizatidine) may prove beneficial, especially in patients with gastric acid hypersecretion. H_2 antagonist therapy must be combined with H_1 antagonist therapy as feedback inhibition of mast cell degranulation is mediated via H_2 receptors on MCs. Ketotifen, which has both antihistamine and mast cell-stabilizing properties, has been effective in combination with ranitidine in controlling symptoms of mast cell disease, as has the tricyclic antidepressant doxepin, which has activity at both H_1 and H_2 histamine receptors. Oral disodium cromoglycate (400 to 1000 mg/day) may alleviate gastrointestinal, cutaneous, and central nervous system symptoms associated with mast cell disease, especially in children.

Omalizumab, which is a humanized murine monoclonal antibody to IgE approved for the treatment of asthma and chronic urticaria, has proven effective in controlling the symptoms of some adult mastocytosis patients who were recalcitrant to combined antihistamine/antileukotriene therapy. It appears, however, that continued therapy is necessary for symptom control.

Psoralen combined with ultraviolet A (PUVA) therapy given four times a week is helpful in controlling the pruritus and cutaneous whealing in mast cell disease patients. However, it does not alter other symptoms associated with this disorder, and does not permanently eliminate cutaneous mast cell infiltrates. In contrast to oral PUVA, bath PUVA is not beneficial for symptomatic mast cell disease patients. Despite early enthusiasm UVA-1 therapy is not as effective as oral PUVA therapy.

Topical corticosteroids under occlusion for 6 weeks or more can greatly reduce the skin mast cell content as well as symptoms associated with mast cell disease. Intralesional injections of triamcinolone acetonide also have been successful in clearing mast cell infiltrates in the skin of mast cell disease patients. Systemic corticosteroids are usually of little benefit in most patients with mast cell disease, but may provide relief of cutaneous and gastrointestinal symptoms in patients with more advanced disease. Cyclosporine A has been used in combination with systemic corticosteroids in a patient with advanced mast cell disease, resulting not only in relief of symptoms but also in a decline in serum tryptase and urinary histamine metabolite levels.

The subcutaneous administration of interferon-α_{2b} (IFN-α_{2b}) also has been used with variable success in patients with more aggressive forms of SM. In a prospective study, six patients with ISM were treated with IFN-α_{2b}; however, only a modest decline in bone marrow MCs and urinary MeImAA levels was noted, and no change in serum tryptase levels was observed. The side effects of the IFN therapy can be significant and include anaphylaxis, hypothyroidism, thrombocytopenia, and depression, which seem to outweigh the benefit of the therapy.

Some mast cell disease patients experience recurrent life-threatening episodes of hypotension resulting from mast cell mediator release. These patients should be supplied with a premeasured epinephrine (adrenaline) preparation (EpiPen). In some instances they may experience recurrent similar attacks within hours of the initial event. The administration of prednisone (20 to 40 mg/day for 2 to 4 days) can often abort or eliminate these recurring episodes.

Numerous chemotherapeutic agents have been used unsuccessfully in the treatment of advanced mast cell disease. Recently, however, 2-chlorodeoxyadenosine has been reported effective in eliminating skin lesions and markedly reducing the numbers of bone marrow MCs in patients with widespread systemic disease. Chemotherapeutic approaches, on the other hand, are important, and can be effective for the treatment of associated hematologic disorders seen in patients with SM-AHNMD. Local radiation therapy (approximately 2000 to 30,000 cGy) may provide relief of bone pain. In some instances pain relief can be achieved during treatment or shortly thereafter, thereby reducing the frequency and amount of oral analgesics required for pain control. Splenectomy may be indicated for mast cell disease patients who experience hypersplenism leading to significant cytopenia, and it appears to improve survival in patients with more aggressive disease.

Imatinib mesylate is a tyrosine kinase inhibitor that blocks KIT and PDGF receptors, as well as the BCR-ABL oncoprotein associated with chronic myelogenous leukemia. The active site for imatinib within the KIT receptor is proximal to the most common mutation at the 816 condon, thus rendering patients with *c-KIT* 816 mutations unresponsive to this agent. On the other hand, imatinib is capable of alleviating the signs and symptoms of mastocytosis in patients with rare *c-KIT* mutations (e.g., del419, K509I, F522C, and V560G) as well as those expressing the *FIP1L1-PDGFRA* fusion gene who are D816-negative. Dasatinib, nilotinib, and midostaurin are multitarget BCR-ABL and SRC family kinase inhibitors, capable of limiting proliferation and facilitating apoptosis in vitro in D816V-expressing mastocytosis mast cell lines. Unfortunately, these tyrosine kinase inhibitors also have proven ineffective for the long-term management of mastocytosis patients, further suggesting that this disorder involves both *c-KIT* and non-*c-KIT* mutations. In the future, it is likely that the treatment of advanced mastocytosis will include a combination of drugs directed at specific mutations.

SUGGESTED READINGS

Akin C, Valent P. Diagnostic criteria and classification of mastocytosis in 2014. Immunol Allergy Clin North Am 2014;34(2):207–18.

Andrew SM, Freemont AJ. Skeletal mastocytosis. J Clin Pathol 1993;46:1033–5.

Bodemer C, Hermine O, Palmerini F, Yang Y, Grandpeix-Guyodo C, Leventhal PS, et al. Pediatric mastocytosis is a clonal disease associated with D816V and other activating c-KIT mutations. J Invest Dermatol 2010;130(3):804–15.

Borgeat A, Ruetsch YA. Anesthesia in a patient with malignant systemic mastocytosis using a total intravenous anesthetic technique. Anesth Analg 1998;86:442–4.

Butterfield JH. Response of severe systemic mastocytosis to interferon-alpha. Br J Dermatol 1998;138:489–95.

Caplan RM. The natural course of urticaria pigmentosa. Arch Dermatol 1963;87:146–57.

Escribano L, Alvarez-Twose I, Sanchez-Munoz L, Garcia-Montero A, Nunez R, Almeida J, et al. Prognosis in adult indolent systemic mastocytosis: a long-term study of the Spanish Network on Mastocytosis in a series of 145 patients. J Allergy Clin Immunol 2009;124(3):514–21.

Kasper C, Freeman RG, Tharp MD. Diagnosis of mastocytosis subsets using a morphometric point counting technique. Arch Dermatol 1987;123:1017–21.

Keyzer JL, DeMonchy JGR, vanDoormaal JJ, et al. Improved diagnosis of mastocytosis by measurement of urinary histamine metabolites. N Engl J Med 1983;309:1603–5.

Kolde G, Frosch P, Czarnetzki B. Response of cutaneous mast cells to PUVA in patients with urticaria pigmentosa: histomorphometric, ultrastructural, and biochemical investigations. J Invest Dermatol 1984;83:175–8.

Lange M, Niedoszytko M, Renke J, Glen J, Nedoszytko B. Clinical aspects of paediatric mastocytosis: a review of 101 cases. J Eur Acad Dermatol Venereol 2013;27(1):97–102.

Longley BJ, Metcalfe DD, Tharp MD, et al. Activating and dominant inactivating c-kit catalytic domain mutations in distinct forms of human mastocytosis. Proc Natl Acad Sci USA 1999;96:1609–14.

Rogers M, Bloomingdale K, Murawski B, et al. Mixed organic brain syndrome as a manifestation of systemic mastocytosis. Psychosom Med 1986;48:437–47.

Sagher F, Even-Paz Z. Mastocytosis and the mast cell. Chicago: Yearbook Medical Publishers; 1967. p. 10–291.

Schwaab J, Schnittger S, Sotlar K, Walz C, Fabarius A, Pfirrmann M, et al. Comprehensive mutational profiling in advanced systemic mastocytosis. Blood 2013;122(14):2460–6.

Tefferi A, Li CY, Butterfield JH, Hoagland HC. Treatment of systemic mast-cell disease with cladribine. N Engl J Med 2001;344(4):307–9.

Valent P, Akin C, Escribano L, et al. Standards and standardization in mastocytosis: consensus statement on diagnostics, treatment recommendations and response criteria. Eur J Clin Invest 2007;37:435–53.

CHAPTER 43

HAIR DISORDERS IN SYSTEMIC DISEASE

Kimberly S. Salkey • Amy McMichael

KEY POINTS

- Hair loss in the setting of systemic disease may occur through one of five mechanisms: telogen effluvium, anagen arrest, hair miniaturization, scarring alopecia, and hair shaft disorders.
- The most common cause of hair loss is telogen effluvium, which can be divided into five subtypes depending on which portion of the hair cycle is pathologically lengthened or shortened.
- Anagen arrest occurs when there is a sudden halt in mitotic activity of the hair matrix cells.
- Hair miniaturization is caused by a complex interplay of genetic and hormonal influences.
- Scarring alopecia results in permanent injury to hair follicles and may be primary or secondary in origin.
- Trichorrhexis nodosa is the most common hair shaft abnormality.
- Systemic disease may cause excess hair in the form of hirsutism or hypertrichosis.

Hair disorders are commonly associated with systemic disease although they may be overlooked by clinicians and dismissed as unimportant, particularly in comparison with the patient's underlying systemic illness. This is an unfortunate reality since hair can be perceived as a critical indicator of health, prosperity, and even social status. One retrospective review on the psychologic impact of alopecia on patients (regardless of cause) indicated that such patients are more likely to suffer from psychiatric illness, low self-esteem, and poor quality of life. Likewise, Americans have been estimated to spend over $2 billion annually on the removal of unwanted hair. In diagnosing and treating diseases that are associated with hair disorders, it is imperative that clinicians are mindful of the unique needs and sensitivities inherent to this group of patients.

FOLLICULAR BIOLOGY

In order to understand the behavior of the hair follicle in the setting of systemic disease, it is first important to appreciate normal follicular biology. At the time of birth, there are approximately 150,000 hair follicles on the scalp. Each undergoes a continuous cyclic pattern of changes (the follicular lifecycle) during the person's lifetime. The first two cycles of hair growth occur synchronously in utero and then shortly after birth. After that, each follicle seems to have a growth cycle independent of those around it.

The duration of hair growth cycles is dependent on varying factors, including location of the hair, the individual's age, nutritional habits, hormonal factors, and health status.

In healthy individuals, scalp hair grows approximately 0.35 mm/day (1 cm per month). It should be noted, however, that data suggest that African textured hair grows more slowly, at approximately 0.77 cm per month. Growth rates are also influenced by the type and anatomic location of hairs. Vellus hairs are widely distributed throughout the body, rooted in the upper dermis. They are nonpigmented, lacking melanin and a medulla, and are finely textured, measuring 0.03 mm or less in diameter and less than 1 cm in length. Growth rates for vellus hairs range from 0.03 to 0.13 mm/day. Hormonal influences at puberty induce vellus hairs to be replaced by terminal hairs in hormone-sensitive areas such as the axillae and pubis. Terminal hairs are medullated and contain melanin and thus are pigmented. They are anchored more deeply in the dermis.

Each hair follicle passes through three cycles: anagen (growth), catagen (involution), and telogen (rest) (Fig. 43-1). A latency or exogen phase is noted in up to 80% of hair cycles. In exogen, the hair shaft is shed without regrowth, and a new anagen phase is turned on. Hair length is determined by the rate and duration of the anagen phase, which is terminated by an internal biologic "clock" built into every follicle. On average, anagen duration on the scalp varies from 2 to 6 years. The catagen phase marks the termination of the growing phase.

Catagen, a transitional phase of acute follicular regression, is irreversible and of relatively short duration, lasting only 2 to 3 weeks. The completion of catagen is marked by formation of the keratinized and depigmented club hair. Only 1% to 2% of scalp hairs are in catagen at any one time.

Telogen, the resting phase, begins when catagen is complete. With an average duration of 3 months, approximately 15% of scalp hairs are in telogen at any given time. Telogen hairs account for the 50 to 100 scalp hairs shed normally each day. The percentage of hairs in the telogen phase, called the telogen count, varies between individuals and even between parts of the scalp. The telogen hair (club hair) is shed during the exogen phase, which may or may not coincide with the new anagen phase. The next anagen phase begins anew from the reservoir of follicular stem cells residing in the bulge area, near where the arrector pili muscle inserts into the hair follicle. These stem cells proliferate rapidly downwards to form a new anagen hair.

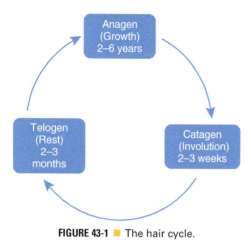

FIGURE 43-1 ■ The hair cycle.

TABLE 43-1	Five Mechanisms for Alopecia in Systemic Disease

Telogen effluvium
Anagen arrest
Androgenetic alopecia/hair miniaturization
Scarring alopecia (cicatricial alopecia)
Hair shaft disorders

TABLE 43-2	Causes of Telogen Effluvium

Injury or physiologic stress
Postfebrile state (extremely high fevers, e.g., malaria)
Severe infection, including HIV
Severe chronic illness
Following a general surgical procedure
Hypothyroidism and other endocrinopathies
Extreme dieting and/or weight loss
Drugs
Heavy metals
Physiologic effluvium of the newborn
Postpartum state
Early stages of androgenetic alopecia

HAIR DISORDERS IN SYSTEMIC DISEASE

The well-oiled machinery that drives the hair cycle can easily be disrupted by systemic disease. In many cases, hair loss (alopecia) is the result, although excess hair growth may also occur.

ALOPECIA

Alopecia has traditionally been subdivided into three main categories: scarring (cicatricial), nonscarring (noncicatricial), and hair shaft disorders. In addition, Solomon proposed the term "biphasic alopecia" to describe forms of alopecia that are nonscarring early in their course, yet result in scarring later in their course. Examples of biphasic alopecia include patterned hair loss and traction alopecia. Another proposed classification scheme divides hair loss into permanent and nonpermanent alopecia. For the purposes of our discussion, we will continue to use the terms scarring and nonscarring, as they are widely accepted and firmly entrenched in the literature.

Hair loss in the setting of systemic disease may occur through one of five mechanisms (Table 43-1): telogen effluvium, anagen arrest, and hair miniaturization (all forms of nonscarring alopecia); scarring alopecia; and hair shaft disorders. An important concept in the evaluation and diagnosis of hair disorders is that more than one mechanism may be operating at a given time. This can amplify the degree of hair loss, modify its pattern, and complicate the clinical picture.

Telogen Effluvium

The most common cause of hair loss associated with systemic disease is telogen effluvium (TE). This form of nonscarring alopecia manifests with diffuse, nonscarring hair shedding, often with an abrupt onset. The shedding is a result of disruption of the normal hair cycle such that a large number of hairs synchronize their growth cycles reaching a catagen and subsequent telogen phase around the same time. This can be triggered by a metabolic or hormonal stress or by drugs (severe illness, infections, medications, surgical procedures or anesthesia, and endocrinopathies). About 3 to 4 months (the time it takes for a hair to move through catagen and the early stages of telogen), after a precipitating event, normal-appearing club hairs begin to fall out in large numbers. Often the patient may recall one of the precipitating events listed in Table 43-2.

According to Headington, telogen effluvium can be further divided into five subtypes, depending on which portion of the hair cycle is pathologically lengthened or shortened. These subtypes are immediate anagen release, delayed anagen release, short anagen, immediate telogen release, and delayed telogen release. There is much overlap between the types, and it is often impossible to distinguish one from another in the clinical setting.

Immediate Anagen Release

Immediate anagen release accounts for most cases of telogen effluvium. Most drugs and physiologic stressors including febrile illness trigger hair loss by this mechanism. As the name suggests, the anagen phase is cut short, and hairs prematurely enter the telogen phase. Immediate anagen release has a rapid onset, usually about 3 to 5 weeks after the inciting event.

Delayed Anagen Release

Delayed anagen release occurs when hairs are retained in the anagen phase longer than usual and then move on to the catagen and telogen phase around the same time. A classic example of delayed anagen release is postpartum telogen effluvium. Metabolic and endocrine changes during pregnancy prolong the anagen phase. Upon normalization of these factors after delivery, hairs enter telogen, and new mothers experience heavy hair shedding. This also accounts for the loss of lanugo hairs in a newborn, which occurs in a synchronous molt shortly after birth. This neonatal shedding is sometimes referred to as a physiologic effluvium.

Short Anagen

Idiopathic shortening of the anagen cycle may result in a mild but persistent increased shedding. Because the duration of anagen is a major factor in determining hair length, short anagen precludes growth of long hair. Some believe that this is the mechanism underlying chronic telogen effluvium. Notably, shedding is typically not noticed until the duration of anagen is reduced by 50%.

Immediate Telogen Release

Immediate telogen release results from a shortening of the normal telogen cycle. There is good evidence that drugs such as minoxidil exert their effect via immediate telogen release, with affected follicles promptly stimulated to enter anagen. Telogen release typically begins within days of the insult, which accounts for the increased shedding some patients experience in the first days and weeks of minoxidil use.

Delayed Telogen Release

Delayed telogen release is far more common in the animal kingdom than in humans. It is by this mechanism that some animals shed their winter fur when spring arrives. Hair is shed synchronously as large numbers of telogen hairs are released, giving way to a new anagen cycle. Although the exact mechanism is not clear, this process is thought to be driven by a neuro-optic signal. Delayed telogen release may also account for the seasonal shedding that some humans experience.

Telogen Effluvium and Drugs

Medications usually cause telogen effluvium in the form of immediate anagen release. Some of the more commonly associated drugs are listed in Table 43-3. While these medications span a wide range of drug classes, cardiovascular medications are heavily represented (anticoagulants, beta blockers, angiotensin-converting enzyme inhibitors). A few (i.e., captopril, quinacrine, nadolol, sulfasalazine) have been associated with a histologically inflammatory telogen effluvium. In the last 10 years, a number of new, biologically targeted, chemotherapeutic agents have become available. Among these new agents are sunitinib, a multitargeted tyrosine kinase inhibitor, associated with alopecia in 6% of patients. Interestingly, sunitinib reportedly causes hair color change in approximately 10% of patients. While the mechanism of alopecia in patients taking sunitinib is not clear, telogen effluvium has been histologically confirmed in a patient taking a similar medication, nolotinib. Similarly, selumetinib, a MEK1 and MEK2 inhibitor, causes alopecia in 9% of patients.

Telogen Effluvium and Androgenetic Alopecia

Telogen effluvium and androgenetic alopecia are both relatively common diagnoses. When the two conditions coexist, patients experience a pattern hair loss that progresses more quickly than the usual course. Early-onset androgenetic alopecia is often accompanied by a brisk and episodic telogen effluvium. Androgenetic telogen effluvium is related to shortened cycle times as large scalp terminal hairs are miniaturized and shortened secondary to decreased matrix volume and reduced duration of anagen, respectively. Hair shedding is obvious only when large terminal hairs are being shed. With ensuing hair cycles, the involved follicles produce progressively miniaturized (vellus) hairs, whose loss is inapparent.

TABLE 43-3 Drugs Associated with Telogen Effluvium

Retinoids (etretinate, isotretinoin)
Anticoagulants (coumadin, heparin)
Antithyroid (propylthiouracil, methimazole)
Anticonvulsants (phenytoin, valproic acid, carbamazepine)
Heavy metals
β-Adrenergic blockers
Amphetamine
Bromocriptine
Captopril
Enalapril
Danazol
Levodopa
Lithium
Pyridostigmine

Chronic Telogen Effluvium

The usual course of telogen effluvium is self-limited. Chronic telogen effluvium occurs when the duration of hair shedding exceeds 6 months. Most common in middle-aged women, this is a diffuse, chronic, fluctuating form of hair loss that affects the entire scalp. Sometimes confused with androgenetic alopecia, chronic telogen effluvium may cause diffuse thinning and bitemporal recession, but severe and obvious balding is rare. Notably, chronic telogen effluvium is a diagnosis of exclusion rather than being linked to an identifiable underlying etiology.

Diagnosis and Treatment

The distinctive history of abrupt onset, diffuse hair shedding and an identifiable inciting event make telogen effluvium a straightforward clinical diagnosis. Despite this, androgenetic alopecia and diffuse alopecia areata should be considered in the differential diagnosis. Patients with telogen effluvium often describe loss of the most hair when showering in addition to finding hairs on clothing, on the bathroom floor, and in their vehicles. Such heavy loss sometimes prompts patients to collect their lost hairs and bring them to an office visit. A patient who presents with a large bag of shed hair is very likely to have telogen effluvium as their diagnosis. Reduced hair volume is typically apparent to the patient after the loss of about 20% of the hair. However, normal hair density may be reduced by up to 50% before thinning is apparent to clinicians. If alopecia is clinically obvious, the loss appears diffuse (Fig. 43-2). In the typical patient with telogen effluvium, the telogen count seldom exceeds 50%. However, in some documented cases, telogen counts can reach up to 80%. Patients with more than 80% telogen hair counts

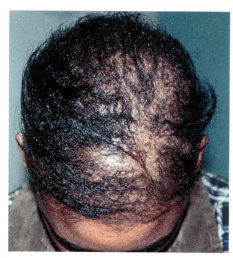

FIGURE 43-2 ■ Young woman with diffusely thin hair from telogen effluvium.

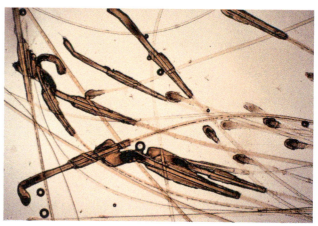

FIGURE 43-4 ■ Forcible hair pluck in a patient with telogen effluvium. A mixture of normal-appearing telogen hairs and anagen hairs is found, but in this case the percentage of telogen hairs exceeds 30%.

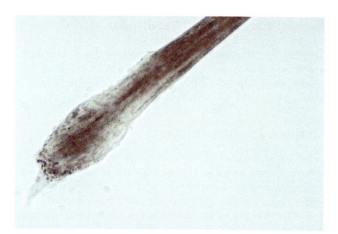

FIGURE 43-3 ■ Spontaneously shed telogen hair. These are increased in a number in patients with telogen effluvium.

probably do not represent a simple case of telogen effluvium. A detailed medical, dietary, and drug history is essential in establishing a diagnosis of telogen effluvium.

Physical examination of any patient with hair loss should begin with an overall inspection of the patient's hair density. The scalp of a patient with telogen effluvium should appear within normal limits, without erythema or scale (unless there is a secondary diagnosis). A hair pull test, in which 25 to 50 hairs are pulled with firm and consistent traction from root to tip, should be done in four quadrants. Patients with telogen effluvium will have a positive result, i.e., more than three hair shafts, the roots of which show the depigmented, keratinized, clubbed morphology of telogen hairs (Fig. 43-3). The patient should not have shampooed for at least one day prior to the hair pull test. A forcible hair pluck extracts a mixture of normal anagen and telogen hairs and an occasional catagen hair. The percentage of telogen hairs is increased, a criterion without which the diagnosis of telogen effluvium cannot be established with certainty (Fig. 43-4). On biopsy, a 4-mm scalp punch specimen should contain 25 to 50 terminal follicles. When more than 12% to 15% of hairs are in telogen, a diagnosis of telogen effluvium is likely.

The cornerstone of telogen effluvium management is reassurance. Once an underlying cause is identified, patients can be advised that this is a self-limiting process that runs a predictable course and then corrects itself. Reassurance can also be facilitated by educating patients about the pathophysiology behind the process including the fact that each shed hair is being replaced by a newly growing hair.

Anagen Arrest

Anagen arrest occurs when there is a sudden halt in the mitotic activity of the hair matrix cells. Hair shafts become severely dystrophic, tapering to a point, like the tip of a sharpened pencil. At this point, even minimal trauma causes breakage of the distal hair shaft. Although anagen arrest is sometimes referred to as anagen effluvium, this is a misnomer because only tapered shafts and not entire anagen hairs are shed. Since this process is not dependent on the hair cycle, breakage occurs quickly after the inciting event, usually within 1 to 2 weeks. Because approximately 85% of hairs are in anagen phase at any time, anagen arrest results in very extensive hair loss.

All therapeutic measures intended to inhibit the proliferation of actively dividing cells can cause the dramatic hair loss seen in anagen arrest. The classic example of noninflammatory anagen arrest occurs in the setting of a chemotherapeutic drug given systemically to treat a malignancy. The various agents may act in different ways (e.g., as antimetabolites or alkylating agents), but they all inhibit metabolism of rapidly dividing anagen matrix cells. Anagen arrest is more common and severe with combination chemotherapy than with the use of a single drug, and the severity is usually dose-dependent. The most severe hair loss occurs with doxorubicin, the nitrosoureas, and cyclophosphamide. Anticancer doses of radiation therapy have a similar effect on hair follicles (Fig. 43-5). Other agents causing anagen arrest are listed in Table 43-4. Of note, both thallium and X-irradiation have been used with the intention of causing total hair depilation for therapeutic purposes. Anagen arrest may also be caused by endocrine diseases, trauma or pressure, and pemphigus vulgaris.

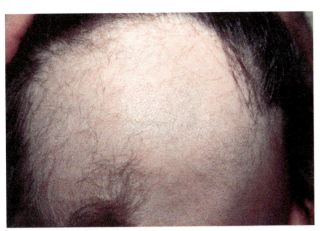

FIGURE 43-5 ■ Anagen arrest secondary to radiotherapy for an intracranial malignancy. Although eventual hair regrowth is expected in such cases, high enough doses of radiation can result in permanent hair loss.

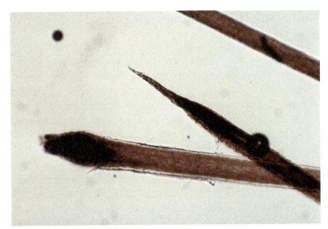

FIGURE 43-6 ■ Spontaneously shed "pencil point" hairs in a patient with anagen arrest who received systemic chemotherapy. Hair shafts taper abruptly to a point and are shed.

TABLE 43-4 Systemic Causes of Anagen Arrest

Noninflammatory
Anticancer chemotherapy
Drugs (colchicine, levodopa, cyclosporine, bismuth)
Radiation therapy
Endocrine diseases
Trauma/pressure
Toxins (poisons, e.g., thallium, boron, arsenic)

Inflammatory
Alopecia areata, totalis, or universalis
Systemic lupus erythematosus (patchy)
Secondary syphilis (patchy or diffuse)

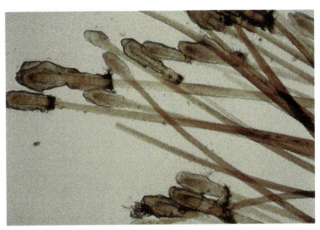

FIGURE 43-7 ■ Forcible hair pluck in a patient who had already experienced massive hair loss from systemic chemotherapy. Only the shafts of telogen hairs remain in the scalp, and so the hair count is 100% telogen hairs.

Anagen arrest may also have an inflammatory etiology. The classic example is alopecia totalis, in which the rapid onset and progression can resemble the hair loss associated with chemotherapy. Presumably, the inflammatory infiltrate surrounding the anagen hair bulb is related to the metabolic shutdown. Although the exact mechanism is unknown, perhaps there is a release of cytokines that inhibit epithelial growth. The patchy hair loss seen in some systemic lupus erythematosus patients and the patchy or diffuse hair loss seen in secondary syphilis are other examples of inflammatory anagen arrest. However, it should be noted that anagen arrest is only one of several mechanisms leading to hair loss in patients with systemic lupus erythematosus or syphilis.

Diagnosis and Treatment

Anagen arrest is a straightforward diagnosis with an appropriate history, extensive hair loss, and a hair pull test productive of dystrophic anagen hairs demonstrating tapered, pencil-point ends (Fig. 43-6). Follicles demonstrate a normal anagen to telogen ratio because of the abrupt onset of anagen arrest. This is demonstrated histologically in horizontal punch biopsy sections. Because hairs are rapidly shed over the course of only a few weeks in anagen arrest, if a cluster of hairs is forcibly plucked late in the course of shedding, virtually all of them will be telogen, as most of the anagen hairs have already shed (Fig. 43-7). This is in contrast to telogen effluvium, where the telogen count rarely exceeds 50% and the remaining hairs are all normal anagen hairs.

Identification and treatment of the underlying cause of hair loss is key to the treatment of anagen arrest. Multiple strategies have been attempted to reduce chemotherapy-induced hair loss including application of a pressure cuff around the scalp and local hypothermia during the infusion of the medication. Use of a topical vasoconstrictor has also been proposed. Each of these techniques is designed to spare the scalp from exposure to the chemotherapeutic agent. It should be noted that because the scalp may act as a safe house for circulating malignant cells, patients with hematologic malignancies are usually not candidates for these procedures. Topical minoxidil has been used unsuccessfully in efforts to prevent chemotherapy-induced alopecia; however, it seems to hasten regrowth once chemotherapy is complete. In most cases, alopecia due to anagen arrest is completely reversible; however, regrown hair sometimes demonstrates a different color or texture than the hair that was lost. In addition, certain chemotherapy regimens such as high-dose busulfan and cyclophosphamide and high-dose radiation are increasingly reported to cause permanent alopecia.

Androgenetic Alopecia/Hair Miniaturization

Androgenetic alopecia is the third nonscarring mechanism by which alopecia can be associated with systemic disease. In androgenetic alopecia, a complex interplay of genetic and hormonal influences combines to result in changes in follicular architecture and deviations in the hair growth cycle. There is shortening of the anagen phase and a reduction in the volume of the hair matrix cells. These two forces in combination result in the conversion of terminal hairs into the short and fine vellus hairs characteristically seen in patterned baldness. In addition, whereas the telogen phase remains stable, the latency between telogen and new anagen is found to increase in androgenetic alopecia.

The mechanisms underlying hair miniaturization in adulthood have been an area of intense study. Initially, the pathophysiology in men and women was thought to be identical. In men with androgenetic alopecia, increased levels of dihydrotestosterone (DHT) and 5α-reductase are found in hair follicles in the frontal region of the scalp. Hair follicles miniaturize under the direct influence of DHT, and its blockade leads to stabilization and sometimes reversal of the miniaturization. Similar blockage of DHT in women does not consistently produce the same results. For this reason, pattern hair loss (male or female) is a more accurate description of this disease. Younger women (ages 20 to 40) who experience pattern hair loss are more likely to have a strong family history of pattern baldness and are more likely to have an underlying androgen excess. The term senescent alopecia has been proposed to describe pattern alopecia in men and women that begins after age 60. This is much more closely attributed to age than to hormone actions.

The cause of hyperandrogenism can be excessive androgen production, hereditary hypersensitivity to androgen action, or a combination of the two. Excessive androgen production may be associated with acne, hirsutism, and irregular menstrual periods. Syndromes of androgen excess include polycystic ovarian syndrome, late-onset congenital adrenal hyperplasia (Fig. 43-8), Cushing's syndrome, and the HAIR-AN syndrome (i.e., hyperandrogenism, insulin resistance, and acanthosis nigricans).

In males, a number of epidemiologic studies have linked androgenetic alopecia to increased risk for ischemic heart disease, hypertension, and the metabolic syndrome. More recently, an association between prostate cancer and androgenetic alopecia has been proposed.

Diagnosis and Treatment

Androgenetic alopecia or pattern hair loss is a clinical diagnosis made in the setting of gradual progressive hair thinning in a typical location on the scalp. In men, the distribution is symmetric and bilateral, affecting the frontotemporal and vertex scalp. In women, the crown is preferentially affected with preservation of the frontal hairline. While some variation in these patterns exists, the classic findings are quantified by using the Norwood–Hamilton scale for men and the Ludwig scale for women. If androgen excess is suspected, serum hormone levels

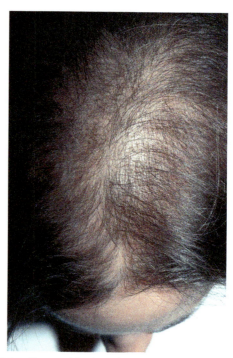

FIGURE 43-8 ■ Severe thinning of the hair on the crown (androgenetic alopecia) in a 14-year-old girl with late-onset congenital adrenal hyperplasia. This patient's hair loss prompted an endocrinologic evaluation.

should be checked. One can easily screen women for hormonal abnormalities by inquiring about cystic acne, irregular menses, infertility, galactorrhea, and virilization. If none of these are present, the patient is unlikely to have a hormonal abnormality.

The only Food and Drug Administration-approved medication for women with androgenetic alopecia is minoxidil. This topically applied medication acts as an arterial vasodilator and enhances DNA synthesis in follicular keratinocytes. This results in thickening of the shafts of miniaturized hairs, although minoxidil's exact mechanism of action is not completely understood. In men, minoxidil is an option as well as finasteride. Finasteride is an orally administered 5α-reductase inhibitor, which exerts its effect by significantly reducing scalp follicle DHT. It is not approved for use in women as it can lead to significant birth defects (genital abnormalities in a male fetus). Finally, surgical hair restoration is a therapeutic option for both men and women. This procedure involves taking hairs from the less androgen-sensitive occipital scalp and redistributing them to the affected vertex or frontal scalp.

Scarring Alopecia (Cicatricial Alopecia)

As the name suggests, scarring alopecia results in the permanent destruction of hair follicles. Scarring alopecia that occurs in the setting of systemic disease can be classified into one of two categories: primary and secondary. In the primary form, hair follicles are destroyed as a result of being a direct target of the process, as in lichen planopilaris, for example (Fig. 43-9) or discoid lupus erythematosus. Intervening dermis is often spared. In secondary scarring alopecia, hair follicles are destroyed as a consequence of nearby activity. Diagnoses causing secondary

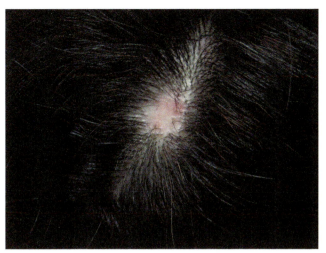

FIGURE 43-9 ■ Scarring alopecia due to lichen planopilaris.

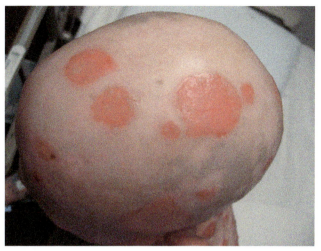

FIGURE 43-11 ■ Patient with active lesions of cutaneous T-cell lymphoma causing scarring hair loss in a multifocal manner across the scalp.

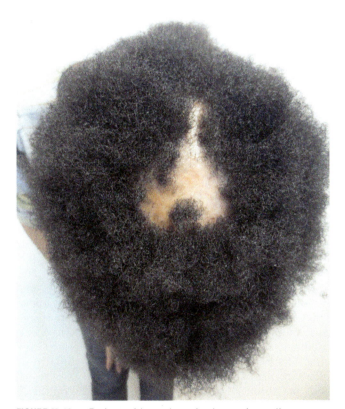

FIGURE 43-10 ■ Patient with an alopecic plaque due to linear morphea involving the scalp.

scarring alopecia are generally infiltrative, infectious, metastatic, or genetic in origin. The exact mechanism of follicular destruction in secondary scarring alopecia may be direct compression, alteration of blood supply, or release of injurious cytokines from infiltrating cells. Some examples of diseases causing secondary scarring alopecia are sarcoidosis, linear morphea of the scalp (en coup de sabre) (Fig. 43-10), and cutaneous T-cell lymphoma (Fig. 43-11). Infectious causes include cutaneous tuberculosis, leprosy, syphilis, and leishmaniasis. Visceral cancers that metastasize to the skin, including renal cell and breast carcinoma, may cause scarring alopecia by crowding out the hair follicles. Likewise, sufficient ischemia or pressure, radiation, and chemotherapy can lead to secondary scarring alopecia, as can bullous disorders such as cicatricial pemphigoid and epidermolysis bullosa. Finally, hereditary disorders such as incontinentia pigmenti or keratitis–ichthyosis–deafness (KID) syndrome have been associated with secondary scarring alopecia (Table 43-5).

Diagnosis and Treatment

The skin overlying a scarring process characteristically demonstrates loss of follicular markings. It may appear smooth or show features of the underlying disease, for example the dyspigmentation seen in discoid lupus erythematosus. A biopsy, which must be taken from an area of active disease rather than from one of old scarring, may be required to determine the underlying disease process. If biopsy is performed, both horizontal and vertical sectioning are recommended. Horizontal (transverse) sections allow for assessment of follicular distribution, number and type, and for visualization of all follicles at different levels. Vertical sections allow for visualization of the dermoepidermal junction and any alterations associated with the infundibular epidermis and the adjacent dermis. Additional tests such as elastin, PAS (periodic acid-Schiff), and mucin stains as well as direct immunofluorescence may also be helpful when the primary diagnosis is unclear.

Treatment options are of limited value once scarring has occurred since the hair cannot regrow once the follicle has been replaced with a scar. Therefore, aggressive therapy early in the disease course of conditions that can result in scarring alopecia is critical. Therapy should be targeted at controlling the underlying process with a goal of halting progression of loss.

Hair Shaft Disorders

Hair shaft disorders, also called trichodystrophies, may be congenital or acquired. Acquired forms include hair

TABLE 43-5 Causes of Scarring Alopecia

Primary
Discoid lupus erythematosus
Lichen planopilaris
Frontal fibrosing alopecia
Central centrifugal cicatricial alopecia
Pseudopalade
Folliculitis decalvans
Dissecting cellulitis
Acne keloidalis nuchae
Alopecia mucinosa

Secondary
Infectious
    Bacterial
    Viral
    Fungal
    Leprosy
    Leishmaniasis
    Tertiary syphilis
Inflammatory/autoimmune
    Cicatricial bullous pemphigoid
    Linear morphea (en coup de sabre)
    Graft-versus-host disease
    Sarcoidosis
Physical/chemical destruction
    Ischemia
    Thermal injury
    Radiation therapy
    Drugs (e.g., high-dose chemotherapy)
Neoplastic
Hereditary (e.g., keratitis–ichthyosis–deafness [KID] syndrome, incontinentia pigmenti)

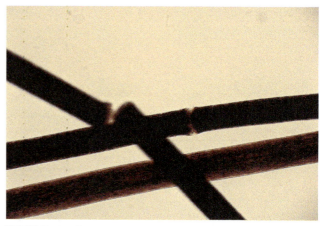

FIGURE 43-12 ■ Trichoschisis in a patient with trichothiodystrophy.

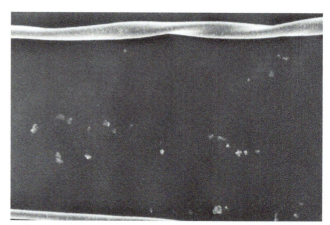

FIGURE 43-13 ■ Pili torti in a patient with Menkes' kinky hair syndrome.

changes seen in individuals with HIV. Straightening of previously curly hair has frequently been reported in this population as well as hair shaft dystrophy ranging from mild to severe with variation in hair shaft diameter, longitudinal ridging, cuticular loss, and trichoschisis. There are many potential mechanisms for these changes including HIV infection itself, secondary infections, immune and endocrine dysfunction, and medications. Nutritional deficiencies may also contribute. Hair loss is common in patients with systemic lupus erythematosus, affecting 70% of patients at some point in their disease course. For those with discoid lesions, hair loss is a scarring process as previously mentioned. For others, hair breakage along the frontal hairline is referred to as lupus hair. Other acquired phenomena that may cause trichodystrophy are excessive grooming (i.e., combing, brushing, heat styling) and chemical application.

There are several congenital syndromes that include hair shaft disorders. In trichothiodystrophy, the hairs are excessively brittle and subject to transverse fractures (trichoschisis) (Fig. 43-12) secondary to reduced sulfur content. The hair shows alternating bright and dark regions (tiger tail hair) with polarizing microscopy. Other features of trichothiodystrophy may include ichthyosis, short stature, mental deficiency, photosensitivity, nail dystrophy, seizures, and infertility. Various names have been associated with different combinations of these physical findings, including Tay syndrome and PIBIDS (photosensitivity, ichthyosis, brittle hair, impaired intelligence, decreased fertility, and short stature). Pili torti, a malformation in which the hair is twisted on its own axis, leads to brittle and easily broken hairs. Classic pili torti, which follows a dominant inheritance pattern, usually starts in early childhood and improves by puberty. However, pili torti has also been associated with trichothiodystrophy, anorexia nervosa, Bjornstad's syndrome, Crandall's syndrome, and isotretinoin and etretinate therapy. Menkes' kinky hair syndrome, a disorder of copper transport, results in abnormal neurodevelopment, connective tissue problems such as skin laxity, and premature death. Psychomotor retardation is noted in the first few months of life, with drowsiness, impaired temperature regulation, and convulsions. The defective gene is located on the X chromosome (Xq13), and encodes a highly evolutionary conserved, copper-transporting P-type ATPase. This gene is expressed in nearly every human tissue, explaining the multisystem nature of the disorder. The hair is pale, brittle, and demonstrates pili torti (Fig. 43-13).

Diagnosis and Management

Some hair shaft disorders can be appreciated with the naked eye; however, microscopic examination of hair shafts is recommended. This evaluation, in addition to a thorough and comprehensive family history, should secure a diagnosis. When in doubt, a genetics consultation may help. Treatment of hair shaft disorders should be targeted toward correcting the primary disorder if possible. In addition, gentle hair care to minimize trauma should be employed. Some hair shaft disorders improve gradually with age.

EXCESSIVE HAIR

There are two mechanisms by which systemic disease may cause increased hair growth: hypertrichosis and hirsutism.

Hypertrichosis

Hypertrichosis is the excessive growth of nonandrogen-dependent hair. Hypertrichosis may be localized or generalized, congenital or acquired. Hypertrichosis may occur via one of two major mechanisms: the conversion of vellus to terminal hairs; or via changes in the hair growth cycle.

Many congenital causes of hypertrichosis exist. One of the most striking forms is congenital hypertrichosis lanuginosa. This is a rare syndrome in which lanugo hair growth persists throughout life instead of being shed in the first few months of life. Patients grow excessively long, fine hairs on all hair-bearing sites. In a variant of this disorder, congenital hypertrichosis terminalis, patients continuously grow terminal hairs all over the body. The latter variant is almost always associated with gingival hyperplasia. Localized patches of hypertrichosis can also occur congenitally, with or without an underlying nevus. These are usually benign and isolated except when located at the base of the spine, which may be an indication of spina bifida. Large congenital melanocytic nevi, which may place the patient at an increased risk for developing malignant melanoma, may be hypertrichotic. Cornelia de Lange syndrome is a congenital disorder in which patients exhibit physical and mental retardation, characteristic facies, and irregular teeth as well as hypertrichotic eyelashes, extensive vellus hypertrichosis on the trunk, posterior neck and elbows, and thick and convergent eyebrows (synophrys). Other causes of congenital hypertrichosis are listed in Table 43-6.

Acquired localized hypertrichosis may be seen in several settings. It can be associated with an underlying disease such as thrombophlebitis, osteomyelitis, or lichen simplex chronicus. It can also occur in skin that has been occluded under a plaster cast. Localized hypertrichosis in the form of trichomegaly (enlarged eyelashes) can be acquired in the setting of HIV or, rarely, systemic lupus erythematosus. Generalized hypertrichosis can be acquired in association with acrodynia, a reaction to chronic mercury exposure, and in children with hypothyroidism. Juvenile dermatomyositis has been associated with hypertrichosis, most prominent on the face and limbs. Generalized hypertrichosis has also been reported in 36% of patients with bulimia nervosa and 77% of patients with anorexia nervosa. Acquired hypertrichosis lanuginosa, also known as "malignant down," is a well-documented cutaneous manifestation of internal malignancy, most commonly cancer of the lung or colon. Drugs associated with hypertrichosis are listed in Table 43-7.

TABLE 43-6 Causes of Congenital Hypertrichosis

Congenital hypertrichosis lanuginosa
Large congenital melanocytic nevi
Cornelia de Lange syndrome
Fetal hydantoin syndrome
Fetal alcohol syndrome
Mucopolysaccharidoses
- Hunter's syndrome
- Sanfilippo syndrome
- Hurler's syndrome

Porphyrias
- Porphyria cutanea tarda
- Erythropoietic protoporphyria
- Erythropoietic porphyria
- Variegate porphyria

TABLE 43-7 Drugs Associated with Hypertrichosis

Dilantin
Streptomycin
Latanoprost
Cyclosporine
Psoralens
Diazoxide
Minoxidil
Acetazolamide

Diagnosis and Treatment

When hypertrichosis is secondary to an underlying condition, management of that condition will often result in its resolution. However, when hypertrichosis is congenital, or when it is a significant cosmetic concern, a number of treatment modalities exist. Albeit temporary, several mechanical and chemical depilatory methods may be used. Electrolysis involves the destruction of the follicle by a direct electric current. Thermolysis involves destruction of the follicle by the heat produced by an alternating electric current. The efficacy of both of these methods is operator-dependent, but considered permanent when performed correctly. Laser hair removal has gained tremendous popularity and can be very effective for dark, coarse hair. Unfortunately, fine, lanugo hairs are not an ideal target for laser hair removal given their light color and do not respond to treatment. Topical eflornithine hydrochloride, an inhibitor of ornithine decarboxylase, is approved for the treatment of increased facial hair in women, but is used off-label by many patients. It slows hair growth, probably by inhibiting cell synthetic or mitotic function. Its use may decrease the frequency with which patients must use mechanical methods of hair removal.

There are circumstances in which hypertrichosis is desired. Agents that provide enhancement of thinning hair include the prostaglandin analogs bimatoprost, for eyelash hypotrichosis, and minoxidil, for pattern hair loss of the scalp.

Hirsutism

Hirsutism is the excessive growth of androgen-dependent terminal body hair. In the clinical realm, hirsutism

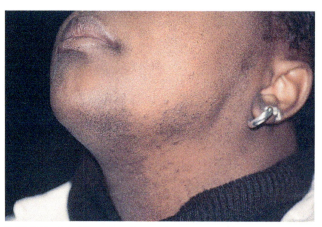

FIGURE 43-14 ■ Hirsutism in the beard area of a woman with polycystic ovarian syndrome.

commonly describes male-patterned body hair growth occurring in a female. The amount of hair growth that is considered abnormal depends on cultural factors and race. Affected patients grow hair in places in which terminal hair is not typically found, such as the face, chest, abdomen, and back in a woman (Fig. 43-14). Hirsutism, acne, and androgenetic alopecia are the cutaneous manifestations of hyperandrogenic states. Alternatively, patients may have normal androgen levels but increased sensitivity to circulating androgens. Hirsutism may be genetic or secondary to adrenal, ovarian, or mixed adrenal and ovarian etiologies (Table 43-8). Polycystic ovarian syndrome is the most common cause of abnormal androgen production, and in addition to the cutaneous signs of hyperandrogenism, may also be characterized by irregular menstrual periods, insulin resistance, hypertension, and dyslipidemia. Hirsutism may also be associated with acromegaly and thyroid dysfunction. Anabolic steroids, androgenic progestins, and glucocorticoids are iatrogenic causes of hirsutism.

Diagnosis and Treatment

Before embarking on a litany of expensive laboratory studies, hirsute patients can be roughly screened for hormonal abnormalities with a thorough history. One should inquire about cystic acne, regular menses, infertility, and galactorrhea. If these are absent and there is a family history of hirsute women, the patient is unlikely to have any underlying hormonal imbalance. If indicated, laboratory studies can be used to rule out serious underlying disorders in the hirsute patient.

The medical treatment of hirsutism consists of suppressing ovarian or adrenal androgen secretion, or of blocking androgen action in the skin. Oral contraceptives and antiandrogens such as spironolactone, cyproterone acetate, and flutamide have been used therapeutically. Glucocorticoids, gonadotropin-releasing hormone agonists such as leuprolide, and insulin-sensitizing agents have also been used. Although the endocrinologic evaluation and treatment of hirsutism are beyond the scope of this chapter, excellent references are available. Cosmetic improvement of hirsutism may be achieved via the previously mentioned modalities.

TABLE 43-8 Etiologies of Hirsutism

Adrenal
Congenital adrenal hyperplasia
Cushing's syndrome
Androgen-secreting adrenal tumors
Severe insulin resistance

Ovarian
Androgen-secreting adrenal tumors

Combined adrenal/ovarian
Polycystic ovarian syndrome
Idiopathic (including increased skin sensitivity to androgens)

Other
Androgen therapy
Anabolic steroids
Androgenic progestins
Glucocorticoids
Hyperprolactinemia
Thyroid dysfunction
Acromegaly

SUGGESTED READING

Blume U, Ferracin J, et al. Physiology of the vellus hair follicle: hair growth and sebum excretion. Br J Dermatol 1991;124(1):21–8.
Drake L, Hordinsky M, Fiedler V, et al. The effects of finasteride on scalp skin and serum androgen levels in men with androgenetic alopecia. J Am Acad Dermatol 1999;41:550–4.
Giles GG, Severi G, Sinclair R, et al. Androgenetic alopecia and prostate cancer: findings from an Australian case-control study. Cancer Epidemiol Biomark Prev 2002;11:549–53.
Headington JT. Telogen effluvium. Arch Dermatol 1993;129:356–63.
Hunt N, McHale S. The psychological impact of alopecia. BMJ 2005;331:951–3.
Khumalo NP. African hair length: the picture is clearer. J Am Acad Dermatol 2006;54:886–8.
Kuster W, Happle R. The inheritance of common baldness: two B or not two B? J Am Acad Dermatol 1984;5:921–6.
McMichael AJ. Hair and scalp disorders in ethnic populations. Dermatol Clin 2003;21:629–44.
Rittmaster RS. Hirsutism. Lancet 1997;349:191–5.
Sellheyer K, Bergfeld WF. Histopathologic evaluation of alopecias. Am J Dermatopathol 2006;28:236–59.
Sinclair R, Jolley J, Mallari R, et al. Morphological approach to hair disorders. J Investig Dermatol Symp Proc 2003;8:56–64.
Soref CM, Fahl WE. A new strategy to prevent chemotherapy and radiotherapy-induced alopecia using topically applied vasoconstrictors. Int J Cancer 2015;136(1):195–203.
van der Donk J, Hunfeld JAM, Passchier J, et al. Quality of life and maladjustment associated with hair loss in women with alopecia androgenica. Soc Sci Med 1994;33:159–63.
Wendelin DS, Pope DN, Mallory SB. Hypertrichosis. J Am Acad Dermatol 2003;48:161–79.
Whiting DA. Chronic telogen effluvium. Dermatol Clin 1996;14:723–31.
Whiting DA. Cicatricial alopecia: clinico-pathological findings and treatment. Clin Dermatol 2001;18:211–25.
Wolfram LJ. Human hair: a unique physiochemical composite. J Am Acad Dermatol 2003;48:S106–14.

CHAPTER 44

NAIL SIGNS OF SYSTEMIC DISEASE

Shari R. Lipner • Richard K. Scher

KEY POINTS

- A complete and detailed history and physical examination of all 20 nails is essential in evaluating patients with suspected manifestations of systemic disease.
- Subacute bacterial endocarditis is the most common systemic cause of splinter hemorrhages, which occur proximally and are typically present in multiple nails.
- Muehrcke lines, half-and-half nails, and Terry nails are all examples of apparent leukonychia, in which there is abnormal nail bed vasculature, thereby changing the translucency of the nail plate. On physical exam, the whiteness disappears with pressure and is unaffected by nail growth.
- Yellow nail syndrome is characterized by the triad of yellow nails, lymphedema, and respiratory tract involvement. Nails are thick and yellow, with an increased transverse curvature, absent cuticles, and slow growth rate.

The nails are unique from other appendages in that they often offer a glimpse into systemic conditions. Therefore, a fundamental understanding of nail unit anatomy is essential to appreciate nail abnormalities and their relationship to systemic diseases (Fig. 44-1). The nail apparatus is composed of a hard and durable nail plate that lies above the nail bed and the distal portion of the nail matrix, which is seen distally as the white "half-moon"-shaped area known as the lunula. The remaining part of the matrix lies below the proximal nail fold. The undersurface of the proximal nail fold forms the eponychium (cuticle). The nail bed lies beneath the nail plate and above the distal phalanx. Due to its rich blood supply, the nail bed appears as a reddish area extending from the lunula to the area just proximal to the free edge of the nail. The proximal and lateral nail folds border the nail plate, and the hyponychium is the area under the free edge and the distal portion of the nail plate. The blood supply to the nail arises from the superficial and deep palmar branches of the digital arteries.

The nail plate is hard and durable due to its composition of keratins and sulfur, the latter in the form of cysteine. The mitotically active nail matrix forms the nail plate keratin. The proximal third of the matrix forms the upper third of the nail plate; the middle part of the matrix, the midportion; and the distal third of the matrix gives rise to the lower third of the plate. Therefore, by using knowledge of this anatomy, melanin in the nail plate may be traced back to its origin in either the distal or proximal matrix to guide an appropriate biopsy if necessary.

A complete and detailed history and physical examination of all 20 nails is essential in evaluating patients with suspected manifestations of systemic disease. While some nail findings may be characteristic of certain diseases, others may narrow the differential diagnosis, allowing an appropriate work-up to be initiated.

ANATOMIC CHANGES OF THE NAIL UNIT (TABLE 44-1)

Nail Matrix and Plate Abnormalities

Beau Lines

Beau lines are transverse grooves in the nail plate that arise due to temporary suppression of nail growth within the nail matrix and occur during periods of acute/chronic stress and/or systemic illness (Fig. 44-2). The precipitating event might be local trauma, paronychia, chemotherapeutic agents that are cytotoxic to the nail matrix, or abrupt onset of systemic disease. These grooves have also been described in association with rheumatic fever, malaria, pemphigus, Raynaud's disease, and myocardial infarction, as well as following deep-sea dives. The distance of the Beau line from the proximal nail fold will give the clinician an estimate of the time of the acute stress, using average growth rates of 3 mm/month for fingernails and 1 mm/month for toenails.

Mees Lines

Mees lines are 1- to 2-mm wide horizontal parallel white bands (leukonychia striata), which span the width of the nail plate, usually affecting all fingernails. They are associated with arsenic poisoning in most instances and may be used to identify the time of poisoning, since they require about 2 months to appear on the fingernails following the initial insult. Mees lines have also been described in association with numerous acute systemic stresses, such as acute renal failure, congestive heart failure, ulcerative colitis, breast cancer, infections such as measles and tuberculosis, systemic lupus erythematosus, and with exposure to other toxic metals such as thallium. Leukonychia striata is also commonly associated with trauma to the nail matrix, such as from manicuring. The clinician can differentiate between leukonychia striata caused by trauma and that associated with systemic disease because in the latter the lines run parallel to the lunula, have smoother borders, are

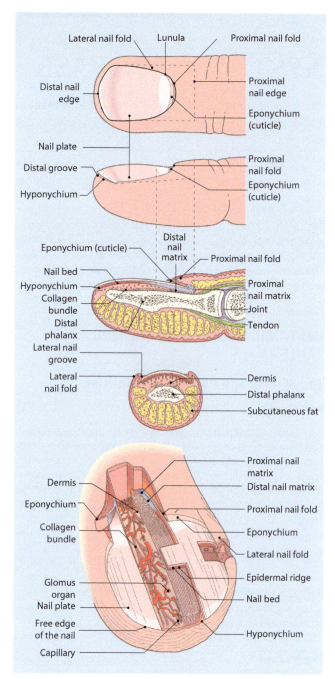

FIGURE 44-1 ■ Anatomic structure of the nail apparatus. (Reproduced with permission from Bologna JL, Jorizzo JL, Rapini RP, editors. Dermatology, 2nd ed. Chicago: Mosby; 2007.)

more homogeneous, span the width of the nail plate, and involve multiple nails. Mees lines are an example of true leukonychia, in which there is abnormal keratinization of the underlying nail matrix, resulting in parakeratosis within the nail plate and an opaque appearance on examination. The white discoloration is unaffected by pressure, and the opacity will move distally as the nail grows out.

Pitting

Nail pitting involves small depressions in the nail plate due to aberrant keratinization within the proximal nail matrix, resulting in clusters of parakeratotic cells within the nail plate. Nail pitting is a nonspecific finding and is associated with diseases affecting the proximal matrix, such as psoriasis, psoriatic arthritis, and reactive arthritis (Fig. 44-3). It has also been reported in association with alopecia areata, atopic dermatitis, Langerhans cell histiocytosis, and junctional epidermolysis bullosa.

Longitudinal Pigmented Bands (Melanonychia)

Longitudinal melanonychia refers to vertical bands of brown-black pigment in the nail plate and may be caused by blood from trauma, bacteria, fungus, HIV infection, drugs, endocrine disorders, exogenous pigment, or melanin. Longitudinal pigmented bands associated with internal disorders are usually present in multiple nails, and have been reported in Addison's disease, systemic sclerosis, leprosy, and following bilateral adrenalectomy for Cushing's disease. Longitudinal pigmented bands may also be caused by many medications, including bleomycin, fluoride, melphalan, cyclophosphamide, doxorubicin, paclitaxel, antimalarials, and zidovudine (Fig. 44-4). Dark transverse bands, on the other hand, may be associated with quinacrine, doxorubicin, and cyclophosphamide. Nitrogen mustard and methotrexate may produce diffuse hyperpigmentation of the nail plate.

Melanin is a pigment produced by melanocytes within the nail matrix and may be caused by benign processes such as benign melanocytic activation, lentigines, and nevi, or by malignant conditions such as melanoma. Fortunately, benign melanocytic activation and benign nevi are the most common causes of longitudinal melanonychia in adults and children, respectively.

Laugier–Hunziker syndrome is a rare acquired disorder characterized by diffuse gray to dark-brown macules, most predominantly located on the lips and oral mucosa. About 50% of patients also have accompanying longitudinal melanonychia of their fingernails.

Brittle Nails

Brittle nails may be a component of the brittle nail syndrome, which is a heterogeneous abnormality characterized by roughness of the surface of the nail plate, fragility or raggedness of the distal nail, splitting, and peeling. While the pathogenesis is not well understood, it is associated with an abnormality of keratin, keratin-associated proteins, water, and/or lipid content. There is also impairment of intercellular adhesion of the corneocytes of the nail plate. The majority of cases are idiopathic, but some are associated with systemic diseases including arterial insufficiency, Raynaud's phenomenon, iron deficiency, bronchiectasis, diabetes mellitus, osteoporosis, amyloidosis, hyper- and hypothyroidism, gout, tuberculosis, hypopituitarism, and sarcoidosis.

Koilonychia

Koilonychia is defined by a concave nail plate with eversion of distal and lateral edges, creating a nail that looks like a spoon. Fingernails are affected more often than toenails, and the second and third fingernails are

TABLE 44-1 Nail Findings and Associations

Nail Condition	Description	Causes/Associated Disease States
Anonychia/Micronychia	Total or partial absence of nail	Trauma; bullous diseases; idiopathic atrophy of the nails; psoriasiform acral dermatitis; ischemia; nail–patella syndrome; epidermolysis bullosa; ectodermal dysplasias; DOOR syndrome; Iso–Kikuchy syndrome
Beau lines	Transverse grooves in nail plate	Nonspecific; acute infection or other metabolic insult; renal failure; myocardial infarction; epilepsy; reflex sympathetic dystrophy or brachial plexopathy (unilateral); deep sea diving/mountain climbing; Heimler syndrome; Guillain–Barré syndrome; local trauma; paronychia; chemotherapy; rheumatic fever; malaria; pemphigus; Raynaud's phenomenon
Brittle nails (fragilitas unguium)	Roughness of nail plate, fragility of distal nail, splitting, peeling	Idiopathic; brittle nail syndrome; nutritional deficiency; thyroid dysfunction; glucagonoma; diabetes mellitus; trichothiodystrophy; drugs; trauma; arterial insufficiency; Raynaud's phenomenon; renal failure; ectodermal dysplasias; deposition disorders (gout, amyloidosis, etc.); osteoporosis; tuberculosis; bronchiectasis; hypopituitarism; sarcoidosis
Bywater's lesions	Hemorrhage/infarct of the nail folds	Rheumatoid arthritis-associated vasculitis
Clubbing	Loss of Lovibond's angle (angle between nail plate and proximal nail fold)	Nonspecific; idiopathic; hereditary; cardiac; pulmonary; gastrointestinal; renal; endocrine; vascular abnormality (aneurysm, fistula, shunt); lymphadenitis; Pancoast tumor; reflex sympathetic dystrophy (unilateral); erythromelalgia; acquired hypertrophic pulmonary osteoarthropathy
Koilonychia	Spoon-shaped nails	Idiopathic; hereditary (autosomal dominant); iron deficiency anemia; fungal infection; psoriasis; high altitude; trichothiodystrophy; Raynaud's phenomenon/ischemia; trauma; liver disease; gastrointestinal malignancies; normal children; infants (temporarily); porphyria; hemochromatosis; occupational
Leukonychia	White discoloration of nails (true or apparent)	True leukonychia (nail plate): zinc deficiency; trauma; chemotherapy; congestive heart failure; altitude changes (increase); infection; diabetes; lymphoma; Heimler's syndrome Apparent leukonychia (nail bed): see Lindsay nails (half-and-half nails); Terry nails; Muehrcke nails; renal; hypoalbuminemia
Lindsay nails/half-and-half nails	White discoloration of proximal half of nail bed, with reddish brown band distally; blanches with pressure	Chronic renal failure; Crohn's disease; Kawasaki disease; cirrhosis; zinc deficiency; chemotherapy; Behçet's disease; pellagra
Lunular color changes	Blue or red lunula	Blue—Wilson's disease; argyria; cyanosis; hereditary benign telangiectasia Red—congestive heart failure; emphysema; chronic obstructive pulmonary disease; chronic bronchitis; carbon monoxide poisoning; systemic lupus erythematosus; alopecia areata; vitiligo; lichen sclerosus; rheumatoid arthritis; psoriasis
Mees lines (Aldrich–Mees lines)	Transverse white bands (usually multiple nails) that grow out with nail plate; unaffected by pressure	Arsenic, thallium, or other heavy metal poisoning; infection; acute renal failure; congestive heart failure; ulcerative colitis; breast cancer; systemic lupus erythematosus
Melanonychia (longitudinal pigmented bands)	Vertical bands of brown or black pigment of the nail plate	Benign melanocytic activation; lentigines; nevi; Laugier–Hunziker syndrome; infection; PUVA therapy; Addison's disease; following adrenalectomy for Cushing's disease; drugs; exogenous pigment; endocrine disorders; trauma; medications; tumors—squamous cell carcinoma, melanoma (Hutchinson's sign = pigment involvement of proximal nail fold, worrisome for melanoma)
Muehrcke lines	Multiple (usually double) transverse white bands, parallel to lunula; unaffected by nail growth, blanch with pressure	Hypoalbuminemia; nephrotic syndrome; postcardiac transplantation; cardiomyopathy; ACTH-dependent Cushing's; Peutz–Jeghers syndrome with hepatic adenoma; chemotherapy; liver disease; malnutrition; HIV/AIDS
Proximal nail fold capillary abnormalities	Distortion of normal capillary architecture	Avascular portions with dilated capillary loops: systemic sclerosis; dermatomyositis Normal vascular density with tortuous capillaries: systemic lupus erythematosus
Onychocryptosis	Ingrown nail	Trauma; neglect; older age; highly active antiretroviral therapy for HIV (especially indinavir, ritonavir); Rubinstein–Taybi syndrome; Turner's syndrome; chemotherapy; epidermal growth factor receptor inhibitors

Continued

TABLE 44-1 Nail Findings and Associations—cont'd

Nail Condition	Description	Causes/Associated Disease States
Onycholysis (Plummer nails; photo-onycholysis)	Separation of the nail plate from the nail bed	Idiopathic; trauma; contact dermatitis; infection; psoriasis; lichen planus; yellow nail syndrome; thyroid disease; porphyria; diabetes mellitus; Raynaud's disease; acrodermatitis continua of Hallopeau; drugs (psoralens, doxycycline, fluoroquinolones)
Onychomadesis (onychoptosis)	Shedding of the nail plate and/or separation of the nail plate from the nail bed at the proximal nail fold	Stevens–Johnson syndrome/toxic epidermal necrolysis; infection; pemphigus vulgaris; epidermolysis bullosa, Kawasaki disease; dialysis; mycosis fungoides; alopecia universalis; critical illness; drugs; immunoglobulin class-switching recombination deficiencies
Onychomycosis/tinea unguium	Infection of the nail plate/bed with dermatophytes, yeasts, or nondermatophyte molds	Nonspecific; immunodeficiency states (HIV/AIDS); diabetes mellitus; older age; previous nail trauma; psoriasis; lichen planus
Onychorrhexis (see also brittle nails)	Longitudinal ridging and occasional splitting of the free nail edge	Older age; brittle nail syndrome; pemphigus vulgaris; psoriasis/psoriatic arthritis; Witkop's tooth and nail syndrome; Darier's disease; palmoplantar keratoderma (punctate); drugs; gasoline exposure
Onychoschizia	Horizontal splitting of the nail plate into layers	Trauma; brittle nail syndrome; chemical exposures; glucagonoma; HIV; pemphigus vulgaris
Paronychia/felon	Inflammation/infection of periungual skin	Nonspecific; Stevens–Johnson syndrome; diabetes mellitus; infection (*Candida, Staphylococcus*, herpes, syphilis, leprosy, leishmaniasis); antiretroviral therapy for HIV; chemotherapy (EGFR inhibitors, capecitabine)
Pseudoclubbing	Overcurvature of the nails transversely and longitudinally, with a normal Lovibond's angle	Hyperparathyroidism; subungual hemangioma; sarcoidosis; systemic sclerosis; nail bed tumors; psoriatic arthritis
Pincer nail (trumpet, plicated, tile-shaped nail)	Transverse overcurvature of the nail plate, pinching the nail bed distally	Systemic lupus erythematosus; colon carcinoma; epidermolysis bullosa (Dowling–Meara type); Kawasaki disease; drugs (β-blocker, SSRI); infection (tinea); psoriasis; tumors of nail unit (exostosis, implantation cyst, myxoid cyst); following placement of *arteriovenous* fistula in forearm; deformity of foot; osteoarthritis
Pitting	Small depressions in the nail plate	Nonspecific; psoriasis/psoriatic arthritis; reactive arthritis; lichen planus; alopecia areata; atopic dermatitis; Langerhans cell histiocytosis; junctional epidermolysis bullosa
Pterygium (dorsal)	Triangular or "wing"-shaped deformity in which the proximal nail fold attaches to the nail bed and/or matrix	Lichen planus; psoriasis/psoriatic arthritis; alopecia areata; porokeratoses; lichenoid graft-versus-host disease; Marfan's syndrome; dyskeratosis congenita; cicatricial pemphigoid; Stevens–Johnson syndrome/toxic epidermal necrolysis; burns; radiation dermatitis; Raynaud's phenomenon; peripheral vascular disease
Pterygium inversum (ventral)	Fusion of hyponychium to distal nail plate	Systemic sclerosis; stroke; acrylate allergy; trauma; systemic lupus erythematosus
Splinter hemorrhages	Thin, longitudinal red-brown lines in the nail plate	Nonspecific; trauma; subacute bacterial endocarditis (proximal may be more specific); mitral stenosis; other infection (trichinosis, fungal, septicemia); pregnancy; renal (dialysis, post-renal transplant, chronic glomerulonephritis); hepatic (cirrhosis, hepatitis); scurvy; vasculitis; juvenile cirrhosis; high altitudes; peptic ulcer disease; anemia; atopic dermatitis; psoriasis; rheumatoid arthritis; systemic lupus erythematosus; antiphospholipid syndrome; malignancy
Terry nails	White discoloration of proximal 80% of nail bed, with reddish brown band distally; blanches with pressure, unaffected by nail growth	Liver disease (cirrhosis, hypoalbuminemia); diabetes; congestive heart failure; thyrotoxicosis; malnutrition; older age; Reiter's syndrome; leprosy; POEMS (Crow–Fukase) syndrome; pulmonary tuberculosis; peripheral vascular disease
Trachyonychia/20 nail dystrophy	Rough, thin nails, longitudinal ridging	Lichen planus; psoriasis; pemphigus vulgaris; alopecia areata; ichthyoses; sarcoidosis; drugs; punctate palmoplantar keratoderma; reflex sympathetic dystrophy (unilateral)
Triangular lunulae	Triangular shape of lunulae	Nail–patella syndrome; cirrhosis; hypoalbuminemia
Whitlow	Enlargement and erythema of the distal digit	Cold painful whitlow: digital ischemia Cold painless whitlow: metastases to bone (fingers, from pulmonary source; toes, from genitourinary source) Warm painful whitlow: infection (herpetic)
Yellow nails	Yellow discoloration of nail plate	Yellow nail syndrome; pulmonary (asthma, tuberculosis, pleural effusion, chronic obstructive pulmonary disease); hypoalbuminemia; hepatic disease; HIV/AIDS; malignancy (laryngeal carcinoma, non-Hodgkin's lymphoma); lymphedema/lymphatic obstruction; rheumatoid arthritis (on gold therapy); medications

DOOR, Deafness, onychdystrophy, osteodystrophy, and mental retardation; PUVA, psoralens and UVA; ACTH, adrenocorticotropic hormone; AIDS, acquired immune deficiency syndrome; EGFR, epidermal growth factor receptor; SSRI, selective serotonin reuptake inhibitor; POEMS, polyneuropathy, organomegaly, endocrinopathy, M-protein, and skin changes.

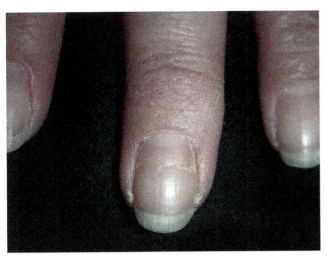

FIGURE 44-2 ■ Beau line.

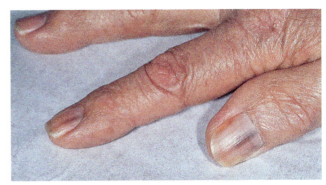

FIGURE 44-4 ■ Longitudinal pigmented bands caused by zidovudine administration in a patient with human immunodeficiency virus.

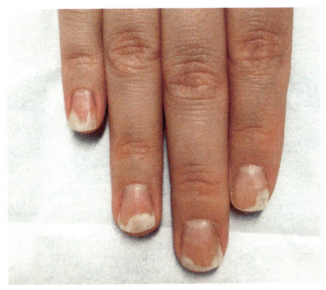

FIGURE 44-3 ■ Onycholysis and pitting (fifth digit) as seen in psoriasis.

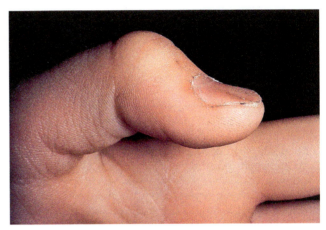

FIGURE 44-5 ■ Koilonychia associated with iron-deficiency anemia. (From Callen JP, Greer KE, Paller A, Swinyer L, editors. Color atlas of dermatology, 2nd ed. Philadelphia: WB Saunders; 2000.)

the most commonly affected. The pathogenesis is not well understood, but may involve the absorption and distribution of iron and protein, or the position of the distal matrix in relation to the proximal matrix.

Koilonychia was originally described in association with iron-deficiency anemia (Plummer–Vinson syndrome) (Fig. 44-5), and the condition normalizes with iron supplementation. It has subsequently been reported in normal children and as a temporary finding in infants, as well as existing in hereditary (autosomal dominant), acquired, and idiopathic forms. The acquired type comprises the largest group of patients with koilonychia and is most commonly seen in psoriasis, fungal infection, distal ischemia (e.g., Raynaud's phenomenon), and trauma. It may also occur in association with porphyrias, hemochromatosis, and occupational exposures (chemical exposure in hairdressers and exposure to organic solvents). Koilonychia has also been reported in association with carcinoma of the upper gastrointestinal tract.

Nail Bed Abnormalities

Splinter Hemorrhages

Splinter hemorrhages arise from extravasation of blood from the longitudinally aligned capillaries of the nail bed (Fig. 44-6) and are usually a result of trauma. Subacute bacterial endocarditis is the most common systemic cause of splinter hemorrhages, which occur proximally in this condition and are typically present in multiple nails. Splinter hemorrhages have also been noted in association with anemia, trichinosis, chronic glomerulonephritis, vasculitis, psoriasis, scurvy, juvenile cirrhosis, high altitudes, eczematous eruptions, fungal nail infections, rheumatoid arthritis, mitral stenosis, septicemia, systemic lupus erythematosus, antiphospholipid syndrome, peptic ulcer disease, pregnancy, malignant tumors, dialysis, and following renal transplantation.

Muehrcke Lines, Half-and-Half Nails (Lindsay nails), and Terry Nails

Muehrcke lines, half-and-half nails, and Terry nails are all examples of apparent leukonychia, in which there is abnormal nail bed vasculature, thereby changing the translucency of the nail plate. On physical exam, the

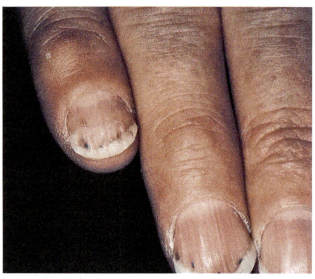

FIGURE 44-6 ■ Splinter hemorrhages of the nail bed.

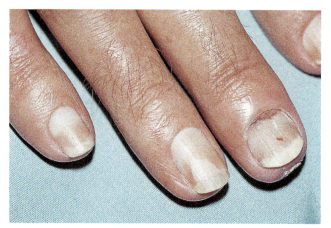

FIGURE 44-7 ■ Half-and-half nails in a patient with renal failure. (Courtesy of Neil Fenske, MD, Tampa, FL.)

whiteness disappears with pressure and is unaffected by nail growth.

Muehrcke lines are paired white transverse bands spanning the width of the nail bed that run parallel to the distal lunula. They were first described in the fingernails of patients with severe hypoalbuminemia, some of whom also had nephrotic syndrome, and resolved with normalization of the serum albumin level. Muehrcke lines have subsequently been reported in patients with liver disease, malnutrition, chemotherapy, organ transplantation, and human immunodeficiency virus/acquired immunodeficiency syndrome (HIV/AIDS). These lines are associated with periods of metabolic stress; times at which the body's capacity to synthesize proteins is diminished.

Half-and-half nails, also known as Lindsay nails, are characterized by a white band proximally, a pink or red-brown band distally, and a sharp demarcation between the two (Fig. 44-7). They were originally described in association with chronic renal disease, and resolve with transplantation, but do not resolve with hemodialysis treatment or change in hemoglobin or albumin levels. Half-and-half nails have subsequently been reported in association with Kawasaki disease, cirrhosis, Crohn's disease, zinc deficiency, chemotherapy, Behçet's disease, and pellagra.

Half-and-half nails should be distinguished from Terry nails. The latter are characterized by leukonychia involving more than 80% of the total nail length. Terry nails were originally reported in association with cirrhosis, usually secondary to alcoholism, but have subsequently been found to be associated with congestive heart failure, adult-onset diabetes, pulmonary tuberculosis, reactive arthritis, older age, leprosy, and peripheral vascular disease.

Onycholysis

Onycholysis is a partial detachment of the nail plate from the nail bed, which may be completely asymptomatic or painful. The most common cause is trauma (from long nails, nail cosmetics), but other causes include psoriasis, infections (dermatophytes, *Candida*, bacteria), irritant or allergic contact dermatitis, lichen planus, and drug reactions. Less frequently, it is a sequela of a systemic disease, such as thyrotoxicosis, hypothyroidism, porphyria, Raynaud's disease, yellow nail syndrome, systemic infection, or diabetes mellitus. In thyrotoxicosis, the nails are typically undulated and curved upwards. With psoriasis and psoriatic arthritis, onycholysis may be accompanied by pitting (Fig. 44-3). When combined with ultraviolet light, tetracyclines, captopril, chlorpromazine, thiazide diuretics, oral contraceptives, and fluoroquinolones, may result in photo-induced onycholysis. Photo-onycholysis is most common in patients undergoing PUVA treatment (psoralens and UVA), but can be prevented by applying colored varnishes to the nails prior to therapy.

Periungual and Distal Digit Abnormalities

Clubbing

Clubbing appears clinically as exaggerated transverse and longitudinal curvature of the nails along with enlargement of the soft tissue structures of the fingertips. It usually involves the thumb and/or index finger of both hands. There is a "spongy" feeling as pressure is applied to the proximal nail fold. Clubbing is defined mathematically; in normal nails, the angle between the nail plate and the proximal nail fold (Lovibond's angle) is less than 180°, usually about 160°, but in clubbing, this angle is greater than 180°. Clubbing must be differentiated from pseudoclubbing, which is an overcurvature of the nails transversely and longitudinally, with a normal Lovibond's angle. While there are many methods to measure clubbing, the simplest way is to oppose the dorsal surfaces of symmetrical digits on each hand. In normal nails, the space created by the distal interphalangeal joint and distal fingertip is diamond-shaped, whereas it is absent with clubbed nails. The pathogenesis of clubbing is likely due to soft tissue fibrovascular hyperplasia between the matrix and the periosteum.

Bilateral clubbing may be hereditary, starting around puberty in otherwise healthy individuals. More frequently, though, bilateral clubbing is acquired and associated with pulmonary (i.e., lung abscess, lung cancer) or cardiovascular (i.e., congestive heart failure, endocarditis) disease, but has also been reported in gastrointestinal (i.e., ulcerative colitis), renal (i.e., chronic pyelonephritis), and endocrine (i.e., Grave's) diseases. Acquired single-digit clubbing is most often associated with vascular lesions in the same extremity, including aneurysms, arteriovenous fistulas, and peripheral shunts. However, lymphadenitis, Pancoast tumors, reflex sympathetic dystrophy, and erythromelalgia have also been shown to cause unilateral clubbing. When only one nail is involved, the cause is often traumatic or, less likely, congenital.

Clubbing is a key sign in the syndrome of acquired hypertrophic pulmonary osteoarthropathy, which also includes muscle weakness, joint pain and swelling, bone pain, acromegalic hypertrophy of the upper and lower extremities, and peripheral neurovascular disease. When all of these signs are present, a malignant thoracic tumor—often bronchogenic carcinoma (Fig. 44-8)—is found in over 90% of cases.

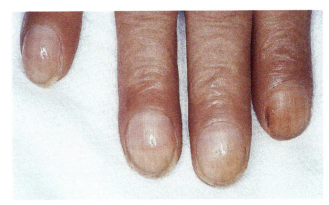

FIGURE 44-8 ■ Clubbing secondary to bronchogenic cancer carcinoma.

Nail Fold Capillary Abnormalities

Distortions of the normal capillary architecture at the proximal nail fold may be seen in diabetes mellitus, cardiovascular disorders, and a number of connective tissue diseases. Dilated capillary loops with avascular areas are often seen in dermatomyositis and systemic sclerosis. Tortuous capillaries with normal vascular density are more specific for systemic lupus erythematosus.

NAIL CHANGES IN SPECIFIC DISORDERS

Cardiovascular and Hematologic Systems

Clubbing and red lunulae may be seen in patients with congestive heart failure, and splinter hemorrhages may be a feature of bacterial endocarditis or pulmonary emboli. The most common findings in patients with Kawasaki disease are periungual desquamation and Beau lines, but these patients may also present with onycholysis, onychomadesis, and pincer nails. A recently described finding in patients with Kawasaki disease is orange-brown chromonychia of the fingernails, which appears between the 5th and 8th days of fever onset and disappears in 7 to 10 days. In hereditary hemorrhagic telangiectasia (Osler–Weber–Rendu syndrome), a consistent nail finding is giant capillary loops of the proximal nail fold. Koilonychia is the most common nail finding in patients with hemochromatosis, who may also have melanonychia (gray, blue, or brown nails), leukonychia, and longitudinal striations. Patients with anemia may have nail bed pallor and, conversely, those with polycythemia may have red nail beds.

Gastrointestinal System

Terry nails are the most common finding reported in patients with cirrhosis. Patients with hepatitis B or C may present with longitudinal striations, nail dystrophy, brittle nails, onychorrhexis, and true leukonychia. Persistent hyperbilirubinemia may cause brown nails due to melanin deposition. Blue lunulae may occur in patients with Wilson's disease and hemochromatosis. Cronkhite–Canada syndrome is characterized by nonfamilial gastrointestinal polyposis, diffuse skin hyperpigmentation, alopecia, and nail changes. Nail dystrophy has been described in 98% of these patients and includes nail thinning, splitting, onycholysis, onychomadesis, leukonychia, and triangular-shaped nail plates. Juvenile polyposis syndrome is an autosomal dominant disorder characterized by multiple juvenile polyps in the gastrointestinal tract. These patients may present with digital clubbing, which may indicate that the patient has coexistent hereditary hemorrhagic telangiectasia.

Endocrine System

Patients with diabetes often have Beau lines, which are likely due to a compromised blood supply. Other common nail changes in patients with diabetes include leukonychia punctata, nail fold dilated and tortuous capillaries (in late-stage disease), onycholysis secondary to *Candida*, onychomycosis, onychogryphosis, and acute and chronic paronychia (Fig. 44-9). Because fusine and fructose-lysine are laid down in the nail plate, nail clippings can be used to assess diabetic control in the preceding 3 to 5 months. Patients with Addison's disease have hyperpigmentation of the mucosa, nipples, genitalia, elbows, and knees and may also have longitudinal pigmented bands. Similar changes have also been described in patients following bilateral adrenalectomy for Cushing's disease. This hyperpigmentation of skin, mucosa, and nails is due to increased production of melanocyte-stimulating hormone.

Patients with acromegaly may present with short, wide, thick, and flat nails. Other findings may include absent lunulae, koilonychia, onychoschizia, and an anchor-like shape of the lateral aspect of the distal phalanges on radiographs. Patients with hypothyroidism may present with brittle nails, slow nail growth, and longitudinal ridges, whereas the most common nail findings in patients with hyperthyroidism are onycholysis and brittle nails. Splinter hemorrhages have been reported with thyrotoxicosis. Plummer nails are a form of onycholysis seen in the setting of thyrotoxicosis in which the free nail edge undulates and curves upwards. The fourth and fifth fingernails are most commonly affected.

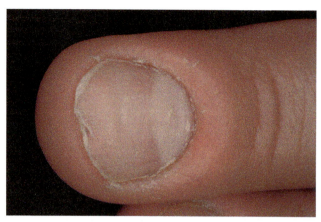

FIGURE 44-9 ■ Chronic candidal paronychia in a patient with diabetes mellitus. (From Mallett RB. Paronychia. In: Lebwohl et al., editors Treatment of Skin Disease, 3rd ed. 2009.)

Infectious Diseases

Most ungual changes associated with infectious diseases are relatively nonspecific. Syphilis has been associated with paronychia, nail thinning, loss of the lunula, nail fragility, fissuring of the free margin, Beau lines, and chancres of the nail folds. Red lunulae have been reported in patients with lymphogranuloma venereum, and pale gray nails in patients with malaria. Loss of the lunula, paronychia, leukonychia, painful subungual abscesses, lilac line of Milan, and pterygium unguium have all been noted in association with leprosy. In addition, paronychia has been reported in patients with cutaneous leishmaniasis.

Patients with AIDS may have yellowing of the nails, onychomycosis (which may be superficial), splinter hemorrhages, as well as ridging. Zidovudine has been shown to cause longitudinal pigmented bands and yellow-brown discoloration of the nails.

Central and Peripheral Nervous Systems

Most nail findings associated with neurologic disorders are nonspecific. In Lesch–Nyhan disease, patients compulsively bite their fingers, which results in destruction of the digital tips and nails (onychotillomania). In central nervous system disease, there may be splinter hemorrhages and onycholysis. Onychogryphosis is associated with spinal cord injuries, whereas Beau lines are associated with epilepsy. Longitudinal striations may be seen in cases of multiple sclerosis, syringomyelia, and hemiplegia.

More specific nail findings are found in patients with neurofibromatosis type I and tuberous sclerosis. Patients with neurofibromatosis type I may present with erythronychia secondary to subungual glomus tumors. Approximately 50% of patients with tuberous sclerosis present with pathognomonic periungual fibromas (Koenen tumors), which are smooth, pedunculated, flesh-colored papules that originate under the proximal nail fold and extend above the nail plate.

Psychiatric Conditions

Onychotillomania is observed in obsessive–compulsive disorder, and findings may include onycholysis, splinter hemorrhages, and hematomas. If severe, scarring, pterygium, paronychia, and ingrown nails may be present. Striated leukonychia can be seen in bipolar disorder, and there is an association between a family history of schizophrenia and visibility of the subcapillary plexus. Double-edged nails are found in some cases of psychosis, and broad white bands of the nails may follow an acute psychotic episode. Finally, brittle nails are seen in patients with anorexia nervosa.

Pulmonary System

The yellow nail syndrome is characterized by the triad of yellow nails, lymphedema, and respiratory tract involvement, which may include asthma, pleural effusion, tuberculosis, bronchiectasis, chronic sinusitis, chronic bronchitis, or chronic obstructive pulmonary disease. Nails are thick and yellow, with an increased transverse curvature, absent cuticles, and slow growth rate (Fig. 44-10). Yellow nail syndrome is linked to an array of underlying diseases including malignancies such as melanoma, sarcoma, lymphoma, and renal carcinoma, as well as diabetes mellitus, thyroid dysfunction, rheumatoid arthritis, myocardial infarction, and nephrotic syndrome. In addition, elevated titanium levels have recently been reported in a few patients with yellow nail syndrome.

Clubbing and red lunulae are seen in association with emphysema, chronic bronchitis, tuberculosis, pneumonia, and chronic obstructive pulmonary disease. Shell nail syndrome is a term used to describe exaggerated longitudinal curvature of the nail plate along with distal nail bed atrophy, resulting in a shell-like space between the thickened nail plate and the thin nail bed. This finding has been reported in association with bronchiectasis and bronchial tumors. Sarcoid may rarely involve the nails (0.2% to 1.5%), but is more likely when there is chronic, systemic disease with bone involvement. Granulomatous lesions of the nail unit and periungual skin, dactylitis, splinter hemorrhages, pterygium, atrophy, onycholysis, subungual hyperkeratosis, and trachyonychia have all been reported.

Renal and Genitourinary Systems

Half-and-half nails (Lindsay nails) (Fig. 44-7), onycholysis, onychogryphosis, yellow or gray discoloration of the nail plates, Mees lines, Muehrcke lines, and splinter hemorrhages have all been reported with renal failure. Hemodialysis patients may also present with splinter hemorrhages, half-and-half nails, absent lunulae, photo-onycholysis, and pseudoclubbing. Since creatinine levels can be measured from nail clippings, they can be used to differentiate between acute and chronic renal failure. Dilated nail fold capillary loops enhanced by capillaroscopy are a common finding in patients with Henoch–Schönlein purpura. Common nail findings in renal transplant recipients include leukonychia, absence of the lunula, onychomycosis, and longitudinal ridging.

In nail–patella syndrome (Fig. 44-11), which involves autosomal dominant inheritance of a mutation in the *LMX1B* gene on chromosome 9, patients present with renal failure along with anonychia, nail plate thinning and/or nail plate discoloration, triangular or poorly formed lunulae, longitudinal ridging, and koilonychia.

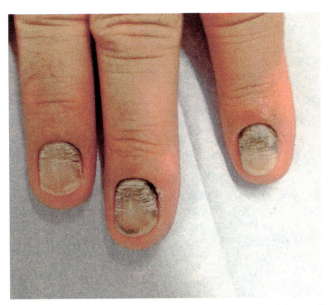

FIGURE 44-10 ■ Yellow nail syndrome, with absent cuticles and yellow discoloration of the nail plate.

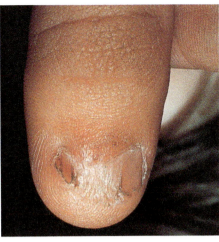

FIGURE 44-11 ■ Triangular lunula in nail–patella syndrome. (Courtesy of Leonard Swinyer, MD, Salt Lake City, UT.)

In some cases of renal adenocarcinoma, there may be accompanying nail bed erythema due to erythropoietin production by the tumor.

Reproductive System

Pregnancy is associated with an increased rate of nail growth and characteristic nail changes including softening, brittleness, Beau lines, onycholysis, subungual hyperkeratosis, and an increased occurrence and severity of ingrown nails. These changes resolve postpartum. Beau lines have also been reported with dysmenorrhea as well as physiologically with each menstrual cycle.

Rheumatologic Diseases

In rheumatoid arthritis, there may be ungual thickening, discoloration, red lunulae, longitudinal ridging with a beaded appearance, splinter hemorrhages, an associated yellow nail syndrome, and periungual hemorrhagic infarcts (Bywater's lesions).

Patients with systemic lupus erythematosus may also present with a range of nail abnormalities, but none are distinctive enough to be used as diagnostic criteria. Onycholysis is the most common nail finding, followed by proximal nail fold erythema. Other potential findings include dilated capillary loops in the proximal nail fold with normal vascular density, splinter hemorrhages, nail plate thinning, and ragged cuticles. Other potential findings include Beau lines, leukonychia, paronychia, oil spots, clubbing, ventral ptygerium, and subungual hyperkeratosis. Changes secondary to Raynaud's phenomenon and distal ischemia may also occur.

Ungual abnormalities are often prominent in patients with dermatomyositis. These may include dilated capillary loops, dropout of capillaries in the nail fold, ragged cuticles, and cuticular hypertrophy. Other potential findings include pitting, splinter hemorrhages, and nail fold erythema.

In reactive arthritis, many of the nail changes are similar to those seen in psoriasis, including yellowing, onycholysis, subungual hyperkeratosis, and pitting.

Raynaud's disease of long duration may produce significant ungual changes. The nail is often thin and brittle, with longitudinal ridging, splitting easily. Discoloration often occurs secondary to an accumulation of debris and infection. There may be onycholysis, koilonychias, and a mild reduction in the growth rate. Excessive cold exposure may produce Beau lines as a result of a temporary interruption of nail growth. Pterygium formation may complicate vasomotor ischemia. Patients with Raynaud's disease often have chronic paronychia as well as fungal infections involving the nail.

The nail changes in systemic sclerosis include erythema and telangiectasia of the proximal nail fold, splinter hemorrhages, ventral ptygerium, and infarcts of the distal digits secondary to ischemia. Other nail findings include clubbing, onychorrhexis, absence of the lunula, onycholysis, ragged cuticles, vesiculation of the periungual area, increased longitudinal and transverse curvature of the fingernails, onychogryphosis, and deep longitudinal sulci.

Nail changes associated with osteoarthritis include leukonychia, concave canaliform dystrophy, "washboard" transverse lines, and longitudinal grooves with beaded ridges. There is also a strong association of digital mucous (myxoid) cysts with radiographic evidence of osteoarthritis.

Multicentric reticulohistiocytosis is another rheumatologic condition with associated ungual changes. These include brittleness, onycholysis, longitudinal ridging, atrophy, and hyperpigmentation, as well as the presence of characteristic papules at the nail folds with a "beaded string" or "coral beading" appearance. The nails are also wider than they are long.

Pitting and onycholysis are features of psoriasis and psoriatic arthritis. With psoriasis, rheumatic fever, and Still's disease, there is a faster than normal nail growth rate. Absent lunulae and reduced cysteine content are found in patients with chronic polyarthritis. Brittleness, leukonychia, crumbling of the nail plate, and longitudinal striations are ungual changes that have been reported in patients with gout.

Nail Changes Associated with Malignancy

Bazex syndrome (acrokeratosis paraneoplastica) is a rare condition characterized by tender, erythematous psoriasiform plaques favoring acral areas, including the ears and nose, in association with internal malignancy. Nail findings are common and include ridging, yellowing, onycholysis, and subungual hyperkeratosis. In severe cases, there may be nail plate atrophy and cuticle loss. A characteristic finding is bulbous enlargement of the distal phalanges with nail dystrophy.

Glucagonoma syndrome is due to a rare glucagon-secreting pancreatic alpha cell tumor that results in elevated glucagon levels, abnormal glucose tolerance, weight loss, anemia, aminoaciduria, diarrhea, thromboembolic disease, and psychiatric disturbances. Necrolytic migratory erythema is the characteristic skin finding, and brittle nails are also common.

Cowden syndrome is a rare, autosomal dominant disorder, with mutations in the tumor suppressor gene *PTEN*. Patients have trichilemmomas, papillomatous papules, acral keratoses, and an increased risk of breast, endometrial, and thyroid cancer. Case reports have demonstrated associated nail findings including Heller-like median canaliform nail dystrophy, subungual fibrotic nodules, and linear subungual hyperkeratosis.

While uncommon, cutaneous metastases may present as subungual tumors. The most common primary malignancies represented are lung cancer, tumors of the genitourinary tract (i.e., kidney), and breast cancer. Subungual metastases are typically painful and may present as a swelling of the distal digit or a red to violaceous nodule that distorts the nail plate and/or the distal digit. The digits of the hands are more commonly involved than those of the feet. Patients with subungual metastases generally have a poor prognosis, with death occurring a few months after the tumor is diagnosed.

Miscellaneous

A variety of other nail abnormalities may occur in association with systemic diseases. Onychomadesis may occur with Stevens–Johnson syndrome, toxic epidermal necrolysis, epidermolysis bullosa, and toxic shock syndrome. In epidermolysis bullosa acquisita, the nail changes are usually more severe than in other bullous disorders. Nail dystrophy, including hyperkeratosis, shedding, hemorrhage, and horizontal ridging, occurs with bullous pemphigoid, and subungual pustules may be a feature of impetigo herpetiformis. Nail findings are common in pemphigus vulgaris and correlate with an increased number of skin bullae and duration of disease. Some findings include pitting, paronychia, nail plate discoloration, transverse lines, onychorrhexis, onychomadesis, subungual hemorrhage, Beau lines, subungual hyperkeratosis, fungal infection, pterygium, and onycholysis.

Onycholysis or disappearing lunulae may be seen in multiple myeloma, whereas Langerhans cell histiocytosis may present with paronychia, purpura, onycholysis, subungual hyperkeratosis, and splinter hemorrhages. Subungual purpura may occur in Letterer–Siwe disease. Mees lines have been reported in Hodgkin's disease and may be related to a poor prognosis. Onycholysis, increased fragility, brittleness, subungual thickening and striations, longitudinal ridging, and crumbling may occur in both primary and myeloma-associated systemic amyloidosis. These changes may resemble lichen planus clinically. On histopathology, amyloid deposits are found in the superficial dermis and surrounding blood vessels. Finally, leukonychia may be present with cryoglobulinemia.

SUGGESTED READINGS

Baran R, Dawber RPR, de Berker DAR, et al. Baran and Dawber's diseases of the nails and their management. 4th ed. Oxford: Blackwell Publishing Ltd. 2012.

Cohen PR. Metastatic tumors to the nail unit: subungual metastases. Dermatol Surg 2001;27(3):280–93.

Cutolo M, Smith V. State of the art on nailfold capillaroscopy: a reliable diagnostic tool and putative biomarker in rheumatology? Rheumatology 2013;52(11):1933–40.

Decker A, Daly D, Scher RK. The role of titanium in the development of yellow nail syndrome. Skin Appendage Disord 2015;1:28–30.

Haneke E. Surgical anatomy of the nail apparatus. Dermatol Clin 2006;24:291–6.

Hinds G, Thomas VD. Malignancy and cancer treatment-related hair and nail changes. Dermatol Clin 2008;26:59–68. viii.

Pappert AS, Scher RK, Cohen JL. Longitudinal pigmented nail bands. Dermatol Clin 1991;9:703–16.

Piraccini BM, Urciuoli M, et al. Yellow nail syndrome: clinical experience in a series of 21 patients. J Dtsch Dermatol Ges 2014;12(2):131–7.

Piraccini BM, Iorizzo M, Starace M, Tosti A. Drug-induced nail diseases. Dermatol Clin 2006;24:387–91.

Scher RK, Daniel CR. Nails: Diagnosis, Therapy, Surgery. 3rd ed. Elsevier Saunders; 2005 (Scher RK, Daniel CR, Rubin AI, Jellinek NJ, 4th edition, in press).

Shah KR, Boland BR, et al. Cutaneous manifestations of gastrointestinal disease: Part I. J Am Acad Dermatol 2013;68(2):189–210.

Tosti A, Iorizzo M, Piraccini BM, Starace M. The nail in systemic diseases. Dermatol Clin 2006;24:341–7.

Tunc SE, Ertam I, Pirildar T, et al. Nail changes in connective tissue diseases: do nail changes provide clues for the diagnosis? J Eur Acad Dermatol Venereol 2007;21:497–503.

Tully AS, Trayes KP, Studdiford JS. Evaluation of nail abnormalities. Am Fam Phys 2012;85(8):779–87.

CHAPTER 45

ORAL DISEASE

Charles Camisa • Jeffrey P. Callen

KEY POINTS

- A thorough examination of the intraoral soft tissues, including palpation, is necessary to detect the subtle signs of systemic disease as well as localized problems such as leukoplakia.
- Autosomal dominant cancer syndromes may present with diverse mucous membrane manifestations: odontogenic keratocysts in nevoid basal cell carcinoma syndrome; papillomatosis in multiple hamartoma and neoplasia syndrome; pigmented macules in Peutz–Jeghers syndrome.
- The mat-like telangiectases of the lips and tongue are morphologically identical in hereditary hemorrhagic telangiectasia syndrome and CREST (calcinosis, Raynaud's phenomenon, esophageal dysmotility, sclerodactyly, and telangiectasia) syndrome (limited scleroderma).
- The most common causes of oral hyperpigmentation are ethnic pigmentation, cigarette-smoking, ingestion of drugs, heavy metals, antimalarials, and minocycline.
- Immunocompromised patients, especially those with very low CD4 counts, are at particularly high risk for oral pathology including necrotic ulcerative gingivitis, periodontitis, and osteitis, as well as oral hairy leukoplakia, Kaposi's sarcoma, and non-Hodgkin's lymphoma.
- The oral lesions of discoid lupus erythematosus and graft-versus-host disease mimic those of lichen planus; differentiation may require knowledge of the clinical situation and biopsy confirmation.
- Gingival hyperplasia is induced by antiseizure drugs, calcium-channel-blocking agents, and cyclosporine. Treatment consists of meticulous personal and professional oral hygiene or stopping the medication.

Pathologic changes in the oral mucous membranes can be involved in the full spectrum of systemic diseases, ranging from developmental disturbances and autoimmune diseases to infectious and neoplastic disorders (Table 45-1; Figs 45-1 to 45-7). A methodic inspection of the soft tissues of the oral cavity with palpation of the gutters, floor of the mouth, tongue, and major salivary glands is necessary to complete a thorough physical examination. Clues to the presenting diagnosis or significant incidental findings, such as leukoplakia or oral carcinoma, may be disclosed. In this chapter, selected oral diseases with systemic implications are discussed and illustrated. The reader is referred to specific chapters for dermatologic diseases with oral mucosal manifestations (e.g., Stevens–Johnson syndrome/toxic epidermal necrolysis, lupus erythematosus, etc.).

NEVOID BASAL CELL CARCINOMA SYNDROME (OMIM #109400)

The nevoid basal cell carcinoma syndrome (NBCCS) is caused by mutations in the *PTCH1* gene on chromosome 9q22, *PTCH2* gene on 1p32, or the *SUFU* gene on 10q24-q25. The autosomal dominant trait has high penetrance and variable expressivity. There is also a high spontaneous mutation rate (about 40% of cases). The major features of NBCCS are numerous basal cell carcinomas (BCCs) at an early age, skeletal anomalies, palmar and plantar pits, and multiple jaw cysts. The jaw cysts, found in about 75% of affected persons, are odontogenic keratocysts (OKCs) that arise from dental lamina remnants or from basal cell components of overlying oral epithelium. They usually occur in the posterior portion of the mandible. An OKC may be the first sign of NBCCS in a child, and if there is more than one, a search for the other stigmata of this syndrome is indicated. The OKC is benign, but its growth may produce lateral bone expansion, displacement of teeth, and pathologic fractures. The histologic findings of OKCs are specific. The cyst cavity is filled with keratin. Surgical excision is the treatment of choice, but there is a high recurrence rate. If one or more major criteria for the diagnosis of NBCCS besides multiple OKCs can be identified, genetic counseling and an aggressive program of skin cancer prevention with vigilant follow-up should be initiated. A novel oral hedgehog pathway inhibitor vismodegib may be a beneficial adjuvant for adult patients who develop numerous or advanced BCCs.

CHEILITIS GRANULOMATOSA (MELKERSSON–ROSENTHAL SYNDROME)

Cheilitis granulomatosa is a distinct clinicopathologic entity of unknown cause that usually affects young adults and is characterized by diffuse, nontender, soft to firm, chronic swelling of one or both lips (Fig. 45-8) and other intraoral sites. Cheilitis granulomatosa is often confused

TABLE 45-1 Systemic Diseases with Mucocutaneous Manifestations

Category	Disease	Oral Manifestations	Cutaneous Findings
Genetic	Nevoid basal cell carcinoma syndrome	Odontogenic keratocysts	Palmar pits, multiple basal cell carcinomas
	Hereditary hemorrhagic telangiectasia (Osler–Weber–Rendu syndrome)	Mat-like telangiectases on the vermilion, tongue, buccal mucosa, and palate	Mat-like telangiectasia on the perioral skin and hands, particularly the fingertips
	Multiple hamartoma syndrome (Cowden's disease)	Papillomatosis (Fig. 45-1) of the gingivae, dorsal tongue, and buccal mucosa	Facial trichilemmomas, acral keratoses, and occasionally palmar or plantar pits
Inflammatory	Behçet's disease	Aphthae—recurrent and severe (Fig. 45-2)	Genital aphthae, pustular "vasculitis," pyoderma gangrenosum-like lesions, erythema nodosum-like lesions, pathergy is common
	Inflammatory bowel disease	Oral aphthae, pyostomatitis vegetans, cobblestone appearance of mucosa (Fig. 45-3), linear ulcers, orofacial granulomatosis	Erythema nodosum, pyoderma gangrenosum
	Lupus erythematosus	Leukoplakic patches, discoid lupus erythematosus lesions (Fig. 45-4), aphthae	Photosensitivity, discoid lupus erythematosus, subacute cutaneous lupus erythematosus, acute "butterfly" rash, bullous systemic lupus erythematosus, leukocytoclastic vasculitis
	Scleroderma (progressive systemic sclerosis)	Reduced oral aperture, mat-like telangiectasia (Fig. 45-5) (particularly in patients with CREST [calcinosis, Raynaud's phenomenon, esophageal dysmotility, sclerodactyly, and telangiectasia] syndrome), xerostomia	Acral or proximal sclerosis, calcinosis cutis, Raynaud's phenomenon, mat-like telangiectasia, murine facies, hypo- and/or hyperpigmentation
	Wegener's granulomatosis	Gingival hyperplasia with petechiae (strawberry gingivitis), oral ulcerations, poorly healing extraction sites	Palpable purpura, cutaneous granulomatous vasculitis
	Sarcoidosis	Infiltrative lesions, orofacial granulomatosis	Papules, nodules, granulomatous lesions in scars
Infectious	Candidiasis	Thrush, angular cheilitis (Fig. 45-6), median rhomboid glossitis	—
	Oral hairy leukoplakia	Corrugated white plaques most commonly on the lateral tongue	—
Neoplastic	Kaposi's sarcoma	Blue to violaceous macular to nodular lesions	Lesions similar to oral cavity
	Leukemia/lymphoma	Infiltrative lesions, boggy, friable gingival surface, erythematous to violaceous nodules of the lateral hard palate (ulceration common)	—
Miscellaneous	Graft-versus-host disease	Reticular lichen planus-like lesions, lichenoid plaques (Fig. 45-7), salivary gland dysfunction, thrush, mucositis, xerostomia	Lichenoid lesions or scleroderma-like changes

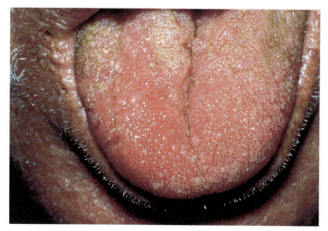

FIGURE 45-1 ■ Papillomatosis of the tongue in a patient with multiple hamartomas and neoplasia.

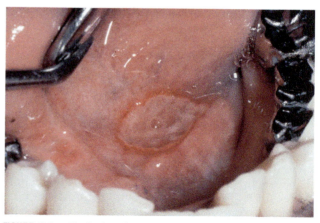

FIGURE 45-2 ■ Typical major aphthous ulceration as seen in Behçet's disease. (Courtesy of Dr. Carl M. Allen.)

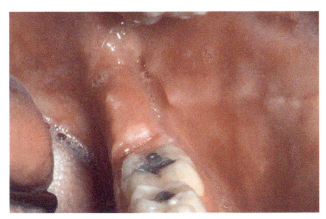

FIGURE 45-3 ■ Cobblestone appearance of oral mucosa in Crohn's disease. (Courtesy of Dr. Carl M. Allen.)

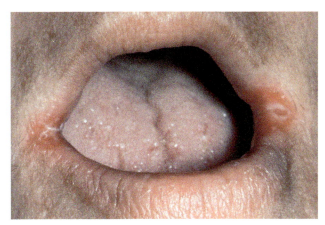

FIGURE 45-6 ■ Angular cheilitis caused by *Candida albicans* infection. (Courtesy of Dr. Carl M. Allen.)

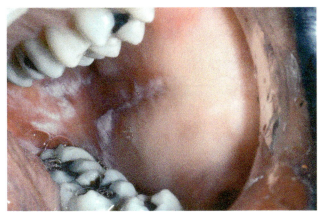

FIGURE 45-4 ■ Discoid lupus erythematosus lesion on the buccal mucosa resembles lichen planus.

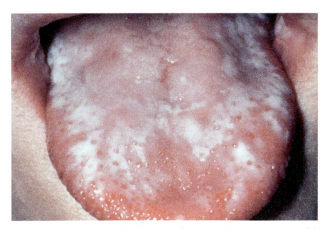

FIGURE 45-7 ■ Lichenoid plaque of tongue in a patient with chronic graft-versus-host reaction. (Courtesy of Dr. Carl M. Allen.)

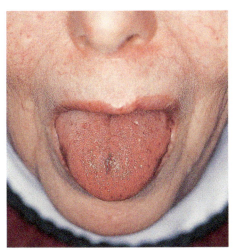

FIGURE 45-5 ■ Mat-like telangiectasia in a patient with CREST (calcinosis, Raynaud's phenomenon, esophageal dysmotility, sclerodactyly, and telangiectasia) syndrome. (From Callen, JC. Color atlas of dermatology. 2nd ed. Philadelphia: WB Saunders; 2000.)

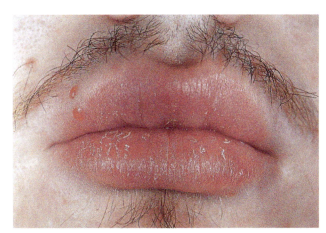

FIGURE 45-8 ■ Asymmetrical swelling of the lips in cheilitis granulomatosa.

with angioedema clinically, but the history of chronicity of the lip swelling is not compatible with angioedema. The biopsy specimen shows nonnecrotizing granulomas, lymphedema, and lymphangiectasia. Crohn's disease and sarcoidosis must be excluded because they also can produce granulomatous cheilitis. Cheilitis granulomatosa together with facial swelling, including periorbital skin, fissured tongue, and facial nerve palsy, constitutes the Melkersson–Rosenthal syndrome. All of these features are infrequently found in patients; therefore, the concept of orofacial granulomatosis has been promulgated to account for a wide array of conditions that show nonspecific granulomatous inflammation in biopsy specimens.

Patients with cheilitis granulomatosa may be treated with intralesional triamcinolone acetonide (10 to 20 mg/mL) injections. Patient comfort is improved by local anesthetic blocks of the lip. The response is usually favorable but temporary, and requires repeated injections at intervals of months or years. Alternative anti-inflammatory medical treatment includes prednisone, hydroxychloroquine sulfate (HCl), sulfasalazine, methotrexate, and tumor necrosis factor (TNF)-α antagonists (antibodies not fusion protein). Surgical reduction of the lips during a quiescent phase may correct persistent macrocheilia and improve function and appearance. Intralesional or systemic corticosteroids have been advocated to reduce the risk of recurrence after surgical treatment.

NECROTIZING ULCERATIVE GINGIVITIS

Necrotizing ulcerative gingivitis (NUG; "trench mouth"; Vincent's infection) is a fairly common oral disease of complex cause that occurs in normal individuals. Contributing factors include the fusospirochetal oral flora, immune deficiency, malnutrition, poor oral hygiene, smoking, and psychologic stress. NUG occurs with increased frequency in human immunodeficiency virus (HIV)-infected patients, in whom it may evolve rapidly to stomatitis, periodontitis, and osteitis if not adequately treated. If the necrotizing infection extends to the facial skin, it is termed noma (cancrum oris). NUG (and oral hairy leukoplakia) are significantly correlated with helper T-cell depletion.

The chief complaint is usually painful bleeding gums. The patient's breath is characteristically fetid, but it is the presence of "punched-out" ulcerated interdental papillae that helps to differentiate NUG from primary herpetic gingivostomatitis. Treatment consists of thorough debridement of the involved tissue and cleaning of the teeth by a dentist, followed by chlorhexidine rinses after meals, and systemic antibiotics such as penicillin, tetracyclines, or metronidazole. In cases that are resistant to standard treatment, it is recommended to screen for nonoral pathogenic enteric bacteria and *Candida albicans* and to rule out infectious mononucleosis and HIV infection.

ORAL PIGMENTATION

The most common form of oral hyperpigmentation is that seen distributed symmetrically in darkly pigmented individuals, although the intensity of the color is not directly related to that of the skin. Antimalarial therapy may produce a bluish-gray discoloration of the palate after long-term use. Bismuth therapy and lead intoxication produce a narrow band of bluish-black pigment along the marginal gingiva. Minocycline may discolor bone, fully developed teeth, and less commonly the oral mucosa. Cigarette smoking is associated with pigmentation of the lip and gingiva. Other causes of intraoral and cutaneous pigmentation include Addison's disease,

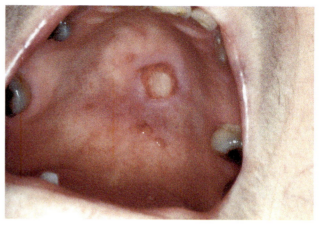

FIGURE 45-9 ■ Ulceration of the palate secondary to dry mouth and trauma in a patient with Sjögren's syndrome.

hemochromatosis, and neurofibromatosis. Peutz–Jeghers syndrome is a highly penetrant, autosomal dominant disorder characterized by gastrointestinal hamartomatous polyps and pigmented macules around the mouth, lips, labial and buccal mucosae, and dorsal and volar aspects of the hands and feet. The pigmentary markers of the syndrome appear early in life allowing for the monitoring of polyps for malignant transformation, which occurs in 2% to 3% of cases. Extraintestinal malignancies are common as well.

XEROSTOMIA

Xerostomia is the subjective sensation of dry mouth caused by a reduction in salivary flow. Patients with xerostomia can be recognized by their ever-present bottles of water or ice chips. A wooden tongue depressor often sticks fast to the dorsum of the tongue. Xerostomia is one cause of glossodynia or the burning mouth syndrome. Drugs with anticholinergic effects, such as antihistamines and antidepressants, and diuretics may contribute to the problem. Hyposalivation is common after radiation therapy of head and neck cancers. Xerostomia and xerophthalmia are symptoms of the sicca complex associated with primary and secondary Sjögren's syndrome. The latter group usually has the sicca complex in addition to a connective tissue disease. The tongue typically has a red, parched, mammillated surface, and keratoconjunctivitis sicca may be present. Oral ulcerations may occur secondary to minor trauma and heal slowly (Fig. 45-9). A biopsy of the labial minor salivary glands or the parotid gland may show foci of lymphoplasmacytic inflammation, which supports the diagnosis of Sjögren's syndrome along with serologic testing.

Patients are particularly prone to dental caries; therefore, sugarless hard candies and saliva substitutes containing carboxymethylcellulose or hydroxyethylcellulose should be used. Oral pilocarpine and cevimeline are recommended for treating hyposalivation and xerostomia, but excessive sweating is the most common side effect.

GINGIVAL HYPERPLASIA

Drug-induced gingival hyperplasia is primarily fibrous and noninflammatory. It typically begins in the interdental papillae of dentate persons and overgrows the teeth. The classic drugs responsible are phenytoin and other anticonvulsants. More recent culprits include cyclosporine and the antihypertensive calcium channel blockers: nifedipine, diltiazem, verapamil, and amlodipine. Meticulous oral hygiene, plaque control, and professional debridement help to prevent gingival hyperplasia, and it may resolve after discontinuation of these drugs. Azithromycin may be used to reduce cyclosporine-induced gingival hyperplasia.

SUGGESTED READINGS

Banks T, Gada S. A comprehensive review of current treatments for granulomatous cheilitis. Br J Dermatol 2012;166:934–7.

Clementini M, Vittorini G, Crea A, et al. Efficacy of AZM therapy in patients with gingival overgrowth induced by cyclosporine A: a systematic review. BMC Oral Health 2008;8:34.

Critchlow WA, Chang D. Cheilitis granulomatosa: a review. Head Neck Pathol 2014;8:209–13.

Daniels TE, Cox D, Shiboski CH, et al. Associations between salivary gland histopathologic diagnoses and phenotypic features of Sjogren's syndrome (SS) among 1726 registry participants. Arthritis Rheum 2011;63:2021–30.

Gaetti-Jardim E, Nakano V, Wahasugui TC, et al. Occurrence of yeasts, enterococci and other enteric bacteria in subgingival biofilm of HIV-positive patients with chronic gingivitis and necrotizing periodontitis. Braz J Microbiol 2008;39:257–61.

Ho AW, Sato R, Ramsdell A. A case of oral melanosis. J Am Acad Dermatol 2014;71:1030–3.

Lazerrini M, Bramuzzo M, Ventura A. Association between orofacial granulomatosis and Crohn's disease in children: systematic review. World J Gastroenterol 2014;20:7497–504.

Macaigne G, Hamois F, Boivin JF, et al. Crohn's disease revealed by a cheilitis granulomatosa with favorable evolution by perfusions of infliximab: report of a case and review of the literature. Clin Res Hepatol Gastroenterol 2011;35:147–9.

Neville BW, Damm D, Allen C, Bouquot J. Oral and maxillofacial pathology. 3rd ed. Philadelphia: WB Saunders; 2009.

Ponti G, Pollio A, Pastorino L, et al. Patched homolog 1 gene mutation (p.G1093R) induces nevoid basal cell carcinoma syndrome and non-syndromic keratocystic odontogenic tumors: a case report. Oncol Lett 2012;4:241–4.

Sasportas LS, Hosford AT, Sodini MA, et al. Cost-effectiveness landscape analysis of treatments addressing xerostomia in patients receiving head and neck radiation therapy. Oral Surg Oral Med Oral Pathol Oral Radiol 2013;116:e37–51.

Tang JY, Mackay-Wiggan JM, Aszterbaum M, et al. Inhibiting the hedgehog pathway in patients with the basal-cell nevus syndrome. N Engl J Med 2012;366:2180–8.

Tincani A, Andreoli L, Cavazzana I, et al. Novel aspects of Sjogren's syndrome 2012. BMC Med 2013;11:93.

Tokgoz B, Sari HI, Yildiz O, et al. Effects of azithromycin on cyclosporine-induced gingival hyperplasia in renal transplant patients. Transpl Proc 2004;36:2699–702.

CHAPTER 46

LEG ULCERS

Katherine L. Baquerizo Nole • Robert S. Kirsner

> **KEY POINTS**
>
> - Venous leg ulcerations are the most common cause of leg ulcers, followed by mixed venous/arterial disease and arterial insufficiency. However, up to 10% of leg ulcers are due to atypical etiologies, infections, metabolic disorders, neoplasms, and inflammatory processes.
> - Venous insufficiency or dysfunction is caused by outflow abnormalities or venous reflux, resulting in sustained ambulatory venous pressures or venous hypertension.
> - Arterial insufficiency results from failure to deliver oxygen and nutrients to the tissue. Progressive atherosclerosis is the most common etiology.
> - Screening for arterial insufficiency should be performed—if clinically relevant—with the measurement of ankle–brachial pressure index (ABI). If ABI is >0.7, compression can be applied safely.
> - Biopsy of the ulcer needs to be considered when atypical etiology is suspected, or when treatment response is not adequate.
> - Wound size and wound duration are the main factors associated with wound healing.
> - Standard of care for venous ulcerations consists of debridement, management of infection, appropriate wound dressings, limb elevation, and compression. If this fails, diagnosis should be reassessed and/or adjunctive therapy should be considered, including autologous skin grafts and tissue-engineered products, among others.
> - Standard of care for arterial ulcerations is revascularization if possible.

Wounds, in particular chronic wounds, represent a clinical challenge to healthcare providers and an unmet medical need for patients. In the United States alone, chronic wounds affect an estimated 7 million patients annually. Leg ulcers are wounds located in the area between the knee and ankle and that is the definition we will use in this chapter.

- The prevalence of leg ulceration is approximately 0.3 to 0.6%, and constitutes a great economic burden to society.
- Venous leg ulcerations are the most common cause of leg ulcers, followed by mixed venous/arterial disease and arterial insufficiency.
- Up to 10% of leg ulcers are due to atypical etiologies, infections, metabolic disorders, neoplasms, and inflammatory processes.

PREVALENCE AND ECONOMIC COST

Leg ulcerations are a common clinical problem with considerable morbidity, high cost to society, and often a dramatic negative impact on a patient's quality of life.

Leg ulcerations have a point prevalence rate of 0.3 to 0.6% and a lifetime cumulative risk of 1.0 to 1.8%. Venous leg ulcerations (VLUs) are the most common cause of leg ulcers, constituting up to 80 to 90%. The average annual incidence rate of VLUs is 2.2% in Medicare-aged populations and 0.5% in younger privately insured patients.

VLUs are associated with increased healthcare costs. Recent data indicate that patients with VLUs utilize significantly more medical resources and have increased annual incremental medical costs compared with matched patients without VLUs. Additionally, working patients with VLUs missed more days from work, resulting in substantially higher work-loss costs.

PATHOPHYSIOLOGY

Overview

Although the differential diagnosis of leg ulcerations is extensive, in the Western world they are most frequently caused by venous insufficiency, arterial insufficiency, or a combination of these (Table 46-1). In one large cohort of patients with leg ulceration, 72% of lesions were attributed to venous insufficiency, 22% to mixed arterial and venous disease, and 6% to predominantly arterial disease.

Atypical wounds are those chronic wounds not secondary to these causes, but rather the result of, among others, infections, metabolic disorders, neoplasms, and inflammatory processes. It is estimated that up to 10% of chronic lower-extremity ulcers are due to these less frequent etiologies. Dermatologists have a particular responsibility to recognize the less common causes due to training in the diagnosis of these conditions.

Appropriate therapy is critically dependent on an accurate diagnosis of the cause of the ulceration. For example, small-vessel disease associated with leg ulcerations may be difficult to recognize and may present as painful pinpoint ulcerations that heal with a white atrophic scar (livedoid vasculopathy; Fig. 46-1). Additionally, for example, care must be taken before establishing a diagnosis of pyoderma gangrenosum (Fig. 46-2) because many other conditions can have similar presentations. Furthermore, it is important to recognize that ulcerations often have several contributing

TABLE 46-1 Causes of Leg Ulcerations

Venous (see Fig. 46-10)
  Deep venous outflow obstruction
  Ineffective venous valves
  Inefficient calf muscle pumps
  Varicose leg veins

Ischemic
  Atherosclerosis with or without superimposed trauma (see Fig. 46-12)
  Atheroemboli (cholesterol emboli)
  Arteriolar disease
  Leukocytoclastic vasculitis (vasculitis of the postcapillary venule)*
  Vascular occlusion
    Coagulopathy (see Fig. 46-11)
    Livedoid vasculopathy (see Fig. 46-1)

Nonvascular
  Trauma
  Pressure
  Injury
  External
  Self-induced or factitious (see Fig. 46-9)
  Burns (chemical, thermal, radiation)
  Cold (frostbite)
  Spider bite (brown recluse spider)

Infection
  Bacterial
  Fungal (deep)
    Blastomycosis
    Cryptococcosis
    Coccidioidomycosis
    Histoplasmosis
    Sporotrichosis
  Viral (herpes simplex)
  Mycobacterial
  Parasitic (leishmaniasis)
  Spirochetal

Osteomyelitis
  Inflammation
    Connective tissue disease
    Lupus erythematosus
    Polyarteritis nodosa
    Rheumatoid arthritis
    Wegener granulomatosis
  Panniculitis
    Infectious
    Noninfectious
      Necrobiosis lipoidica (see Fig. 46-16)
      Pancreatic fat necrosis (malignancy pancreas)
      α_1-Antitrypsin panniculitis

Malignancy (see Fig. 46-7)
  Squamous cell carcinoma
  Basal cell carcinoma
  Melanoma
  Lymphoma
  Metastatic disease
  Sarcoma
  Kaposi
  Angiosarcoma

Metabolic
  Diabetes mellitus
  Gout
  α_1-Antitrypsin deficiency
  Calciphylaxis (see Fig. 46-14)

Hematologic
  Sickle cell anemia (see Fig. 46-13)
  Thalassemia
  Coagulopathy (see Fig. 46-11)
  Cryoglobulinemia

Medication (hydroxyurea) (see Fig. 46-18)
  Pyoderma gangrenosum
    Ulcerative (see Fig. 46-2)
    Bullous
    Pustular
    Vegetative

Multifactorial (any combination of causes)

*Often caused by infection, medication, malignancy, and connective tissue disease.
Modified from Davis MDP. Leg ulcerations. In: Rooke TW, Sullivan TM, Jaff MR, editors. Vascular medicine and endovascular interventions. Malden (MA): Blackwell Futura; 2007. p. 141–148, with permission.

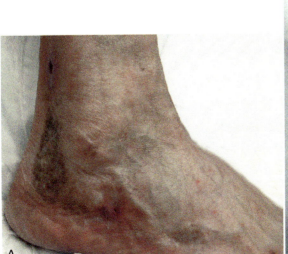
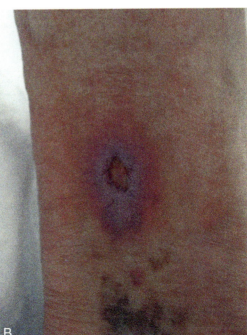

FIGURE 46-1 ■ Ulceration due to livedoid vasculopathy. **A,** Smooth, porcelain-white scars that are surrounded by punctate telangiectasia and hyperpigmentation, in lateral and dorsal aspect of the foot. **B,** Shallow, pinpoint ulceration.

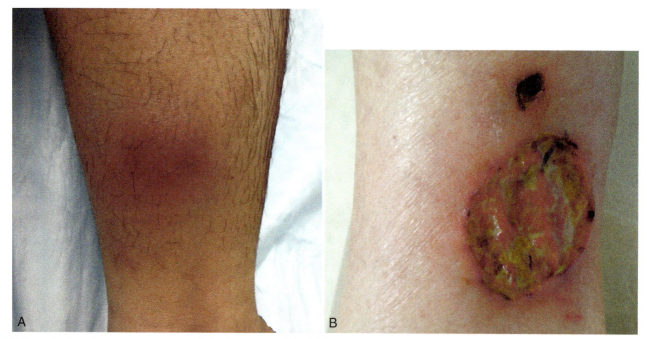

FIGURE 46-2 ■ Pyoderma gangrenosum. **A,** Violaceous nodule, initial lesion. **B,** Ulcerated lesion. Suppurative cutaneous ulcerations have edematous, boggy, blue, undermined, and necrotic borders that can progress rapidly.

factors and different mechanisms of pathogenesis. A patient with pyoderma gangrenosum, for instance, can have arthritis and reduced ankle range of motion that might cause calf muscle pump dysfunction, which leads to venous insufficiency.

Pathophysiology of Chronic Ulcerations

Normal wound healing is a dynamic, integrated process that requires the interplay of numerous factors. An acute wound heals in a series of sequential but overlapping phases known as hemostasis, inflammation, proliferation, and remodeling (Fig. 46-3). A chronic wound fails to progress through this ordered healing process in a timely manner, but rather remains in a dysregulated, asynchronous, and prolonged inflammatory state, and, therefore, does not result in healing. Various factors that contribute to a nonhealing ulceration have been identified. Cells are affected and as an example fibroblasts appear oddly shaped and dysfunctional. Signals are perturbed, for example growth factors are deficient and metalloproteinases are often in excess and are associated with a state of ongoing destruction within the wound. Biofilms (communities of microorganisms in a polysaccharide matrix) can be present in a wound and form a structure that is difficult to penetrate with antibiotics, and they may affect healing. Increasing patient age, nutritional deficiency (especially protein and vitamin deficiency), chronic illness, chronic immunosuppression, hypoxia, vasculopathy, and infection all can contribute to poor wound healing.

We will briefly review the pathophysiology of the most common causes of leg, venous, and arterial ulcerations.

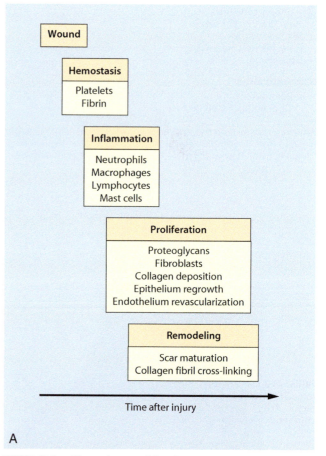

FIGURE 46-3 ■ Normal wound healing. **A,** Timeline of wound-healing events.

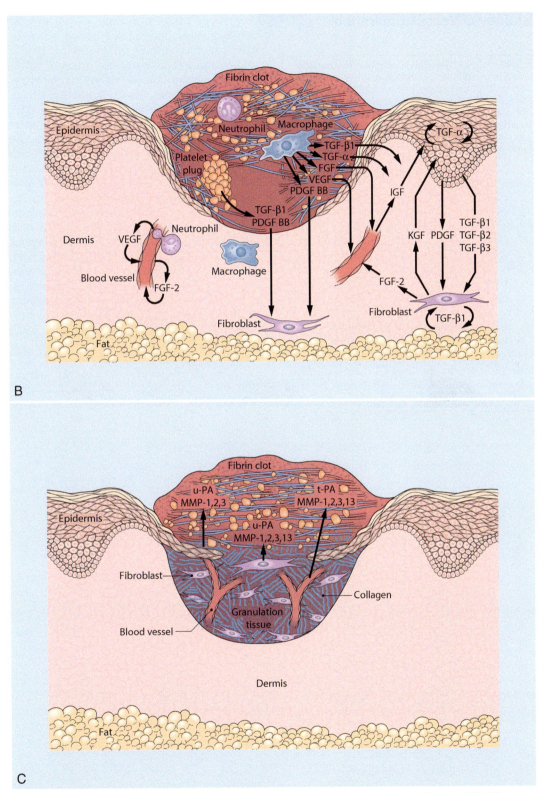

FIGURE 46-3, cont'd ■ **B,** Inflammatory phase (day 3). **C,** Reepithelialization and neovascularization (day 5). *FGF,* Fibroblast growth factor; *IGF,* insulin-like growth factor; *KGF,* keratinocyte growth factor; *MMP,* matrix metalloproteinase; *PDGF,* platelet-derived growth factor; *TGF,* transforming growth factor; *t-PA,* tissue plasminogen activator; *u-PA,* urokinase-type plasminogen activator; *VEGF,* vascular endothelial growth factor. (From Singer AJ, Clark RAF. Cutaneous wound healing. N Engl J Med 1999;341:738–746, with permission.)

Pathophysiology of Venous Ulceration

- Venous insufficiency or dysfunction is caused by outflow abnormalities or venous reflux including either valve dysfunction, deep vein obstruction, calf muscle failure due to muscle disease, or decreased ankle range of motion.
- This results in sustained ambulatory venous pressures or venous hypertension.
- Arterial insufficiency results from failure to deliver oxygen and nutrients to the leg.
- Progressive atherosclerosis is the most common etiology, but any other process that obstructs the arterial flow can result in arterial insufficiency.

Venous blood flow in the lower extremities is dependent on the superficial, communicating, and deep venous systems. The long and short saphenous veins and their tributaries make up the superficial system. The communicating (or perforator) veins connect the superficial veins of the leg with the deep venous system. Communicating veins are equipped with one-way bicuspid valves that direct flow only into the deep system. The deep veins contain valves and are either intramuscular or intermuscular (Figs. 46-4 and 46-5).

When a person is standing, the pressure in the superficial and deep venous systems is roughly equal to the hydrostatic pressure in the legs (80 mm Hg). During the muscle contraction phase of ambulation and with a full range of movement of the ankle, the calf muscle contraction exerts a pressure greater than 80 mm Hg in the deep veins, and blood is propelled cephalad. Proper valve function ensures unidirectional flow and prevents transmission of high venous pressure to the superficial drainage system. After deep venous emptying, calf muscle relaxation, and the muscle relaxation phase of ambulation, deep venous pressure decreases to 0 to 10 mm Hg. Valves open and allow flow from the superficial system to deep venous drainage. Generally, in a healthy person, veins empty and ambulatory venous pressure decreases during exercise; this process requires intact leg veins, intact venous valves, efficient calf muscle pumps, and no deep venous outflow obstruction (Fig. 46-5).

In contrast, in persons with venous insufficiency or dysfunction outflow problems or reflux exist. This is associated with valve dysfunction, deep vein obstruction, and calf muscle failure, at times caused by decreased ankle range of motion. This results in increased sustained ambulatory venous pressure (also known as venous hypertension) during exercise, and it is most often due to obstruction or valvular dysfunction affecting superficial, perforator, or deep veins. As a result, patients develop edema and slow-healing wounds, most commonly on their lower legs, near their ankles.

Although the causes of chronic venous hypertension (venous insufficiency) seem reasonably well understood, the pathophysiology of ulceration in venous

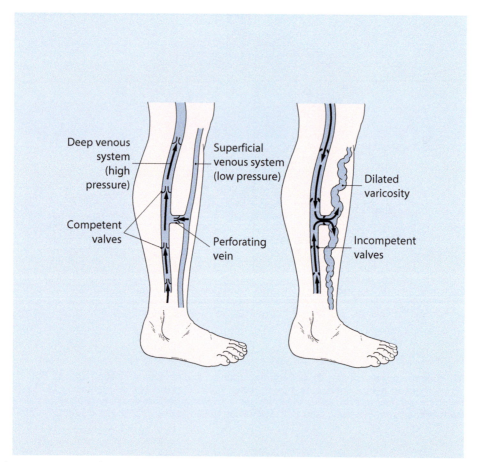

FIGURE 46-4 ■ The low-pressure superficial venous system, which is protected by valves from the high-pressure deep venous system. Venous insufficiency is associated with valvular dysfunction. High pressure is thus transmitted throughout the superficial and deep venous systems. (From Phillips TJ, Dover JS. Leg ulcers. J Am Acad Dermatol 1991;25:965–987, with permission.)

insufficiency is still unknown. One theory postulates that increased intraluminal pressure in the capillaries causes leakage of fibrinogen through capillary walls with deposition of pericapillary fibrin cuffs and impairment of oxygen or nutrient diffusion to tissue; together, these changes may result in tissue necrosis and ulceration (Fig. 46-6). A second theory regarding the mechanism of injury posits that the known sludging of white blood cells in venous insufficiency causes capillary obstruction. Trapped white blood cells may become activated and release proteolytic enzymes that promote ulceration. A third theory, the "trap" hypothesis, suggests that the leakage of fibrin and other macromolecules into the dermis traps or binds growth factors and reduces the amount available for tissue repair.

Pathophysiology of Arterial Ulceration

Arterial insufficiency results in local ulceration and skin, digital or even limb necrosis, depending on the severity of ischemia; the failure to deliver oxygen and nutrients to the leg results in tissue breakdown. Progressive atherosclerosis is the most common etiology, where the arteries become stenotic as a resultant of deposits of lipid and plaque deposition in arterial vessel walls. While some restrict the term to large vessel disease, any other process that obstructs the arterial flow can result in an arterial ulceration. Diseases associated with arterial insufficiency and formation of ischemic ulcers include large-vessel disease (thromboangiitis obliterans, arteriovenous malformations), small-vessel disease (Raynaud's phenomenon), microthrombotic disease (antiphospholipid syndrome, cryoglobulinemia, and cholesterol emboli), vasculitis, sickle cell disease, and polycythemia vera, among others.

PATIENT HISTORY AND PHYSICAL EXAMINATION FINDINGS

- Thorough examination of arterial supply is essential in patients with leg ulcerations.
- Physical examination should include palpation for dorsalis pedis and posterior tibialis pulses.
- Screening for arterial insufficiency should be performed if clinically relevant, with the measurement of ankle–brachial pressure index (ABI).
- If ABI is >0.7, compression can be applied safely.

History

An adequate history must be obtained to establish the cause of ulceration (Table 46-2). A history of ulcerations may be predictive of future ulcerations. Medications, family history, social history, and review of systems also may provide important information. For example, a long-standing, nonhealing ulceration has less probability to heal, especially if older than 6 months. Atypical etiologies often suffer from delayed diagnosis including malignant etiologies (Fig. 46-7). Contact allergy to topical medications used on the leg is a common aggravating factor (up to 65% of patients in some studies). A family history of ulcerations could be attributable to coagulopathy disorders; a social history of intravenous drug abuse may indicate that ulcerations could be caused by infection, or

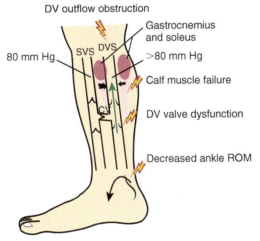 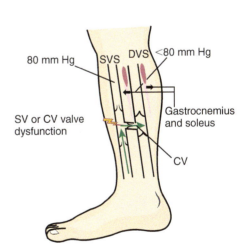

FIGURE 46-5 ■ Calf muscle pump and venous insufficiency. Venous blood return to the heart results from blood flowing from the SVS to the DVS via the action of the calf muscle pump. At rest in the standing position, the hydrostatic pressure in the SVS and DVS systems is approximately 80 mm Hg and net flow equals 0. **A,** Muscle contraction during ambulation: with full ROM of the ankle during ambulation and resultant contraction of the gastrocnemius and soleus muscles, a pressure >80 mm Hg is exerted on the DVS and venous blood flows cephalad, whereas the SVS and CV valves close to prevent retrograde flow into the SVS. **B,** Muscle relaxation in ambulation: with relaxation of calf muscles following the emptying of the DVS, pressure therein decreases below 80 mm Hg and blood from the SVS empties into the DVS through the patent SV and CV valves. A combination of pathologies may occur resulting in venous insufficiency. SVS or CV valve dysfunction, calf muscle failure, decreased ROM at the ankle, DVS outflow obstruction, and DVS valve dysfunction can all cause venous hypertension or more appropriately termed sustained ambulatory venous pressures (venous pressure that does not reduce with walking). Calf muscle: gastrocnemius and soleus muscles. *CV,* Communicating veins; *DVS,* deep venous system; *ROM,* range of motion; *SV,* superficial veins; *SVS,* superficial venous system. Arrows toward DVS, calf muscle contraction; arrows away from DVS, calf muscle relaxation. Blue arrows, venous flow. (From Kirsner RS, Baquerizo Nole KL, Fox JD, Liu SN, Healing refractory venous ulcers: new treatments offer hope. J Inv Dermatol 2015;135:19–23.)

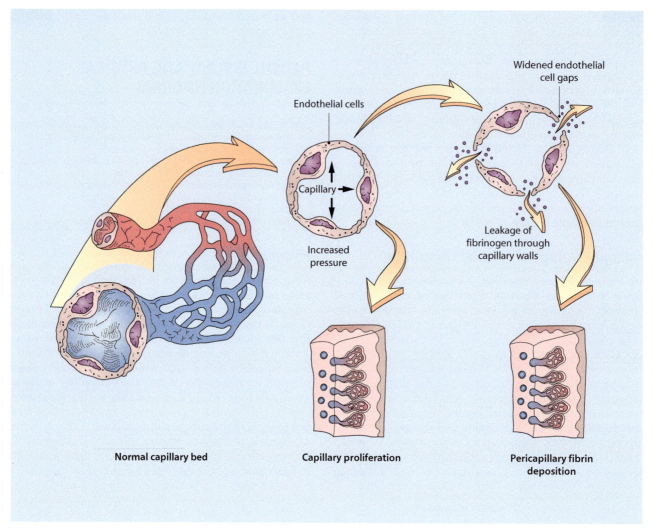

FIGURE 46-6 ■ Venous insufficiency. The high venous pressure is transmitted to the capillary circulation. The endothelial pores widen, allowing the escape of fibrinogen into the extracellular fluid, with deposition around the capillaries. Capillary proliferation also occurs. (From Phillips TJ, Dover JS. Leg ulcers. J Am Acad Dermatol 1991;25:965–987, with permission.)

by injection of foreign material. On the other hand, past medical history of uncontrolled hypertension could be a clue to the diagnosis of Martorell ulcers (Fig. 46-8), and a history of injections for cosmetic purposes may indicate a lipogranuloma. Patients may also have factitious or self-inflicted ulcerations (Fig. 46-9).

Physical Examination

A focused physical examination could give us clues for diagnosis. For instance, paleness and jaundice in a patient could indicate the coexistence of sickle cell, and the absence of pedal pulses indicates arterial insufficiency. Key elements of the ulceration that can provide diagnostic information are outlined in Table 46-3. The size of the ulcer should be documented at each visit with photographs and by noting dimensions of greatest length and perpendicular width and depth. Size and depth may be important prognostically because larger ulcerations are slower to heal. Any undermining, sinuses, or tunneling must be determined. The pattern of the ulcerations may also provide important clues. Characteristics of the ulcer base (color, presence of necrosis) can affect healing. The moisture level (dry, moist, or wet) and the presence or absence of exudate helps elucidate the cause of the ulceration and affect management decisions. The surrounding skin may suggest causes of ulceration (e.g., red, hot skin may indicate cellulitis).

For all patients with leg ulcers, thorough examination of arterial supply is essential. Part of a physical examination should include palpation for dorsalis pedis and posterior tibialis pulses. Screening for arterial insufficiency should be performed in most patients if clinically relevant, starting with the measurement of ABI. The inter-Society Consensus for the Management of Peripheral Arterial Disease defines a cutoff ABI value of 0.90 or less for diagnosing *peripheral vascular disease* at rest. In elderly patients or in patients with diabetes mellitus, a falsely elevated ABI (>1.1) may require additional testing to evaluate for arterial disease. This measurement can be easily done in the office. If ABI is >0.7, compression can be applied safely. Ruling out of sensory neuropathy can be accomplished through the use of nylon monofilament (10 g). Sensory neuropathy is more common with plantar foot ulcers than leg ulcers. Patients who are unable to feel anything when

TABLE 46-2 Important Historical Features for Diagnosis of Ulcerations

Pain
    Usually severe when associated with ischemic ulcerations, pyoderma gangrenosum, calciphylaxis, hydroxyurea-induced ulcerations
    Less severe when associated with venous ulcerations
Rate of progression (rapid vs. slow)
    Pyoderma gangrenosum ulcerations progress rapidly
Duration of ulceration
    Long duration of ulceration is a predictor of poor healing
Prior therapy
    Systemic
    Topical
Medical and surgical history
    History of ulcerations (predictive of future ulcerations)
    Venous disease, arterial disease, lymphedema
    Neurologic disease
    Diabetes mellitus
    Hematologic disease (sickle cell anemia, thalassemia, coagulopathy)
    Gastrointestinal tract disease (inflammatory disease may underlie pyoderma gangrenosum)
    Renal disease (calciphylaxis)
    Rheumatologic disease (connective tissue disease)
    Skin disease
    Psychiatric disease
Medications (hydroxyurea)
Family history
    Ulcerations
    Metabolic disorders
    Coagulopathy
Social history
    History of picking at skin
    Psychologic or psychiatric factors
    Smoking (exacerbates ischemic ulcerations)

From Davis MDP. Leg ulcerations. In: Rooke TW, Sullivan TM, Jaff MR, editors. Vascular medicine and endovascular interventions. Malden (MA): Blackwell Futura; 2007. p. 141–148, with permission.

sufficient pressure is applied to buckle the filament are at increased risk for neuropathic foot injury. Table 46-4 shows investigations that may be performed when determining the cause of leg ulcerations.

COMMON CAUSES OF ULCERATION

- Most venous ulcerations occur in the gaiter area, typically over the medial malleolus, may have an irregular, shaggy border, and are superficial.
- Symptoms include aching and swelling in the legs that are exacerbated by dependency and relieved by elevation of the limb.
- Arterial ulcerations typically have a "punched-out" appearance, and occur over sites of pressure or trauma, or at distal points. They are usually dry, with a gray/black base that may be covered with necrotic debris. There is occasional exposure of vital structures, e.g., tendon, bone.
- Arterial ulcerations typically present with symptoms of intermittent claudication. Pain is usually severe, often worsening when the legs are elevated but improving with dependency.
- Atypical etiology needs to be suspected if an ulcer presents in an atypical location, with atypical appearance or symptoms, or if it does not respond to conventional therapy in a timely manner.

Venous Ulcerations

Venous ulcerations increase in prevalence with age, peaking between ages 60 and 80 years. The first episode of venous ulceration may occur much earlier than this, however: 13% are affected by age 30 years, 22% by age 40 years. Studies suggest a somewhat increased risk in women, with a female:male ratio of 1.6:1.

Most venous ulcerations occur in the area between the ankle and the lower calf (the gaiter area), classically over the medial malleolus, and characteristically have an irregular, shaggy border (Fig. 46-10). VLUs are typically superficial, and thus rarely extend to bone or tendon. While patients are at high risk for skin and soft tissue infection such as cellulitis, bone infection is rare, the prevalence of osteomyelitis is low, and, in the absence of concomitant arterial insufficiency, so is their risk of amputation.

Patients with venous ulcerations typically describe aching and swelling in the legs that are exacerbated by dependency and relieved by elevation of the limb. Ulcerations themselves are classically painless but when associated with pain, it is usually described as a burning sensation or ache. Edema of the lower limbs is common. Brown or brown-red hemosiderin pigmentation occurs because of extravasation of red cells into the dermis, collection of hemosiderin within macrophages, and melanin deposition and increased production. Eczematous changes with erythema, scaling, pruritus, and sometimes weeping are common.

Lipodermatosclerosis or sclerosing panniculitis (woody induration and fibrosis of the dermis and subcutaneous tissue) often develops in patients with venous insufficiency, and often precedes venous ulceration. After ulceration is well established, repeat episodes of infection and cellulitis can damage the lymphatic system and result in chronic lymphedema. Ultimately, fibrous or bony ankylosis at the ankle may develop because of immobility. However, ankle immobility may also be a cause as well as a consequence of venous ulcerations.

Patients may be predisposed to the development of a venous thrombosis if they have coagulation disorders (Fig. 46-11), antithrombin III deficiency, activated protein C resistance (mainly factor V Leiden mutation), antiphospholipid antibody and lupus anticoagulant, protein C or S deficiencies, prothrombin G20210A mutation, some dysfibrinogenemias, hereditary or acquired hyperhomocysteinemia, and elevated levels of procoagulant factors IX, X, and XI. A higher risk of venous thrombosis is associated with an increased risk of venous insufficiency, and patients with venous insufficiency are more likely to have venous ulceration.

Medical conditions associated with the development of VLUs are outlined in Table 46-5.

Patients with venous ulcerations seem to have an increased incidence of contact dermatitis and are especially sensitive to lanolin, topical antibiotics (e.g., gentamicin, neomycin, and bacitracin), and components of Unna boots. Contact dermatitis can also occur with almost any of the occlusive or semiocclusive dressings, despite improvements in wound care technology.

Poor prognostic factors include a large wound area, long wound duration, poor compliance with compression, history of knee or hip replacement, ABI <0.8, and

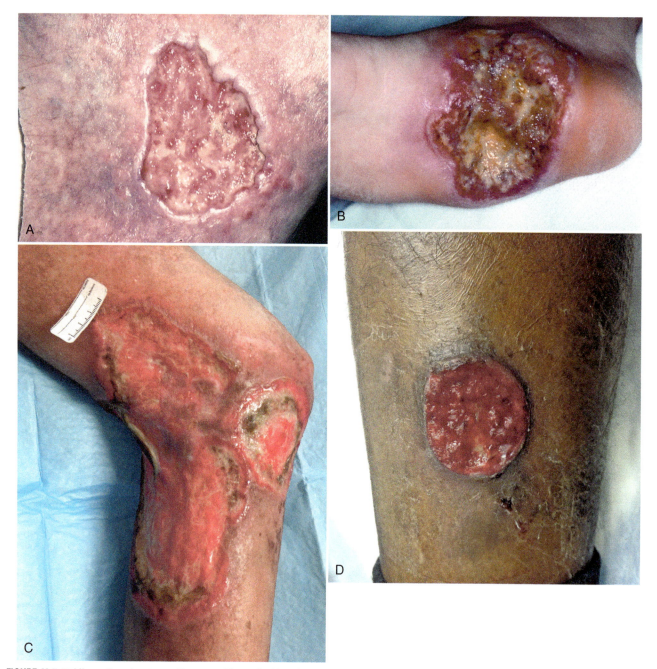

FIGURE 46-7 ■ Ulceration due to malignancy. The rolled border, necrotic tissue, and edge hypergranulation are suggestive of malignancy. **A,** Basal cell carcinoma. **B,** Clear cell sarcoma. **C** and **D,** Cutaneous T-cell lymphoma.

fibrin on 50% or more of the wound surface. One recent study showed that 72% of ulcerations with surface areas <5 cm² at baseline had complete healing, whereas those ≥5 cm² healed at only a 40% rate using the same treatment regimen. Likewise, ulceration duration less than 1 year was associated with a 65% healing rate, and ulcerations of 1 year or longer duration healed at a rate of less than 29%. Others have found 6 months' duration also to be indicative of a refractory ulcer.

Arterial Ulcerations

Patients with arterial ulcerations are usually older than 45 years. They typically present with symptoms of intermittent claudication and pain that initially occur with moderate exercise but are eventually present even at rest as the occlusive disease progresses. The pain from ulceration is usually severe and difficult to control, often worsening when the legs are elevated but improving with dependency. Cigarette smoking, diabetes mellitus, hypertension, hyperlipidemia, family history of vascular disease, coronary disease, hyperhomocysteinemia, obesity, and a sedentary lifestyle are risk factors for arterial ulcerations because of atherosclerosis of the lower limbs.

Arterial ulcerations typically have a "punched-out," sharply demarcated border and occur over sites of pressure or trauma (e.g., bony prominences, heel, anterior aspect of lower leg) (Fig. 46-12) or at distal points

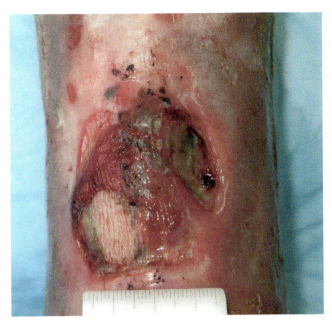

FIGURE 46-8 ■ Martorell ulcer. Posterior ankle location, violaceous border, necrotic tissue, and undermining are diagnostic clues.

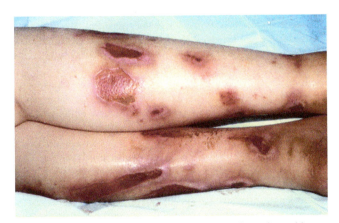

FIGURE 46-9 ■ Factitious or self-inflicted ulceration. Linear, superficial ulcerations in accessible areas suggest external trauma as a cause.

(e.g., toes). They usually appear dry and have a gray or black base that may be covered with necrotic debris, and occasionally present with exposure of vital structures, e.g., tendon, bone.

They can be associated with diminished or absent peripheral pulses, although mild peripheral arterial disease (PAD) in up to 80% of cases can have a palpable pulse as previously discussed. A prolonged capillary filling time (>4 to 5 seconds) and change in limb color with elevation are common findings. Despite the wide belief that lower extremity hair loss is associated with PAD, this fact has not been corroborated.

Atypical Wounds

Although most chronic leg ulcerations have a vascular etiology (venous and/or arterial), up to 10% of leg ulcers may have an atypical etiology. Briefly, if an ulcer

TABLE 46-3 Physical Examination Findings and Clinical Significance

Location
  Ulcerations in the "gaiter" area (between the lower third of the calf and 1 inch below the malleolus) are characteristic of venous disease
  Ulcerations on the lateral malleolus, bony prominences, and distal regions are characteristic of arterial disease
  Thigh ulcerations are characteristic of polyarteritis nodosa, calciphylaxis, or factitious causes

Size
  Smaller ulcerations (<1.5 cm) are more likely to heal within 20 weeks
  Larger ulcerations are slower to heal

Pattern
  Linear ulcerations are likely to be factitial

Base
  Color
    Beefy red appearance preferred; dusky red base may indicate poor blood supply
    Necrotic yellow or brown fibrinous slough or debris inhibits wound healing (needs debridement)
  Depth
    Superficial: likely to heal
    Deep (muscle, bone): difficult to heal
      Osteomyelitis may be suspected clinically if the ulceration reaches the bone
      Undermining: pocket of "dead space" may be a nidus for recurrence of ulceration or infection
  Moisture level
    Moist environment: preferred for healing
    Dry or wet wounds: slow to heal
      Desiccation of tissue occurs with dry wounds
      Maceration of tissue occurs with wet wounds
  Exudate
    Clear: edema
    Yellow: infection
  Odor: fishy odor indicates likely *Pseudomonas* infection

Edges of ulceration
  Sloping: characteristic of venous ulceration
  Vertical: characteristic of arterial ulceration
  Rolled: characteristic of basal cell carcinoma
  Undermined, violaceous: characteristic of pyoderma gangrenosum
  Stellate: livedoid vasculopathy

Surrounding skin
  Skin disease
    Cellulitis
    Dermatitis: eczema, xerosis, allergic contact dermatitis
    Dry skin (asteatosis, xerosis)
    Panniculitis
    Other skin condition
  Color
    Pale: ischemic disease
    Postinflammatory hyperpigmentation
    Yellow plaques: necrobiosis lipoidica
  Edema
    Venous disease
    Lymphedema
    Systemic (cardiac, pulmonary, or renal) disease
  Induration: lipodermatosclerosis
  Patterned
    Livedo reticularis (due to polyarteritis nodosa)
    Livedoid vasculopathy

Diminished pulse: large-vessel disease
Varicose veins: predispose patients to ulceration
Abnormal sensation and motor function: neurologic disease

Modified from Davis MDP. Leg ulcerations. In: Rooke TW, Sullivan TM, Jaff MR, editors. Vascular medicine and endovascular interventions. Malden (MA): Blackwell Futura; 2007. p. 141–148, with permission.

TABLE 46-4 Investigations of Leg Ulcerations (If Clinically Indicated)

Arterial studies
    Ankle–brachial index
    Exercise ankle–brachial index
    Toe–brachial index
    Pulse volume recordings
    Arterial duplex ultrasonography
    Magnetic resonance angiography
    CT angiography
    Conventional angiography
    Transcutaneous oximetry measurements
    Laser Doppler flowmetry
Venous studies
    Duplex ultrasonography to exclude deep vein thrombosis
    Contrast venography
    Functional testing (plethysmography)
Lymphatic studies
    Lymphangiogram
    Lymphoscintigraphy
    Abdominal or pelvic computed tomography or magnetic resonance imaging
Neurologic studies
    Electromyography
    Small-fiber nerve testing
        Autonomic reflexes (Valsalva, table tilting, quantitative sudomotor axon reflex test)
Blood tests to identify potential underlying disorders
    Complete blood count
    Erythrocyte sedimentation rate, C-reactive protein
    Blood chemistry (liver, kidney, thyroid function tests)
    Protein electrophoresis
    Rheumatologic investigations (antinuclear factor, antineutrophil cytoplasmic antibodies)
    Special coagulation studies (factor V Leiden, cryofibrinogens, proteins C and S, cryoglobulins, anticardiolipin antibody, antiphospholipid antibody screening)
Wound swab (usefulness is debated)
    Gram stain, fungal stain, acid-fast stain, *Nocardia* smear
    Culture or polymerase chain reaction assays (to identify virus, bacteria, mycobacteria, fungi)
Biopsy of the edge of ulceration
    Elliptical incisional biopsy (preferred over punch biopsy)
        Specimen should include edge of ulceration to depth of subcutaneous fat
        Routine histologic examination (hematoxylin and eosin stain)
            Special stains (Gram, Periodic acid–Schiff–diastase, methenamine silver, Fite) to detect microorganisms
        Culture in appropriate medium (bacteria, fungi, mycobacteria)
Radiologic studies to exclude osteomyelitis
    Radiograph of underlying bone
    Magnetic resonance image
    Bone scan

Modified from Davis MDP. Leg ulcerations. In: Rooke TW, Sullivan TM, Jaff MR, editors. Vascular medicine and endovascular interventions. Malden (MA): Blackwell Futura; 2007. p. 141–148, with permission.

is present in an atypical location for a common chronic wound, its clinical appearance or ulcer symptoms vary from that of a common chronic wound, or if it does not respond to conventional therapy in a timely manner, then suspecting an atypical etiology is warranted.

For example, a wound on the medial aspect of the leg but extending deep to the tendon would be considered atypical despite being in a common location because the depth of this wound is atypical for VLU. Finally, any wound that is not healing after several weeks (8 to 12 weeks) of appropriate treatment should raise the consideration of an atypical cause, even if the distribution and clinical appearance are classic for a common chronic wound.

Some of the most commonly encountered etiologies for an atypical wound include inflammatory causes, infections, vasculopathy, metabolic and genetic factors, malignancies, and external causes (Fig. 46-13).

Table 46-6 describes the most common atypical leg ulcers, a brief clinical description, management, and associated conditions.

DIAGNOSTIC TESTS

Laboratory Tests

Laboratory investigations are not necessary for all patients with leg ulcerations. However, for those with nonhealing ulcers, a routine blood cell count and measurement of the blood glucose level help exclude clinically significant hematologic disorders, such as anemia, sickle cell disease (Fig. 46-13), or diabetes mellitus. A high erythrocyte sedimentation rate may indicate osteomyelitis or a connective tissue disorder. Low serum albumin or transferrin levels may suggest nutritional deficiencies. A high creatinine level may suggest calciphylaxis (Fig. 46-14). A positive antinuclear factor may be associated with ulcerations attributable to connective tissue disease.

Evaluation of underlying coagulation disorders should probably be limited to patients younger than 50 who have a history of recurrent venous thrombosis and to patients with a single thrombotic event and a positive family history of coagulopathy or recurrent venous thromboses. Coagulation testing can also be considered for patients in whom underlying coagulopathy may be present, such as livedoid vasculopathy (see Fig. 46-1), calciphylaxis, or other particular situations. Importantly, measurement of plasma antithrombin, protein C, protein S, or procoagulant levels may be falsely low or high within 6 months of a thrombotic event, so they should be investigated with caution in the acute setting. However, antiphospholipid antibodies or lupus anticoagulant can be measured immediately, and identification of gene mutations in factor V and prothrombin can be performed at any time. In rare instances, cryoglobulinemia may be a cause of leg ulcerations.

Vascular Studies

A summary of laboratory vascular tests that may be performed is given in Table 46-4.

Venous Studies

Physiologic tests and ultrasonography are used to evaluate venous disease. Currently, ultrasonography is used most frequently to assess acute and chronic venous disease. Physiologic tests are used to evaluate chronic venous disorders by measuring alterations in blood pressure, flow, and other parameters that indirectly assess the location

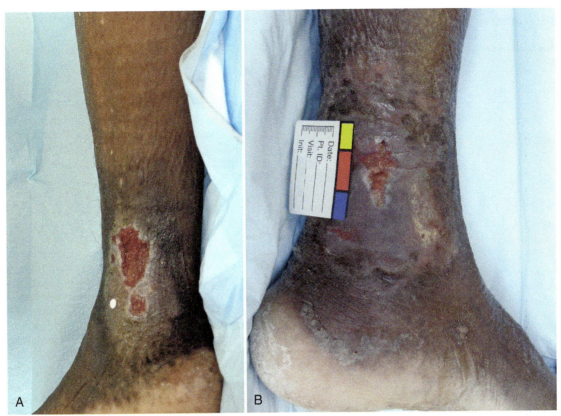

FIGURE 46-10 ■ Venous ulceration. **A,** Venous ulceration over the medial malleoli. **B,** Ulceration on the "gaiter" area of the leg shows an irregular and ill-defined border and a shallow wound bed. Ulceration is surrounded by brown pigmentation, which is characteristic of venous insufficiency.

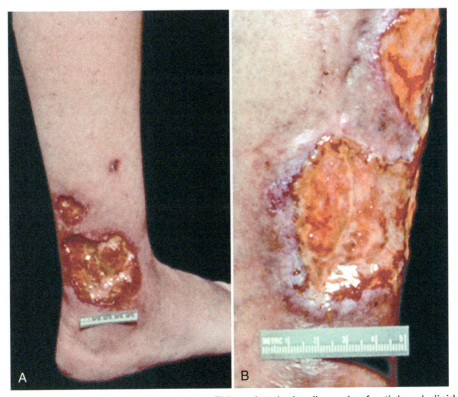

FIGURE 46-11 ■ Ulceration due to hypercoagulable syndrome. This patient had a diagnosis of antiphospholipid syndrome, but the ulcerations resembled those of pyoderma gangrenosum. (From Weenig, RH, Davis MDP, Dahl PR, Su WPD. Skin ulcers misdiagnosed as pyoderma gangrenosum: clinicopathologic correlation and proposed diagnostic criteria. N Engl J Med 2002;347:1412–1418, with permission.)

TABLE 46-5 Conditions Associated with Venous Chronic Insufficiency

Mechanism	Associated Conditions
Valve dysfunction	Primary: • Congenital defect • Idiopathic Secondary: • Physical injury to valves • Phlebitis • Venous distension: hormonal effects, high pressure • Valve damage secondary to deep venous thrombosis
Vein obstruction	• Thrombotic • Nonthrombotic
Calf muscle failure	• Obesity • Immobilization • Neuromuscular conditions • Muscle-wasting syndromes
Decreased ankle range of motion	• Osteoarthritis • Rheumatoid arthritis • Secondary to trauma

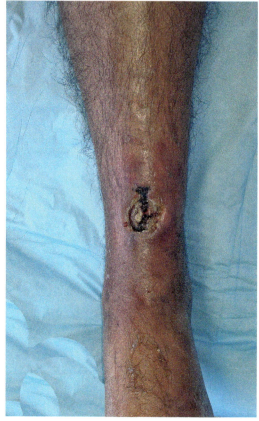

FIGURE 46-12 ■ Arterial ulceration. Ulceration is round with a sharply demarcated border. Note the necrotic debris at the base of the ulceration.

and severity of lesions. Other tests for venous insufficiency include duplex ultrasonographic scanning, photoplethysmography, air plethysmography, strain gauge plethysmography, light reflux rheography, foot volumetry, and phlebography. Duplex ultrasonographic scanning allows direct visualization of the veins, identifies venous flow, and maps superficial and deep veins. It perhaps can be considered the diagnostic standard, but this method also requires the most technical proficiency.

Arterial Studies

The measurement of systolic blood pressure in the ankle is the most sensitive method of detecting large-vessel disease. The ABI is determined by dividing the systolic pressure in the ankle by that in the arm. Patients with moderate to severe arterial disease will have an ABI <0.7. In patients whose peripheral pulses are not palpable, a Doppler flowmeter should be used to hear the arterial pulsations over the dorsalis pedis and posterior tibial arteries. Any patient whose Doppler studies suggest arterial disease should have arteriography and surgical assessment for the feasibility of arterial reconstruction. In patients with diabetes mellitus, noninvasive vascular studies (including the ABI) are frequently poor indicators of the severity of arteriosclerotic disease. Consequently, if ischemia is suspected in such patients, additional tests should be performed such as the toe–brachial index.

Patients with leg ulcerations attributable to rheumatoid arthritis or systemic sclerosis may have arterial or venous insufficiency that contributes to ulcer formation and failure to heal. Calf muscle failure may predispose these patients to venous ulcerations. A study of 15 consecutive patients with leg ulcerations together with one of these conditions showed that all but one had vascular insufficiency that markedly contributed to their ulcer formation, despite the clinical diagnosis of connective tissue disease-associated ulceration. Therefore, patients with rheumatic diseases and ulcerations that respond poorly to appropriate therapies might need vascular assessment to look for complicating disease.

Additional noninvasive tests (pulse waves from the toes and transcutaneous oximetry) may be helpful when assessing the risk of amputation in patients with skin lesions and arterial disease. Pulse waves from the toes can be recorded quickly and easily with photoplethysmography, and the wave amplitude is indicative of blood flow. These measurements may help guide decisions about arterial reconstruction.

Transcutaneous oximetry (the amount of oxygen diffusing through the skin from the capillaries) can be measured with an electrode applied to the skin surface. Oximetry can be used to predict wound healing and the most appropriate level for amputation. In one study, successful healing of below-knee amputations occurred in 96% of patients with a calf transcutaneous oxygen pressure >20 mm Hg, but successful healing occurred in only 50% of patients with a calf transcutaneous oxygen pressure of ≤20 mm Hg.

Biopsy

- Biopsy of the ulcer needs to be considered when atypical etiology is suspected, or when treatment response is not adequate.
- An incisional biopsy involving the wound edge is preferred.
- Tissue is to be sent to histology and tissue culture. If clinically relevant immunofluorescence testing can be added.

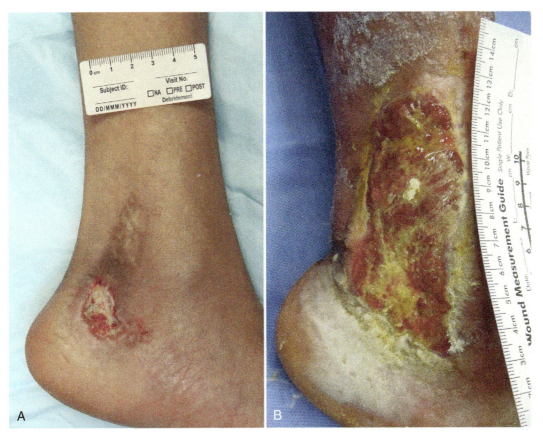

FIGURE 46-13 ■ Sickle cell ulcer. **A,** Small ulceration, fibrinous slough in medial ankle. **B,** Large ulceration in medial aspect of lower leg.

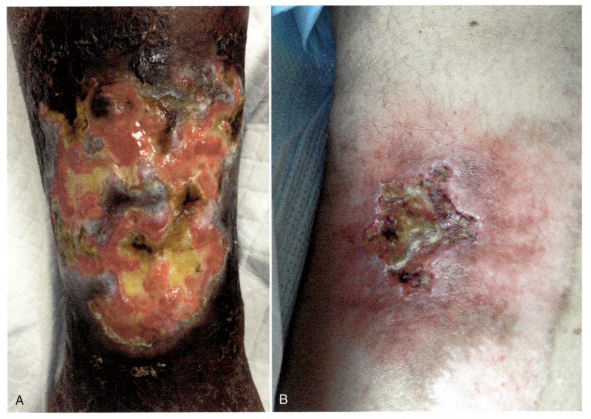

FIGURE 46-14 ■ Ulceration due to calciphylaxis. **A,** Atypical shape wound with necrotic tissue. **B,** Ulcerations on the lower leg show subcutaneous tissue that is tender and hard to palpation.

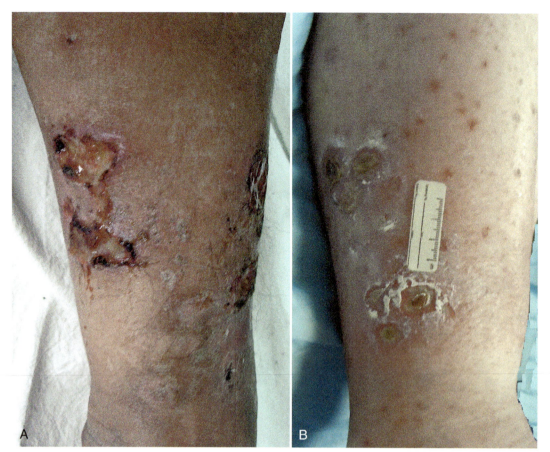

FIGURE 46-15 ■ Ulceration due to vasculitis. **A,** Irregular ulcers with necrotic tissue. **B,** Multiple violaceous papules and necrotic tissue with ulceration.

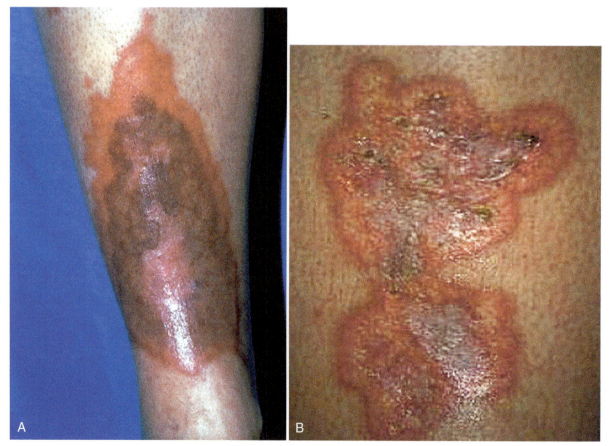

FIGURE 46-16 ■ Necrobiosis lipoidica. **A,** Pretibial plaque, orange hue, and atrophic center. **B,** Central areas of ulceration.

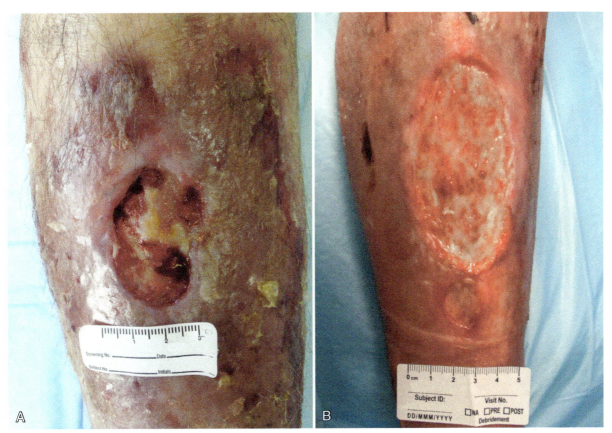

FIGURE 46-17 ■ Ulceration due to radiation. **A,** Patient with past medical history of squamous cell carcinoma, receiving radiation 5 years ago. Note epidermal changes in periulcer area. **B,** Postradiation ulcer in anterior aspect of leg.

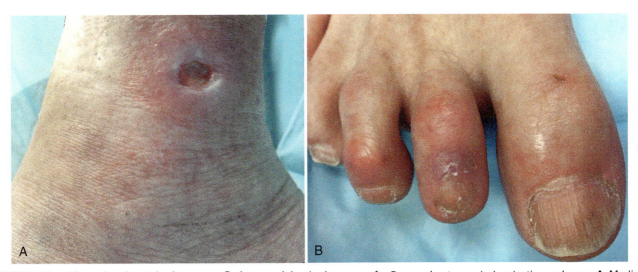

FIGURE 46-18 ■ Ulceration due to hydroxyurea. Patient receiving hydroxyurea for 5 years due to myelodysplastic syndrome. **A,** Medial ankle ulcer. **B,** Redness and atrophy in distal toes.

TABLE 46-6 Differential Diagnosis, Management, and Associated Conditions to Leg Ulcerations

Etiology	Condition	Clinical Description	Specific Management	Associated Conditions
Inflammatory	Vasculitis (see Fig. 46-15)	Wedge-shaped, irregular borders, necrotic tissue. Usually bilateral. Presence of palpable purpura and livedo reticularis	Topical steroids Systemic steroids Dapsone Colchicine Potassium iodide Stanozolol Immunosuppressant Plasmapheresis	Infections Connective tissue disorders Malignancies
	Pyoderma gangrenosum (see Fig. 46-2)	Papule/pustule evolving to an irregular, necrotic ulcer Violaceous rolled up and undermined borders Cribriform scarring wounds may display pathergy Extremely painful	Topical steroids Tacrolimus Nicotine patch Intralesional steroids Dapsone Minocycline Cyclosporine Other immunosuppressant medications TNF-α antagonists	Inflammatory bowel disease Rheumatoid arthritis Connective tissue disease Myeloproliferative disease Monoclonal gammopathy
Infectious	Buruli ulcer	Nodules, papules, plaque, or edema Painless ulcer, undermined edges Massive ulceration over joints, may lead to contractures	Antibiotic therapy Excision followed by skin grafts Amputation in extreme cases	
	Vibrio vulnificus	Contaminated seawater: pustular lesions, lymphangitis, lymphadenitis, and cellulitis Ingestion of raw oysters: septicemia Fever/hypotension	Combination of doxycycline and ceftazidime	Liver disease Diabetes Renal failure Immunosuppression
	Necrotizing fasciitis	Bullous cellulitis/necrotic skin ulcers Hemorrhagic bullae Overlying skin shiny and tense Frank cutaneous gangrene Extremely painful	Surgical debridement Intravenous antibiotics Hyperbaric oxygen therapy	Very ill patients Immunosuppression Diabetes mellitus AIDS Malignancy Obesity
Vasculopathy	Microthrombi-related ulcers (see Fig. 46-1)	Multiple, small, necrotic, painful punched out ulcers. Presence of livedo reticularis, splinter hemorrhages, superficial thrombophlebitis, cyanosis, gangrene	Directed to underlying cause Aspirin Warfarin Prednisone Fibrinolytic agents: stanozolol, streptokinase, streptodornase	Peripheral vascular disease Primary hypercoagulable states Factor V Leiden Antithrombin III deficiency Prothrombin gene mutation Protein C/S deficiency Antiphospholipid antibody Cryoglobulinemia Cryofibrinogenemia Cholesterol emboli

Metabolic and genetic	Calciphylaxis (see Fig. 46-14)	Extensive, irregular, necrotic, and painful ulcers on fatty areas such as thighs, abdomen, breasts	Phosphate binders Cinacalcet Bisphosphonates Sodium thiosulfate Parathyroidectomy Skin grafting	End-stage chronic kidney disease Secondary hyperparathyroidism
	Hypertensive ulcer (Martorell ulcer) (see Fig. 46-8)	Rapidly progressive, extremely painful. Shallow ulcer with purple edges and black eschar located on lateral-dorsal calf or Achilles tendon Commonly misdiagnosed as pyoderma gangrenosum	Debridement followed by skin grafts Blood pressure control Smoking cessation Sporadic success: Anticoagulation therapy Hyperbaric oxygen Prostaglandin E1 Becaplermin Spinal cord stimulation	Local subcutaneous atherosclerosis: • Hypertension • Diabetes
	Necrobiosis lipoidica diabeticorum (see Fig. 46-16)	Plaque-like reddened areas, predominantly in anterior shins The center is a brown-yellow, waxy atrophic texture. Often blood vessels visible Large lesions are most likely to undergo ulceration (35% of patients)	Topical and intralesional corticosteroids Systemic corticosteroids Topical mycophenolate mofetil Perilesional heparin Stanozolol Ticlopidine Pentoxifylline Infliximab Cyclosporine, Clofazimine, Pioglitazone PUVA Excision and grafting Bioengineered skin	Diabetes mellitus
	Sickle cell ulcer (see Fig. 46.13)	Shallow ulcer over medial malleolus Many associated venous insufficiency and frequent infections Exquisitely painful	Keep hemoglobin above 10g/dL Pentoxifylline Hydroxyurea, Erythropoietin Surgical grafts and flaps Bioengineered tissue Pain control	Sickle cell anemia
Malignancies	Squamous cell carcinoma Basal cell carcinoma lymphoma Kaposi's sarcoma (see Fig. 46-7)	Longstanding nonhealing ulcer. Usually exophytic with exuberant granulation tissue and friable center	Surgical excision Topical 5-fluorouracil Topical retinoids Imiquimod Radiotherapy Photodynamic therapy	
External	Radiation (see Fig. 46-17)	With exposure to high doses (>10 Gy), intense erythema, vesiculation, erosion, and superficial ulceration Common postinflammatory pigmentary abnormalities, telangiectasia, and atrophy	Hyperbaric oxygen Surgical excision followed by flaps Pentoxifylline	
Drug-induced	Hydroxyurea (see Fig. 46-18)	Reported in 10% of patients treated for myelodysplastic disorders Painful, well-demarcated wounds Commonly on lateral or medial ankle	Usually cessation of drug Dextranomer dressing Prostaglandins E1, E2 Topical granulocyte-macrophage colony-stimulating factor Human skin equivalent Topical basic fibroblast growth factor Bovine collagen Hyaluronate and collagenase	Myelodysplastic disorders

Features of an ulceration that should prompt a biopsy include an atypical clinical appearance such as vegetative, indurated, undermining border, and atypical location, an atypical presentation such as rapid increase in size or a tendency to bleed, or a failure to respond to therapy. Biopsy of all ulcerations that have not improved after several weeks of adequate treatment should be considered to identify malignancy, vasculitis, vasculopathy, or other inflammatory disorders as possible causes. This can be done by performing an incisional biopsy from the wound edge toward the center of the wound, or multiple punch biopsies of both wound bed and edge. Tissue should be sent to histology with special stains, tissue culture, and immunofluorescence testing if an immune-based cause is suspected.

Histology can be especially helpful in determining ulcers of vasculitic or vasculopathic etiologies, as well as infectious and malignant causes, but are less specific in pyoderma gangrenosum. Depending on the biopsy result, further laboratory testing assessing for underlying and associated disease may be warranted.

Malignancy is identified in chronic wounds in roughly 0.33% of cases, and squamous cell carcinoma and basal cell carcinoma are the most commonly cited. Squamous cell carcinoma arising in a chronic ulceration tends to behave much more aggressively with metastatic disease than with the usual skin-derived squamous cell carcinoma.

Wound Swabs

Bacteria are present on almost all wounds, and swabs may show only colonizing (not causative) microorganisms. In the case of clinical suspicion of infection, a culture from wound swabs would help to direct antimicrobial therapy but does not determine the presence or absence of infection.

Radiographic Studies

Although VLUs are unlikely to predispose to osteomyelitis, other causes of leg ulcerations can. As a rule, if bone is palpated at the base of a chronic ulceration, osteomyelitis must be suspected. Characteristic findings of osteomyelitis can be confirmed through radiographic studies (X-rays), but this method is not very sensitive. Further investigations such as a bone scan, computed tomography scan, gallium scan, or bone biopsy may be necessary to confirm a diagnosis of osteomyelitis. The relative values of magnetic resonance imaging and three-phase bone scans have been debated, but either of these methods can be used to detect osteomyelitis.

PROGNOSIS

Although it is difficult to establish prognoses for all causes of leg ulcers, for VLUs, two risk factors inversely correlated with ulcer healing prognosis are wound size and wound duration. For example, a VLU with a wound size $<5\,cm^2$ and a duration <6 months is more likely to heal with compression therapy than larger and more chronic wounds. Compliance with adequate therapy greatly affects the outcome in patients with lower extremity ulcers. Patient and staff education are important for achieving successful outcomes. In patients with VLUs, recurrence rates are high and patients should be educated on the importance of preventive measures. This includes rigorous use of compression stockings after complete healing and possible venous intervention through endovascular procedures.

GENERAL PRINCIPLES OF WOUND CARE

Wound care is a critical part of patient management and is essential to prevent unnecessary morbidity and death. Leg ulcerations are common (up to 2% of individuals will be affected in their lifetime), and, as outlined above, the associated costs of care are extremely high. Many factors can be associated with delayed wound healing, including vascular insufficiency, diabetes mellitus, neurologic defects, nutritional deficiencies, and local factors (e.g., exudate, venous insufficiency, infection, and edema). Identification and correction of these factors is essential.

The most important aspect of wound care is recognition and appropriate management of underlying disease. For example, arterial disease should be managed with revascularization, venous disease with compression, inflammatory conditions with immunosuppressant medications, and infectious disease with appropriate antimicrobial agents. General principles of wound care include appropriate debridement of devitalized tissue, prompt treatment of any supervening wound infection, maintenance of a moist and clean healing environment, and compression therapy for leg ulcers not associated with PAD.

Debridement of Devitalized Tissue

Debridement is the removal of slough, exudate, eschar, bacterial biofilms, and abnormal cells from wound bed and edge to permit healing (Table 46-7; Fig. 46-19). These elements generally are considered impediments to wound healing and most clinicians agree that they should be removed, unless the ulceration is ischemic (ischemic tissues tend to desiccate after debridement and may be associated with ulcer enlargement) or the diagnosis of pyoderma gangrenosum is suspected (due to possible pathergy). In theory, debridement converts a chronic wound to an acute wound and triggers the acute wound healing response. It may also directly stimulate the underlying granulation tissue by initiating bleeding.

Management of Infection

All open wounds are colonized by microorganisms. Systemic antibiotic therapy should be used only if a wound has clinical evidence of infection (e.g., cellulitis). Culture results from either biopsies or wound swabs will in most cases identify the infectious organism and direct antibiotic therapy. Empiric therapy is appropriate early in the course of care; regimens might include cephalexin, clindamycin, sulfamethoxazole/trimethoprim, and fluoroquinolones.

The use of antibiotics is not appropriate to treat what is grown on wound cultures because these organisms

TABLE 46-7 Methods of Debridement

Method	Description
Surgical	Most commonly performed debridement procedure Uses a curette or scissors and forceps. Can be performed in the outpatient setting Extensive debridement is usually an inpatient procedure requiring local or general anesthesia
Mechanical	Performed by placing wet gauze on an ulceration and allowing to air dry until moist (preferred) or completely dry. Gauze and adhered debris are then removed Frequently changed saline dressings are safe. Wound surface remains moist, surface bacteria are removed, and ulceration surfaces are debrided Other methods include high-pressure irrigation, pulsed lavage, and hydrotherapy
Autolytic	The body's innate enzymes separate slough and necrotic tissue from the wound bed. Best achieved in a moist wound environment
Biological	Sterile maggots of the green bottle fly (*Lucilia sericata*) are placed directly into wound bed. Larvae ingest necrotic material while avoiding newly formed healthy tissue
Enzymatic	Several enzymatic debriding agents are available in the United States (collagenase, papain–urea preparations) Enzymatic debriding agents may affect adjacent healthy tissue and cause ulceration enlargement

are usually colonizing the wounds. Systemic, antibiotic therapy does not decrease biofilm formation, nor does it increase healing rates in noninfected ulcers. Studies also have shown that topical antibiotics do not improve the probability of treatment success; in fact, topical antiseptic solutions are generally ineffective against infection and can damage granulation tissue. Still, antiseptic solutions are frequently used in the care of leg ulcerations, and recently interest in antimicrobial dressings with slow-release iodine has renewed due to their positive effect in reepithelization.

To summarize, systemic antibiotic treatment should generally be started only if there is evidence of tissue infection.

Wound Dressings

For hundreds of years, therapeutic efforts focused on drying wounds and absorptive gauzes were the mainstay of management. Nevertheless, since the 1960s, clinicians have understood that moist wounds heal more rapidly than dry ones (e.g., a wound exposed to air), and most currently available dressings are designed to maintain a moist environment for optimal healing. In general, absorbent dressings (e.g., alginates, foams) are used on exudative wounds; dressings that moisturize (e.g., hydrogels, hydrocolloids) are used on dry wounds. Care must be taken to avoid an excessively moist wound, however, because the surrounding skin may macerate and result in a larger ulceration.

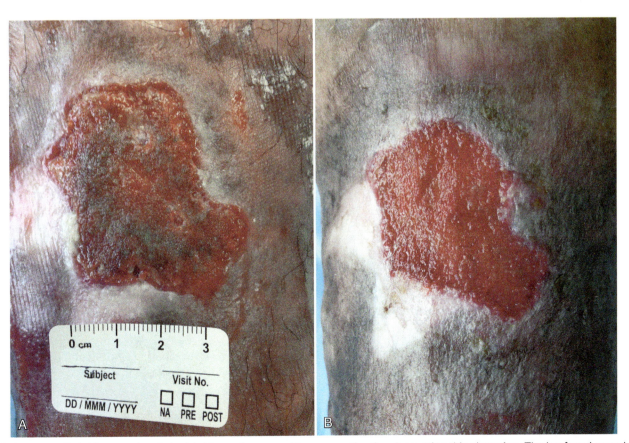

FIGURE 46-19 ■ Debridement. Autolytic debridement was used to remove the slough covering this ulceration. The beefy red granulation tissue at the base is considered optimal for wound healing.

Dressings can do more than provide a moist environment: they can help debride the wound, change the bacterial flora, and change the biochemical environment. Moisture-retentive dressings have the additional advantages of providing local pain relief, promoting granulation tissue formation, and reducing the frequency of dressing changes. Functionally different wound dressings are combined in commercial products (e.g., silver combined with alginate, collagen with hydrocolloid). The best combinations for exudative wounds are alginates, foams, and dry gauze. The best for dry wounds are hydrogels, hydrocolloids, and impregnated gauze.

Limb Elevation

Control of edema is extremely important for healing venous ulcerations, and probably to any cause of leg ulcerations. This can be achieved primarily through limb elevation and compression. The simplest method of leg elevation is to get patients off their feet and into bed when possible; elevating the affected leg 18 cm above the level of the heart for 2 to 4 hours during the day and at night is most effective. If this is not possible, patients should understand that the ankle must be elevated higher than the level of the knee to be of any benefit. Leg elevation should be encouraged in all patients with venous insufficiency, unless they have concomitant arterial insufficiency.

Compression

Compression is as important as elevation in the management of venous ulcerations and should be applied on arising and maintained at least until bedtime. Raising the local hydrostatic pressure and reducing the superficial venous pressure reduce the leak of solutes and fluid into the interstitial space, thus reducing edema. Compression also improves lymphatic drainage, reduces bacterial load, and improves fibrinolysis.

The optimal pressure of the compression bandaging for most patients without arterial disease is 35 to 40 mm Hg and typically is changed weekly unless an excessive amount of drainage requires more frequent changes. Methods of compression include support stockings, elastic and nonelastic single-layer bandages, multilayer bandages, and intermittent pneumatic compression.

Elastic Support Stockings

Elastic support stockings should be comfortable and may be removed at night and before bathing or sleeping. Their major disadvantages are inadequate control of drainage, and the difficulty of application and removal, particularly for elderly patients. However, stockings with a zipper and several similar devices are commercially available to facilitate the process.

Unna Boot

The Unna boot is an inelastic compression bandage that consists of a zinc-oxide-impregnated gauze wrap that is applied from the toes to the knee, covered with a layer of cotton, and wrapped with an elastic compression dressing. Given its inelastic nature, it only works in ambulatory patients. When correctly applied, however, Unna boots are helpful in treating elderly patients, especially those with concomitant mild arterial insufficiency.

Elastic Multilayer Bandaging Systems

A Cochrane systematic review determined that compression therapy was more effective than noncompressive dressings for the treatment of VLUs. Furthermore, high-compression systems were more effective than low-compression systems. No significant differences in the effectiveness of different high-compression systems were observed.

Multilayered bandage systems additionally provide cushioning, have absorptive capacity, and require less frequent dressing changes. However, this system requires trained personnel for adequate application.

Adjunct Wound Care Techniques
Growth Factors

Animal models of chronic wounds have shown that growth factors can improve healing, but overall, results from clinical trials studying growth factors to accelerate wound healing have been disappointing. To date, the US Food and Drug Administration has approved only recombinant platelet-derived growth factor BB (becaplermin, in gel form) for adjunct treatment of diabetic neuropathic foot ulcerations. However, an available hematopoietic stimulant, granulocyte-macrophage colony stimulating factor, when used intralesionally, has shown to improve wound healing in VLUs. The main disadvantage that precludes its use is pain both locally and with the occurrence of bone pain.

Skin Grafts

Surgical skin grafts may be beneficial for some patients with recalcitrant ulcerations. Split-thickness and full-thickness grafts can be used, with split-thickness grafts being more common. The main disadvantages of their use are donor site morbidity and limited tissue availability. A relatively recent technique, epidermal grafting, has been used in the management of chronic wounds. The main advantage is that the donor site heals completely within a few days without scarring, and may be used in future procedures.

Tissue-Engineered Products

Tissue-engineered skin equivalents have been approved by the US Food and Drug Administration for use in treating venous ulcerations. Skin substitutes are effective in healing larger and deeper ulcerations and those of long duration. They can be classified as acellular and cellular products.

Currently available is a product composed of human growth-arrested keratinocytes and fibroblasts, and bovine collagen type I. A study of 240 patients with venous ulcerations showed that a higher proportion were healed 24 weeks after treatment with this product and compression, compared with compression alone (57% vs. 40%, respectively).

Among the acellular products, porcine-derived small intestine submucosa healed 55% of VLUs treated when compared with 34% in the compression-alone group at 12 weeks. In a randomized controlled trial with VLUs that used as an endpoint 40% wound closure after 4 weeks, 62% of the group that received dehydrated human amnion/chorion membrane allografts achieved the endpoint when compared with 32% in the control group.

Pentoxifylline

Pentoxifylline, a substituted xanthine derivative, has been shown to improve wound healing associated or not with compression. Usually higher doses (800 mg every 8 hours) are associated with better outcomes; however, gastrointestinal adverse events are the limiting factor for its use. Possible mechanisms of action include reduction of leukocyte adhesion to vascular endothelium, fibrinolytic activity, reduction of thrombus formation by reducing blood viscosity, increasing red cell deformability, increasing collagenase expression, inhibiting platelet aggregation, and anti-TNF-α activity.

Aspirin

Aspirin 300 mg/daily has been shown to decrease by 46% the time to heal when associated with compression therapy. It is believed that it works due to reduction of inflammation and inhibition of platelet activity.

Venous Surgery

Although surgical correction of venous pathology does not improve healing, it has been shown to prevent ulceration recurrence along with the use of compression stockings.

OTHER ASPECTS TO CONSIDER

Wound Care Centers

It is important to ascertain the home circumstances of each patient and determine who is available to help cleanse the ulcerations and apply dressings. Patients with recalcitrant wounds may have considerable benefit if they are referred to a multispecialty wound care or wound healing center, where many specialists and state-of-the-art therapies are available.

Pain Management

In general, pain management is an often neglected aspect of wound care. Many leg ulcerations are associated with disabling pain that consequently affects activities of daily living and disrupts sleep. Because chronic wounds may persist for months or years, patients can develop a chronic pain syndrome. For patients with venous ulcerations, quality-of-life measures, mental health, and social function are reduced compared with age-equivalent scores. A flurry of recent publications, primarily from the nursing literature, have described the inadequacy of prevalent pain management protocols and revived interest in pain management for chronic wounds. However, no evidence-based studies have been conducted to date.

Sometimes, simply covering a wound with a moisturizing dressing can reduce pain substantially. Topical analgesics such as lidocaine also may be effective. Systemic and local measures may be taken to control pain.

Management of Arterial Ulcerations

The goals of treatment of ischemic ulcers are to relieve pain, establish adequate circulation, and prevent amputation. This can only be achieved by providing an increase in blood supply; therefore the presence of an ischemic ulcer is an indication for intervention. Patients should be referred to vascular surgery or interventional radiology to be evaluated for potential surgical or endovascular revascularization. Any reversible risk factor should be controlled, and exercise should be encouraged to promote the development of collateral circulation. Many ischemic ulcerations are precipitated by trauma, so the patient should therefore be given detailed instructions regarding care of the lower limbs. Regular use of analgesics may be required to relieve ischemic pain.

Percutaneous balloon angioplasty or stent placement and laser angioplasty are used in conjunction with surgical revascularization. In the event of failure or presence of progressive gangrene or severe rest pain amputation of the involved limb may be necessary.

If the patient is not a candidate for revascularization, or if ischemia is not causing severe pain or gangrene, arterial ulcerations can be managed conservatively.

The use of systemic agents to promote healing of arterial ulcerations remains controversial. Pentoxifylline, cilostazol, and certain prostaglandins have been advocated in some patients but have limited evidence.

Acknowledgment

The editors would like to acknowledge Mark D.P. Davis for his contribution to the fourth edition of this chapter.

SUGGESTED READINGS

Alavi A, Mayer D, Hafner J, Sibbald RG. Martorell hypertensive ischemic leg ulcer: an underdiagnosed entity. Adv Skin Wound Care 2012;25:563–72.

Baquerizo Nole KL, Yim E, Van Driessche F, Davidson JM, Martins-Green M, Sen CK, et al. Wound research funding from alternative sources of federal funds in 2012. Wound Rep Regen 2014;22(3):295–300.

Brueseke TJ, Macrino S, Miller JJ. Lack of lower extremity hair not a predictor for peripheral arterial disease. Arch Dermatol 2009;145:1456–7.

Collins TC, Suarez-Almazor M, Peterson NJ. An absent pulse is not sensitive for the early detection of peripheral arterial disease. Fam Med 2006;38:38–42.

Davis MDP. Leg ulcerations. In: Rooke TW, Sullivan TM, Jaff MR, editors. Vascular medicine and endovascular interventions. Malden (MA): Blackwell Futura; 2007. p. 141–8.

Eberhardt RT, Raffetto JD. Chronic venous insufficiency. Circulation 2014;130:333–46.

Goyal S, Huhn KM, Provost TT. Calciphylaxis in a patient without renal failure or elevated parathyroid hormone: possible aetiological role of chemotherapy. Br J Dermatol 2000;143:1087–90.

Kirsner RS, Baquerizo Nole KL, Fox JD, Liu SN. Healing refractory venous ulcers: new treatments offer hope. J Inv Dermatol 2015;135:19–23.

Phillips TJ, Machado F, Trout R, et al. Prognostic indicators in venous ulcers. J Am Acad Dermatol 2000;43:627–30.

Quattrone F1, Dini V, Barbanera S, Zerbinati N, Romanelli M. Cutaneous ulcers associated with hydroxyurea therapy. J Tissue Viability 2013;22:112–21.

Quattrone F, Dini V, Robetorye RS, Rodgers GM. Update on selected inherited venous thrombotic disorders. Am J Hematol 2001;68:256–68.

Rice JB, Desai U, Cummings AK, Birnbaum HG, Skornicki M, Parsons N. Burden of venous leg ulcers in the United States. J Med Econ 2014;17(5):347–56.

Serena TE, Carter MJ, Le LT, Sabo MJ, DiMarco DT. EpiFix VLU Study Group. A multicenter, randomized, controlled clinical trial evaluating the use of dehydrated human amnion/chorion membrane allografts and multilayer compression therapy vs. multilayer compression therapy alone in the treatment of venous leg ulcers. Wound Repair Regen 2014;22:688–93.

Shiman MI, Pieper B, Templin TN, Birk TJ, Patel AR, Kirsner RS. Venous ulcers: a reappraisal analyzing the effects of neuropathy, muscle involvement, and range of motion upon gait and calf muscle function. Wound Repair Regen 2009;17:147–52.

Singer AJ, Clark RA. Cutaneous wound healing. N Engl J Med 1999;341:738–46.

Smiley CM, Hanlon SU, Michel DM. Calciphylaxis in moderate renal insufficiency: changing disease concepts. Am J Nephrol 2000;20:324–8.

Tang JC, Vivas A, Rey A, Kirsner RS, Romanelli P. Atypical ulcers: wound biopsy results from a university wound pathology service. Ostomy Wound Manage 2012;58:20–2. 24, 26-9.

Trent JT, Falabella A, Eaglstein WH, Kirsner RS. Venous ulcers: pathophysiology and treatment options. Ostomy Wound Manage 2005;51:55.

Valencia IC, Falabella A, Kirsner RS, Eaglstein WH. Chronic venous insufficiency and venous leg ulceration. J Am Acad Dermatol 2001;44:401–21.

Weenig RH, Davis MDP, Dahl PR, Su WPD. Skin ulcers misdiagnosed as pyoderma gangrenosum: clinicopathologic correlation and proposed diagnostic criteria. N Engl J Med 2002;347:1412–8.

CHAPTER 47

CUTANEOUS DRUG ERUPTIONS

Kara Heelan • Neil H. Shear

KEY POINTS

- Prevent harm: Be aware of high-risk drugs and always consider a drug reaction as part of a differential diagnosis.
- Monitoring: Monitor for systemic involvement.
- Diagnosis: Determine the morphology of the eruption and decide if it is simple or complex.
- Management and treatment: After a causality assessment, stop most likely potential drugs when clinically appropriate.

INTRODUCTION

Cutaneous drug reactions account for a large proportion of adverse drug reactions. Cutaneous drug reactions can be very challenging to diagnose. They can mimic many other skin diseases; this is especially evident during childhood when viral exanthems are commonplace. If a patient is taking numerous medications, establishing causality to a specific drug can be difficult.

This chapter includes a review of general principles, mechanisms, and clinical manifestations of cutaneous drug eruptions. We have classified different types of drug eruptions by morphology: exanthematous, urticarial, pustular, and bullous. Within each of these groups we have divided them into simple, benign, or nonfebrile and complex or febrile reactions. We also include a miscellaneous group to ensure a methodical review. Diagnostic maneuvers are discussed, and an algorithm is presented to enable the clinician to attain an idea about the possible responsible drug.

There are a number of ways to classify drug reactions. Our classification is a widely accepted and simplified approach based on morphology and subdivided into simple and complex to take into account systemic features. Alternative common methods of classification are either to divide reactions into Type A (predictable, acute, related to mechanism of action) or Type B (idiosyncratic, unpredictable, and not related to mechanism of action), versus classifying reactions based on the type of immunologic response (immediate IgE-mediated hypersensitivity reactions, cytotoxic reactions, immune-complex-mediated reactions, and T-cell-mediated/delayed type reactions).

EPIDEMIOLOGY OF CUTANEOUS DRUG REACTIONS

Cutaneous adverse drug reactions (CADRs) are a commonly reported type of adverse drug reaction (ADR) and can lead to frequent clinical visits and discontinuation of therapy. Dermatologic reactions are the most common manifestation of systemic drug hypersensitivity. Up to 2% to 3% of all hospitalized patients experience either an urticarial or an exanthematous drug eruption. Up to 5% of patients who receive certain antibiotics while hospitalized experience either urticarial or exanthematous reactions. During hospital admission 10% to 20% of patients have a drug reaction, and they represent the fifth most common cause of death in hospital.

When a combination of trimethoprim–sulfamethoxazole is given to human immunodeficiency virus (HIV)-infected patients a hypersensitivity reaction may develop in as many as 50%. The risk of severe drug eruptions such as Stevens–Johnson syndrome (SJS) and toxic epidermal necrolysis (TEN) is increased in HIV-positive patients and also in SLE, allo/BMT patients, and other immune dysregulated/immune abnormal states. Fatal anaphylaxis from intramuscular penicillin and fatal anaphylactoid reactions from radiocontrast each occur in about 1:50,000 exposed patients. In hospitalized children, cutaneous eruptions are the most common type of drug reaction seen. Around 2.5% of children receiving medication in the outpatient setting will experience a drug eruption, and this figure rises to 12% if the drug is an antibiotic.

DRUG-INDUCED SKIN INJURY

The International Serious Adverse Event Consortium in collaboration with other stakeholders initiated the Phenotype Standardization Project. The goal was to develop standardized phenotypic definitions for three types of ADRs including cutaneous reactions caused by drugs: "drug-induced skin injury" (DISI). While the majority of DISIs are mild, the more serious entities including drug-induced hypersensitivity syndrome (DIHS), which is also known as drug reaction with eosinophilia and systemic symptoms (DRESS), SJS/TEN, and acute generalized exanthematous pustulosis (AGEP) form a more complex scenario within which genetics are an emerging factor.

APPROACH TO THE PATIENT WITH A SUSPECTED DRUG ERUPTION

Making the correct diagnosis is a vital element in the assessment process of possible CADRs prior to introducing treatment or recommendations. Diagnosis can be difficult because drug eruptions can closely mimic other diseases (e.g., exanthematous drug reaction vs. a viral

TABLE 47-1 Characteristics of Major Cutaneous Drug Eruptions

Type of Eruption	Morphology	Mucous Membrane Involvement	Time to Onset	Common Implicated Drugs
Exanthematous	Erythematous No blistering Generalized	Absent	4–14 days	Penicillins, sulfonamides Anticonvulsants
Drug-induced hypersensitivity syndrome/drug reaction with eosinophilia and systemic symptoms	Severe exanthematous rash Facial involvement Edema	Infrequent	2–8 weeks	Anticonvulsants Sulfonamides Allopurinol Minocycline
Urticaria	Wheals Pruritus	Absent	Minutes to hours	Penicillins, opiates Aspirin/nonsteroidal anti-inflammatory drugs (NSAIDs) Sulfonamides Radiocontrast media
Angioedema	Swollen deep derma and subcutaneous tissue	Present or absent	Minutes to hours	Angiotensin-converting enzyme inhibitors Aspirin NSAIDs
Acneiform	Inflammatory lesions No comedones Atypical sites	Absent	Variable	Iodides, isoniazid Corticosteroids Androgens Lithium, phenytoin Epidermal growth factor-receptor inhibitors
Acute generalized exanthematous pustulosis	Nonfollicular, sterile pustules arising on background of edematous erythema	Present or absent	<4 days	β-Lactam antibiotics Macrolides Other antimicrobial agents Calcium channel blockers Rarely radiocontrast dye or dialysates
Stevens–Johnson syndrome	Atypical targets Mucosal inflammation <10% body surface area	Present	1–3 weeks	Anticonvulsants Sulfonamides Allopurinol NSAIDs
Toxic epidermal necrolysis	Confluent and extensive epidermal detachment >30% body surface area	Present	1–3 weeks	Anticonvulsants Sulfonamides Allopurinol NSAIDs
Fixed drug eruption	One or more round, well-circumscribed erythematous edematous plaques Sometimes central bullae	Absent	First exposure: 1–2 weeks Reexposure: <48 hours, usually within 24 hours	Trimethoprim/Sulfamethoxazole NSAIDs Tetracyclines Pseudoephedrine

exanthem, toxin-mediated erythema, or acute graft-versus-host disease, and AGEP vs. pustular psoriasis). Identification of the causative drug can be complicated if the patient is taking several different drugs concomitantly. For accurate diagnosis a rational approach is required. This includes an initial clinical impression, forming a differential diagnosis, analysis of drug exposure (including timing of new medications, dose adjustments or increases, drug–drug interactions, and metabolic changes and their impacts on drug levels, such as renal or hepatic insufficiency), laboratory results, diagnostic tests, and utilization of the available literature. Prioritization of the diagnosis includes a causality assessment.

An initial clinical impression is based principally on the morphology of the eruption. The four main categories described, based on the primary lesion, are exanthematous, urticarial, blistering, or pustular. Systemic signs (e.g., malaise, fever, hypotension, tachycardia, lymphadenopathy, synovitis, dyspnea, etc.) allow for refinement of the primary clinical impression (Table 47-1). These systemic signs may aid in differentiating a benign or simple cutaneous drug eruption from a severe or complex drug eruption (Table 47-2). Establishment of the diagnosis is the final step in diagnosis. Table 47-3 identifies the target organs potentially involved in complex reactions.

A careful analysis of drug exposure should ensue. All medications should be included, regardless of route of administration, and incorporate prescription drugs, over-the-counter, and herbal remedies. Patients or caregivers should be asked specifically about vitamins, pain medications, sedatives, laxatives, oral contraceptive pills, and any medications that may not be on a pharmacy list (e.g., infliximab, radiocontrast dye). In the Boston collaborative drug study most cutaneous reactions occurred after the first week of exposure. The onset of

TABLE 47-2 Morphologic Classification of Drug Eruptions

Exanthematous
Simple	Exanthematous drug eruption
Complex	Drug-induced hypersensitivity syndrome/drug reaction with eosinophilia and systemic symptoms

Urticarial
Simple	Urticaria
Complex	Serum sickness-like reaction

Pustular
Simple	Acneiform
Complex	Acute generalized exanthematous pustulosis

Bullous
Simple	Pseudoporphyria Fixed drug eruption
Complex	Drug-induced pemphigus Drug-induced bullous pemphigoid Drug-induced linear immunoglobulin-A disease Stevens–Johnson syndrome Toxic epidermal necrolysis

Miscellaneous
Fixed drug eruption	Purpura (nonvasculitis)
Neutrophilic eccrine hidradenitis	Photosensitivity
Eruptions from biologic agents	Erythema nodosum
Drug-induced lupus	Lichenoid
Sweet's syndrome	Alopecia
Vasculitis	Hirsutism
Warfarin-induced necrosis	Hyperpigmentation
Dermatomyositis	Systemic allergic contact dermatitis

TABLE 47-3 Target Organs with High-Risk Drug Eruptions

Target	Types of Reaction
Upper airway	Anaphylaxis, anaphylactoid reactions
Cardiovascular system	Anaphylaxis, anaphylactoid reactions, erythroderma
Lung	Anaphylaxis, anaphylactoid reactions, TEN, vasculitis
Liver	Drug hypersensitivity syndrome/Drug reaction with eosinophilia and systemic symptoms
Kidney	Vasculitis, serum sickness, TEN, drug hypersensitivity syndrome
Gastrointestinal system	Vasculitis, TEN
Skin (burn-like complications)	SJS/TEN, pemphigus, pemphigoid, severe photosensitivity (sepsis, fluid/electrolyte abnormalities)
Mucosa (eyes, mouth, genital)	SJS/TEN
Thyroid	Drug hypersensitivity syndrome

SJS, Stevens–Johnson syndrome; *TEN*, toxic epidermal necrolysis.

TABLE 47-4 Diagnostic Tests used Selectively in Drug Reactions

In vitro Tests
IgE assays: radioallergosorbent test, immunoenzymatic assays
Basophil activation test
Lymphocyte transformation test
Lymphocyte activation test

In vivo Tests (Caution—Testing by Experienced Personnel in an Appropriate Clinical Setting)
Prick, scratch, or intradermal skin tests
Epicutaneous patch test
Histopathologic examination
Rechallenge/provocation

---

the cutaneous reaction should be carefully documented as well as the effect of previous patient-initiated rechallenge and dechallenge. Each drug, its dose, and duration along with relevant signs and symptoms should also be recorded.

A literature search may provide helpful information. Laboratory tests can aid a diagnosis. A complete blood count and differential, liver and renal function should be requested. Cutaneous biopsies can be useful to differentiate between differential diagnoses but biopsies do not allow for confirmation of a causative drug. Histopathologic findings may help clarify the drug reaction pattern, but they do not identify the responsible drug. Histopathologic examination can confirm the diagnosis of SJS, fixed drug eruption, vasculitis, and erythroderma, and may support the clinical diagnosis of urticarial or morbilliform drug reactions. Eosinophils are widely believed to be major participants in many cutaneous drug reactions. The microscopic presence of eosinophils certainly suggests a drug cause; however, the absence of eosinophils does not exclude a drug as a possible etiologic agent nor does the presence of eosinophils confirm a drug as a possible etiologic agent.

There is no single diagnostic test that can be employed across the board in cases of cutaneous drug hypersensitivity. This is because of the variability of pathogenetic mechanisms operating in the different morphologic variants, the possibility that drug–virus interactions were important clinically, or that nonpharmacologic additives or excipients were responsible.

A list of available in vitro and in vivo diagnostic tests for drug hypersensitivity is found in Table 47-4. In vitro testing includes lymphocyte transformation test, lymphocyte toxicity assay, histamine release test, basophil degranulation test, passive hemagglutination lymphocyte transformation test, leukocyte and macrophage migration inhibition factor tests, and radioallergosorbent test. Specific IgE assays, such as the radioallergosorbent test, are the most commonly employed for evaluating immediate hypersensitivity reactions. These include urticaria, angioedema, and anaphylaxis. Only a few drugs can be tested this way, such as the β-lactams and insulin. Although IgE assays are still less sensitive than scratch tests, they should be used together with scratch testing under proper supervision in patients at risk for anaphylaxis. The basophil activation test uses flow cytometry to detect markers of response to drug allergens. It has been employed in cases of immediate hypersensitivity to β-lactams, muscle relaxants, and nonsteroidal anti-inflammatory drugs (NSAIDs).

The lymphocyte transformation test measures the proliferative response of a patient's T cells in vitro to a suspected drug culprit. It has been reported to be more sensitive for diagnosis than patch testing, but has some limitations. First, although it has been found to be positive in the majority of cases of exanthematous reactions, the drug hypersensitivity syndrome, and AGEP, it is only rarely positive in cases of TEN, fixed drug eruption, and vasculitis. Second, timing of the test is important, with cases of the drug hypersensitivity syndrome showing a negative test in the first few weeks after onset of the eruption. Finally, the test is not available at most clinical centers.

In vivo tests include skin testing and provocation or oral rechallenge and also patch testing. Prick tests have been found to be a useful diagnostic tool in cases of sensitivity to β-lactams and muscle relaxants used in anesthesia. Intradermal testing can be performed when prick tests are negative. To date, penicillin is the most widely used systemic drug for which intradermal skin testing is significantly reliable. Patients with the majority of important drug reactions, including SJS and TEN, exanthematous reactions, vasculitis, and erythroderma, should not undergo this form of testing.

Patch testing for cutaneous drug reactions has been studied the most vigorously of all the skin tests. Sensitivity varies depending on the type of reaction, the putative drug, the concentration of drug tested, and, for fixed drug eruptions, the site at which the patch is placed. Positive results have been obtained in cases of exanthematous reactions, fixed drug eruption, AGEP, and the drug hypersensitivity syndrome. Sensitivity has varied between 30% and 50%. The specificity and negative predictive value have not been determined.

Establishment of the final diagnosis is the final step in the diagnosis. If a definite diagnosis is not possible then a prioritization diagnosis must be completed by combining the information gathered. The traditional approach of highly probable, probable, possible, unlikely, and almost excluded are helpful. The Naranjo assessment classifies a drug reaction as definite, probable, and possible. To fulfill the criteria for a definite reaction four components must be met. These include (1) temporal relationship, (2) a recognized response to the suspected drug, (3) improvement after drug withdrawal, and (4) reaction on rechallenge. A probable reaction includes parts 1 to 3 but does not include rechallenge and a possible reaction only requires a temporal relationship.

Discontinuation of drug therapy and resumption of therapy with the drug in question at a later time may allow immunologic effector mechanisms to "recharge" fully, making large-scale discontinuation of all drugs the patient is receiving worthy of careful scrutiny. The potential for the disease being treated to worsen after drug discontinuation has to be considered in dechallenge decisions. Each case should be handled individually, with a consideration of the risks and benefits of discontinuing drug therapy. In managing patients with high-risk reaction patterns, rechallenge with the drug in question should be carried out only in very rare circumstances, when the need to know the responsible drug exceeds the risk of a severe reaction with the rechallenge. Intentional rechallenge can be performed only when a clinical presentation meets the criteria in Table 47-5. Reports of patients with accidental rechallenge provide useful information on drug causes, but it is essential to avoid such accidental rechallenge. It is important to note that rechallenge is not optimally sensitive or specific. Despite these limitations, rechallenge, when indicated, is the best way to identify accurately the causative drug in the clinical setting. The presence or absence of drug–drug and drug–virus interactions should always be considered in this diagnostic step.

TABLE 47-5 Criteria for Intentional Drug Rechallenge with Potentially Serious Drug Reactions

Drug in question is essential for treatment of the specific medical condition
No suitable alternative drug(s) is available
Illness to be treated is potentially serious
Rechallenge occurs ideally at least 1–2 months after reaction subsides
Appropriate informed consent is obtained
Undertaken in hospital setting, preferably with an oral form of the drug in question
Pretreatment with corticosteroids, antihistamines, or desensitization protocol, if applicable, is considered

The technique of "reverse challenge" seems most reasonable and practical when there is one drug of high suspicion and several others of lower suspicion that were started simultaneously prior to the cutaneous drug eruption. The failure to reproduce the reaction when the patient receives the low-suspicion drugs increases the likelihood that the high-suspicion drug (which is not rechallenged) is responsible for the drug reaction. This method essentially clears from responsibility the drugs that were actually rechallenged.

A negative result with oral rechallenge can mean that the drug tested was not responsible for the reaction; that it was perhaps administered at too low a dose; or that the rechallenge did not reproduce all the clinical conditions for the prior cutaneous drug eruption. A positive rechallenge can be regarded with reasonable certainty as indicating that the drug tested was responsible for the cutaneous drug reaction. Again, rechallenge is not endorsed for high-risk drug reaction patterns, except in the most exceptional circumstances.

In order to exclude (to a reasonable degree of certainty) nondrug causes for the reaction pattern present the clinician should use appropriate historic and physical examination findings, along with well-directed laboratory tests. Most commonly, a variety of infectious agents can mimic the majority of cutaneous drug eruptions discussed.

MECHANISMS OF CUTANEOUS DRUG ERUPTIONS

The patient's genetic background may be significant. Human leukocyte antigen (HLA) molecules play an important role in drug reactions, as they present antigen

TABLE 47-6	Sources for Information on Specific Cutaneous Drug Eruptions and Responsible Drugs

Dermatology Texts
General dermatology texts
Specific monographs on drug reactions
Kauppinen K, Alanko K, Hannuksela M et al. Skin reactions to drugs. Informa Healthcare, 1998
Breathnach SM, Hintner H. Adverse drug reactions and the skin. Oxford: Blackwell Scientific Publications; 1992
Litt's drug eruption and reaction manual, 21st ed. CRC Press; 2015

Major Clinical Studies
Boston Collaborative Drug Surveillance Program
Finnish studies (see Suggested Readings)
RegiSCAR studies (see Suggested Readings)

Periodicals
The Medical Letter on Drugs and Therapeutics
WHO Pharmaceuticals Newsletter
WHO Drug Information

Other Resources
FDA Medwatch (http://www.fda.gov/medwatch/)
Package insert for a given drug
PDR Guide to Drug Interactions, Side Effects and Indications, 2008. Thompson Healthcare (updated yearly)
Pharmaceutical company data
USP DI. Drug Information for the Health Care Professional. Greenwood Village, CO: Thomson Micromedex (published annually)

to T cells. Specific HLA genotypes have been shown to confer a greater susceptibility to various drug eruptions, e.g., HLA B*1502 and carbamazepine-induced SJS, HLA B*5701, and abacavir-induced hypersensitivity syndrome. Defective detoxification of reactive metabolites (with anticonvulsants, by epoxide hydroxylases) is thought to be responsible for a familial predisposition to aromatic anticonvulsants and sulfonamides hypersensitivity syndrome. In drug-induced lupus the acetylator phenotype is important: slow acetylators have a higher risk. Key information sources on specific cutaneous eruptions and responsible drugs are listed in Table 47-6.

Most drugs that induce cutaneous drug eruptions have a molecular weight of less than 1000 Da, therefore they must serve as haptens for an immunologic response. A cell-based or soluble carrier protein is necessary for a drug of this size to become a complete antigen. In most instances, drug metabolites, and not the parent drug, induce the immunologic hypersensitivity. Most allergic (immunologic hypersensitivity) drug reactions should demonstrate the following features: (1) they occur in a small percentage of patients; (2) there is a history of prior exposure to the drug or a chemically related compound; and (3) there was a latency of 1 to 2 weeks between the initial exposure and the onset of the reaction and a latency of 1 to 2 days with rechallenge. Allergic drug reactions are not dose-dependent. The reaction differs from the drug's pharmacologic effects and from other established signs of drug intolerance. The eruption should resolve with dechallenge and reappear after rechallenge with the drug in question.

Cutaneous drug eruptions that have no specific sensitization to a drug hapten are known as "pseudoallergic" or anaphylactoid reactions. Drugs such as opiates and radiocontrast material directly degranulate mast cells without prior specific antigen sensitization. Aspirin and NSAIDs may induce urticaria by effects on the arachidonic acid pathway, leading to nonspecific mast cell degranulation. Idiosyncratic reactions can lead to either organ-specific (such as the skin) or generalized hypersensitivity.

Reactivation of viruses has been observed in drug reactions, especially in the drug hypersensitivity syndrome. Whether the reactivated virus further stimulates the immune system, leading to a more severe clinical course, or whether the virus is an innocent bystander that is reactivated by drug-induced immune stimulation, is controversial.

The most common mode of drug administration leading to sensitization is topical exposure. Oral exposure leads to specific sensitization more commonly than does parenteral (intramuscular or intravenous) exposure. After specific sensitization has occurred, rechallenge by parenteral routes is significantly more risky than by oral administration. Topical exposure presents the least risk of serious reactions with rechallenge.

Cross-reactions between chemically related drug groups are important to consider when assessing cutaneous drug reactions. Most notable are the many potential cross-reactions between drugs with a β-lactam nucleus, such as the original penicillins, aminopenicillins, semisynthetic penicillins, and probably cephalosporins; this holds true for certain groups of anticonvulsant medications as well. After the patient is sensitized to one member of this broad group of drugs, other related drugs should be considered to have a potential for cross-reaction. Aspirin and the various NSAIDs may cross-react, usually by nonallergic mechanisms. Cross-reactivity between antibacterial and nonantibacterial sulfonamides, on the other hand, is extremely unlikely based on their divergent chemical structures.

MORPHOLOGIC SUBTYPES

Exanthematous Eruptions

Simple Exanthematous Eruptions

Exanthematous drug eruptions (synonyms: morbilliform, maculopapular, or scarlatiniform eruptions) are the most common drug-induced eruptions (Fig. 47-1). They occur in 1% to 5% of first-time users of most drugs. This type of drug reaction is increased in the presence of viral infections, e.g., a near 100% incidence of exanthematous reaction in patients who have Epstein–Barr virus taking penicillin. Patients with human immunodeficiency virus infections or bone marrow transplant are at increased risk. The most common classes of drugs implicated include penicillins, sulfonamides, cephalosporins, and antiepileptic medications. Exanthematous drug eruptions are characterized by erythematous macules and/or papules, usually beginning 7 to 14 days after the initiation of a new medication, and sometimes after drug discontinuation. The eruption is usually

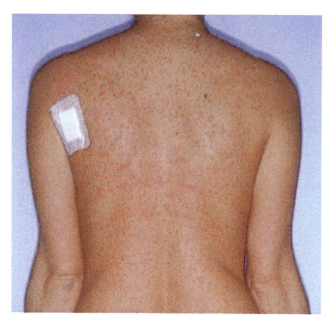

FIGURE 47-1 ■ Exanthematous drug eruption on the trunk.

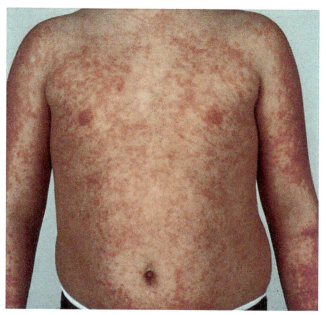

FIGURE 47-2 ■ Drug-induced hypersensitivity syndrome (aka drug reaction with eosinophilia and systemic symptoms) due to carbamazepine. Fever, pharyngitis, exanthem, and nephritis.

symmetrical, beginning on the trunk, becoming generalized and is without blistering or pustulation. Mucous membranes are usually spared, and facial involvement is uncommon, but palms and soles are often involved. Pruritus is the main symptom.

Pathology is nonspecific and consists of eosinophils, a mild perivascular lymphocytic infiltrate, and associated necrotic keratinocytes at the basal layer. The differential diagnosis of exanthematous rashes is very broad. Viral exanthems tend to be indistinguishable from exanthematous drug eruptions and are more common in the pediatric population. Symptoms and a comprehensive history that includes timelines are very important in helping to establish the diagnosis. Toxic shock syndrome, scarlet fever, acute graft-versus-host disease, Kawasaki disease, and juvenile idiopathic arthritis should be excluded on the basis of clinical features. A number of tests can be performed to further evaluate the patient. These include laboratory tests to evaluate internal organ involvement and rapid strep test/throat bacterial culture. Skin biopsy is generally not useful in this setting. To further complicate issues exanthematous rashes can be exacerbated by concomitant viral infections.

The eruption is self-limited, therefore the management is largely supportive. A decision whether to discontinue the implicated drug must be made. This is based on the availability of an unrelated substitute, or if the drug is of paramount importance a decision can be made to continue it and offer symptomatic treatment. The risk:benefit ratio of this option has to be carefully weighed and the evolution of the eruption meticulously monitored. Whether continuation of a drug can lead to SJS is debatable. Oral antihistamines, bland emollients, and topical corticosteroids can be used to treat pruritus. The eruption often turns to a brownish-red and fades within 7 to 14 days of discontinuation of the offending drug. Scaling or desquamation may follow. Rechallenge may lead to the reaction appearing within a few days.

Complex Eruption: Drug-Induced Hypersensitivity Syndrome

Drug-induced hypersensitivity syndrome (DIHS, also referred to as DRESS) should be suspected when an exanthematous drug reaction occurs with associated fever and internal organ involvement (Fig. 47-2). DIHS has cutaneous, hematologic, and internal organ manifestations, is severe, and leads to mortality in up to 10% of individuals. It occurs usually on first exposure to the offending drug with first symptoms 2 to 8 weeks after exposure. The reaction occurs in approximately 1:3000 exposures. The most commonly associated drugs are the aromatic anticonvulsants including phenytoin, carbamazepine, and phenobarbital. Other offending drugs are lamotrigine, sulfonamides, antibiotics, dapsone, minocycline, allopurinol, and nevirapine.

Fever and malaise are usually the first symptoms and can be accompanied by cervical lymphadenopathy and pharyngitis. While cutaneous eruption associated with DIHS can be mild it is more often extensive and severe. It often begins on the face, frequently periorbitally, initially with edema and subsequently erythema and pruritus. It then spreads caudally. Facial edema and lymphadenopathy are common; hand edema has been reported in one-third of patients. The lack of mucosal involvement is a useful distinguishing feature from SJS. Reports of DIHS in the literature describe many different morphologies and include exanthematous eruptions, purpura, cheilitis, vesicles, bullae, and targets.

Atypical lymphocytosis and/or eosinophilia are typically seen early in the course. Regarding visceral involvement, the liver is the most commonly involved internal organ (about 50%); hepatitis may be fulminant and could necessitate liver transplantation. Lymphadenopathy, joint pain, and inflammation of the kidneys, central nervous system, heart and lungs have all frequently been described. Cardiac inflammation can be either acute or delayed, and concerning symptoms should prompt immediate organ reassessment. Thyroiditis can occur but is usually not noticed for 2 to 3 months after onset; other forms of delayed autoimmunity can occur following this eruption, including diabetes, vitiligo, and lupus-like syndromes. The eruption persists for weeks to months after withdrawal. During the recovery period an initial period of improvement may be followed by flare of the cutaneous and visceral manifestations. Rechallenge with the offending drug leads to reactivation of fever and erythroderma within hours. Anticonvulsants metabolized by the cytochrome P450 system can cross-react. A patient who reacts to phenobarbital, phenytoin, or carbamazepine should avoid all three medications.

Patients with DIHS should have a battery of laboratory tests to consider visceral involvement including thyroid testing, which should be repeated at 2- to 3-month intervals. In the management of DIHS prompt withdrawal of the offending drug is vital. The role of systemic corticosteroids is controversial but generally in patients with visceral involvement or severe symptoms, treatment with prednisone (1 to 2 mg/kg per day) is usually ensued; patients often require months of systemic corticosteroid treatment (50 days on average). Antihistamines and topical corticosteroids have also been used to alleviate symptoms. Intravenous immunoglobulin (IVIG) has also been used in the management of DIHS and there are some reports also of the use of cyclosporine. First-degree relatives have a higher risk of developing the same drug reactions, so counseling of family members should be considered.

Urticarial Eruptions

Simple Urticaria

Urticaria is characterized by transient pruritic wheals of the skin and mucous membranes (Fig. 47-3). Drug-induced urticaria represents approximately 5% of all cutaneous drug eruptions. The majority (80%) of cases of new-onset urticaria resolve in 2 weeks and >95% resolve within 3 months.

Complex Urticarial: Serum Sickness-Like Reaction

True "serum sickness" is a probable immune complex mediated (Arthus) reaction that occurs when antibody–antigen complexes deposit and activate a complement cascade. Tissue damage follows. In contrast "serum sickness-like reactions" (SSLRs) do not exhibit immune complexes, hypocomplementemia, vasculitis, or renal lesions that are seen with a true serum sickness reaction. An SSLR is characterized by cutaneous eruption that is usually urticarial sometimes morbilliform, which may favor distal extremities with lesions prominent over joints (Fig. 47-4), malaise, low-grade fever, and arthralgias. Lymphadenopathy and eosinophilia may be present. SSLRs usually occur 1 to 3 weeks after drug exposure and resolve soon after drug discontinuation.

Epidemiologic data on SSLRs are scarce but this reaction is known to occur more often in infants and children. The estimated pooled incidence of cefaclor-related SSLRs has been calculated in the range 0.02% to 0.2% per drug course in pediatric patients. Studies

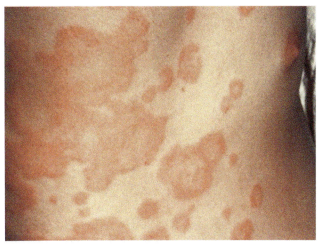

FIGURE 47-3 ■ Urticarial drug eruption.

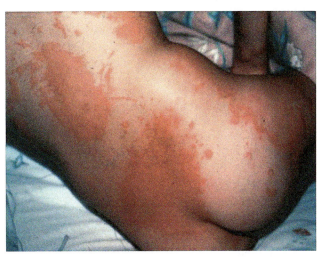

FIGURE 47-4 ■ Serum sickness-like reactions from cefaclor fever, arthralgia, and rash. Urticaria with major itch—dermographism.

have also suggested that the risk of SSLR is greater with cefaclor than with any other antibiotic therapy including other cephalosporins. However, bacterial resistance to cefaclor has reduced its use in pediatric infections and therefore SSLR may be less common than it was in the past. Other drugs that have been implicated include biological agents (efalizumab, omalizumab, rituximab, infliximab), antibiotics (cefuroxime, cefazolin, meropenem, minocycline, ciprofloxacin, rifampicin), antimycotics (griseofulvin, itraconazole), and other agents such as bupropion, clopidogrel, fluoxetine, insulin detemir, immunoglobulin, mesalamine, or streptokinase.

SSLR is a self-limiting disease that subsides within 2 to 3 weeks after discontinuation of the causative agent. The causative drug should be avoided in the future. As the underlying cause of SSLRs remains unknown, treatment is purely symptomatic, consisting of identifying and discontinuing the offending drug, antihistamines if urticaria is the case, and NSAIDs for patients with arthralgia and/or arthritis. It is unclear whether a short course of systemic glucocorticoids is a suitable treatment for those patients who have persisting symptoms despite antihistamines.

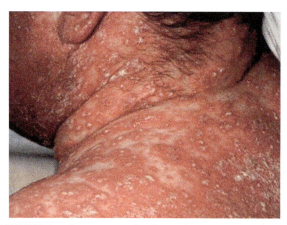

FIGURE 47-5 ■ Acute generalized exanthematous pustulosis.

Pustular Eruptions

Simple: Acneiform

Drug-induced acne often affects the arms and legs; this is in contrast to typical acne vulgaris. The lesions are usually monomorphous and heal without scarring. They have been reported to occur with iodides, bromides, adrenocorticotropic hormone, corticosteroids, isoniazid, androgens, lithium, actinomycin D, EGFR inhibitors, and phenytoin. Corticosteroids can precipitate steroid acne within 2 weeks of starting the medication. The risk appears to be directly proportional to the dose and duration of the therapy and is higher in those with a history of severe acne. Topical medications that are oil-based can also lead to a type of acne known as pomade acne. Cases of testosterone-induced acne fulminans in adolescent boys being treated for excessively tall stature have been reported. Treatments include topical benzoyl peroxide, topical antibiotics, and topical tretinoin.

Complex: Acute Generalized Exanthematous Pustulosis

AGEP is a serious pustular drug hypersensitivity reaction occurring with an incidence of 1 to 5 cases per million per year in the general population. It is rare in the pediatric population; however, it has been observed in children treated with aminopenicillins, cefixime, clindamycin, paracetamol, bufexamac, cytarabine, vancomycin, and possibly labetalol. Recently described cases have attributed AGEP to exposure to radiocontrast dye or dialysates, including peritoneal dialysates. In rare cases AGEP has also been described to occur in the course of viral infections (e.g., parvovirus, Coxsackievirus, cytomegalovirus) and bacterial infections (*Chlamydia pneumoniae*, *Mycoplasma pneumoniae*). It is thought that drug-specific, HLA-expressing CD+ and CD8+ T cells play a central role in the pathogenesis of AGEP.

AGEP usually has a rapid onset during the first week of drug exposure (often the first 1 to 2 days). The skin rash consists of an erythematous edema exhibiting an intertriginous predilection, which is followed by the appearance of hundreds to thousands of nonfollicular, often coalescing, sterile pustules (Fig. 47-5). The majority of affected patients develop fever; however, in children in particular, cases have been reported where fever has been absent. Mild nonerosive mucous membrane involvement occurs in approximately 20% and internal organ involvement is rare. There is a preponderance of peripheral leukocytosis with a neutrophil count often exceeding 7000/μL. The differential diagnosis includes subcorneal pustulosis, candidiasis, and pustular psoriasis. Some patients may display additional cutaneous lesions, e.g., facial edema, atypical target lesions, blisters, and mucosal erosions.

AGEP is self-limited and once the offending drug is withdrawn is characterized by spontaneous resolution over 15 days with fine desquamation and without scarring. There is a favorable prognosis. Treatment should include withdrawal of implicated drug and in severe cases corticosteroids at a dose 1 to 2 mg/kg per day can be given until resolution.

BULLOUS ERUPTIONS

Simple Bullous Eruptions

Pseudoporphyria

Pseudoporphyria is characterized by erythema, skin fragility, blistering, and scarring on photoexposed skin. In contrast to erythropoietic porphyria and porphyria cutanea tarda, milia formation, hypertrichosis, and waxy skin changes do not occur and plasma porphyrins are not elevated. Pseudopophyria has been linked to NSAID use, particularly naproxen, antibiotics (doxycycline, nalidixic acid), diuretics, retinoids, oral contraceptives, and kidney dialysis.

Complex Bullous Eruptions

Drug-Induced Pemphigus

Pemphigus is an autoimmune bullous disease that affects the skin and mucous membranes. Drug-induced pemphigus is a well-established variety of pemphigus. There have been many drugs that have reportedly been involved, e.g., D-penicillamine and captopril.

Drug-Induced Bullous Pemphigoid

The incidence of bullous pemphigoid (BP) increases with age. In general drug-induced BP occurs in a younger population than the idiopathic condition. Implicated drugs include analgesics, antibiotics, diuretics, captopril, D-penicillamine, PUVA, gold, and potassium iodide. Other reported cases include after hepatitis B vaccination and after the combined diphtheria–tetanus–pertussis and polio vaccination.

Drug-Induced Immunoglobulin-A Bullous Dermatosis

Linear immunoglobulin-A (IgA) bullous disease is an autoimmune subepidermal blistering disease that has been described in both children and adults. Characteristically blisters form in an annular fashion. In adults reports have shown that as many as two-thirds of occurrences may be drug-induced. The offending drugs include antibiotics, predominantly vancomycin, nonsteroidal anti-inflammatory agents, and diuretics. Reports in children most commonly include infections and drugs, although an idiopathic form of childhood linear IgA bullous dermatosis exists as well.

Stevens–Johnson Syndrome and Toxic Epidermal Necrolysis

SJS and TEN are clinical variants of the same severe bullous drug reaction. The annual incidence of SJS and TEN is 1.2 to 6 and 0.4 to 1.2 per million individuals, respectively. The annual incidence of SJS and/or TEN in HIV patients is estimated at 1 to 2 per 1000 individuals, approximately 1000-fold higher than that of the general population. The incidence of SJS/TEN increases with age; children less than 15 years of age account for only 10% of the samples in most studies. It is characterized by widespread keratinocyte apoptosis resulting in extensive epidermal detachment. SJS and TEN are differentiated quantitatively, depending on the extent of epidermal detachment. By definition SJS affects <10% and TEN >30%; those affecting 10 to 30% are classified as SJS/TEN overlap. The distinction between these entities is crucial as TEN has a mortality of 25 to 30% whereas SJS has a mortality of 1 to 5%.

Drug exposure is the most common cause of SJS/TEN, with more than 200 drugs identified. Other causes include infections (*M. pneumoniae*, dengue fever, cytomegalovirus, and *Yersinia enterocolitica*), contrast media, and vaccinations. Fuchs syndrome is a unique type of SJS involving the mucosal membranes without skin lesions, which was reported to be associated with *M. pneumoniae* predominantly in children and adolescents; some authors consider this a separate and distinct syndrome, as those patients often display a better prognosis.

Symptoms usually start within 4 to 28 days of the drug initiation. The prodrome phase lasts approximately 48 to 72 hours; nonspecific symptoms including malaise, fever, and anorexia can occur. Shortly thereafter, a symmetrical, erythematous rash consisting of dusky, tender macules on the trunk and extremities develops, which rapidly evolves into atypical lesions with central bulla formation. Nikolsky's sign is positive. A fulminant exfoliative dermatitis evolves (Figs. 47-6, 47-7, and 47-8). Symptoms of epidermal barrier breakdown including hypothermia, dehydration, and sepsis can ensue. Long-term sequelae include skin dyspigmentation, onychodystrophy, and scarring. Severe ocular complications can lead to permanent visual impairment. Other complications include strictures of anogenital mucosa with associated dysuria and painful defecation. Pulmonary mucosal damage leading to severe respiratory symptoms including acute respiratory distress syndrome occurs in up to 30% patients. Severe colitis, hepatitis, and nephritis can also occur.

The SCORTEN was developed by Bastuji-Garin and coworkers to help predict mortality in adults. It comprises seven criteria found to be independent predictors of outcome, age >40 years, total body surface area >10%, serum urea >28 mg/dL, glucose level >252 mg/dL, bicarbonate level <20 mEq/L, heart rate >120 beats per minute,

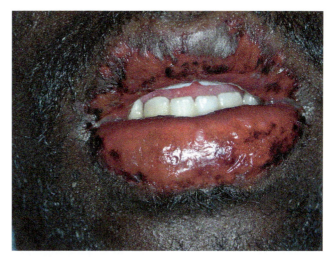

FIGURE 47-6 ■ Painful erythema, hemorrhagic erosion, and epidermal apoptosis from cotrimoxazole.

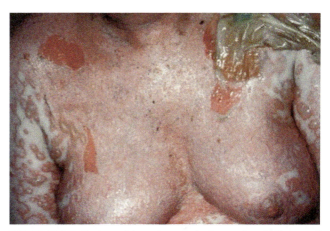

FIGURE 47-7 ■ Toxic epidermal necrolysis: active bullae and erosions.

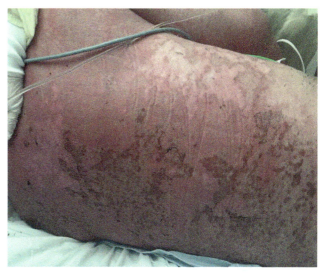

FIGURE 47-8 ■ Toxic epidermal necrolysis: early reepithelialization.

presence of visceral or hematological malignancy. Due to its age dependency this score cannot be used in the pediatric population and to date a modified scoring system has not been developed.

While the pathogenesis is not known, evidence has found a genetic predisposition toward the development of SJS in Han Chinese individuals given carbamazepine (HLA-B*1502). It is therefore extremely important to test for HLA B*15:02 before prescribing carbamazepine to those from East-Asian ancestry. If SJS/TEN is suspected, the incriminating drug and any other medications that are not imperative should be discontinued. Patients should be treated in an intensive care unit setting and retrospective uncontrolled evidence has shown that treatment in a burns care center may shorten overall length of hospital stay and could also reduce risk of systemic infections and subsequently infection-related mortality in some patients.

Treatment should include supportive measures such as hydration, wound care, and nutritional support. Antibiotics can be commenced if there are positive blood cultures or clinical signs of systemic infection. Prophylaxis is not recommended. Ophthalmological care is critical at the acute stage to help minimize potential complications and ophthalmological consultation should occur early in the disease course. Potential systemic treatments include systemic IVIG, corticosteroids, cyclosporine, cyclophosphamide, tumor necrosis factor-alpha antagonists, pentoxifylline, plasmapheresis, and ulinastatin. Many uncontrolled studies, the majority retrospective, have yielded conflicting results with regards the benefits of these. When dosed early, at high doses (1 g/kg/day on 4 consecutive days), IVIG may show a tendency to reduce mortality compared to SCORTEN predictions. Cyclosporine use is expanding, particularly in Europe, with promising results in observed mortality compared to SCORTEN predicted outcomes. Corticosteroids may be helpful in some cases at high doses, administered early in disease course; however, there are numerous cases of TEN developing in patients while on corticosteroids and of patients progressing despite corticosteroid therapy. ALDEN, an Algorithm for the Assessment of Drug Causality in SJS and TEN, was developed by the RegiSCAR study group as a reference tool for assessing drug causality in the diseases. ALDEN uses six parameters in order to potentially identify the offending drug. Drug causality is attributed either as very unlikely, unlikely, possible, probable, or very probable.

Miscellaneous

Fixed Drug Eruption

Fixed drug eruptions (FDEs) are characterized by mucocutaneous lesions that recur at the same site upon re-administration of the causative medication. Responsible drugs include tetracycline and sulfonamide antibiotics, barbiturates, phenolphthalein-containing laxatives, and NSAIDs. Phenolphthalein may also be present in maraschino cherries and other nontraditional exposures. In Finnish studies, FDEs rank in frequency below exanthematous reactions, and above urticaria and angioedema. In other series they are relatively less common. The exact pathogenic mechanisms remain unknown; however, there is evidence that it is a lymphocyte CD8-mediated reaction, wherein the offending drug may induce local reactivation of memory T-cell lymphocytes localized in epidermal and dermal tissues and targeted initially by the viral infection.

The lesions appear as pruritic, well-demarcated erythematous, sometimes bullous macules and plaques. Typically solitary but can be multiple, they heal with a dusky brown hyperpigmentation when the offending drug is discontinued. With rechallenge of the drug a flare is noticed usually within 1 to 8 hours. The sites of predilection include the lips, trunk, legs, arms, and genitals. Genitals are affected particularly in male adolescents. Generalized bullous FDE mimics SJS/TEN. Pathology reveals hydropic degeneration of the basal layer resulting in pigmentary incontinence. In the epidermis dyskeratotic cells may be found. Dermal edema and superficial or deep perivascular lymphohistiocytic infiltrates with scattered eosinophils can be seen. Subepidermal bullae may be present. Rechallenge remains the gold standard for diagnosis. Management is supportive and topical steroids may hasten resolution.

Neutrophilic Eccrine Hidradenitis

This eruption is characterized by erythematous and edematous patches, papules, and/or plaques localized to the extremities, trunk (particularly the axilla), and face. It is usually asymptomatic and begins after chemotherapy but has also been reported to occur in individuals not receiving chemotherapy. Neutrophilic eccrine hidradenitis resolves spontaneously in most patients without treatment. Dapsone has been used prophylactically to prevent recurrences during chemotherapeutic regimens.

Eruptions Caused by Biologic Treatments

Epidermal growth factor receptor inhibitors have been associated with cutaneous eruptions, namely, skin rash, folliculitis, acneiform eruptions, and pruritus. Tumor necrosis factor-alpha antagonists, rituximab (a monoclonal antibody directed against CD20 antigen on B lymphocytes), and tyrosine kinase inhibitors all have the potential to cause cutaneous eruptions. Sorafenib and sunitinib have been shown to cause hand–foot skin reactions. Cutaneous reactions are the most common toxicity to BRAF inhibitors affecting 74% of patients and may display a wide array of cutaneous reactions (including squamous cell carcinoma development, warty growths, keratosis pilaris-like eruptions, palmoplantar thickening, curling of the hair, and more).

Drug-Induced Lupus

A number of medications have been reported to cause a drug-induced lupus syndrome. The more commonly associated ones in adults include hydralazine, procainamide, methyldopa, isoniazid, quinidine, chlorpromazine, anticonvulsants, and antithyroids. Many drugs have been implicated in causing subacute cutaneous lupus especially thiazides, naproxyn sodium (as over-the-counter Aleve), terbinafine, antitumor necrosis factor agents, and others.

Vasculitis

Drug-induced vasculitis (also known as hypersensitivity vasculitis) is relatively uncommon. This is usually a small-vessel vasculitis. Typically, palpable purpura is present. Commonly, these lesions are admixed with nonpalpable purpura, hemorrhagic bullae, erosions, and cutaneous infarcts with necrosis. Mucosal involvement is seldom present.

Drug-induced vasculitis results from circulating antigen–antibody immune complexes that deposit in the affected vessels and activate complement and other inflammatory mediators. Target organs include the joints, kidneys, and gastrointestinal tract, with significantly less frequent involvement of the central nervous system and lungs. Although deaths are infrequent, the risk of death is greatest when there is renal, central nervous system, or pulmonary involvement. Drugs commonly responsible include antibiotics, thiazide diuretics, furosemide, propylthiouracil, and phenytoin.

A subset of patients develop p-ANCA positivity in association with small-vessel vasculitis in the skin. Hydralazine, propylthiouracil, and allopurinol are the common offenders here, and may induce glomerulonephritis, upper respiratory tract disease, and pulmonary hemorrhage. Cocaine abuse, particularly when tainted with levamisole, may induce a mixed cutaneous vasculitis/vasculopathy, and patients may display dual ANCA positivity. Minocycline rarely induces p-ANCA positivity, which presents with fever, arthralgias, livedo reticularis, and subcutaneous nodules.

Other Miscellaneous

There are many other drug reactions that are outside the scope of this chapter. Sweet's syndrome can be drug-induced, most associated with granulocyte colony stimulating factor. Other examples include warfarin-induced necrosis, dermatomyositis, purpura (nonvasculitis), photosensitivity, erythema nodosum, lichenoid, alopecia, hirsutism, hyperpigmentation, and systemic allergic contact dermatitis.

CONCLUSIONS

A high index of suspicion needs to be maintained when a cutaneous drug eruption is suspected. The management of drug eruptions in the emergency department is also worth considering. For those professionals not managing drug eruptions on a usual basis, Table 47-7 provides what we think are the important and critical steps that should be taken if such a diagnosis is suspected. In order to reduce risks of potentially fatal reactions offending drugs need to be withdrawn in a timely fashion. If a cutaneous drug eruption is diagnosed the follow-up and aftercare of these patients become important. It is crucial to provide clear information to the patient concerning his/her drug rash. The name of the medication and any potential medications that could cross-react need to be supplied. In addition, drugs that are safe to be taken should be emphasized. Follow-up in outpatients may be necessary, e.g., in drug hypersensitivity syndrome thyroid function tests need to be evaluated. The presence of a genetic component of some drug reactions needs to be considered and family counseling should be part of a comprehensive assessment.

SUGGESTED READINGS

Alanko K, Stubb S, Kauppinen K. Cutaneous drug reactions: clinical types and causative agents. A five year survey of inpatients (1981–1985). Acta Dermatol Venereol Stockh 1989;69:223–6.

Barbaud A. Drug patch testing in systemic cutaneous drug allergy. Toxicology 2005;209:209–16.

Bigby M. Rates of cutaneous reactions to drugs. Arch Dermatol 2001;137:765–70.

Cacoub P, Musette P, Descamps V, Meyer O, Speirs C, Finzi L, et al. The DRESS syndrome: a literature review. Am J Med 2011;124(7):588–97.

Dodiuk-Gad RP, Laws PM, Shear NH. Epidemiology of severe drug hypersensitivity. Semin Cutan Med Surg 2014;33(1):2–9.

Genin E, Schumacher M, Roujeau JC, Naldi L, Liss Y, Kazma R, et al. Genome-wide association study of Stevens-Johnson syndrome and toxic epidermal necrolysis in Europe. Orphanet J Rare Dis 2011;6:52.

Genin E, Chen DP, Hung SI, Sekula P, Schumacher M, Chang PY, et al. HLA-A*31:01 and different types of carbamazepine-induced severe cutaneous adverse reactions: an international study and meta-analysis. Pharmacogenomics J 2013. http://dx.doi.org/10.1038/tpj.2013.40. [Epub ahead of print].

Haddad C, Sidoroff A, Kardaun SH, Mockenhaupt M, Creamer D, Dunant A, et al. Stevens-Johnson syndrome/toxic epidermal necrolysis: are drug dictionaries correctly informing physicians regarding the risk? Drug Saf 2013;36(8):681–6.

Kardaun SH, Sekula P, Valeyrie-Allanore L, Liss Y, Chu CY, Creamer D, et al. The RegiSCAR study group. Drug Reaction with Eosinophilia and Systemic Symptoms (DRESS): an original multisystem adverse drug reaction. Results from the prospective RegiSCAR study. Br J Dermatol 2013;169(5):1071–80.

Knowles S, Shear NH. Clinical risk management of Stevens-Johnson syndrome/toxic epidermal necrolysis spectrum. Dermatol Ther 2009;22(5):441–51.

Lee HY, Dunant A, Sekula P, Mockenhaupt M, Wolkenstein P, Valeyrie-Allanore L, et al. The role of prior corticosteroid use on the clinical course of Stevens-Johnson syndrome and toxic epidermal necrolysis: a case-control analysis of patients selected from the multinational EuroSCAR and RegiSCAR studies. Br J Dermatol 2012;167(3):555–62.

Li K, Haber RM. Stevens-Johnson syndrome without skin lesions (Fuchs syndrome): a literature review of adult cases with Mycoplasma cause. Arch Dermatol 2012;148(8):963–4.

Lipowicz S, Sekula P, Ingen-Housz-Oro S, Liss Y, Sassolas B, Dunant A, et al. Prognosis of generalized bullous fixed drug eruption: comparison with Stevens-Johnson syndrome and toxic epidermal necrolysis. Br J Dermatol 2013;168(4):726–32.

Mittmann N, Knowles SR, Koo M, Shear NH, Rachlis A, Rourke SB. Incidence of toxic epidermal necrolysis and Stevens-Johnson syndrome in an HIV cohort: an observational, retrospective case series study. Am J Clin Dermatol 2012;13(1):49–54.

Naranjo CA, Shear NH, Lanctot KL. Advances in the diagnosis of adverse drug reactions. J Clin Pharmacol 1992;32(10):897–904.

Nigen S, Knowles SR, Shear NH. Drug eruptions: approaching the diagnosis of drug-induced skin diseases. J Drugs Dermatol 2003;2(3):278–99.

TABLE 47-7	Important Steps in the Emergency Department

Be suspicious and suspect an adverse event as a differential diagnosis
Stop drugs immediately
Be familiar with patterns
Know the high-risk drugs
Determine if simple or complex: check temperature, complete blood count (CBC), urea and electrolytes (U&E), liver function tests (LFTs)
Drug history—if you are not familiar with a drug look it up
Check records (MD, pharmacy, hospital)
If in doubt—admit
Call for help
Transfer to burns unit/intensive care unit as soon as possible if required
Consult other teams early, e.g., dermatology, ophthalmology

Paquet P, Pierard GE. New insights in toxic epidermal necrolysis (Lyell's syndrome): clinical considerations, pathobiology and targeted treatments revisited. Drug Saf 2010;33(3):189–212.

Phillips EJ, Chung WH, Mockenhaupt M, Roujeau JC, Mallal SA. Drug hypersensitivity: pharmacogenetics and clinical syndromes. J Allergy Clin Immunol 2011;127(3 Suppl):S60–6.

Pirmohamed M, Friedmann PS, Molokhia M, Loke YK, Smith C, Phillips E, et al. Phenotype standardization for immune-mediated drug-induced skin injury. Clin Pharmacol Ther 2011;89(6):896–901.

Reyes-Habito CM, Roh EK. Cutaneous reactions to chemotherapeutic drugs and targeted therapy for cancer: Part II. Targeted therapy. J Am Acad Dermatol 2014;71(2):217.

Romano A, Demoly P. Recent advances in the diagnosis of drug allergy. Curr Opin Allergy Clin Immunol 2007;7:299–303.

Roujeau JC, Stern RS. Severe adverse cutaneous reactions to drugs. N Engl J Med 1994;331(19):1272–85.

Sekula P, Liss Y, Davidovici B, Dunant A, Roujeau JC, Kardaun S, et al. Evaluation of SCORTEN on a cohort of patients with Stevens-Johnson syndrome and toxic epidermal necrolysis included in the RegiSCAR study. J Burn Care Res 2011;32(2):237–45.

Sekula P, Dunant A, Mockenhaupt M, Naldi L, Bouwes Bavinck JN, Halevy S, et al. Comprehensive survival analysis of a cohort of patients with Stevens-Johnson syndrome and toxic epidermal necrolysis. J Invest Dermatol 2013;133(5):1197–204.

Shiohara T. Fixed drug eruption: pathogenesis and diagnostic tests. Curr Opin Allergy Clin Immunol 2009;9(4):316–21.

Star K, Noren GN, Nordin K, Edwards IR. Suspected adverse drug reactions reported for children worldwide: an exploratory study using VigiBase. Drug Saf 2011;34(5):415–28.

Stern RS. Clinical practice. Exanthematous drug eruptions. N Engl J Med 2012;366(26):2492–501.

Struck MF, Hilbert P, Mockenhaupt M, Reichelt B, Steen M. Severe cutaneous adverse reactions: emergency approach to non-burn epidermolytic syndromes. Intensive Care Med 2010;36(1):22–32.

Valeyrie-Allanore L, Sassolas B, Roujeau JC. Drug-induced skin, nail and hair disorders. Drug Saf 2007;30:1011–30.

CHAPTER 48

PRINCIPLES OF SYSTEMIC DRUG USE

Cindy England Owen • Stephen E. Wolverton

KEY POINTS

- Systemic medications used for dermatologic conditions are associated with risks.
- The choice of systemic medication requires assessment of the disease severity and the performance of a risk–risk analysis balancing the risk of the disease with the risks of the medication.
- Patients should be made aware of the Food and Drug Administration indications for the selected systemic medication and the basis for off-label use.
- Systemic drug choices should take into account the expense, regimen, other medications used by the patient, pharmacogenomic screening results (where indicated), in addition to patient preferences.
- Informed consent should be obtained and documented. Handouts in lay language about the medication can help with this process and improve safety monitoring.
- Appropriate baseline tests and well-defined monitoring can allow early detection of adverse effects. Particularly strict monitoring may be necessary for critical toxicities. Assistance from other medical specialties may be helpful in monitoring certain high-risk medications.
- Preventive approaches are described that can limit predictable adverse effects.

Although the subject of systemic drug therapy for dermatologic conditions is vast, in this chapter we will review the important principles that guide safe use. Supporting concepts and important clinical examples follow each principle. Two broad categories overriding these principles are drug selection and monitoring.

PRINCIPLES OF DRUG SELECTION

Principle 1. Systemic Drugs with an Element of Risk Are Essential in the Management of Numerous Dermatoses

Many dermatologic therapies are administered through relatively safe topical routes. In addition, there are a number of systemic drugs for which there are few significant risks and which therefore require little or no routine monitoring for adverse effects (Table 48-1). This chapter focuses on the systemic drugs with a significant element of risk that are commonly used to treat more serious dermatologic conditions (Table 48-2).

Principle 2. It Is Important Initially to Make a Reasonable Estimation of the Cutaneous Disease "Severity"

There are a number of dermatologic conditions in which disease severity and associated risks are self-evident. Blistering diseases such as pemphigus vulgaris and blistering drug reactions such as toxic epidermal necrolysis (TEN) have well-established risks. Malignancies that are multicentric at the outset, such as cutaneous T-cell lymphoma (mycosis fungoides), represent another example of high-risk dermatoses. At times, the dermatologic risk is a function of the systemic findings associated with the dermatologic signs of internal disease. Systemic lupus erythematosus, sarcoidosis, drug reaction with eosinophilia and systemic symptoms (DRESS), and dermatomyositis are appropriate examples. The severe irreversible ocular mucosal morbidity with mucous membrane pemphigoid also presents a noteworthy risk.

It is more difficult to determine disease severity and risk in conditions without life-threatening potential and without severe irreversible morbidity. Dermatologists are commonly confronted with the psychosocial risk and/or functional impairment presented by patients with severe acne vulgaris or psoriasis. In these cases the patient and physician collectively will have to determine if appropriate systemic drug therapy with an element of risk is warranted.

Dermatologic conditions in which the morbidity results in a loss of work can also justify potentially risky systemic therapy. Pyoderma gangrenosum is an example of such a condition.

Principle 3. "Risk–Risk" Analysis Is Performed by Comparing the Risk(s) of a Given Disease (As Defined Earlier) with the Inherent Risk(s) of the Proposed Systemic Drug Therapy. The Treatment Risks Should Not Exceed the Inherent Untreated Disease Risk

The risk–risk analysis may be preferable to the risk–benefit ratio, which is traditionally discussed. Even after considering conditions deemed severe by the criteria cited earlier,

TABLE 48-1	Some Systemic Agents Used in Dermatology that Require Little or No Routine Monitoring

Antibiotics
Penicillins
Cephalosporins
Tetracycline
Doxycycline
Trimethoprim-sulfamethoxazole
Erythromycins
Fluoroquinolones

Antivirals
Acyclovir
Valacyclovir
Famciclovir

Antifungal
Griseofulvin

Antihistamines

Vasoactive drugs
Pentoxifylline
Nifedipine
Aspirin
Dipyridamole

Miscellaneous
Potassium iodide
Niacinamide
Finasteride
Apremilast

TABLE 48-2	Some Important Dermatoses Selectively Requiring Systemic Medications with an Element of Risk*

Psoriasis—acitretin, anti-IL-12/23 agents, cyclosporine, methotrexate, PUVA, T-cell modulating agents, tumor necrosis factor-alpha (TNF-α) antagonists, ustekinumab, secukinumab
Acne vulgaris—isotretinoin, minocycline, oral contraceptives, spironolactone
Vasculitis—azathioprine, colchicine, corticosteroids, dapsone
Lupus erythematosus—antimalarials (hydroxychloroquine, chloroquine, quinacrine), azathioprine, corticosteroids, cyclosporine, dapsone, methotrexate, mycophenolate mofetil, retinoids, thalidomide
Pyoderma gangrenosum—adalimumab, anti-TNF-α agents, corticosteroids, cyclosporine, dapsone, infliximab, intravenous immunoglobulin, mycophenolate mofetil, thalidomide
Pemphigus vulgaris—azathioprine, corticosteroids, cyclosporine, intravenous immunoglobulin, mycophenolate mofetil, rituximab
Bullous pemphigoid—azathioprine, corticosteroids, cyclosporine, dapsone, methotrexate, rituximab
Dermatitis herpetiformis—dapsone, sulfapyridine
Mycosis fungoides—bexarotene and other retinoids, methotrexate, PUVA romidepsin, vorinostat, denileukin diftitox
Disorders of keratinization—systemic retinoids
Atopic dermatitis, severe—azathioprine, corticosteroids, cyclosporine, mycophenolate mofetil, PUVA
Severe cutaneous adverse reactions:
DRESS—systemic corticosteroids, intravenous immunoglobulin, cyclosporine
SJS/TEN—intravenous immunoglobulin, cyclosporine, anti-TNF-α agents, systemic corticosteroids
Hemangioma of infancy—propranolol

*The drugs listed under each heading are those on which this chapter focuses and are not an exhaustive list of therapeutic options. The listing of drugs is alphabetical, and does not imply a therapeutic sequence.
PUVA, Psoralen–ultraviolet A therapy; DRESS, drug reaction with eosinophilia and systemic symptoms; SJS, Stevens–Johnson syndrome; TEN, toxic epidermal necrolysis.

dermatologists predominantly face conditions with less risk of death and severe morbidity than do most other specialists in medicine. In most cases, there is a significant subjective element to this risk–risk analysis. The patient has a central role in this decision-making process.

Principle 4. It Is Important to Be Aware of a Given Drug's Official Food and Drug Administration (FDA)-Approved Indications, and the Generally Accepted but "Unapproved" or "Off-Label" Indications for That Drug

Official FDA approval means that there has been an application for a specific use of a drug and that sufficient safety and efficacy data have been presented to warrant use of the drug for that specific disease indication. Safety data are usually applicable to generally accepted but "off-label" indications. What is lacking in these off-label indications is efficacy data officially submitted by the pharmaceutical company to the FDA. Considerable expense is associated with applications for each "new use." Usually, the decision to use systemic medications for off-label indications is based either on significant personal experience or evidence from the medical literature.

Systemic drug therapy is commonly associated with some element of risk. The patient ideally should be notified when the drug will be used for an off-label indication.

Principle 5. The Priority Sequence of Systemic Drug Choices Should Be Individualized for Each Specific Patient. Factors Such As Drug Cost, Simplicity of the Therapeutic Regimen, Inherent Drug Risk, and Patient Preference Enter into the Decision

When all other factors are equal, a drug that is relatively inexpensive, simple to use, and relatively safe should be prescribed. Ideally, such a drug should be supported by an FDA indication or sufficient clinical data and experience to justify its use. If such therapy is not appropriate or is not successful, then more costly, complicated, or novel treatments with an element of risk can be tried. Frequently, patient preferences are shaped by logistics, such as drug cost, patient income, time, travel, and the patient's tolerance of risk.

For female patients of childbearing potential, plans for pregnancy should be discussed before prescribing systemic medications. For potentially teratogenic medications, birth control methods should be discussed and documented in the chart. Physicians should also inquire if the patient is breastfeeding prior to initiating systemic therapy.

Principle 6. Be Aware of Pharmacogenomics Biomarkers Required to Assess Drug Safety for Individual Patients

Pharmacogenomics plays an important role in identifying patients at risk for specific adverse events and in identifying potential nonresponders. Two examples of important pharmacogenomics tests in dermatology are glucose-6-phosphodehydrogenase (G6PD) level to assess for G6PD deficiency in patients prescribed dapsone, and thiopurine methyltransferase testing to assess for intermediate or poor metabolizers in patients prescribed azathioprine (see the FDA website listed in Suggested Readings for available pharmacogenomics biomarkers).

Principle 7. Be Cognizant of Important Drug–Drug Interactions when Prescribing Systemic Therapy for Cutaneous Diseases

An increasing number of patients who present to the dermatologist are already receiving a wide variety of systemic medications for nondermatologic medical problems. An awareness of the patient's complete medication profile helps enhance the safety of prescribing systemic drugs, particularly for patients who are receiving cyclosporine or methotrexate. A systematic way of recording and updating the patient's complete medication profile helps minimize the risk of these potential interactions. It is our suggestion that current drug therapy be monitored and recorded at each patient visit. Electronic medical records have helped decrease the risk of drug–drug interactions by alerting physicians to potential interactions between medications prescribed and those recorded in the chart. This should not replace an effort on the part of the dermatologist to be alert to potential drug–drug interactions when prescribing systemic medications. It is also important to notify the patient of key interactions and medications to avoid during therapy.

MONITORING PRINCIPLES

Principle 1. Informed Consent Is a Communication Process and Not Merely a Signature on a Piece of Paper. Appropriately Thorough Informed Consent Is an Essential Step toward the Safe Use of Systemic Drugs

There is an important medicolegal basis for informed consent. This communication is usually documented by noting that the patient is aware of the risks, benefits, and alternatives to the proposed therapy. Generally, chart documentation of this discussion by the physician is sufficient. Experimental protocols require a signed consent form. In addition, consent forms for the use of isotretinoin in both men and women as part of the iPledge program are mandated by the FDA.

The medical basis for the informed consent communication process is even more important. This discussion enables the patient to be more aware of specific areas of risk and the patient's role in reporting important signs and symptoms. Occasionally, a patient decides not to use a specific drug after learning about the risks. This is probably preferable to treating a patient who continually focuses on the potential risks of therapy, however remote.

Principle 2. A Patient Information Handout Specific to the Drug Being Prescribed Can Be an Important Measure to Reinforce All Aspects of the Monitoring Process

A patient information handout should reinforce all elements of the informed consent process described earlier. More importantly, a clear listing of the signs and symptoms the patient should report allows the patient to know when to be concerned regarding problems that may arise later in therapy. These patient information handouts should clarify the follow-up visits required, laboratory testing, X-ray procedures, and nondermatologist specialty examinations required for a given drug therapy.

Sources of such handouts include the American Academy of Dermatology, National Psoriasis Foundation, American College of Rheumatology, various pharmaceutical companies, the patient (lay) volume of the United States Pharmacopeia Drug Information annual booklet, and the American Medical Association Patient Medical Instruction sheets. Clinicians with sufficient experience with a given drug can develop their own patient information handouts. The distribution of a patient handout should be documented in the medical record.

Principle 3. Monitoring for Adverse Effects Associated with Systemic Drugs Used in Dermatology Is Largely Based on Risk Reduction through Preventing and Detecting Drug-Induced Abnormalities at an Early Reversible Stage

The complete elimination of risks from systemic drugs is not possible, although more favorable "risk–risk" ratios, as defined previously, are definitely achievable. The monitoring process is most important when there are subclinical findings that have serious potential consequences. A classic example is the low-grade fibrosis and potential for subsequent cirrhosis in patients receiving long-term methotrexate therapy. In addition, mild asymptomatic leukopenia or transaminase elevations may herald serious complications if left undetected. Lastly, corticosteroid-induced osteoporosis should be detected early with dual-energy X-ray absorptiometry scans and, where possible, prevented with vitamin D, calcium, and bisphosphonates (see American College of Rheumatology guidelines referenced in the Suggested Readings). As with corticosteroid-induced osteoporosis, adverse effects that are common or predictable can be prevented by pretreatment or cotreatment for the anticipated adverse effect, especially in high-risk patients. One example of this would be the recommendation to normalize triglycerides and thyroid levels prior to initiating therapy with bexarotene.

Principle 4. Virtually All Tests and Examinations to Be Used in the Monitoring Process Should Have a Baseline Determination

Baseline laboratory testing can often aid in the following issues:
- To determine which patients should *not* receive a given drug.
- To determine which patients are at high risk and require closer subsequent surveillance.
- To allow the clinician to avoid assigning blame to the drug therapy for a preexisting condition(s).
- To serve as a basis of comparison for subsequent follow-up testing.

Principle 5. "Critical Toxicities" Are Defined as Any Drug-Induced Adverse Effect that May Result in Either Loss of Life or Potentially Irreversible Significant Morbidity. These Adverse Effects Receive the Highest Priority in Systemic Drug Monitoring

The following adverse effects meet this definition of "critical toxicities":
- Hepatotoxicity
- Hematologic toxicity (agranulocytosis, aplastic anemia, or thrombocytopenia)
- Induction of malignancy
- Teratogenicity
- Drug reactions with systemic features such as Stevens–Johnson syndrome
- Opportunistic infections (such as reactivation or dissemination of tuberculosis)
- Hypothalamo–pituitary–adrenal axis suppression
- Growth suppression
- Renal toxicity
- Hyperlipidemia
- Ocular toxicity (retinopathy, cataracts)
- Bone toxicity (osteoporosis or osteonecrosis)

Principle 6. Risk Reduction Can Be Optimized through the Use of Well-Defined Monitoring Guidelines

Both patient and physician benefit when consistent monitoring guidelines are used. Systematic ordering of laboratory tests, X-ray procedures, and specific examinations minimize the potential for oversights leading to inadequate monitoring. For example, before treating with a tumor necrosis factor-alpha (TNF-α) inhibitor, testing for tuberculosis is recommended at baseline and periodically by *purified protein derivative of tuberculin* (or by interferon gamma release assay), in addition to checking a hepatitis B surface antigen. A well-trained nurse can assist in the tracking and recording of these values.

Specific guidelines can be found in the reference cited in the Suggested Readings section. These guidelines were derived from consensus articles that discussed single or multiple drugs, and from pharmaceutical company or FDA guidelines proposed for specific drugs.

Principle 7. Monitoring Guidelines Are Based on Data from Low-Risk Patients with Normal Test Results. More Frequent Surveillance Is Necessary for High-Risk Patients and for Those Patients with Significantly Abnormal Test Results

An example of a high-risk patient is an individual who might be receiving methotrexate and who has any of the following: mildly abnormal baseline liver function test results, increased probability of nonalcoholic steatohepatitis (as a result of obesity, ethanol abuse, or diabetes mellitus), prior hepatitis, renal disease, or immunosuppression. Patients at very high risk should usually not receive the drug at all.

Subsequent abnormal test results also warrant more frequent surveillance. An example would be mild to moderate retinoid-induced elevations of triglycerides. Mild to moderate dapsone-induced hemolysis is another example.

Principle 8. Particularly Close Follow-up Is Required for "Critical Toxicities" that Are Idiosyncratic and Have A Potential for Rapid and Severe Changes in the Patient's Status

Toxic hepatitis and agranulocytosis are two critical toxicities that stand out in this regard. Toxic hepatitis may be preceded by mild to moderate asymptomatic elevations of liver transaminase levels, whereas agranulocytosis may be preceded by relatively mild leukopenia. Significant laboratory abnormalities of either type require careful follow-up and, in many cases, drug discontinuation. Drugs prescribed by dermatologists that are most likely to induce toxic hepatitis include methotrexate, azathioprine, itraconazole, dapsone, and minocycline. Dapsone and methotrexate present the greatest risk of agranulocytosis among the systemic dermatologic drugs. Azathioprine may also produce significant depression of the white blood cell count, although this effect is much more likely to be predictable by measuring thiopurine methyltransferase levels and by avoiding concomitant use of allopurinol.

These toxicities can be significantly contrasted with low-grade indolent changes that may have significant implications. Examples include cirrhosis from low-dose methotrexate, ocular toxicity from antimalarials, and the risk of nonmelanoma and melanoma skin cancer in patients treated with photochemotherapy (psoralen with UVA light [PUVA]). Long-term surveillance through special examinations and procedures is used when prescribing these drugs.

Principle 9. Share the Responsibility of Monitoring for Adverse Effects with Other Appropriate Specialists

The practice of medicine is in many instances a team effort, requiring coordinated management by various physicians. Monitoring for adverse effects of systemic drugs frequently requires the application of this principle. Ophthalmologic consultation for patients receiving antimalarial therapy is an example. Consultation with an appropriate specialist is important for decisions regarding abnormal liver function test results and assessment of liver fibrosis in patients receiving methotrexate. The patient's primary care physician plays a significant role in monitoring for potential malignancy induction from immunosuppressive therapy.

Less well clarified is the need for comanagement with dermatologists from an academic center. We believe that in many situations systemic drug therapy with an element of risk can be orchestrated through an academic dermatologist, with the patient's primary dermatologist playing the major role in the ongoing surveillance process.

Principle 10. Minimize the Risk of Systemic Drug Therapy through Adjunctive Therapy with Other Systemic Drugs and Topical or Local Therapy, and by Modifying Disease Precipitators when Possible

The classic addition of corticosteroid-sparing agents, such as azathioprine and methotrexate, serves to reduce the dose and the associated risk of systemic corticosteroid therapy. A combination of oral retinoids and PUVA therapy for patients with psoriasis is another example of systemic drug combination therapy with a lower overall treatment risk.

In situations requiring systemic corticosteroid therapy, concomitant use of topical and/or intralesional corticosteroid therapy may reduce the systemic corticosteroid dose requirement. Modifying disease precipitators in patients with psoriasis, atopic dermatitis, and acne may improve the efficacy and safety of systemic drug therapy.

SUGGESTED READINGS

Grossman JM, Gordon R, Ranganath VK, Deal C, Caplan L, Chen W, et al. American College of Rheumatology 2010 recommendations for the prevention and treatment of glucocorticoid-induced osteoporosis. Arthritis Care Res Hoboken November 2010;62(11):1515–26.

Wolverton SE, editor. Comprehensive dermatologic drug therapy. 3rd ed. London: Elsevier 2012. Table of Pharmocogenomic Biomarkers in Drug Labeling. http://www.fda.gov/Drugs/ScienceResearch/ResearchAreas/Pharmacogenetics/ucm083378.htm.

Index

A

A533D mutation, mast cell disease, 370
Abatacept, for rheumatoid arthritis, 54
ABCC6 mutation, 243
Abscess, 272–273, 273f
Acanthamoeba, 288, 288f, 338
Acantholysis, 117–121
Acanthosis nigricans (AN), 205, 206f
    malignancy and, 131–132, 132f
Achilles tendon, xanthomas in, 224
Acitretin, for psoriasis, 48
Acne, in pregnancy, 360–361
Acne rosacea, 203
Acne vulgaris, 230
    drug selection principles, 438t
Acneiform eruption, 426t, 432
Acoustic neurofibromatosis, 346
Acquired hypertrichosis lanuginosa, 385
Acquired hypertrophic pulmonary osteoarthropathy syndrome, 393
Acquired ichthyosis
    malignancy and, 135
    in systemic lymphomas, 168
Acquired immunodeficiency syndrome (AIDS)
    see also Human immunodeficiency virus (HIV)
    herpes zoster in, 266
    HIV-1 and HIV-2 retroviruses, 289–304
    Muehrcke's lines and, 394
    syphilis in, 301
Acquired perforating dermatoses (APD), 205–206, 327, 327f
ACR. *see* American College of Rheumatology (ACR).
Acral petechiae, in meningococcemia, 274
Acroangiodermatitis, 200f
Acrochordons (skin tags), 211
    in pregnancy, 362
Acrocyanosis, 173
Acrodermatitis chronica atrophicans, in Lyme disease, 274–275
Acrodermatitis enteropathica (AE), 248–250, 249f, 365
Acrokeratosis paraneoplastica, 132, 132f, 396
Acromegaly, 232–233, 233f
Acropachy, thyroid, in Graves' disease, 219
Actinic keratoses (AKs), 340–341
Actinic purpura, 113
Activated charcoal, for intrahepatic cholestasis of pregnancy, 367
Acute cutaneous lupus erythematosus (ACLE), 7–8, 8f
Acute febrile neutrophilic dermatosis. *see* Sweet's syndrome.
Acute generalized exanthematous pustulosis (AGEP), 425, 426t, 432, 432f
Acute GVHD, 341–342
Acute monocytic leukemia, 185

Acute retroviral syndrome, 290
ACVRL1 gene, in HHT, 245
Acyclovir
    for erythema multiforme, 92
    for herpes simplex, 330–331
    for herpes zoster, 331
Adalimumab
    for psoriasis, 48
    for rheumatoid arthritis, 54
    for sarcoidosis, 314
Addison's disease, 229, 230f
    nail disorders, 388
    systemic sclerosis and, 26
Adenocarcinoma, gastric, 131–132
Adenoma, pituitary, 233
Adenoma sebaceum, 351
Adenomatous polyposis syndromes, 246–248
Adjunctive therapy, 441
Adrenal disorders, 228–230
Adrenal insufficiency, 229
Adrenaline. *see* Epinephrine (adrenaline).
Adrenocorticotropic hormone (ACTH), pituitary, 228
Adrenogenital syndromes, 232
Adverse effects
    see also Drug eruptions; Drug selection principles
    drugs indicated
        dapsone, 434
        NSAIDs, 427–428
    gingival hyperplasia, 401
    longitudinal pigmented bands, 388
    monitoring for, 441
AESOP syndrome, 175
    in systemic lymphomas, 169
Afamelanotide, for erythropoietic protoporphyria and X-linked dominant protoporphyria, 241
African-Americans, punctate keratoses in, 136
Age, in myositis and malignancy, 18
AGel amyloidosis, 180
Aggressive systemic mastocytosis (ASM), 370–371
AIDS. *see* Acquired immunodeficiency syndrome (AIDS).
Aldrich-Mees' lines, 389t–390t
Algorithm
    erythroderma, 107f
    pruritus, 101f
Alkyl sulfonates, 143
Alkylating agents, for cancer therapy, 141–146
All-trans retinoic acid (ATRA), 149
Allergies
    see also Urticaria
    contact, 407–408
    drug, in SJS and TEN, 91–92
Allopurinol, 314, 435
    for erythroderma, 105

Alopecia, 230, 248, 325, 378–385
    see also Telogen effluvium
    androgenetic, 320
    categories, 378
    in dermatomyositis, 15, 16f
    erythroderma and, 105–106
    five mechanisms for, 378t
    and hyperthyroidism, 218
    male pattern, 361
    nonscarring, 378
    scarring, 378, 382–383, 383f
        causes of, 384t
    or nonscarring, in sarcoidosis, 306, 310f
    in SLE, 8
Alopecia areata, 221
Alopecia neoplastica, 156–157
Alopecia totalis, 381
Alpha-1 antitrypsin deficiency panniculitis, 97
Amebic infections, 287
American College of Rheumatology (ACR)
    on RA, 51
    on SLE, 1, 1t, 6, 8
    on systemic sclerosis, 26–27
    on vasculitis, 31
American trypanosomiasis, 287, 287f
Amiodarone, for linear IgA bullous dermatosis, 129
Amlodipine, and gingival hyperplasia, 401
Amphotericin B, 212
    for aspergillosis, 283
Ampicillin, for linear IgA bullous dermatosis, 129
Amputations, below-knee, 414
Amyloidosis, 177–182
    epidermolysis bullosa acquisita and, 126
    familial syndromes of, 180
    hemodialysis-related, 179–180
    light chain-related systemic, 113, 178–179
    nail disorders, 396
    and purpura, 178–179, 179f
    reactive or secondary, 179
    senile and mutant transthyretin, 180
    skin-limited, 179
    subcutaneous fat aspiration in, 181
    systemic, characteristics of, 178t
Amyopathic dermatomyositis, 13, 17–18
Anagen, 377
    short, 379
Anagen arrest, 380–381, 381f
    systemic causes of, 381t
Anagen release, 378
Anakinra
    for CAPS, 60
    for DIRA, 63
    for PAPA syndrome, 66
    for rheumatoid arthritis, 54
    for SAPHO syndrome, 67
    for TRAPS, 64
Anaphylactoid reactions, 429

Note: Page numbers followed by "t", and "f" refer to tables, and figures respectively.

Anastrozole, 153
Anchoring filaments, hemidesmosome and, 117
Androgen activity
  deficient, 232
  excessive, 230–232, 231f
Androgen insensitivity syndrome, 232
Androgen-related disorders, 230–232
Androgenetic alopecia, 379, 382, 382f
Androgens, 153
Anemia
  microangiopathic, 116
  pernicious. see Pernicious anemia
Aneurysms, coronary, and Kawasaki disease, 56
Angioedema, 426t
  urticaria and, 77–80, 78f, 82–83, 85
Angiofibromas, facial, 351, 351f
Angiogenesis, errors in, 200
Angiogenesis inhibitors, for cancer therapy, 151–152
Angioid streaks, 243, 355
  differential diagnosis of, 245t
Angiokeratomas, 200
Angiolupoid sarcoidosis, 307–308
Angiomas, 354–355
  eruptive, malignancy and, 134
Angiomyolipomas, 352, 354
Angiosarcoma, 203–204, 203f
Angiotensin-converting enzyme (ACE), in sarcoidosis, 305–306, 311–313
Angiotensin-converting enzyme (ACE) inhibitors, 6–7, 28, 120
  in urticaria, 80
Ankylosis, ankle, 409
Annular subacute cutaneous lupus erythematosus (SCLE-A), 5–6, 5f
Anonychia, 389t–390t
Anorexia nervosa, 384
Anthracyclines, 148
Anti-La (SS-B) antibodies, in SCLE, 7
Anti-Ro (SS-A) antibody, in cutaneous LE and subsets, 6, 9–10
Antiandrogens, 153
Antibiotics
  see also specific antibiotics
  broad-spectrum, causing candidiasis, 336
  for erythroderma, 108
  for wound infections, 420–421
Antibodies
  ANA system. see Antinuclear antibody (ANA) titer
  antiphospholipid, 8, 116, 315
  in bullous pemphigoid, 123–125
  in LE and subsets, 6, 9–10, 9t–10t
  myositis and, 13–14, 19
  in pemphigus, 118–122
  in systemic sclerosis, 27
Anticancer agents, for cancer therapy, 153–154
Anticancer therapies, targeted, 149–153
Anticentromere autoantibody, in systemic sclerosis, 27
Anticonvulsants, 430–431
Anticyclic citrullinated peptide, 51
Antidiabetic therapy, complications, 213–214
Antigen-binding profiles, in bullous pemphigoid, 124
Antihistamines, 363, 369
  for urticaria, 84–85, 85t
Antimalarials
  lobular panniculitis and, 96
  for lupus erythematosus, 2, 11
  for porphyria cutanea tarda, 240
  for sarcoidosis, 314

Antimetabolite agents, for cancer therapy, 146–147
Antimicrotubule agents, for cancer therapy, 148
Antineoplastic agents, 313
Antineutrophil cytoplasmic antibody (ANCA), vasculitis associated with, 31, 34
Antinuclear antibody (ANA) titer, 2, 9–10, 10t
Antiphospholipid antibodies, 8, 116, 315
Antiphospholipid antibody syndrome, 315, 319f
Antiphospholipid syndrome, 407, 413f
Antiviral infections, in transplant recipients, 330–333
Aphthae
  genital, 39, 40f
  oral, in metastatic Crohn's disease, 251
Aphthous stomatitis, 121, 290–291
Aphthous ulceration, 398f
Apocrine gland activity, in pregnancy, 360–361
Apremilast
  for lupus erythematosus, 11
  for psoriasis, 48
APUDomas, 137
Aromatase inhibitors, 153
Arrhythmias, 320
Arsenic trioxide (ATO), 149
Arsenical keratoses, of palms and soles, 136
Arsenicals, for cancer therapy, 149
Arterial studies, 414
Arterial ulceration, 410–411, 414f
Arteriovenous malformations (AVMs), 193, 199–200
Arthralgias, 16, 79
Arthritis
  Behçet's disease and, 39
  in dermatomyositis, 16
  juvenile idiopathic, 53
  psoriatic. see Psoriatic arthritis
  and pyoderma gangrenosum, 43
  rheumatoid. see Rheumatoid arthritis
  and sarcoidosis, 311
Arthritis mutilans, psoriatic, 50f
Ash leaf macules, 351, 351f
L-Asparaginase, 154
Aspergillosis, 282–283, 282f
  in transplant recipients, 337, 337f
Aspirin
  see also Nonsteroidal anti-inflammatory drugs (NSAIDs)
  drug eruptions, 429
  for leg ulcers, 423
  for purpura, 116
  in urticaria, 78
Astrocytomas, 348
Ataxia-telangiectasia, 192, 356–357
Ataxia telangiectasia mutation (ATM), 356
Atopic dermatitis, 221
  erythroderma and, 104–106, 108
  in pregnancy, 362–363
  severe, drug selection principles, 438t
"Atopic eruption of pregnancy", 367, 369
Atypical measles, 262
Atypical mycobacterial infections, 335
Atypical pyoderma gangrenosum, 41, 42f
Atypical wounds, 411–412
Autoimmune connective tissue diseases (AI-CTD), 194
Autoimmune diseases
  blistering, 117
  see also Bullous pemphigoid; Pemphigus
  in pregnancy, 365
  thyroid disorders, 215–216, 221

Autoimmune progesterone dermatitis (APD), 363
Autoinflammatory syndromes, 59–68, 60f, 61t
Autosomal recessive lipoprotein lipase deficiency, 223
5-Azacitidine (5-AzaC), 149
Azathioprine
  for Behçet's disease, 40
  for bullous pemphigoid, 125
  for dermatomyositis/polymyositis, 20
  for lupus erythematosus, 11
  for pemphigoid gestationis, 368
  for pemphigus, 122
  for sarcoidosis, 314
  for vasculitis, 36
Aziridines, 143

B

B-cell lymphomas
  body cavity-related, 200
  primary cutaneous. see Primary cutaneous B-cell lymphomas
Bacillary angiomatosis, 196
  HIV and, 292–293, 292f–293f
Bacteria, 271–276
Bacterial diseases, 271–276
Bacterial infections
  in diabetes mellitus, 212–213
  in human immunodeficiency syndrome (HIV), 292–293, 292f–293f
  in transplant recipients, 334–335
Balamuthia, 288
Bandages, compression, 422
Bannayan-Ruvalcaba-Riley syndrome, 138
Barbiturates, 105
Bartonella spp., 196
Basal cell carcinoma (BCC), 410f
  lymphoma, 418t–419t
  in transplant recipients, 338–341, 339f–343f
Basal cell vacuolization, 120
Baseline determination, 440
Basement membrane zone (BMZ), 117
Bazex syndrome, 396
  malignancy and, 132, 132f
Beau's lines, 389t–390t, 391f
  nails, 327, 387
Behçet's disease, 39–40, 39t, 40f
  erythema nodosum and, 95
  superficial migratory thrombophlebitis and, 96
Bence Jones protein, 174
Benign cephalic histiocytosis, 186t–187t
Benign familial pemphigus (Hailey-Hailey disease), 121
Benzoyl peroxide, for pruritic folliculitis of pregnancy, 369
Bexarotene, 149
Bicalutamide, 153
Bilateral hilar adenopathy, sarcoidosis and, 310
Bile acid-binding resins, 226
Biofilms, in leg ulcers, 404
Biopsy
  amyloidosis, 180–181
  blistering disorders, 121
  Cryptococcus infection, 337–338
  dermatitis herpetiformis, 250
  dermatomyositis, 16
  erythema nodosum, 95
  erythroderma, 106
  glucagonoma, 254
  leg ulcers, 414–420, 414t

Biopsy *(Continued)*
  POEMS syndrome, 175
  pseudoxanthoma elasticum, 244
  sarcoidosis, 306, 312–313
  scalp, 380
  systemic sclerosis, 27
  vasculitis, 36
Birt-Hogg-Dubé syndrome, 138, 138f
Bismuth, and anagen arrest, 381t
Bjornstad's syndrome, 384
Bladder, transitional cell cancer of, 129
Bland occlusion syndromes, in purpura, 112–113, 115–116
Blastic plasmacytoid dendritic cell neoplasm (BPDCN), 166
Blastomycosis, 280–281, 280f, 338
Bleomycin, 154, 203
Blistering diseases, RA and, 53
Blood hypereosinophilia, 69
Blood pressure, arterial studies, 414
Blue rubber bleb nevus syndrome, 199–200, 200f
Blueberry muffin baby, 157
Boceprevir, for hepatitis C, 260
Borrelia-associated lymphocytoma cutis, 167
Borrelia organisms, 163–164
Bortezomib, 149
Botulinum toxin, for Raynaud's phenomenon, 29
Bourneville's disease (tuberous sclerosis complex), 350–354
Bowel-associated dermatosis-arthritis syndrome, 43–44, 44f
Bowen's disease, 339–340
BP230, BP180 and, 117, 122–123
BPAG1, antibodies to, 123
BPAG2, antibodies to, 123
BRAF inhibitors, for cancer therapy, 152
Brazil, pemphigus in, 119
Breast cancer, 155
  metastatic, 156–157, 157f
Brittle nails, 388, 389t–390t
Bronchiolitis obliterans, 120–121
Bronchoalveolar lavage, 309–310
Bronze diabetes, 258
Brunsting-Perry type, cicatricial pemphigoid, 124
Buerger's disease, 173
Bullous dermatoses, malignancy and, 132–133, 133f
Bullous diseases, 117–130, 118f
  see also Bullous pemphigoid; Dermatitis herpetiformis; Epidermolysis bullosa acquisita (EBA); Pemphigushemodialysis and, 329f
  linear IgA bullous dermatosis, 129–130, 129f
  pemphigus, 117–122, 119f, 121f, 121t
  renal disease and, 329, 329f
Bullous eruptions, 432–435
Bullous impetigo, 272, 272f
Bullous lupus erythematosus, 8–9, 9f
Bullous mastocytoma, 372f
Bullous pemphigoid, 122–125, 122f, 124f
  associated conditions, 221
  drug selection principles, 438t
  malignancy and, 132
  nail disorders, 396
  urticaria and, 82, 85
Bullous pyoderma gangrenosum, 41
Bürger-Grütz disease, 223
Burning mouth syndrome, 400
Buruli ulcer, 418t–419t
Busulfan, 143
"Butterfly" rash, 7–8
Bywater's lesions, 53, 389t–390t, 395

C

c-KIT mutations, mast cell disease, 370
C nerve fibers, 100, 103
C-reactive protein (CRP)
  in CAPS, 59–60
  in DIRA, 63
  in HIDS, 66
  in Schnitzler's syndrome, 62
C1 esterase inhibitor deficiency, in urticaria, 80, 85
Café-au-lait macules, 216–217, 346, 347f, 347t, 352
Calcification, in Sturge-Weber syndrome, 354–355
Calcinosis cutis, 325, 326f
  in dermatomyositis, 17, 21
Calciphylaxis, 325–327, 326f–327f, 412, 415f, 418t–419t
Calcipotriene, for circumscribed morphea, 25
Calcium channel blockers, 6–7, 401
  for Raynaud's phenomenon, 29
Calf muscle pump, 407f
Canakinumab
  for CAPS, 60
  for TRAPS, 64
Cancer therapy, dermatologic adverse events of, 141–154
  agents/inhibitors
    alkylating, 141–146
    angiogenesis, 151–152
    anticancer, 153–154
    antimetabolite, 146–147
    antimicrotubule, 148
    arsenicals, 149
    BRAF, 152
    cytotoxic chemotherapeutic, 141–149
    demethylating, 148–149
    endocrine, 153–154
    epidermal growth factor receptor, 149–151, 149f–150f
    histone deacetylase, 148–149
    mammalian target of rapamycin, 152
    miscellaneous, 154
    monoclonal antibodies, 152–153
    multikinase, 151
    proteasome, 148–149
    retinoids, 149
    topoisomerase, 147–148
  targeted anticancer therapies, 149–153
    dermatologic adverse events from, 144t–145t
Candidal paronychia, chronic, 394f
Candidiasis, 137–138, 283, 283f
  in transplant recipients, 336–337, 336f
Capecitabine, 146, 147f
Capsaicin, topical, 103
Captopril, for linear IgA bullous dermatosis, 129
Carbamazepine, for erythroderma, 105
Carbon monoxide poisoning, 389t–390t
Carboxymethylcellulose, 400
Carcinoid syndrome, 315–319
  malignancy and, 137
Carcinoma
  see also Malignant disease specific types
  HIV infection and, 291, 292f
Carcinoma erysipeloides, 156–157
Cardiac disease
  in dermatomyositis, 17
  hemochromatosis and, 320
  in sarcoidosis, 312
Cardiac involvement, in tuberous sclerosis complex, 353
Cardiovascular diseases, 315–322, 316t–319t

Cardiovascular system, nail disorders, 393
Carmustine, 146
"Carney complex", 320
Carotenemia, in hypothyroidism, 220
CASPAR (Classification of Psoriatic Arthritis), 49–50, 50t
Castleman's disease, 175
  PNP and, 120
Cat scratch disease, 274
Catagen, 377
Catheters, and *Candida* infection, 336
Cavernous hemangioma, 196
CD4+ T-cells
  in HIV, 202
  in pemphigus, 118
  in psoriasis, 45
  in sarcoidosis, 305
CD8+ T-cells
  in EM, SJS, and TEN, 87
  in polymyositis, 13–14
  in psoriasis, 45
  in sarcoidosis, 305
CD10 positivity, in renal cell carcinoma, 157
CD34+ precursor cells, 330
Celiac disease, 127–128, 130
Cellulitis, 213, 272, 334
Central nervous system (CNS)
  cryptococcosis and, 337–338
  herpes simplex infections and, 331
  malignancy of, 138
  nail disorders, 394
  neurofibromatosis and, 348–349
  tuberous sclerosis complex and, 352
Cephalosporins, for cellulitis, 272
Certolizumab, for rheumatoid arthritis, 54
Cetirizine, 374–375
Chadwick's sign, in pregnancy, 361
Chagas' disease. *see* American trypanosomiasis.
Chancroid, 301, 301f, 302t
Chapel Hill Consensus Conference (CHCC), on vasculitis, 31, 32t
Chediak-Higashi syndrome, 189t
Cheilitis granulomatosa, 397–400, 398f–399f
Cheiroarthropathy, diabetic, 211
Chemotherapy
  anagen arrest, 381
  for glucagonoma, 254
Cherry angiomas, 196
Chest imaging studies, 313
Chicken pox, 265
Chiclero ulcer, 285
Chikungunya, 269
Chilblains lupus, 5, 5f
Children
  Hand-Schuler-Christian disease, 184
  infantile hemangiomas, 196
  lipid metabolism disorders, 223
  mast cell disease, 372–373
  papular acrodermatitis of, 259
Chlorambucil, 143
  for dermatomyositis/polymyositis, 20
  for sarcoidosis, 314
Chloroquine, for dermatomyositis/polymyositis, 20
Chloroquine phosphate
  for lupus erythematosus, 11
  for sarcoidosis, 314
Cholecalciferol (vitamin D3), for erythropoietic protoporphyria and X-linked dominant protoporphyria, 241
Cholelithiasis, 241
Cholestasis, pruritus of, 101–102
Cholesterol, 225
Cholestyramine, 367

Chronic bullous disease of childhood (CBDC), 129
Chronic GVHD, 342–343
Chronic mucocutaneous candidiasis, 283
Chronic otitis media, 184
Chronic plaque psoriasis, 45–46, 46f
Chronic telogen effluvium, 379–380, 380f
Chronic ulcerations, pathophysiology of, 404, 404f–405f
Chronic urticaria, in intestinal amebiasis, 287
Churg-Strauss syndrome, 110
　defined, 71t
Churg-Strauss vasculitis, 34
Chylomicrons, 223
Cicatricial alopecia, 382–383, 383f
Cicatricial pemphigoid, 123–125, 124f, 132
"Cigarette paper" scars, in Ehlers-Danlos syndrome, 320
Cilostazol, for leg ulcers, 423
Cimetidine, in urticaria, 85
Circulating immune complex-mediated disease, 93–95
Circulating immune complexes, 53
Circumscribed morphea, 22
　treatment for, 25
Cirrhosis, 255–257, 256f–257f
　of hereditary hemorrhagic telangiectasia, 246
Cladribine, 147
Clindamycin, for erythrasma, 213
Clotrimazole, for erythrasma, 213
Clubbing, 389t–390t, 392–393, 393f
　in acropachy, 219
　in pachydermoperiostosis, 137
Coagulation cascade problems, in hemostasis, 110
Coagulation disorders, 412
Cobb syndrome, 356
Coccidioidomycosis, 279–280, 280f
Colchicine
　anagen arrest, 381t
　for Behçet's disease, 40
　for epidermolysis bullosa acquisita, 127
　for FMF, 65
　for linear IgA bullous dermatosis, 130
　for Schnitzler's syndrome, 62
　for Sweet's syndrome, 41
　in urticaria, 85–86
　for vasculitis, 36
Cold agglutinin disease, 172–174
Cold sensitivity, 172
Colectomy, for adenomatous polyposis syndromes, 248
Collagen VII, 126
Collagen XVII, 123, 129
Colonoscopy, for Gardner's syndrome, 247–248
Combination immunosuppressive therapy, for dermatomyositis/polymyositis, 20
Complement cascade, activation of, in urticaria, 77–78
Complex bullous eruptions, 432–434
Complex urticarial eruption, 431
Complications, drug. see Adverse effects.
Compression, leg ulcer, 422
Computed tomography (CT), 309–310, 353
Conduction abnormalities, in myositis, 321
Condyloma lata, secondary syphilis and, 299, 299f
Condylomata acuminata, 291, 333, 364
Congenital erythropoietic porphyria (CEP), 235–236, 241–242
Congenital hypothyroidism, 220–221
Congenital rubella syndrome, 263
Congenital self-healing reticulocytosis, 184
Congenital syphilis, 300

Congenital varicella syndrome, 364
Congestive heart failure, 321, 392–393
Conjunctival granulomas, 310
Conjunctivitis, 90f
Connective tissue disease, 176
　see also Rheumatoid arthritis (RA); Systemic lupus erythematosus (SLE)autoimmune, 194
Constipation, in neurofibromatosis, 349
Contact allergy, 407–408
Coproporphyria, hereditary, 242
Cornelia de Lange syndrome, 385
Coronary aneurysms, and Kawasaki disease, 56
Coronary artery disease (CAD), 319, 321
Corticosteroids
　for Behçet's disease, 40
　for bowel-associated dermatosis-arthritis syndrome, 44
　causing candidiasis, 335–336
　for circumscribed morphea, 25
　for dermatomyositis/polymyositis, 19–20
　for erythroderma, 108
　for GVHD, 343
　for impetigo herpetiformis, 363
　for mast cell disease, 375
　and monoclonal protein production disorders, 177
　for necrobiosis lipoidica, 209
　for PAPA syndrome, 66
　for pemphigoid gestationis, 368
　in pemphigus, 119–120, 122
　for pruritic folliculitis of pregnancy, 369
　for relapsing polychondritis, 320
　for rheumatoid arthritis, 54
　for SAPHO syndrome, 67
　for sarcoidosis, 313
　for TRAPS, 64
　in urticaria, 82, 85
　for vasculitis, 36
Cortisol, 228–229
Corynebacterium minutissimum, 213
Cowden disease, 138, 216–217
Coxsackie virus, 263–264
Crandall's syndrome, 384
Cranial imaging, in tuberous sclerosis complex, 354
Cretinism, 220
"Critical toxicities", 440
　close follow-up for, 440–441
Crohn's disease, 126, 129
　metastatic, 251, 251f
Cronkhite-Canada syndrome, 248, 393
Crow-Fukase syndrome, 174–175
Crowe's sign, 347
Cryofibrinogenemia, 173
Cryoglobulinemia, 126, 172
　mixed, 110, 173
　nail disorders, 396
　treatment of, 174
　type 1, in systemic lymphomas, 169, 169f
Cryoglobulinemic vasculitis, 34–35
Cryoglobulins, 34–35, 171–172, 174
Cryopyrin-associated periodic syndrome (CAPS), 59–60, 61t, 62f
Cryptococcosis, 281, 281f
Cryptococcus, 337–338
Crystal storing histiocytosis (CSH), in systemic lymphomas, 169
Cullen's sign, 252, 253f
Cushing syndrome, 137, 228–229, 229f, 382
Cutaneous adverse drug reactions (CADRs), 425
Cutaneous anaplastic large cell lymphoma (cALCL), 162–163, 162f

Cutaneous angioimmunoblastic T-cell lymphoma (cAITL), 167–168
Cutaneous Assessment Tool, 21
Cutaneous atrophy, 228
Cutaneous B-cell chronic lymphocytic leukemia (B-CLL), 167
Cutaneous B-cell lymphomas (CBCLs), 163–164, 164f–165f
Cutaneous cryptococcosis, HIV infection and, 293, 293f
Cutaneous Dermatomyositis Area and Severity Index, 21
Cutaneous diffuse large B-cell lymphoma, leg-type (cDLBCL-LT), 166
Cutaneous disease, 437
　associated with gastrointestinal abnormalities, 243–254, 244t
　associated with viral hepatitis, 259–260, 259f–261f
Cutaneous drug eruptions, 425–436
　caused by biologic treatments, 434
　drug-induced skin injury and, 425
　epidemiology of, 425
　important steps in emergency department, 435t
　major, characteristics of, 426t
　mechanisms of, 428–429
　miscellaneous, 434–435
　morphological subtypes of, 429–432
Cutaneous follicle center lymphoma (cFCL), 165–166
Cutaneous Hodgkin's lymphoma (HL), 168
Cutaneous leishmaniasis, 285, 286f
Cutaneous lesions, 372–373
Cutaneous lupus erythematosus, 9–10
　agents used to treat, 11t
　evaluation for, 10t
Cutaneous Lupus Erythematosus Disease Area and Severity Index (CLASI), 10
Cutaneous lymphomas, 159–170
　primary, 159–166
　in WHO classification, 159t
Cutaneous marginal zone lymphoma (cMZL), 166
Cutaneous metastasis, 216
Cutaneous myelogenous leukemia (cML), 167
Cutaneous sclerosis
　morphea and, 24
　systemic sclerosis and, 26–27
Cutaneous T-cell lymphoma (CTCL), 159–160
　see also Primary cutaneous T-cell lymphomaserythroderma and, 105–106, 108
　malignancy and, 135
Cutaneous vasculitis (CV), 31
Cutaneous xanthomas, 225–226
Cuticular hypertrophy, in dermatomyositis, 15, 15f
Cutis marmorata, 220–221, 360
Cyclophosphamide, 143
　and anagen arrest, 380
　for Behçet's disease, 40
　for bullous pemphigoid, 125
　for pemphigoid gestationis, 368
　for pemphigus, 122
　for sarcoidosis, 314
　for systemic sclerosis, 28
　for vasculitis, 37
Cyclosporine
　for Behçet's disease, 40
　for dermatomyositis/polymyositis, 20
　for epidermolysis bullosa acquisita, 127
　and gingival hyperplasia, 401

Cyclosporine *(Continued)*
  for graft-*versus*-host disease, 342
  for impetigo herpetiformis, 363
  for pemphigoid gestationis, 368
  for psoriasis, 48
  for sarcoidosis, 314
  for TEN, 92
Cyproterone, for androgen-related disorders, 386
Cystatin C-derived amyloid, 180
Cysts, renal, 352–353
Cytarabine, 146
Cytokines
  in bullous pemphigoid, 123
  mast cell disease, 371–372
  in pemphigus, 118
  in sarcoidosis, 305–306
Cytolytic degranulation, of eosinophils, 70
Cytomegalovirus (CMV), 267–268
  HIV and, 291
  in transplant recipients, 332
Cytotoxic agents
  for monoclonal protein disorders, 174
  for monoclonal protein production disorders, 177

D

Dabrafenib, 152
Dacarbazine, 146
Danazol, for monoclonal protein disorders, 174
Danger-associated molecular patterns (DAMPS), 59, 60f
Dapsone
  adverse effects, 434
  for bullous pemphigoid, 125
  for dermatitis herpetiformis, 128
  for linear IgA bullous dermatosis, 130
  for lupus erythematosus, 11
  for pemphigus, 122
  for relapsing polychondritis, 320
  in urticaria, 85–86
  for vasculitis, 36
Darier disease, 121
Darier's sign, 373, 373f
"Darrier-Roussy" sarcoidosis, 306
Dasatinib, 151
Debridement, 427f
  of devitalized tissue, 420
  methods of, 421t
  surgical, 338
Dechallenge decisions, drugs, 428
Decitabine, 149
Deficiency of interleukin-1 receptor antagonist (DIRA), 61t, 62–63, 63f
Degos disease (malignant atrophic papulosis), 319
Demethylating agents, for cancer therapy, 148–149
Demodex mites, 338
Dengue, 268–269
Dermal-epidermal junction, 118f
Dermatitis herpetiformis, 127–129, 127f, 250–251
  bullous pemphigoid and, 124
  drug selection principles, 438t
  malignancy and, 133
  and polyclonal IgA gammopathy, 177
  and thyroid disorders, 221
Dermatographism, urticaria and, 78, 82, 82f
Dermatomyositis, 13–21, 194, 195f
  associated diseases with, 13–14
  cutaneous manifestations of, 14–16
  definition and classification of, 13, 14t

Dermatomyositis *(Continued)*
  evaluation of patient with, 18–19, 19t
  malignancy and, 13, 18, 133–134
  muscle disease in, 16
  in pregnancy, 365
  systemic features of, 16–17
Dermatomyositis Skin Severity Index, 21
Dermatoses, numerous, 437, 438t
Desloratadine, 85
Desmoglein, in pemphigus, 118, 120
Desmoid tumors, 248
Desmosomes, in bullous diseases, 117
Desquamative gingivitis, 123–124
Dexamethasone, 367
Diabetes insipidus, 184, 311
Diabetes mellitus, 205–214
  bullous pemphigoid and, 124–125
  cutaneous manifestation of, 205–211
  dermatologic diseases associated with, 213
  epidermolysis bullosa acquisita and, 126
  eruptive xanthomas as, 226
  pruritus in, 102
  uncontrolled, 213
Diabetic bullae, 206
Diabetic cheiroarthropathy, 211
Diabetic dermopathy, 206–207, 207f
Diabetic foot, 207–208, 207f
Diabetic neuropathy, 212
Diabetic thick skin, 211
Diascopy, 114, 306–307, 306f
Diclofenac, for linear IgA bullous dermatosis, 129
Dietary restriction, dermatitis herpetiformis and, 127
Diffuse cutaneous systemic sclerosis (dSSc), 25
Diffuse plane xanthomas, 226, 226f
Digit abnormalities, periungual and distal, 392–393
Digital ulcers, in Raynaud's phenomenon, 29
Dihydrotestosterone (DHT), 382
Dimethyl sulfoxide, 182
Dimorphic fungi, 338
Direct fluorescent antibody (DFA) test, for lymphogranuloma venereum, 302–303
Direct immunofluorescence
  see also Immunofluorescence
  bullous pemphigoid and, 123–124
  dermatitis herpetiformis and, 128
  epidermolysis bullosa acquisita and, 126–127
  linear IgA bullous dermatosis and, 129–130
  pemphigus and, 120–121
  in scarring alopecia diagnosis, 383
  for vasculitis, 36
Direct testing, for syphilis, 300
Discoid lupus erythematosus (DLE), 2, 3f
  oral, 2, 4f
  palmar/plantar, 2, 3f
Disease-modifying antirheumatic drugs (DMARDs), 54
Disseminated candidiasis, 336
Disseminated gonococcal infection, 302t, 303, 303f
Disseminated granuloma annulare, in diabetes mellitus, 213
DNA, damaged in Louis-Bar syndrome, 356
Docetaxel, 148
Doppler flowmeter, 414
Doxepin, for urticaria, 85
Doxorubicin, 380
DRESS (drug reaction with eosinophilia and systemic symptoms), 255, 261f, 425, 426t
  drug selection principles, 438t

Dressings, wound, 421–422
Drug-drug interactions, 439
Drug eruptions, 425–436
  approach to patient with suspected, 425–428
  criteria for intentional drug rechallenge, 428t
  diagnostic tests, 427t
  morphologic classification of, 427t
  specific cutaneous, 429t
  target organs with high-risk, 427t
Drug-induced bullous pemphigoid, 432
Drug-induced hypersensitivity syndrome, 426t, 430–431, 430f
Drug-induced immunoglobulin-A bullous dermatosis, 432–433
Drug-induced lupus, 434
Drug-induced pemphigus, 432
Drug-induced SCLE (DI-SCLE), 6–7, 7t
Drug-induced skin injury, 425
"Drug Safety Database", 242
Drug selection principles, 437–439
  monitoring, 439–441
Drugs
  antibiotics. *see* Antibiotics
  anticonvulsants. *see* Anticonvulsants
  antihistamines. *see* Antihistamines
  complications. *see* Adverse effects
  DMARDs. *see* Disease-modifying antirheumatic drugs (DMARDs)
  effects of, in transplant recipients, 343, 343t
  hypersensitivity reaction, 104
  NSAIDs. *see* Aspirin; Nonsteroidal anti-inflammatory drugs (NSAIDs)
  overview of, for various cancers, 142t
  for rheumatoid arthritis, 54
  telogen effluvium and, 379
Duhring disease, 127–129
Dupuytren's contracture, in diabetic hand syndrome, 210
Dyshidrosis, in pregnancy, 360–361
Dysphagia, in dermatomyositis, 16–17, 19

E

Earlobe creases, 319, 320f
EBA. *see* Epidermolysis bullosa acquisita (EBA).
Ebola, 269–270
Ecchymosis, in purpura, 109, 113f, 116
Echocardiogram, 312
Echocardiography, 193–194
Ecthyma gangrenosum, 274
Ectopic adrenocorticotropic syndrome, 137
Eczema, 103
Eczema herpeticum, 267
Eczematous plaque, 136
Edema
  in erythroderma, 105–106
  facial, 105
  laryngeal, 84
  of leg ulcer, 422
  in pregnancy, 360
Ehlers-Danlos syndrome (EDS), 113, 320, 321f
  in pregnancy, 365
Eicosanoids, 371–372
Elastic multilayer bandaging systems, 422
Elastic support stockings, 422
Elastosis perforans serpiginosa, 258, 259f
Electrocardiography, in sarcoidosis, 312
Electrodesiccation, 226
Electroencephalography, 311
Electrolysis, excessive hair, 385

Electromyography (EMG), for dermatomyositis, 16
Elevation, limb, in leg ulcers, 422
EM. *see* Erythema multiforme (EM).
Embolic phenomena, 320
Emollients, 103, 363
  for Sjögren's syndrome (SS), 57
En coup de sabre, 22–23, 24f
End-stage renal disease pruritus, 101
Endemic mycoses, 279
Endemic typhus, 275
Endocrine abnormalities, sarcoidosis and, 311–312
Endocrine agents, for cancer therapy, 153–154
Endocrine disease, pruritus in, 102
Endocrine system, nail disorders, 393
Endogenous familial hypertriglyceridemia, 223
Endoglin, 245
Enzyme-linked immunosorbent assay (ELISA) testing, 123
Eosinophil-associated dermatoses, 72, 73t
Eosinophilia myalgia syndrome (EMS), 29–30
  defined, 71t
Eosinophilic fasciitis (EF), 28–29
Eosinophilic folliculitis, HIV infection and, 295, 296f
Eosinophilic granuloma, 184
Eosinophilic granulomatosis with polyangiitis (EGPA), 34
  defined, 71t
Eosinophils, 69
  classification of, 69–70
  dermatological diseases associated with, 69–76
    differential diagnosis of, 72, 75t
    histopathology of, 72, 74f
    pathogenesis of, 70–72, 70t–71t
    treatment of, 72–76
  flame figures of, 72, 74f, 74t
  tissue involvement of, 70
Epidemic typhus, 275
Epidermal growth factor receptor, drug eruption and, 434
Epidermal growth factor receptor inhibitors, for cancer therapy, 149–151, 149f
Epidermal necrosis, in SJS and TEN, 91
Epidermal nevus syndrome, 358, 358f
Epidermal transglutaminase (TG3), dermatitis herpetiformis and, 127
Epidermodysplasia verruciformis, 333
Epidermolysis bullosa acquisita (EBA), 8, 126–127, 126f, 178–179
  blistering, 117
  malignancy and, 133
  and RA, 53
Epinephrine (adrenaline), 84
Epomediol, for intrahepatic cholestasis of pregnancy, 367
Epoxides, 143
Epstein-Barr virus (EBV), 264–265, 265f
  HIV and, 291
  in transplant recipients, 332–333
Erdheim-Chester disease, 190t, 191f
Ergotism, 173
Eruptive xanthoma, 223–224, 226, 226f
Eruptive xanthomatosis, 208, 208f
Erysipelas, 213, 272, 272f
Erysipelas-like erythema (ELE), 64, 65f
Erythema
  annular, and Sjögren's syndrome (SS), 57
  diffuse, in erythrodermic psoriasis, 46–47
  palmar, 212

Erythema annulare centrifugum, SCLE distinguished from, 5–6
Erythema elevatum diutinum (EED), 35–36, 36f, 177
Erythema gyratum repens, 132f, 134, 134f
Erythema induratum, 96
Erythema infectiosum, 263
Erythema marginatum, 271
Erythema migrans, in Lyme disease, 274–275
Erythema multiforme (EM), 87–92, 89f
  bullous pemphigoid and, 124
  causes of, 88t
  purpura and, 110, 115
  urticaria and, 82
Erythema nodosum (EN), 93–95, 94t, 95f, 252
  in pregnancy, 365–366
  RA and, 53
  and sarcoidosis, 306
Erythrasma, 213
Erythrocyte sedimentation rate (ESR)
  in DIRA, 63
  in Schnitzler's syndrome, 62
Erythroderma, 104–108, 105f–107f, 105t
  in drug eruptions, 430–431
  malignancy and, 134
  in SCLE, 5–6
Erythrodermic psoriasis, 46–47, 47f
Erythromycin, 213
Erythropoietic protoporphyria, 240–241
Esophageal disease, in dermatomyositis, 16–17
Esophageal dysmotility, in systemic sclerosis, 26
Essential cryoglobulinemia, 115
Estramustine phosphate sodium, 148
Estrogen receptor downregulators, 153
Etanercept
  for necrobiosis lipoidica, 209
  for psoriasis, 48
  for rheumatoid arthritis, 54
Etoposide, 148
Everolimus, 152
Exanthem subitum, 264
Exanthematous eruptions, 429–431
Excisional biopsy, for vasculitis, 36
Exemestane, 153
Exfoliative dermatitis. *see* Erythroderma.
Exophthalmos, in Graves' disease, 219, 219f
Extracorporeal photopheresis
  for NSF, 328
  for Sézary syndrome, 162
Eye, involvement of, in bullous pemphigoid, 123–124
Eye disease, in sarcoidosis, 310

F

Fabry's disease, 324t–325t
Facial angiofibromas, 351, 351f
Facial edema, drug eruptions, 430
Factitious ulceration, 411f
Factor X depletion, in amyloidosis, 178–179
Famciclovir
  erythema multiforme and, 92
  for herpes simplex, 331
  for herpes zoster, 331
Familial adenomatous polyposis (FAP), 246–247
Familial apoprotein CII deficiency, 223
Familial cerebrotendinous xanthomatosis, 224
Familial combined hyperlipidemia, 223
Familial dysbetalipoproteinemia, 224
Familial glucocorticoid resistance, 232
Familial Hibernian fever, 63

Familial hypercholesterolemia, 223–225
Familial Mediterranean fever (FMF), 61t, 64–65, 65f
Familial syndromes of systemic amyloidosis, 180–181
Fas/Fas ligand, interaction of, 88
Felty's syndrome, rheumatoid nodules in, 51–52
Fentanyl, in mast cell disease, 374
Ferriman-Gallwey scale, for hirsutism, 230, 231f
Fever, TRAPS and, 64
Fexofenadine, 85, 374–375
Fibrates, 226
Fibroblasts, 356, 404
Fibrofolliculoma, 138
Fifth disease, 263
Figurate erythemas, malignancy and, 134, 134f
Finasteride, alopecia, 382
Finger pebbles, in diabetes mellitus, 211
Fingernails, 388–391
Fite stain, in sarcoidosis, 312
Fixed drug eruptions (FDE), 426t, 434
Flame figure, in eosinophils, 72, 74f, 74t
Fludarabine, 147
Fluorescent treponemal antibody absorption (FTA-ABS), 299–300
5-Fluorouracil, 146, 341
Fluoxetine, for Raynaud's phenomenon, 29
Fluoxymesterone, 153
Flushing
  in carcinoid syndrome, 315–319
  pheochromocytoma and, 230
Flutamide, 153
  for hirsutism, 231–232
Fogo selvagem, 117–118, 120
Folate antagonists, 146
Follicular biology, hair, 377
Follicular dendritic cell sarcoma, 188
Follicular dystrophy of immunosuppression (trichodysplasia spinulosa), 341
Folliculitis, 213
  in AIDS, 294
  in transplant recipients, 338
Food and Drug Administration (FDA) approval, drugs, 438
Foot, diabetic, 207–208, 207f
Forschheimer spots, 263
Fox-Fordyce disease, in pregnancy, 360–361
Fragilitas unguium, 389t–390t
Fulminant exfoliative dermatitis, 433
Fumarate hydratase, mutations in, 138–139
Fungal disease, 277–284
Fungal infections
  deep, 336–338
  in diabetes mellitus, 212
  superficial fungi, 335–336, 335f
  in transplant recipients, 335–338
Furosemide, 435
Furunculosis, 272–273, 273f

G

Gabapentin, 329
Gadolinium, 328
Gadolinium-based contrast agents (GBCAs), 29–30
Ganciclovir, for cytomegalovirus, 332
Gangrene, and cryoglobulinemia, 172
Gardner-Diamond syndrome, 110, 114, 114f
Gardner syndrome, 216–217, 246–247, 247f
  malignancy and, 138
Gastrointestinal abnormalities, cutaneous diseases associated with, 243–254, 244t

Gastrointestinal disorders
 neurofibromatosis and, 349
 urticaria and, 79–80
Gastrointestinal hemorrhage, 243–246
Gastrointestinal system, nail disorders, 393
Gelsolin protein, 180
Gemcitabine, 146, 147f
Generalized eruptive histiocytoma, 186t–187t, 188f
Generalized granuloma annulare, 221
Generalized morphea, 23, 23f
 treatment for, 25
Generalized plane xanthomatosis, 176
Genes, sarcoidosis and, 305–306
Genetic disorders, causing chronic renal disease, 323, 324t–325t
Genetic predisposition, in polymyositis/dermatomyositis, 13–14
Genetic testing, 350, 354
Genitourinary system, nail disorders, 394–395
German measles (Rubella), 263
Gianotti-Crosti syndrome, 255, 259
 Epstein-Barr virus and, 264–265
Giant cell reticulohistiocytoma, 186t–187t
Gigantism, 232–233
Gingival hyperplasia, 401
Gingivitis, 361
Glaucoma, in Sturge-Weber disease, 355
Gleich's syndrome, defined, 71t
Gliadin, in dermatitis herpetiformis, 127
Glossodynia, 400
Glucagonoma, 253–254
Glucagonoma syndrome, 137–138, 396
Glucocorticoid activity
 excessive, 228–229, 229f
 insufficient, 229, 230f
Glucocorticoids
 eosinophil receptors for, 70
 for HES, 72
Glucose-6-phosphate dehydrogenase levels, in dermatitis herpetiformis, 128
Glucose transporter protein-1 (GLUT-1), 196
Gluten-free diet, in dermatitis herpetiformis, 127–128
Goiter, dermatitis herpetiformis and, 127–128
Gold, 368
 for erythroderma, 105
Golimumab, for rheumatoid arthritis, 54
Gonococcal infection, disseminated, 302t, 303, 303f
Goodell's sign, in pregnancy, 361
Gottron's papules, in dermatomyositis, 14, 14f–15f
Gout, 57–58, 58f
Graft-versus-host disease (GVHD), 105
 and systemic sclerosis, 27
 in transplant recipients, 330, 341–343
Gram-negative infection, 274–276
Gram-negative rods, 334, 338
Granulocyte-macrophage colony-stimulating factor (GM-CSF), eosinophils and, 70
Granuloma annulare
 disseminated, in diabetes mellitus, 213
 HIV infection and, 296, 296f
Granuloma gravidarum, 362
Granuloma inguinale, 301, 302t, 303f
Granulomas, 310–311
Granulomatosis with polyangiitis (GPA), 34
Granulomatous slack skin, 162
Graves' disease, 217–219
 and atopic dermatitis, 221
 and pemphigoid gestationis, 368
Griscelli syndrome, 190t

Grover disease, 121
Growth factors, 205, 422
Guanosine triphosphatase-activation protein (GTPase), 346
Guttate psoriasis, 46, 47f

H
Hailey-Hailey disease, 121
HAIR-AN syndrome, 382
Hair cycle, 378f
Hair disorders, 377–386
 see also Alopecia; Telogen effluviumexcessive hair, 391
 in systemic disease, 378
Hair shaft, 377
Hair shaft disorders, 383–385
Hairy cell leukemia, 133–134
Half-and-half nails (Lindsay's nails), 327, 389t–390t, 392f, 394
Halogenoderma, 177
Hamartomatous polyposis syndromes, 248
Hand, foot, and mouth syndrome, 263–264, 264f
Hand-foot skin reaction (HFSR), 151
Hand-Schuler-Christian disease, 184
Hashimoto-Pritzker disease, 184
Hashimoto's thyroiditis, 218
Heart disease, 321
Heerfordt-Waldenström syndrome, 306, 311
Heliotrope eruption, in dermatomyositis, 14–15, 14f
Hemangioma of infancy, drug selection principles, 438t
Hemangiomas, 196
Hematologic disease, pruritus in, 102
Hematologic system, nail disorders, 393
Hematopoietic stem cell transplantation, 177
Hemidesmosomes, in bullous diseases, 117
Hemifacial atrophy, 24f
Hemochromatosis, 258, 258f, 320
Hemodialysis, pruritus and, 101
Hemodialysis-related amyloidosis, 179–180
Hemorrhage
 see also Purpuraintracranial, 366
 periorbital, 178–179
 simple, 109–114
 splinter, 389t–390t, 391, 392f
Hemosiderin, 112, 114, 409
Henoch-Schönlein purpura, 110
 and vasculitis, 31, 34
HEp-2 (human epithelium) substrate, in SCLE, 7
Hepatic disease
 pruritus of, 255, 256f
 skin and, 255–261
Hepatic sarcoidosis, 311
Hepatitis B, 259
Hepatitis C, 259
 dermatitis and, 261f
 leukocytoclastic vasculitis and, 260f
 lichen planus and, 260f
 necrolytic acral erythema and, 259f
 porphyria cutanea tarda and, 259f
 pruritus in, 101–102
 purpura and, 115
Hepatitis C virus (HCV)
 and cryoglobulinemic vasculitis, 34–35
 malignancy and, 133
Hepatocellular carcinoma, porphyria cutanea tarda and, 239
"Hepatoerythropoietic porphyria", 235–236
Hepatolenticular degeneration. see Wilson's disease.
Hepatosplenomegaly, 223

Hereditary coproporphyria, 242
Hereditary hemorrhagic telangiectasia (HHT), 193, 194f, 245–246, 245f
 in pregnancy, 366
Hereditary hypereosinophilia, 69
Hereditary nonpolyposis colorectal cancer (HNPCC) Lynch syndrome II, 135
Hereditary progressive mucinous histiocytosis, 186t–187t
Herpangina, 264
Herpes simplex virus (HSV), 266–267, 267f
 erythema multiforme and, 87, 91–92
 HIV infection and, 290–291, 290f
 in pregnancy, 364
 in transplant recipients, 330–331, 331f
Herpes zoster, 266, 266f, 331
 HIV infection and, 290–291, 290f
Heterozygosity loss, and malignant tumors, 346, 350
HHV-8 DNA, in Kaposi's sarcoma, 200
High-density lipoproteins (HDLs), 222
High-resolution CT scans, 18–19
Highly active antiretroviral combination therapy (HAART), 289
Higouménakis' sign, 300
Hirsutism, 230, 385–386, 386f, 386t
 in pregnancy, 361
Histamine
 in mast cell disease, 371–372, 374–375
 in urticaria, 77, 84
Histiocytic sarcoma, 188
Histiocytosis, cutaneous manifestations of, 183–191
 class I. see Langerhans cell histiocytosis
 class II, 185–188
  clinical manifestations of, 185–188, 186t–187t
  differential diagnosis of, 188
  evaluation of, 188, 189t–190t
  pathogenesis and pathology of, 185
  treatment for, 188
 class III, 188
Histone deacetylase inhibitors, for cancer therapy, 148–149
Histoplasmosis, 279, 338
HLA alleles
 bullous pemphigoid and, 123
 dermatitis herpetiformis and, 127
 pemphigus and, 119
HLA genotypes, drug eruptions, 428–429
Hodgkin disease
 CTCL and, 135
 linear IgA bullous dermatosis and, 129
Hodgkin's lymphoma
 amyloidosis, 178
 cutaneous, 168
 pruritus in, 102
Holster sign
 in Gottron's papules, 14
 in poikiloderma, 15f
Hormone-secreting syndromes, 137–138
Hot flashes, androgen deficiency and, 232
Hot tub folliculitis, 274
HSV. see Herpes simplex virus (HSV).
Human herpesvirus 6 (HHV-6), 264
 in transplant recipients, 332
Human herpesvirus 8 (HHV-8), 332–333
Human immunodeficiency virus (HIV), 289–297
 see also Acquired immunodeficiency syndrome (AIDS)bacterial infections in, 292–293, 292f–293f
 cutaneous manifestations of
  infectious, 289–294
  inflammatory, 294–296, 294f–296f

Human immunodeficiency virus (HIV) (Continued)
  miscellaneous, 297, 297f
  neoplastic, 296–297, 296f–297f
 fungal infections in, 293–294, 293f–294f
 and Kaposi's sarcoma, 200
 parasitic/ectoparasitic infections in, 294
 pruritus of, 102
 syphilis in, 301
 viral infections in, 290–292, 290f–291f
Human leukocyte antigen (HLA), 250, 428–429
 Behçet's disease and, 39
Human papillomavirus, 333–334, 333f
Human parvovirus B19, 263
Human T lymphotropic virus 1 (HTLV-1), 163
Human trypanosomiasis, 287
Hunter's syndrome, 385t
Huntley papules, in diabetes mellitus, 211
Hurler's syndrome, 385t
Hutchinson's sign, 266
Hutchinson's triad, 300
Hydralazine, drug eruptions, 435
Hydrazines, 146
Hydrochlorothiazide, anti-Ro (SS-A) antibody induced by, 6–7
Hydrogels, dry wounds, 422
Hydroquinone, for melasma, 359–360
Hydroxychloroquine
 for dermatomyositis/polymyositis, 20
 for graft-*versus*-host disease, 343
Hydroxychloroquine sulfate
 for lupus erythematosus, 11
 for sarcoidosis, 314
Hydroxyethylcellulose, 400
Hydroxyurea, 146, 417f, 418t–419t
Hydroxyzine, 84–85
Hyper-IgE syndromes, defined, 71t
Hyperandrogenism, 382
Hyperbaric oxygen, 327
Hypercalcemia, 311
Hypercalciuria, 311
Hypercholesterolemia, 225
Hyperchylomicronemia, 223
Hypercoagulable syndrome, 413f
Hypercortisolism, 228
Hypereosinophilia, 69
Hypereosinophilia of undetermined significance, 69
Hypereosinophilic syndromes (HES), 70
 clinical manifestations of, 71t
 defined, 71t
 mucocutaneous manifestations in, 72t
Hyperestrogenemia, 193
Hypergammaglobulinemic purpura, 110, 112, 177
Hyperglycemia, 336
Hyperhidrosis, in pregnancy, 360–361
Hyperimmunoglobulinemia D syndrome (HIDS), 61t, 65–66, 65f
Hyperinsulinemia, 205
Hyperkeratosis, 119, 177
Hyperlipidemias, 223
 secondary, 225
Hyperlipoproteinemia
 primary, 222, 223t
 secondary, 223t, 224
Hyperparathyroidism, pruritus in, 102
Hyperpigmentation, 148f, 150, 151f, 229, 230f
 in café-au-lait macules, 346
 in hemochromatosis, 258, 258f
 in hyperthyroidism, 218
 in pregnancy, 359–360
 in systemic sclerosis, 26

Hyperpituitarism, 232–233, 233f
Hypersensitivity syndrome, drug, 428
Hypersensitivity vasculitis, 31, 32f
Hypertension
 in neurofibromatosis, 349
 pheochromocytoma and, 230
 pseudoxanthoma elasticum and, 321
Hypertensive ulcer, 418t–419t
Hyperthyroidism, 100, 102, 127–128, 217–219, 218t, 221
 causes of, 217t
Hypertrichosis, 385
 drugs associated with, 385t
 hirsutism and, 230
Hypertrichosis lanuginosa (malignant down), malignancy and, 134–135, 134f
Hypertriglyceridemia, 208, 223, 226
Hypertrophic cardiomyopathy, 320–321
Hypertrophic (verrucous) lupus erythematosus (HLE), 2, 3f
Hyperviscosity syndrome, 171–173
Hypoalbuminemia, 128
Hypocomplementemia, in LE, 10
Hypocomplementemic urticarial vasculitis (HUV), 35, 35f
Hypolipoproteinemia, 224
Hypomelanosis of Ito, 357, 357f
Hypomelanotic macules, 351, 351f
Hypomyopathic dermatomyositis, 17
Hypopigmentation, in sarcoidosis, 309
Hypopituitarism, 233
Hypothyroidism, 219–221
 causes of, 220t
 congenital, 220–221
 dermatitis herpetiformis and, 127–128
 dermatological manifestations of, 220t
 hemangiomas, 196
 pruritus in, 102

I

Iatrogenic thyroid ablation, 219
Ibritumomab tiuxetan, 152–153
Ibuprofen, for Schnitzler's syndrome, 62
Ichthyosis, acquired, in systemic lymphomas, 168
Ichthyosis-associated syndromes, 358
Ichthyosis-like lesions, 309
Idelalisib, 152
Ifosfamide, 143
IgA deposition, dermatitis herpetiformis and, 250–251
IgA/IgG pemphigus, 117–118, 120, 122
IgA vasculitis (IgAV), 34
IgG paraprotein-associated disorders, 177
IgG4-related diseases, 72
 defined, 71t
IL1RN gene, 62
Imatinib, 151
Imatinib mesylate, for HES, 73–74
Imiquimod, 341
Immune checkpoint inhibitors, 153
Immune reconstitution inflammatory syndrome (IRIS), 290–291
Immunofixation techniques, 174, 178
Immunofluorescence
 direct. *see* Direct immunofluorescence
 erythema multiforme and, 91
 monoclonal protein disorders, 173
 for pemphigus, 120
Immunoglobulin, intravenous
 burn management, 431
 for dermatomyositis/polymyositis, 20
 for lupus erythematosus, 11
 for pemphigoid gestationis, 368

Immunoglobulin, intravenous (Continued)
 pemphigus and, 122
 TEN and, 88
Immunohistochemistry, for metastatic disease, 157
Immunosuppressants
 for dermatomyositis/polymyositis, 20
 for lupus erythematosus, 11
 in myositis and malignancy, 18
 in pemphigus, 119, 122
 for relapsing polychondritis, 320
 for vasculitis, 37
Impetigo, 272, 272f
Impetigo herpetiformis (IH), 363, 396
Inclusion bodies, in sarcoidosis, 312
Inclusion body myositis, dermatomyositis and, 13
Incontinentia pigmenti (IP), 357, 357f
Indeterminate cell histiocytosis, 186t–187t
Indolent systemic mastocytosis (ISM), 370–371
Infantile hemangiomas, and congenital hypothyroidism, 221
Infections
 bacterial. *see* Bacterial infections; Mycobacteria
 in diabetes mellitus, 212–213
 fungal. *see* Fungal infections
 management of, 420–421
 parasitic, 338, 338f–339f
 in pregnancy, 364–365
 ulceration due to, 421f
 viral. *see* Viral infections
Infectious diseases
 nail disorders and, 394
 skin, causing pruritus, 100t
Inflammation, 59
 erythroderma and, 106–107
 in purpura, 114–115
Inflammatory bowel disease, 251–252
 cutaneous associations of, 251t
 epidermolysis bullosa acquisita and, 126
Inflammatory myopathies. *see* Dermatomyositis; Myositis; Polymyositis.
Infliximab
 complications of, 20
 for necrobiosis lipoidica, 209
 for psoriasis, 48
 for rheumatoid arthritis, 54
 for sarcoidosis, 314
Informed consent, 439
Insect bites, urticaria and, 82
Insulin, allergy to, 214
Insulin growth factor (IGF-1), 205
Intellectual disability, in neurofibromatosis, 348–349
Interdigitating dendritic cell sarcoma, 188
Interferon-γ, for linear IgA bullous dermatosis, 129
Interferons, in dermatomyositis/polymyositis, 13–14
Interleukin-2, for linear IgA bullous dermatosis, 129
Interleukin (IL)-3, eosinophils and, 70
Interleukin (IL)-5, eosinophils and, 70
Intermediate density lipoproteins (IDLs), 222
 elevated, 224
International Dialysis Outcomes and Practice Patterns study, 101
Interstitial granulomatous dermatitis, RA and, 54–55
Intertrigo, and glucagonoma syndrome, 137–138

Intestinal amebiasis, 287–288
Intracellular signaling hypothesis, in pemphigus, 119
Intrahepatic cholestasis of pregnancy (ICP), 366–367, 369
Intrathoracic disease, in sarcoidosis, 309–310
Iodine, for linear IgA bullous dermatosis, 129
Ipilimumab, 153
Irinotecan, 147
Isolated bone marrow mastocytosis (IBMM), 370–371
Isotretinoin
 and pili torti, 384
 for sarcoidosis, 314
Ivermectin, for scabies, 294
IVIg. *see* Immunoglobulin, intravenous.
Ixodes scapularis, in Lyme disease, 274

J

Jaundice, 360
Jo-1 antibody, in myositis, 13–14
Juvenile gastrointestinal polyposis, 193–194
Juvenile idiopathic arthritis (JIA), 53, 53f
Juvenile myelomonocytic leukemia, 349
Juvenile rheumatoid arthritis, 53
Juvenile xanthogranuloma (JXG), 188, 188f, 224, 349

K

K5091 mutation, mast cell disease, 370
Kaposiform hemangioendotheliomas, 196
Kaposi's sarcoma, 200–203, 201f–202f, 398t, 418t–419t
 in AIDS, 296–297, 296f–297f
 in transplant recipients, 332, 338
Kaposi's varicelliform eruption, 267
Kasabach-Merritt syndrome, 113, 196
Kawasaki disease, 55–57, 56f, 56t
Kayser-Fleischer ring, 258, 259f
Keratinization, disorders of, drug selection principles, 438t
Keratinocytes, in bullous diseases, 117
Keratoacanthoma, malignancy and, 135
Keratoconjunctivitis sicca, 176
Keratoses, seborrheic, malignancy and, 134
Keratosis pilaris, 211, 212f
Ketoconazole, 229
Ketotifen, for mast cell disease, 374–375
Kidney disease, 323, 324t–326t
 see also Renal cell cancer; Renal failure
  disorders and, 396
 polycystic, 352–353
 tuberous sclerosis complex and, 352–353
KIT, mast cell disease, 370
Klippel-Trenaunay syndrome, 199f
Klippel-Trenaunay-Weber syndrome, 355
Koenen's tumors, 351–352, 351f
KOH (potassium hydroxide) preparation, 335
Koilonychia, 388–391, 389t–390t, 391f
Koplik spots, 262
Kyrle disease, 327, 327f

L

Laboratory tests, leg ulcers and, 412
Laënnec's cirrhosis, 255–256
LAMB syndrome, 320
Lamotrigine, drug eruptions, 430
Langerhans cell histiocytosis, 183–185, 185f
Langerhans cell sarcoma, 188
Langerhans cells, 183
Lanugo hair, 378
Laser technology, for Sturge-Weber syndrome, 356
Laser therapy, for xanthomas, 226
Latanoprost, 385t
LDLs (low density lipoproteins), 222
 increased, 223–224
Leflunomide
 for rheumatoid arthritis, 54
 for sarcoidosis, 314
Leg ulcers, 402–424
 arterial, 410–411
 causes of, 403t
 diabetic neuropathic, 422
 diagnostic tests of, 412–420
 differential diagnosis, management, and associated conditions to, 418t–419t
 investigations of, 412t
 lupus erythematosus and, 8
 pathophysiology of, 402–407
 patient history and physical examination findings and, 407–409, 407t
 prevalence and economic cost of, 402, 402t
 prognosis of, 420
 vascular studies, 412–414, 412t
 venous, 409–410
Leiomyomatosis, hereditary, 138–139, 139f
Leishmaniasis, 285–287, 286f
Lenalidomide, 154
LEOPARD syndrome, 320–321, 321f
Leprosy, 364
Lesch-Nyhan syndrome, 394
Leser-Trélat, sign of, 134–135
Letrozole, 153
Letterer-Siwe disease, 183–184, 184f, 396
Leukemia
 see also Lymphomaacute monocytic, 185
 hairy cell, 133–134
 lymphocytic, 120
 myeloid, 136–137
 pruritus in, 102
 recurrent, in transplant patients, 341
Leukocytoclastic angiitis, 31
Leukocytoclastic vasculitis
 hepatitis C infection and, 260f
 and mixed cryoglobulins, 172
 and monoclonal protein disorders, 173
 purpura and, 110, 113–116
 urticaria and, 79–80
Leukonychia, 389t–390t
Leuprolide, 153
Levocetirizine, 85
Levodopa, and anagen arrest, 381t
Lhermitte-Duclos disease, 138
Lichen amyloidosis, 180–181
Lichen myxedematosus, 176f
Lichen planus
 bullous pemphigoid and, 123–124
 and diabetes mellitus, 213
 oral, 255
  hepatitis C infection and, 260f
 SCLE and, 5–6, 6f, 9
Lichen planus pemphigoides, 124
Lichen sclerosus, morphea and, 23–24
Lichenoid GVHD, 342–343
Lidocaine, 374
Light chain-related systemic amyloidosis, 113, 178–179
Limited cutaneous systemic sclerosis (lSSc), 25
Lindsay's nails, 327, 389t–390t, 392f, 394
Linear IgA bullous dermatosis (LABD), 129–130, 129f, 177
 hemidesmosomal interactions, disruption of, 117
Linear immunoglobulin-A (IgA) bullous disease, 432–433
Linear morphea, 22–23, 23f
 treatment for, 25
Lipemia retinalis, 223
Lipid disorders, cutaneous manifestation of, 222–227
Lipids, 222
Lipoatrophy
 in diabetes mellitus, 214
 panniculitis and, 97–98
Lipodermatosclerosis, 409
 morphea and, 24
Lipodystrophy, in highly active antiretroviral combination therapy, 297, 297f
Lipogranuloma, and leg ulcers, 407–408
Lipohypertrophy, in diabetes mellitus, 214
Lisch nodules, 348
Lithium, 432
 for linear IgA bullous dermatosis, 129
Livedo racemosa, lupus erythematosus and, 8, 9f
Livedo reticularis
 associated conditions, 172
 biopsy for, 36
 lupus erythematosus and, 8
 and RA, 53
 vasculitis associated with, 35
Livedoid vasculopathy, 173–174, 173f, 403f, 412
Liver disorder, intrahepatic cholestasis of pregnancy and, 366
Lobo's disease, leishmaniasis and, 285
Lobular panniculitis, 96–98
Local anesthetics, for pruritus, 103
Loeys-Dietz syndrome, 316t–318t
Löfgren's syndrome, 306, 311–312
Longitudinal pigmented bands, nails, 388, 389t–390t, 391f
Loratadine, 85, 374–375
Louis-Bar syndrome, 356–357
Low density lipoproteins (LDLs), 222
 increased, 223–224
Low-pressure superficial venous system, 406f
Lubricating drops, for Sjögren's syndrome (SS), 57
Lues. *see* Syphilis.
Lumbar puncture, for neurosarcoidosis, 311
Lung cancer, pachydermoperiostosis and, 137
Lunular color changes, 389t–390t
Lupus erythematosus, 1–12
 acute cutaneous, 7–8, 8f
 antibody subsets in, 9t
 antiphospholipid antibody syndrome and, 315
 bullous pemphigoid and, 124
 chronic cutaneous, 1–5
 cutaneous changes associated with, 8–9
 DLE-SLE subset of, 5
 drug selection principles, 438t
 laboratory phenomena in, cutaneous, 9–10
 mucocutaneous lesions in, classification of, 2t
 neonatal, 7, 7f
 photosensitivity in, 8
 and polymyositis/dermatomyositis, 14
 subacute. *see* Subacute cutaneous lupus erythematosus (SCLE)
 and Waldenström's hypergammaglobulinemic purpura, 176
Lupus panniculitis (LEP), 4, 4f
Lupus pernio, 307–308, 308f
Lupus tumidus, 2–4, 4f

Luteinizing hormone-releasing hormone agonists, 153
Lyme disease, 274–275
Lymph nodes, sarcoidosis and, 306, 310–311
Lymphadenopathy, 310–311
  in erythroderma, 105–106
Lymphangiomyomatosis (LAM), 353
Lymphedema, 409
Lymphoblasts, in Louis-Bar syndrome, 356
Lymphocyte transformation test, 428
Lymphocytic leukemia, 120
Lymphogranuloma venereum, 302–303, 302t
Lymphoma
  see also Leukemia; Mycosis fungoides; Sézary syndromeassociated conditions, 224
  B-cell. see B-cell lymphomas
  dermatitis herpetiformis and, 128
  epidermolysis bullosa acquisita and, 126
  erythroderma and, 104–105
  Hodgkin's. see Hodgkin's lymphoma
  intestinal, 133
  non-Hodgkin's. see Non-Hodgkin's lymphoma
  pruritus in, 102
  recurrent, in transplant patients, 341
  sarcoidosis-lymphoma syndrome, 306
  T-cell. see T-cell lymphomas
Lymphomatoid granulomatosis, 121
Lymphomatoid papulosis, 162–163, 163f
Lymphoproliferative disorder, post-transplant, 332
Lymphoreticular system, tumors of, 133–134
Lynch syndrome II, 135

M

Macrocephaly, in neurofibromatosis, 349
Macrophage activating syndrome (MAS), 53
Macular amyloidosis, 180–181, 216–217
Macular telangiectases, 193
Maffucci syndrome, 196, 199f
Magnetic resonance imaging (MRI)
  for dermatomyositis, 16
  for neurosarcoidosis, 311
  for Sturge-Weber syndrome, 355
  T2, 348
Majocchi's granuloma, 335f
Major histocompatibility complex (MHC) class I antigens, 13–14
Malabsorption, 248–251
Male pattern androgenic alopecia, 361
Malignancy
  bullous pemphigoid and, 124
  in erythroderma, 105–106, 106f, 108
  internal, skin signs of, 131–140, 131t
    hormone-secreting syndromes, 137–138
    inherited syndromes, 138–140
    proliferative and inflammatory dermatoses, 131–137
  in polymyositis/dermatomyositis, 13, 18
Malignant disease
  see also Leukemia; Lymphoma; Metastatic disease; Tumorsreticuloendothelial system, 224
Malignant down, 385
  malignancy and, 134f
Malignant lymphomas, pruritus in, 102
Malignant otitis externa, 213
Malignant tumors, and heterozygosity loss, 346
Mammalian target of rapamycin (mTOR), 350–351
Marburg, 269–270
Marenostrin-encoding fever (MEFV) gene, 64

Marfan syndrome, 366
Martorell ulcer, 411f, 418t–419t
"Mask of pregnancy", 359
Mast cell disease, 370–376, 371t
Mast cell leukemia (MCL), 370–371
Mast cells, 123, 370
  mediators, 371t, 373f
  urticaria and, 77–78, 80, 84
Mastocytosis (mast cell disease), 370
  adult, 373f
  diagnostic tests for patients with, 374t
  symptoms and signs of, 372t
Mat telangiectasia, in scleroderma, 195f
Matrix and plate abnormalities, nails, 387
Measles (rubeola), 262–263
Mechlorethamine, 141–143
Mees' lines, nails, 387–388, 389t–390t
Megestrol acetate, 153
Melanocytic nevus, in pregnancy, 361
Melanoma, 394
  in pregnancy, 362
Melanonychia, 388, 389t–390t
Melasma (chloasma), in pregnancy, 359
Melatonin, for sarcoidosis, 314
Melkersson-Rosenthal syndrome, 397–400
Melphalan, 143
Meningococcemia, 274
Menkes' kinky hair syndrome, 384, 384f
Mental defect, 355
Mental retardation, 385
Mepolizumab, for HES, 73–74
Mercaptopurine, 147
MERLIN (negative growth regulator), 346
Metabolic abnormalities, 311–312
Metabolic syndrome, 321
Metastatic disease, 155–158
  see also Malignant diseaseappearance of, 156–157, 156f–157f
  carcinoma, cutaneous involvement by, 156t
Methemoglobinemia, 128
Methicillin-resistant Staphylococcus aureus (MRSA), 213
Methotrexate, 146
  for Behçet's disease, 40
  for cheilitis granulomatosa, 400
  for dermatomyositis/polymyositis, 20
  for erythroderma, 108
  for graft-versus-host disease, 342
  for linear morphea, 25
  for lupus erythematosus, 11
  for pemphigoid gestationis, 368
  for pemphigus, 122
  for psoriasis, 48
  for rheumatoid arthritis, 54
  for sarcoidosis, 314
  for systemic sclerosis, 28
  for vasculitis, 36
Methotrexate-induced cirrhosis, 257
Methylprednisolone, for Sweet's syndrome, 41
Mevalonic aciduria (MA), 65
MF. see Mycosis fungoides (MF).
Microangiopathy, in diabetic dermopathy, 207
β_2-microglobulin, hemodialysis-related amyloidosis, 179–180
Micronychia, 389t–390t
Microscopic polyangiitis (MPA), 34
Microthrombi-related ulcers, 418t–419t
Microvascular syndromes, minimally inflammatory, 110
Miescher's radial granulomas, 95
Migratory thrombophlebitis, malignancy and, 135
Mikulicz syndrome, 306

Miliaria, in pregnancy, 360–361
Milroy's disease, 203
Miniaturization, hair follicles, 382, 382f
Minocycline
  drug eruptions, 435
  for pemphigoid gestationis, 368
Minoxidil, alopecia, 382
Mitomycin C, 143
Mitoxantrone, 148
Mixed connective tissue disease (MCTD), 29
Mixed organic brain syndrome, 373
Modifying genes, 346
Mohs' technique, 341
Moisturizers, for pruritus, 103
Mollusca contagiosum (MC), 334
Molluscum fibrosum gravidarum, 362
Monoclonal antibodies, for cancer therapy, 152–153
Monoclonal cryoglobulinemia, 115
Monoclonal gammopathies, platelet function and, 110
Monoclonal gammopathy of undetermined significance (MGUS), 171
Monoclonal protein, disorders directly related to, 171–174, 172f–173f
Monoclonal protein production, disorders associated with, 174–177
Mononucleosis, cytomegalovirus, 268
Montelukast, for urticaria, 85
Montgomery tubercles, 360–361
Morphea, 22–25, 23f–24f, 24t
mTOR. see Mammalian target of rapamycin (mTOR).
Muckle-Wells syndrome, 180
Mucocutaneous lymph node syndrome, 55–57, 56f, 56t
Mucocutaneous manifestations, systemic diseases with, 398t
Mucormycosis, 212, 213f, 281
Mucosal neuromas, 216–217
Muehrcke's lines, 389t–390t, 391–392
Muir-Torre syndrome, 139
Multicentric reticulohistiocytosis, 188, 189t, 191f
  malignancy and, 135, 135f
Multikinase inhibitors, for cancer therapy, 151
Multiple endocrine neoplasia (MEN), 139, 139f, 180, 216–217
Multiple hamartoma syndrome, 216–217
Multiple lentigines, 320–321
Multiple myeloma
  amyloidosis, 178
  epidermolysis bullosa acquisita and, 126
  keratotic lesions in, 177f
  and MGUS, 171
  nail disorders, 396
  POEMS syndrome, 174–175
  and purpura, 179f
  and secondary hyperlipoproteinemia, 224
Muscle disease, in dermatomyositis, 16, 19
Musculoskeletal disorders, 349
MVK gene, 65
Myalgia, TRAPS and, 64
Myasthenia gravis, pemphigus in, 120–122
Mycobacteria, 334–335
Mycophenolate mofetil
  for bullous pemphigoid, 125
  for dermatomyositis/polymyositis, 20
  for graft-versus-host disease, 342–343
  for linear morphea, 25
  for lupus erythematosus, 11
  for pemphigus, 122
  for vasculitis, 36

Mycosis fungoides (MF), 159–162
  see also Sézary syndromedrug selection principles, 438t
  early phases of, precise characterization of, 160
  malignancy and, 135
  morphology of, 160
  plaques of, 160–161
  staging of, 161, 161t
Myelodysplastic syndromes (MDS), 167
Myeloid leukemia, 136–137
Myeloma
  see also Multiple myelomamalignancy and, 133
Myeloperoxidase (MPO)-ANCA, 34
Myeloproliferative disease, 110
Myiasis, 75f
Myopathies, inflammatory, classification of, 13, 14t
Myositis
  see also Dermatomyositis; Polymyositisand cardiovascular diseases, 321
  evaluation of patient with, 18–19, 19t
  inclusion body, 13
  Jo-1 antibody in, 13–14
  and malignancy, 18
Myositis-specific autoantibodies, 19
Myxedema, 220
  pretibial, 218, 218f

N

Nail bed, 387
Nail bed abnormalities, 391–392
Nail changes
  in hyperthyroidism, 218
  in pregnancy, 361
  in renal disease, 327, 328f
Nail disorders
  see also Periungual telangiectasesclubbing. see Clubbing
  in Graves' disease, 219
Nail fold capillary abnormalities, 393
Nail matrix and plate abnormalities, 387
Nail-patella syndrome, 394, 395f
Nail plate, 387
Nail psoriasis, 45–46, 46t
Nail signs
  changes associated with malignancy, 396
  findings and associations, 389t–390t
  of systemic disease, 387–396
Nailfold changes, in dermatomyositis, 15, 15f
Nails
  anatomy of, 388f
  pruritus in, 99
Naltrexone, for pruritus, 329
NAME syndrome, 320
Necrobiosis lipoidica, 208–209, 209f, 416f, 418t–419t
Necrobiotic xanthogranuloma, 177, 185, 189t
  malignancy and, 135–136
  with paraproteinemia, 176, 176f
Necrolytic acral erythema, hepatitis C infection and, 259f
Necrolytic migratory erythema, 137–138, 254
Necrosis
  of fingertips, in polyarteritis nodosa, 33f
  in inflammatory myopathies, 13–14
  keratinocyte, 120
  purpura and, 115–116
Necrotizing fasciitis, 213, 418t–419t
Necrotizing ulcerative gingivitis (NUG), 400
Neonatal jaundice, 255

Neonatal lupus erythematosus, 7, 7f, 365
Neoplasms
  in pregnancy, 361–362, 361t
  in transplant recipients, 338–341
Nephrogenic systemic fibrosis (NSF), 29–30, 328, 328f
Neuralgia, postherpetic, 99–100
Neurocutaneous disease, 345–358, 346t
Neurofibromas, 216–217, 347–348, 348f, 362
Neurofibromatosis (von Recklinghausen disease), 346–350, 347f
  and endocrine disorders, 349
Neurofibromin, 346
Neuropathic itch, 102–103
Neuropathy, diabetic, 212
Neurosarcoidosis, 311
Neurosyphilis, diagnosis of, 300–301
Neutropenia, 336
Neutrophilic dermatoses, 39–44
  malignancy and, 136–137, 136f
Neutrophilic eccrine hidradenitis, 434
Neutrophilic vasculitis, 34
Neutrophils, in Sweet's syndrome, 41
Nevi araneus, 360
Nevirapine, drug eruptions, 430
Nevoid basal cell carcinoma syndrome (NBCCS), 397
Nevoid lesions, 352
Nevoxanthoendothelioma, 224
NF1 gene, neurofibromatosis and, 346, 349
Nicotinamide, for linear IgA bullous dermatosis, 130
Nicotinic acid, 226
Nifedipine, 401
Nikolsky sign
  in pemphigus, 119
  in TEN, 89–90, 90f, 92
Nilotinib, 151
97-kDa protein antigen, in linear IgA bullous dermatosis, 129
Nitrogen mustards, 141–143, 388
Nitrosoureas, 146
  and anagen arrest, 380
Nivolumab, 153
NK/T-cell lymphomas, 163
NLRP3, 59
Nocardiosis, in transplant patients, 334
Nod-like receptors (NLRs), 59
Nodular cutaneous amyloidosis, 180
Nodular vasculitis, 96
Non-Hodgkin's lymphoma
  CTCL and, 135
  PNP and, 120
Nonhormone secreting pancreatic carcinoma, 254
Nonsteroidal anti-inflammatory drugs (NSAIDs)
  drug eruptions, 427–428
  for SAPHO syndrome, 67
  for sarcoidosis, 313
  for Schnitzler's syndrome, 62
  in urticaria, 78, 82
  for vasculitis, 36
Noonan syndromes, 320–321
Normolipemic xanthomatosis, 224
Norwegian scabies, 294
NSAIDs. see Nonsteroidal anti-inflammatory drugs (NSAIDs).
Nuclear medicine imaging, on SAPHO syndrome, 67

O

Occlusive dressings, 29
Octreotide acetate, 153–154

Ocular sarcoidosis, 314
Oculoglandular syndrome of Parinaud, 274
Odontogenic keratocysts (OKCs), 397
Omenn syndrome, defined, 71t
Oncostatin M-specific receptor β gene, 180
Onychocryptosis, 389t–390t
Onycholysis, 218, 327, 391f, 392
Onychomadesis, 389t–390t
Onychomycosis, 389t–390t
Onychoptosis, 389t–390t
Onychorrhexis, 389t–390t
Onychoschizia, 389t–390t
Onychotillomania, 394
Oophorectomy, for pemphigoid gestationis, 368
Opportunistic fungal infections, 281
Opportunistic mycoses, 338, 338f–339f
  emerging, 283–284
Oral candidiasis, 283, 283f
  HIV infection and, 293, 293f
Oral contraceptives
  for androgen-related disorders, 386
  for hirsutism, 231–232
Oral discoid lupus erythematosus, 2, 4f
Oral disease, 397–401
Oral disodium cromoglycate, mast cell disease, 374–375
Oral hairy leukoplakia, 291, 291f
Oral mucous membranes, 397
Oral pigmentation, 400
Organomegaly, in POEMS syndrome, 174–175
Oropharyngeal candidiasis, 283
Oropharyngeal erosions, in pemphigus, 117–118
Osler-Weber-Rendu syndrome, 192
Osteoarticular disease, SAPHO syndrome and, 66–67
Osteomyelitis, 409
Osteoporosis, 373
Osteoprotegerin, for calciphylaxis, 327
Otitis externa, malignant, 213
Oximetry, transcutaneous, 414

P

p53 signaling pathway, 356
Pachydermoperiostosis, malignancy and, 137
Paclitaxel, 148
Paecilomyces lilacinus, 283–284
Paget's disease of breast, extramammary Paget's disease and, malignancy and, 136, 136f
Pain
  management, leg ulcers, 423
  neuropathic itch and, 102
Palisaded neutrophilic granulomatous dermatitis (PNGD), 55, 55f
Palmar discoid lupus erythematosus, 2, 3f
Palmar erythema, 212
  cirrhosis and, 256–257
  in pregnancy, 360
  systemic lupus erythematosus and, 8
Pancreatic disease, 252–254, 253t
Pancreatic panniculitis, 96–97, 97f
Pancreatitis, 252–253, 253f
Panhypopituitarism, 233, 311
Panniculitis, 93–98, 252–253, 253f
  alpha-1 antitrypsin deficiency, 97
  classification of, 94t
  connective tissue-associated, RA and, 53
  erythema induratum and, 96
  erythema nodosum and, 93–95, 94t, 95f
  lipoatrophy and, 97–98
  lobular, 96–98

Panniculitis (Continued)
  nodular vasculitis and, 96
  pancreatic, 96–97, 97f
  septal, 93–96
  superficial migratory thrombophlebitis and, 96
Pansclerotic morphea, 23
Papillary adenocarcinomas, 216
Papillomatosis, 119, 398f
Papular acrodermatitis, of children, 259
Papular mucinosis. *see* Scleromyxedema.
Papular telangiectasias, 193, 194f
Papular xanthoma, 186t–187t
Papulosquamous subacute cutaneous lupus erythematosus (SCLE-P), lesions of, 5–6, 6f
Paracoccidioidomycosis, 281
Paraneoplastic autoimmune multiorgan syndrome (PAMS), 133
Paraneoplastic conditions, and systemic sclerosis, 27–28
Paraneoplastic disorders, malignancy and, 140t
Paraneoplastic pemphigus (PNP), 120
  malignancy and, 133, 133f
  in systemic lymphomas, 168
Paraproteinemia
  with necrobiotic xanthogranuloma, 176, 176f
  in systemic lymphomas, 169
Parasitic infections, in transplant recipients, 338, 338f–339f
Parathyroidectomy, for calciphylaxis, 327
Paronychia, 150, 150f, 389t–390t
Paroxysmal attacks, pheochromocytoma and, 230
Paroxysmal nocturnal hemoglobinuria, 174
Parry-Romberg syndrome, 22–23, 24f
Pastia's lines, 271
Pathergy, 39
Pathogen-associated molecular patterns (PAMPs), 59, 60f
Patient information handout, 439
PCT. *see* Porphyria cutanea tarda (PCT).
Pembrolizumab, 153
Pemetrexed, 146
Pemphigoid gestationis (PG), 367–368, 367f
Pemphigus, 117–122, 119f, 121f, 121t
  see also specific forms
  malignancy and, 133
  and thyroid disorders, 221
Pemphigus erythematosus, 117–118, 120
Pemphigus foliaceus, 105, 117–118, 119f, 120, 365
Pemphigus vegetans, 117–119, 365
Pemphigus vulgaris, 117–118, 118f, 120–123, 125
  drug selection principles, 438t
  nail disorders, 396
  in pregnancy, 365
Penicillamine, autoimmune disorders and, 120
Penicillin
  for erythroderma, 105
  in urticaria, 83–84
Penicillin G, for linear IgA bullous dermatosis, 129
Pentoxifylline
  for leg ulcers, 423
  for Raynaud's phenomenon, 29
  for sarcoidosis, 314
Pericardial effusions, 319
Pericarditis, 319
Perifollicular hemorrhage, 113–114, 114f
Perifollicular hyperkeratosis, 211

Periodic acid-Schiff stain, in sarcoidosis, 312
Peripheral arterial disease (PAD), 411
Peripheral blood eosinophilia, 69
Peripheral nervous system, nail disorders, 394
Peripheral vascular disease, 408–409
Peristomal pyoderma gangrenosum, 42, 42f
Periungual telangiectases, 212
  in dermatomyositis, 15, 15f, 195f
  systemic lupus erythematosus and, 8
Pernicious anemia, 121, 124
Petechia, 109, 110f
Petechial simple hemorrhage, 109–110
Peutz-Jeghers syndrome, 139–140, 139f, 248, 400
"Phakomatoses", 345
Pharmacogenomics biomarkers, 439
Phenobarbital, 367
Phenytoin, for linear IgA bullous dermatosis, 129
Pheochromocytoma, 216–217, 230
  in neurofibromatosis, 349
Phlebitis, nonhormone secreting pancreatic carcinoma and, 254
Phosphatase and tensin homolog (PTEN) hamartoma tumor syndrome, 248
Phosphate binders, calcium-containing, 325
Photosensitivity, in SLE, 8
Phototherapy
  for generalized morphea, 25
  for necrobiosis lipoidica, 209
Pigmentary alteration, 329
Pili torti, 384, 384f
Pimecrolimus, 20, 103
Pincer nail, 389t–390t
Piroxicam, for linear IgA bullous dermatosis, 129
Pitting, 389t–390t
  of nails, 388
Pituitary disorders, 228–234
  with cutaneous manifestations, 232–233
Pityriasis lichenoides, purpura and, 110
Pityriasis rotunda, 177
  malignancy and, 136
Pityriasis rubra pilaris (PRP), 104–107
Planar xanthomas, 225–226, 225f–226f
Plantar discoid lupus erythematosus, 2
Plasma transthyretin protein, in amyloidosis, 178
Plasmacytomas, cutaneous, 175, 177
Plasmacytosis, cutaneous and systemic, 175–176
Plasmapheresis
  monoclonal protein disorders, 174
  for NSF, 328
  for pemphigoid gestationis, 368
  for pemphigus, 122
Platelet defects, hyperviscosity syndrome, 173
Platelet dysfunction, purpura and, 109–110
Plexiform neurofibromas, 347–348
Plummer's nails, 389t–390t, 393
Pneumonia
  measles and, 262
  in pregnancy, 364
Podagra, 57–58
POEMS syndrome, 174–175, 175f, 177
  in systemic lymphomas, 169
Poikiloderma, 194, 194f
  in dermatomyositis, 15, 15f
Polyangiitis, microscopic, 34
Polyarteritis nodosa (PAN), 31, 33–34, 33f
Polyarthralgia, Chikungunya and, 269
Polyarthritis, symmetric, 53–54
Polycystic kidney disease (PKD1), 352–353

Polycystic ovary syndrome, elevated androgen levels in, 231
Polycythemia vera, 102
Polymerase chain reaction (PCR), 335
Polymorphic eruption of pregnancy (PEP), 368–369, 368f
Polymyositis
  see also Dermatomyositisbullous pemphigoid and, 124
  course and treatment of, 19–21
  defined, 13
  and dermatomyositis, 13
  evaluation of patient with, 18–19, 19t
  as multisystem disorder, 16
  pathogenesis of, 13–14
  prognosis of, 21
Polyomavirus, 268
Polyposis syndromes, 246–248
Pomalidomide, 154
Porphyria cutanea tarda (PCT), 125, 235–240, 238f–239f
  and amyloidosis, 178–179
  conditions and precipitating/aggravating factors associated with, 239t
  hepatitis C infection and, 259f
  malignancy and, 133
  in pregnancy, 366
  and renal disease, 329
Porphyrias, 235–242, 236t, 329
  see also Porphyria cutanea tarda (PCT)characteristic biochemical finding in, 235, 237t
Porphyrin, in renal disease, 329
Porphyrin-heme pathway, 235, 236f
Port-wine stain, in Sturge-Weber syndrome, 354f
Postherpetic neuralgia (PHN), herpes zoster and, 266
Potassium hydroxide (KOH) preparation, 335
Potassium iodide, for Sweet's syndrome, 41
Pramoxine, 103, 182
Prednisone
  bullous pemphigoid and, 125
  for dermatomyositis/polymyositis, 19–20
  erythema multiforme and, 92
  for graft-*versus*-host disease, 343
  for hirsutism, 231–232
  for impetigo herpetiformis, 363
  for Langerhans' cell disease, 185
  for linear IgA bullous dermatosis, 130
  pemphigus and, 122
  for Sweet's syndrome, 41
Pregnancy, 359–369
  connective tissue changes in, 360
  cutaneous neoplasms affected by, 361–362, 361t
  dermatomyositis during, 17
  glandular changes in, 360–361
  hair changes in, 361
  mucous membrane changes in, 361
  nail changes in, 361
  physiologic skin changes in, 359–361
  pigmentary changes in, 359–360
  preexisting skin diseases in, 362–366, 362t
  pruritus in, 102, 366–367
  specific dermatoses of, 367–369
  tuberous sclerosis in, 366
  vascular changes in, 360
Pregnancy epulis, 362
Pressure spikes, intravascular, in purpura, 110
Pretibial myxedema, 218, 218f
Prick tests, 428
Primary biliary cirrhosis, 224f, 257–258, 258f

Primary cutaneous B-cell lymphomas, 163–166, 164f–165f
Primary cutaneous CD30+ lymphoproliferative disorders (pcCD30+LD), 162–163, 162f
Primary cutaneous small/medium CD4+ T-cell lymphoma, 163
Primary cutaneous T-cell lymphomas, 159–163
  mycosis fungoides, 159–162
  other, 163
  primary cutaneous CD30+ lymphoproliferative disorders (pcCD30+LD), 162–163, 162f
  Sézary syndrome, 159–162
Primary hypereosinophilia, 69
Primary (neoplastic) hypereosinophilic syndromes, 70–71
Primary syphilis, 297–298, 298f, 298t
Primary varicella, 364
PRKRA1A gene mutations, in Carney complex, 316t–318t
Probucol, 226
Procarbazine, 146
Progressive nodular histiocytosis, 186t–187t
Prolonged partial thromboplastin time (PTT), 116
Propofol, in mast cell disease, 374
Prostanoids, for Raynaud's phenomenon, 29
Protease inhibitors, for Hepatitis C, 260
Proteasome inhibitors, for cancer therapy, 148–149
Protozoal diseases, 285–288
Proximal nail fold capillary abnormalities, 389t–390t
Proximal subungual onychomycosis, 293
Prurigo of pregnancy (PP), 369
Pruritic folliculitis of pregnancy (PFP), 369
Pruritic urticarial papules and plaques of pregnancy (PUPPP), 368
Pruritus, 99–103, 100t, 101f
  cause of, 100t
  of cholestasis, 101–102
  chronic, skin signs of, 99
  and dermatomyositis, 21
  diabetes-related, 211
  end-stage renal disease, 101
  endocrine disease and, 102
  erythroderma and, 105–106, 108
  HIV infection and, 102, 295
  itch and, cause of, 100t
  lymphomas, leukemia, and hematologic disease, 102
  neuropathic itch and, 102
  in pregnancy, 102, 366–367
  renal, 328–329
  in systemic lymphomas, 168
  in thyroid disorders, 221
  in urticaria, 78, 80
Pseudo-Cushing syndrome, 228–229
Pseudoarthrosis, in neurofibromatosis, 349
Pseudoclubbing, 389t–390t
Pseudomonas aeruginosa, 212–213, 334
Pseudomonas aeruginosa folliculitis, 274
Pseudoporphyria, 239, 240f, 329, 329f, 432
  medications associated with, 240t
Pseudoxanthoma elasticum (PXE), 113, 243–245, 244f, 321
  in pregnancy, 366
Psoriasis, 45–50, 46f, 46t, 48t
  bullous pemphigoid and, 124
  and diabetes mellitus, 213
  drug selection principles, 438t
  and heart disease, 321
  HIV infection and, 295, 295f

Psoriasis (Continued)
  LE and, 9
  SCLE and, 5–6
  skin disease and, 104
  and thyroid disorders, 221
Psoriasis vulgaris, 45–46, 46f
Psoriatic arthritis, 49–50, 50f, 50t
Psoriatic arthritis mutilans, 50f
PSTPIP1 gene, 66
Psychiatric conditions, nail disorders, 394
Psychiatric diseases, pruritus in, 99
Psychogenic purpura, 110
PTCH/PTCH2 genes, mutations, 397
Pterygium, 389t–390t
Pterygium inversum, 389t–390t
PTPN11 gene mutations, in LEOPARD and NOONAN syndromes, 320–321
Pulmonary arterial hypertension (PAH), systemic sclerosis and, 27
Pulmonary arteriovenous fistulae, hereditary hemorrhagic telangiectasia and, 246
Pulmonary disease
  blastomycosis and, 281
  in dermatomyositis, 17
  urticaria and, 79–80
Pulmonary function tests, 309–310, 313
Pulmonary involvement, tuberous sclerosis complex and, 353
Pulmonary system, nail disorders, 394
Pulse methylprednisolone therapy, for dermatomyositis/polymyositis, 20
Punch biopsy
  amyloidosis, 180
  in panniculitis, 93
  for vasculitis, 36
Punctate keratoses, 136
Purine analogs, 147
Purpura, 109–116
  in amyloidosis, 178–179, 179f
  benign hypergammaglobulinemic purpura of Waldenström. *see* Waldenström, benign hypergammaglobulinemic purpura of
  chronic pigmented, 112f
  cryofibrinogenemia, 173
  cryoglobulinemia, 172, 172f
  differential diagnosis, 111t, 115
  lesion, 114
  noninflammatory retiform, 112f
  palpable, 110, 112–116, 112f
    in vasculitis, 33
  pigmented, 212
  simple hemorrhage and, 109–114
  urticaria and, 79–80, 82
  vasculitis, 53
Purpura fulminans, 113f, 115
Pustular eruptions, 432
Pustular psoriasis, 47, 48f
PUVA, for systemic sclerosis, 28
PUVA (psoralens and ultraviolet A)
  amyloidosis, 180
  for graft-*versus*-host disease, 343
  for impetigo herpetiformis, 363
  mast cell disease, 375
Pyoderma gangrenosum, 41–43, 42f, 251–252, 252f
  associated conditions with, 43, 43t
  atypical or bullous, 41, 42f
  drug selection principles, 438t
  IgA association, 177
  leg ulcers and, 404f, 413f, 418t–419t
  malignancy and, 136–137, 136f
  peristomal, 42, 42f
  pyostomatitis vegetans and, 41
  RA and, 53
  in systemic lymphomas, 168

Pyoderma gangrenosum-like leg ulcerations, lupus erythematosus and, 8
Pyogenic arthritis, pyoderma gangrenosum, and acne (PAPA) syndrome, 61t, 66, 67f
Pyogenic bacteria, 334, 334f
Pyogenic granuloma, 196, 199f
  of pregnancy, 362
Pyostomatitis vegetans, 41
Pyrimidine analogs, 146
Pyrin, 64

Q
QuantiFERON-TB Gold test, 335
Quinacrine
  for dermatomyositis/polymyositis, 20
  for lupus erythematosus, 11

R
RA. *see* Rheumatoid arthritis (RA).
Radiation, 417f, 418t–419t
Radiation-induced morphea, 24
Radiation therapy, and anagen arrest, 380
Radioallergosorbent test (RAST), 427–428
Radiographic studies, leg ulcers, 420
Radiological studies, on SAPHO syndrome, 67
Raloxifene, 153
Ranitidine, for urticaria, 85
Rapamycin, for tuberous sclerosis complex, 354
Rapamycin inhibitors, mammalian target of, for cancer therapy, 152
Rapid plasma reagin (RPR), 299–300
Rash
  in DIRA, 62–63, 63f
  in FMF, 64, 65f
  in HIDS, 65–66, 65f
  in TRAPS, 64f
Raynaud's phenomenon, 29, 29f
  and cryoglobulinemia, 172
  and hyperviscosity syndrome, 173
  nail disorders, 388
  and POEMS syndrome, 175
  in pregnancy, 365
  systemic lupus erythematosus and, 8
  in systemic sclerosis, 26–27
Reactive perforating collagenosis, 327
Recombinant platelet-derived growth factor, 422
Red blood cell aplasia, pemphigus and, 121
Relapsing polychondritis, 320, 320f
Renal cell cancer, malignancy and, 138–139
Renal cell carcinoma
  CD10 positivity in, 157
  metastatic, 156–157, 156f
Renal disease, 323–329
Renal failure, 323
  sarcoidosis and, 313
Renal system, nail disorders, 394–395
Renal transplantation, 206
Reproductive system, nail disorders, 395
Reslizumab, for HES, 73–74
Reticuloendothelial system, malignancies of, 224
Retinitis, 291
Retinoic acid, for amyloidosis, 182
Retinoids
  for cancer therapy, 149
  for HLE, 2
  for impetigo herpetiformis, 363
  for PAPA syndrome, 66
Rhabdomyosarcoma, 349
Rheb (Ras homolog), 350–351

Rheumatic fever, 271
Rheumatoid arthritis (RA), 51–53
    bullous pemphigoid and, 124
    cutaneous manifestations of, 51, 52t
    definition of, 51
    dermatologic conditions associated with, 53
    diagnosis of, 51
    epidemiologic data on, 51
    leg ulcers, 414
    pemphigus and, 119, 121
    purpura and, 110
    symmetric polyarthritis, 53–54
    and vasculitis, 35
Rheumatoid factor (RF)
    and cryoglobulinemic vasculitis, 34–35
    and mixed cryoglobulins, 172
    in RA, 51
    Waldenström's hypergammaglobulinemic purpura, 176
Rheumatoid neutrophilic dermatitis, RA and, 53
Rheumatoid nodules, 51–52, 52f
Rheumatoid vasculitis, 35, 53
Rheumatologic diseases, nail disorders, 395
Rhinocerebral infection, in mucormycosis, 282
Rickettsia, 275
Rickettsial diseases, 271–276
Rickettsial pox, 275
Rifampin, for linear IgA bullous dermatosis, 129
Rilonacept, for CAPS, 60
"Risk-risk" analysis, 437–438
Ritodrine, for pemphigoid gestationis, 368
Rituximab, 152–153
    for dermatomyositis/polymyositis, 20
    for pemphigus, 122
    for rheumatoid arthritis, 54
    for vasculitis, 37
Rocky Mountain spotted fever, 275
Romidepsin, 148–149
Rosacea, 192
Rosai-Dorfman disease, 185, 189t
Roseola infantum, 264
Rubella, 263
Rubeola. *see* Measles (rubeola).
Rubeosis, faciei, 212
Russell viper venom test, purpura and, 116

S
S-adenosyl-1-methionine, for intrahepatic cholestasis of pregnancy, 367
Sacroileitis, SAPHO syndrome and, 66–67
Sand fly, 285, 286f
Sanfilippo syndrome, 385t
SAPHO syndrome, 61t, 66–67
Saprophytic fungi, 338
Sarcoidal granulomas, in systemic lymphomas, 168–169
Sarcoidosis, 305–314
    acquired ichthyosis, 135
    cutaneous and systemic disease, 312
    cutaneous manifestations of, 306–309, 306f–310f
    and erythema nodosum, 306
    musculoskeletal manifestations of, 311, 311f
    ocular manifestations of, 310, 310f
    Waldenström's hypergammaglobulinemic purpura, 176
Scabies, in AIDS, 294
Scalp, involvement of, in dermatomyositis, 15

Scar, in sarcoidosis, 308–309
Scarlet fever, 271
Scarring alopecia, 378
    in sarcoidosis, 306, 310f
Scarring ocular disease, in bullous pemphigoid, 124f
SCC. *see* Squamous cell carcinoma (SCC).
Schistocytes, in purpura, 116
Schnitzler's syndrome, 60–62, 61t, 82, 173, 177
    in systemic lymphomas, 169
Scleredema, 209–210, 210f
    and systemic sclerosis, 27
Sclerodactyly, 210
    in systemic sclerosis, 25, 28
Scleroderma, 22–28
    CREST variant, 194
    and dermatomyositis, 15
    localized. *see* Morphea
    malignancy and, 133
    pemphigus and, 119
    telangiectasias in, 195f
Scleroderma-like skin changes, in diabetes, 210–211, 210f–211f
Sclerodermoid GVHD, 343
Scleromyxedema, 176–177, 176f
    and systemic sclerosis, 27
Sclerosing panniculitis, 409
Scrub typhus, 275–276
Sea-blue histiocytositic syndrome, 190t
Seborrheic dermatitis, HIV infection and, 294, 294f
Seborrheic keratoses, malignancy and, 134
"Second hit" mutation, in malignant tumors, 346, 350
Secondary hypereosinophilia, 69
Secondary hyperlipoproteinemia, 223t, 224–225
Secondary (reactive) hypereosinophilic syndromes, 71
Secondary syphilis, 298–300, 298t, 299f, 381
Secukinumab, for psoriasis, 48
Seizures, in Sturge-Weber syndrome, 355
Selective estrogen receptor modulators (SERMs), 153
Self-inflicted ulceration, 411f
Senear-Usher syndrome, 120
Senile and mutant transthyretin amyloidoses, 180
Sensory neuropathy, ulcers, 408–409
Serology tests, for syphilis, 300–301
Sertoli cell testicular tumors, 139–140
Serum amyloid A (SAA)
    in CAPS, 59–60
    in HIDS, 66
    in TRAPS, 64
Serum autoantibody titers, in pemphigus, 118–119
Serum-free light chain assay, 174, 178, 182
Serum sickness-like reaction, 431, 431f
Serum sickness-like signs and symptoms, erythema nodosum and, 93–95
Sexually transmitted infections, 289–304
Sézary syndrome, 102, 105–107, 162
    see also Mycosis fungoidesShagreen patch, tuberous sclerosis complex and, 352, 352f
Shins, acquired ichthyosiform changes, 211
Short stature, in neurofibromatosis, 349
Sickle cell ulcer, 415f, 418t–419t
Side effects. *see* Adverse effects
Silymarin, for intrahepatic cholestasis of pregnancy, 367
Simple bullous eruptions, 432
Simple exanthematous eruptions, 429–430, 430f

Simple urticaria, 431
Simulium black flies, in fogo selvagem, 120
Simvastatin, for HIDS, 66
Single-organ cutaneous small vessel vasculitis (SoCSVV), 31, 36
Sirolimus, 341
    for graft-*versus*-host disease, 342
    for tuberous sclerosis complex, 354
Sister Mary Joseph's nodule, 156, 254
Sjögren-Larsson syndrome, 358
Sjögren's syndrome, 57, 57f
    purpura and, 112
    SCLE and, 6
    secondary, 8, 400, 400f
    and vasculitis, 34–35
    and Waldenström's hypergammaglobulinemic purpura, 176
Skin
    cardiovascular diseases and, 315–322, 316t–319t
    hepatic disease and, 255–261
    renal disease and, 323–329
    thick, diabetic, 211
Skin biopsy, amyloidosis, 181
Skin fold freckling, 347, 347f
Skin grafts, 422
Skin-limited amyloidosis, 179
Skin substitutes, leg ulcers, 422
Skin tags (acrochordons), 211
    in pregnancy, 362
SLC39A4 gene, 248–249
SLE. *see* Systemic lupus erythematosus (SLE).
Slit lamp evaluation, Lisch nodules and, 348
SMAD4 gene, mutations in, 193–194
Small-vessel vasculitis, 34–35, 133–134
    drug eruptions, 435
Smoking cessation
    in Graves' disease, 219
    for lupus erythematosus, 11
    for Raynaud's phenomenon, 29
Smoldering myeloma, 171
Smoldering systemic mastocytosis (SSM), 370–371
SMT. *see* Superficial migratory thrombophlebitis (SMT).
Snedden-Wilkinson disease, 120
Sodium thiosulfate (STS), for calciphylaxis, 327
Solitary mastocytoma, 372f
Somatostatin, for linear IgA bullous dermatosis, 129
Somatostatin analogs, 153–154
Sorafenib, 152
Spider angiomas, 193
    cirrhosis and, 256–257, 256f
    in pregnancy, 360
Spindle cell hemangiomas, 196, 199f
Spirochetes, 274
Spironolactone
    for androgen-related disorders, 386
    for hirsutism, 231–232
Splenomegaly, 373
Splinter hemorrhages, 389t–390t, 391, 392f
Spoon-shaped nails, 389t–390t
Sporotrichosis, 277–278, 278f
Squamous cell carcinoma (SCC), 418t–419t
    Bazex syndrome and, 132
    cutaneous, invasive, 152f
    and DLE, 9
    and leg ulcers, 417f
    in transplant recipients, 338–341, 339f–343f
Square biopsy, in morphea, 24

SSSS. *see* Staphylococcal scalded skin syndrome (SSSS).
Staging
 in mycosis fungoides, 161, 161t
 in pulmonary sarcoidosis, 309–310
Stanozolol, for monoclonal protein disorders, 174
Staphylococcal scalded skin syndrome (SSSS), 273, 273f
Staphylococcus aureus, in transplant recipients, 334
Stasis ulceration, 413f
Statins, 226
Steroid hormone receptors, disorders of, 232
Steroids
 see also Prednisonefor Sweet's syndrome, 41
Stevens-Johnson syndrome (SJS), 87–92, 89f–90f, 426t
 see also Toxic epidermal necrolysis (TEN)causes of, 88t
 drug eruptions, 433–434, 433f
 drug selection principles, 438t
 nail disorders, 396
 PNP and, 120
Stewart-Treves syndrome, 203
Still's disease
 see also Juvenile idiopathic arthritis (JIA)adult, 53–54
Streptococcal infections, 271–274
Streptococcus pyogenes, in transplant recipients, 334
Streptozocin, 146
Striae gravidarum, in pregnancy, 360
Strongyloides stercoralis, HES and, 72
Sturge-Weber syndrome (SWS), 354–356, 354f
Subacute cutaneous lupus erythematosus (SCLE), 5–7
 see also Acute cutaneous lupus erythematosus (ACLE); Lupus erythematosusannular (SCLE-A), 5–6, 5f
 anti-La (SS-B) antibodies in, 7
 anti-Ro (SS-A) antibody in, 6
 and DLE, 1
 drug-induced, 6–7, 7t
 immune complexes in, 10
 papulosquamous (SCLE-P), 5–6, 6f
Subcorneal pustular dermatosis, 177
Subcutaneous fat aspiration, in amyloidosis, 181
Subcutaneous mycoses, 277
 other, 278–279
 with systemic manifestations, 277–278
Subcutaneous nodules, of rheumatic fever, 271
Subcutaneous panniculitis-like T-cell lymphoma (SPLTCL), 163
Subcutaneous sarcoidosis, 308–309
Sulfas, for erythroderma, 105
Sulfasalazine, 85–86, 400
 for FMF, 65
Sulfonamides, drug eruptions, 430
Sulfonylureas, allergies to, 213–214
Sunscreens/sun avoidance, for cutaneous LE, 10
Superficial migratory thrombophlebitis (SMT), 96
Suprabasilar acantholysis, 120
Suprabasilar cleft formation, in pemphigus, 119
Surveillance, Epidemiology, and End Results program, 135

Sweet's syndrome, 40–41, 41f
 neutrophilic dermatoses and, 136–137
 in systemic lymphomas, 168
 and thyroid disorders, 221
Symmetric polyarthritis, 53–54
Syphilis, 297–303
 congenital, 300
 diagnosis of, 300–301
 in HIV infection and AIDS, 301
 nail disorders, 394
 primary, 297–298, 298f, 298t
 secondary, 298–300, 298f, 299f, 381
 tertiary, 300
Systemic candidiasis, 283
Systemic disease, psoriasis and, 45–50
Systemic drug therapy, 438
 adverse effects associated with, 439–440
 priority sequence of, 438–439
Systemic drug use, principles of, 437–441
Systemic lupus erythematosus (SLE)
 see also Lupus erythematosusACR criteria for, 1, 1t, 6, 8
 alopecia in, 8
 hair loss, 381
 immune complexes in, 10
 nail disorders, 395
 in pregnancy, 365
 prevalence of, 1
 purpura and, 110
 and Raynaud's phenomenon, 8
 and telangiectasias, 194
 ulcerations in, 2
 urticaria, 77–78, 80
 and vasculitis, 34–35
Systemic lymphomas
 cutaneous signs of, 159–170, 160t
 nonspecific signs of, 168–169, 169f
 specific manifestations of, 166–169
Systemic mast cell disease, 370–371, 371t
Systemic mastocytosis with an associated clonal hematologic nonmast cell lineage disease (SMAHNMD), 370–371
Systemic mycoses, 277, 279
Systemic sclerosis, 25f–26f, 26t–27t
 ACR classification criteria for, 26t
 eosinophilic fasciitis distinguished from, 28
 leg ulcers, 414

T
T-cell leukemia, 102
T-cell lymphomas
 see also Mycosis fungoides; Sézary syndromecutaneous, malignancy and, 135
 erythroderma and, 104–105
 primary cutaneous. *see* Primary cutaneous T-cell lymphomas
 pruritus in, 102
 in transplant recipients, 332
Tacrolimus
 for circumscribed morphea, 25
 for dermatomyositis/polymyositis, 20
 for graft-*versus*-host disease, 342–343
 for pruritus, 103
Takatsuki syndrome, 174–175
Takayasu arteritis, and vasculitis, 33
Tamoxifen, 153
Tangier disease, 224
Taxanes, 148, 203
Tay syndrome, 384
^{99}Tc scan, on SAPHO syndrome, 67
"Tel Hashomer" Criteria, for FMF, 64–65

Telangiectases, 192–194, 192f–193f, 193t
 in cirrhosis, 256–257, 256f
 malignancy and, 134
Telangiectasia macularis eruptiva perstans (TMEP), 192–193, 372–373
Telangiectatic mats, in systemic sclerosis, 28
Telaprevir, for hepatitis C, 260
Telogen, 377
Telogen effluvium, 378–379
 see also Alopeciacauses of, 378t
 drugs associated with, 379t
 in pregnancy, 361
 in SLE, 8
Telogen hair, 377
Telogen release
 delayed, 379
 immediate, 379
Temozolomide, 146
Temsirolimus, 152
Tendinous xanthomas, 225–226
Teniposide, 148
Terbinafine, 6–7
Terminal hairs, 377
Terry's nails, 175, 257, 257f, 389t–390t, 391–392
Tertiary syphilis, 300
Testicular feminization syndrome, 232
Testosterone, hirsutism and, 230–231
Tetracycline
 for linear IgA bullous dermatosis, 130
 for sarcoidosis, 314
Thalidomide, 154
 for Behçet's disease, 40
 for FMF, 65
 for lupus erythematosus, 11
 for monoclonal protein production disorder, 177
 for sarcoidosis, 314
 in TEN, 92
Thallium, 380
Thermally dimorphic mycoses, 279
Thermolysis, 385
Thioguanine, 147
Thiopurine methyl transferase testing, 20
ThioTEPA, 143
Thrombocytopenia, in purpura, 109–110
Thrombophlebitis
 migratory, malignancy and, 135
 superficial migratory, panniculitis and, 96
Thrombosis, venous, 409
Thymoma, pemphigus and, 120–122, 133
Thyroglossal duct cysts, 216
Thyroid cancer, dermatologic syndromes associated with, 216–217, 217t
Thyroid disorders, 215–221
 dermatitis herpetiformis and, 127–128
Thyroid gland
 description and function of, 215
 evaluation of, 215–216, 216t
Thyroid-stimulating hormone (TSH), 215–216, 219–220
Thyroiditis, 124, 126, 219
Thyromegaly, in Graves' disease, 219
Thyrotoxicosis. *see* Hyperthyroidism.
Thyroxine (T_4), 215
Tinea, HIV infection and, 293, 294f
Tinea pedis, 212
Tinea unguium, 389t–390t
Tissue-engineered products, 422–423
Tissue hypereosinophilia, 69
TNF inhibitors, for psoriasis, 49
TNFRSF1A gene, 63–64
Toenails, 387
Tofacitinib, for rheumatoid arthritis, 54
Toll-like receptors, 59

Tongue, papillomatosis of, 398f
Tophi, 57–58, 58f
Topoisomerase I inhibitors, 147
Topoisomerase II inhibitors, 148
Topoisomerase inhibitors, for cancer therapy, 147–148
Topotecan, 147
Toremifene, 153
Total body irradiation, for dermatomyositis/polymyositis, 20
Toxic epidermal necrolysis (TEN), 87–92, 89f–90f, 426t, 433f
see also Stevens-Johnson syndrome (SJS)causes of, 88t
  drug eruptions, 433–434, 433f
  drug selection principles, 438t
  nail disorders, 396
  in SCLE, 5–6, 6f
Toxic oil syndrome (TOS), 29–30
  defined, 71t
Toxic shock syndrome, 273–274
  nail disorders, 396
Toxoplasmosis, 288
Trachyonychia, 389t–390t
Transaminitis, in Schnitzler's syndrome, 62
Transcutaneous oximetry, 414
"Transplant elbow", 334
Transplant recipients
  cutaneous manifestations observed in, 330–344
  infections and, 330–338
Transplantation, renal, 326t, 329
Trastuzumab, 152
Trastuzumab emtansine (T-DM1), 152
Triamcinolone acetonide
  cheilitis granulomatosa, 400
  for lupus erythematosus, 11
Triangular lunulae, 389t–390t
Triazine derivatives, 146
Trichilemmomas, in Cowden disease, 138
Trichloroacetic acid, 226
Trichodiscoma, 138
Trichodysplasia-associated polyomavirus, 268
Trichodystrophies, 383–384
Trichomegaly, 150, 150f
  in AIDS, 297, 297f
Trichomoniasis, 285
Trichoschisis, 384f
Triiodothyronine (T$_3$), 215
Trimethoprim-sulfamethoxazole, 425
  for linear IgA bullous dermatosis, 129
Tripe palms, malignancy and, 137, 137f
Trombiculid mites, 275
Trousseau syndrome, malignancy and, 135
Trypanosomiasis, human, 287
TSC1 and TSC2 genes, in tuberous sclerosis, 350, 352–354
Tsutsugamushi fever, 275
Tuberculosis
  in erythema induratum, 96
  in transplant recipients, 334–335
Tuberin/hamartin complex, 350–351
Tuberous sclerosis complex (TSC), 350–354, 353f
Tuberous xanthomas, 224–225, 225f
Tumid lupus erythematosus, 2–4, 4f
Tumor necrosis factor inhibitors
  for erythroderma, 108
  for lupus erythematosus, 11–12
  for rheumatoid arthritis, 54
Tumor necrosis factor receptor associated periodic syndrome (TRAPS), 61t, 63–64, 64f

Tumor necrosis factor (TNF)-α antagonists, cheilitis granulomatosa, 400
Tumors
  see also Malignant disease; Metastatic diseaseanaplastic, 216
  Koenen's, 351–352, 351f
  Sertoli cell testicular, 139–140
  vascular, 195–200, 196t–198t, 199f, 204f
Turcot syndrome, 138
Turner's sign, 252, 253f
20 nail dystrophy, 389t–390t
Typhus
  endemic, 275
  epidemic, 275
  scrub, 275–276
Tzanck smear
  oral mucosal blisters and, evaluation of, 91
  viral infections and, 331f

U

U1 small nuclear ribonucleoprotein autoantigen, 29
Ulcerations
  see also Leg ulcersarterial, 414f
  of chancroid, 301
  common causes of, 409–412, 409t
  due to malignancy, 410f
  foot, 207
  historical features for diagnosis of, 409t
  in LE, 8
  mucocutaneous, in CMV infection, 332
  in necrobiosis lipoidica, 208–209, 209f
  on penile chancre, 297, 298f
  in pyoderma gangrenosum, 41
  of sarcoid lesions, 309
  in SLE, 2
  venous, 409–410, 411t
Ulcerative colitis, 251
Ultrasound, in tuberous sclerosis complex and, 353
Ungual fibromas, 351–352, 351f
Unidentified bright objects, 348
Unna boots, 409, 422
Uremia, dermatologic manifestations of, 323–329, 325t
Uremic frost, 329
Urinalysis, in purpura, 116
Uroporphyrinogen decarboxylase (UROD), 235–236
Ursodeoxycholic acid, for intrahepatic cholestasis of pregnancy, 367
Urticaria, 77–86, 78f, 426t
  acute, 77
  antihistamines for, 85t
  cause of, 79t
  chronic
    alternative therapies for, 86t
    classification of, 80t
    management of, 84f
    pruritus in, 99, 103
  classification of, 78–82, 82f
  disease related to, 79–80, 82f
  distinctive, 80–82
  eruptions, 431, 431f
  patient evaluation, 83, 83t
  physical, comparison of, 81t
  in thyroid disorders, 221
Urticaria pigmentosa, 192–193, 372f
Urticarial vasculitis, 35, 77–80, 82, 82f, 85
  and Waldenström's macroglobulinemia, 173
Ustekinumab, for psoriasis, 48
UVA-1, for systemic sclerosis, 28
UVB, for systemic sclerosis, 28

UVB phototherapy, for psoriasis, 49
Uveitis, 310, 313
  posterior, Behçet's disease and, 39

V

Vaccine, live attenuated, for measles, 262
Valacyclovir
  erythema multiforme and, 92
  for herpes simplex, 331
  for herpes zoster, 331
Valganciclovir, for cytomegalovirus, 332
Valley fever. see Coccidioidomycosis.
Valsalva-like maneuvers, 110
  hemorrhage, 178–179
Vancomycin, for linear IgA bullous dermatosis, 129
Varicella, 265–266, 265f
Varicella-zoster virus (VZV), 265
  HIV infection and, 290–291, 291f
  in transplant recipients, 331, 332f
Varicosities, in pregnancy, 360
Variegate porphyria, 242
Vascular endothelial growth factor (VEGF), 151, 175
Vascular malformations, 195–200, 196t–198t
Vascular morphogenesis, errors in, 195
Vascular neoplasms and malformations, 192–204
  angiosarcoma, 203–204, 203f
  telangiectases, 192–194
  vascular tumors and malformations, 195–200, 197t–198t
Vasculitis, 31–38, 416f, 418t–419t
  ANCA-associated, 34
  autoimmune systemic diseases, associated with, 35
  classification criteria for, 31
  clinical manifestations of, 32–35
  cutaneous, in LE, 8
  diagnostic approach to, 36
  drug eruptions, 434–435
  epidemiology of, 31–32
  general concepts in, 32–33, 32f–33f
  and Henoch-Schönlein purpura, 31
  hypersensitivity, 31
  leukocytoclastic. see Leukocytoclastic vasculitis
  medium-sized vessel in, 32–33
  nodular, 96
  nomenclature for, 31, 32t
  rheumatoid, 35, 53
  secondary, 32t
  small-vessel, 34–35, 435
    malignancy and, 133–134
  spectrum of, in systemic vasculitides, 33–35
  treatment of, 36–37, 37f
  urticarial, 77–80, 82, 82f, 85, 173
  variants of, 35–36
Vecuronium, in mast cell disease, 374
VEGF receptor (VEGFR), 151
Vellus hairs, 377
Vemurafenib, 152
Venous blood flow, in lower extremities, 406
Venous insufficiency, 402, 403t, 406t, 407f–408f
  chronic, conditions associated with, 414t
  and thrombosis risk, 409
Venous leg ulcerations (VLUs), 402
Venous studies, 412–414
Venous surgery, 423
Venous thrombosis, 409
Venous ulceration, 413f
  pathophysiology of, 406–407, 406t
  studies, 412–414

Verapamil, and gingival hyperplasia, 401
Verrucae vulgaris, 333
Very-low-density lipoproteins (VLDLs), 222
    increased, 223
Vibrio vulnificus, 418t–419t
Vinblastine, 148, 185, 203
Vinca alkaloids, 148
Vincristine, 148, 203
Vindesine, 148
Vinflunine, 148
Vinorelbine, 148
Viral-associated trichodysplasia (VAT), 268
Viral diseases, 262–270
Viral hepatitis, cutaneous disease associated with, 259–260, 259f–261f
Viral infections
    see also Viral hepatitis
    human immunodeficiency syndrome (HIV), 290–292, 290f–292f
Vitamin K, 367
Vitiligo
    and diabetes mellitus, 213
    malignancy and, 137
VLDLs (very-low-density lipoproteins), 222
    increased, 223
Vogt-Koyanagi-Harada syndrome, 358
von Hippel-Lindau syndrome, 357
Von Recklinghausen disease (neurofibromatosis), 140, 346–350
von Willebrand syndrome, 178–179
Voriconazole, for fungal infections, 337
Vorinostat, 148–149
Vulvovaginal candidiasis (VVC), in pregnancy, 364–365

W

Waardenburg syndrome (WS), 357
Waldenström, benign hypergammaglobulinemic purpura of, 110, 112, 176
Waldenström's macroglobulinemia, 173
Warthin-Starry staining, 196
Wegener's granulomatosis, 34, 110
Werner's syndrome, 316t–318t
Whitlow, 389t–390t
Wilms' tumor, 349
Wilson's disease, 119, 258, 259f, 393
Wolff-Parkinson-White syndrome, 353
Woronoff's rings, 45–46
Wound care
    adjunct techniques, 422–423
    general principles of, 420–423
    swabs, 420
Wound care centers, 423
Wound healing, normal, 404, 404f–405f
Wounds, atypical, 411–412

X

X-linked dominant protoporphyria, 240–241
Xanthelasmas, 225, 225f
Xanthogranuloma
    juvenile, 188, 188f
    necrobiotic, 185, 189t
        with paraproteinemia, 176, 176f
Xanthoma disseminatum, 176, 189t, 224
Xanthoma striatum palmare, 226

Xanthomas
    cutaneous, 225–226
    diffuse plane, 226, 226f
    eruptive, 223–224, 226, 226f
    planar, 225–226, 225f–226f
    primary biliary cirrhosis and, 257–258, 258f
    tendinous, 225
Xanthomatosis, 135–136
    eruptive, 208, 208f
Xenopsylla cheopis, 275
Xerophthalmia, 400
Xerosis, 329
    and Sjögren's syndrome (SS), 57
Xerostomia, 400

Y

Yellow nail syndrome, 394, 395f
Yellow nails, 389t–390t
    in diabetes mellitus, 212
Yellow skin, in diabetes mellitus, 212

Z

Zidovudine, 394
Zinc deficiency
    causes of, 249, 249t
    oral supplementation for, 250
Zostavax, 266